MW01641049

Cervical Spine Trauma

Cervical Spine Trauma

Alexander R. Vaccaro, MD, PhD

The Rothman Institute at Jefferson University Hospital
Philadelphia, Pennsylvania

Paul Anderson, MD

University of Wisconsin Hospitals
Department of Orthopedic Surgery and Rehabilitation
Madison, Wisconsin

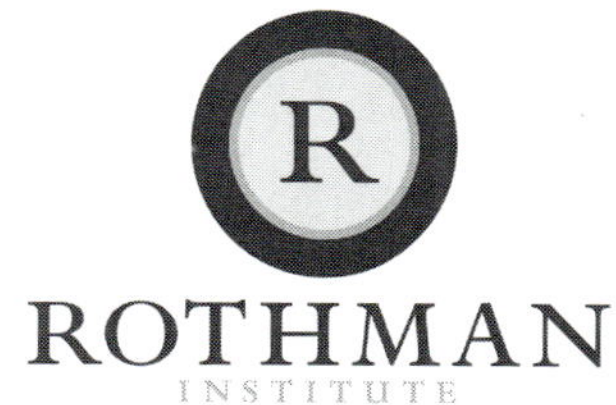

Product Manager: Jennifer Jett
Production Service: Maryland Composition Inc.

925 Chestnut Street
Philadelphia, PA 19107

Published by Wolters Kluwer Pharma Solutions.

Printed in The United States of America

Library of Congress Cataloging-in-Publication Data

Vaccaro, Alexander R.
Cervical spine trauma / Alexander R. Vaccaro, Paul Anderson.
p. ; cm.
Includes bibliographical references.
ISBN-13: 978-0-7817-6702-6
ISBN-10: 0-7817-6702-4
1. Cervical vertebrae—Wounds and injuries. 2. Surgical emergencies. I. Anderson, Paul, 1952- II. Title.
[DNLM: 1. Cervical Vertebrae—injuries. 2. Cervical Vertebrae—surgery. 3. Orthopedic Procedures—instrumentation. 4. Spinal Cord Injuries—therapy. WE 725 V114c 2009]
RD531.V33 2009
617.5′6059—dc22

2009010546

I would like to dedicate this book to my wonderful family and friends who have stood with me during trying times in the completion of this project, especially my parents, Sue and Alex, my sister Susie, and brothers, Richard and Andrew.

Alexander Vaccaro

CONTENTS

PREFACE

Cervical Spine Trauma, edited by Alex Vaccaro, MD, PhD, and Paul Anderson, MD, is yet another important contribution from the two editors. They have created an extremely useful, comprehensive book on the topic. It spans the breadth of cervical spine trauma from basic science, pathophysiology, and biomechanics of injury as they relate to clinical conditions, and discuss treatment and controversies in the management. Additionally, and importantly, it highlights new ideas in this up-to-date compendium.

The authors include anatomists, researchers, and experienced clinicians. There is a mix of orthopaedic surgeons and neurosurgeons, in addition to neurologists/neurophysiologists and rehabilitation specialists. This will prove to be a helpful book for spine surgeons, and more so for residents and spine fellows. I commend the editors for their vision in putting this together, and the authors for their contributions.

Dr. Steve Garfin
Professor and Chair, Department of Orthopaedics
University of California, San Diego
San Diego, California

ACKNOWLEDGMENTS

Great works, such as the efforts put forth by the contributors of this text, are inspired by leadership, dedication, perseverance, and the support of many people ranging from the members of the Spine Trauma Study Group and the Cervical Spine Study Group, to their supporting staff and close personal associates (H.H.).

Alexander R. Vaccaro, MD, PhD
Paul Anderson, MD

CONTRIBUTING AUTHORS

Bizhan N.M.N. Aarabi, MD, FACS, FRCSC
Professor of Neurosurgery
University of Maryland School of Medicine
Baltimore, Maryland

Kuniyoshi Abumi, MD
Professor of Medicine
Department of Orthopaedic Surgery
Hokkaido University Hospital
Sapporo, Japan

Todd J. Albert, MD
Richard H. Rothman Professor and Chairman
Department of Orthopaedic Surgery
Professor of Neurosurgery
The Rothman Institute
Thomas Jefferson University Hospital
Philadelphia, Pennsylvania

Joseph T. Alexander, MD
Wake Forest University
Department of Neurosurgery
Winston-Salem, North Carolina

Neel Anand, MD
Institute for Spinal Disorders
Cedars Sinai Medical Center
Los Angeles, California

D. Greg Anderson, MD
Associate Professor of Orthopaedic Surgery
Thomas Jefferson University and The Rothman Institute
Philadelphia, Pennsylvania

Paul A. Anderson, MD
University of Wisconsin Hospitals
Department of Orthopedic Surgery and Rehabilitation
Madison, Wisconsin

Paul M. Arnold, MD
Professor of Neurosurgery
University of Kansas Hospital
Kansas City, Kansas

Nazih Assaad, MB, BS (Hons), FRACS
Department of Neurosurgery and Spinal Injuries Unity
Royal North Shore Hospital
Australian School of Advanced Medicine
Macquarie University
Sydney, Australia

Darryl C. Baptiste, BSc, PhD
Scientific Associate
Department of Genetics & Development
Toronto Western Hospital
Toronto, Ontario, Canada

Bryan B. Barnes, MD
Georgia Neurological Surgery
Athens, Georgia

Natalie M. Best, MD
Resident Physician
Department of Anesthesiology
University of Utah
Salt Lake City, Utah

Sumon Bhattacharjee, MD
Neuroscience Group of North East Wisconsin
Neenah, Wisconsin

Christopher M. Bono, MD
Assistant Professor of Orthopaedic Surgery
Harvard Medical School
Chief, Orthopaedic Spine Service
Brigham and Women's Hospital
Boston, Massachusetts

Michael C. Boyd, MD, MSc, FRCSC
Clinical Associate Professor
Department of Surgery
Division of Neurosurgery
University of British Columbia
Vancouver, British Columbia, Canada

Darrel S. Brodke, MD
Professor and Vice Chairman
Department of Orthopaedics
University of Utah
Salt Lake City, Utah

Mark G. Burnett, MD
Department of Neurosurgery
NeuroTexas Institute
Austin, Texas

Kyle Cabbell, MD
Orthopaedic Resident
Boston University School of Medicine
Boston, Massachusetts

Carson Campe, MD
Resident
Department of Radiology Residency
Massachusetts General Hospital
Boston, Massachusetts

Steven Casha, MD, PhD, FRCSC
Assistant Professor
Department of Clinical Neurosciences
University of Calgary
Calgary, Canada

Steve Chang, MD
Division of Neurological Surgery
Barrow Neurological Institute
St. Joseph's Hospital and Medical Center
Phoenix, Arizona

Gordon K.T. Chu, MD, MSc, FRCSC
Division of Neurosurgery and Spinal Program
Toronto Western Hospital
University of Toronto
Toronto, Ontario, Canada

Andrew T. Dailey, MD
Associate Professor of Neurosurgery
University of Utah Medical Center
Salt Lake City, Utah

Michael Daubs, MD
Assistant Professor
Department of Orthopaedic Surgery
University of Utah
Salt Lake City, Utah

Charles Davis, MD
Fellowship-Trained Spine Specialist
Chesapeake Orthopaedic and Sports Medicine Center
Glen Burnie, Maryland

Michael A. DeLuca, BS
Department of Orthopaedics and Rehabilitation
Yale University School of Medicine
New Haven, Connecticut

Sanjay S. Dhall, MD
Assistant Professor
Department of Neurosurgery
Emory University
Atlanta, Georgia

John R. Dimar, MD
Professor
Department of Orthopedics
University of Louisville
Louisville, Kentucky

Christian P. DiPaola, MD
Fellow
University of British Columbia
Vancouver General Hospital
Vancouver, British Columbia, Canada

Derek J. Donegan, MD
Resident
Department of Orthopaedic Surgery
University of Pennsylvania Health System
Philadelphia, Pennsylvania

Marcel Dvorak, MD, FRCSC
Professor of Orthopaedics
University of British Columbia
Vancouver General Hospital
Vancouver, British Columbia, Canada

Kurt M. Eichholz, MD
Assistant Professor
Department of Neurosurgery
Vanderbilt University
Nashville, Tennessee

Hossein Elgafy, MD, MCh, FRCS Ed, FRCSC
Fellow
Combined Orthopaedic and Neurosurgical Spine Program
Department of Orthopaedic Surgery
University of British Columbia
Vancouver, British Columbia, Canada

Daniel Fassett, MD, MBA
Interim Head of Neurosurgery
Illinois Neurological Institute
University of Illinois College of Medicine Peoria
Peoria, Illinois

Michael G. Fehlings, MD, PhD, FRCSC, FACS
Professor of Neurosurgery
Director, Neuroscience Program
Department of Surgery and Spinal Program
University of Toronto
Toronto, Ontario, Canada

Richard G. Fessler, MD, PhD
Professor
Department of Neurosurgery
Northwestern University
Chicago, Illinois

Charles Fisher, BSc, MHSc
Assistant Professor
Division of Spine
Department of Orthopaedics
University of British Columbia
Vancouver Coastal Health
Vancouver, British Columbia, Canada

Stacey L. Forsythe
Spine Colorado
Mercy Regional Medical Center
Durango, Colorado

John C. France, MD
Professor of Orthopaedic and Neurosurgery
Chief of Spine Surgery and Orthopaedic Surgery
West Virginia University
Morgantown, West Virginia

Christian Fras, MD
Department of Orthopaedic Surgery
University of Pennsylvania
Philadelphia, Pennsylvania

Peter G. Gabos, MD
Co-Director, Division of Spine and Scoliosis Surgery
Alfred I. duPont Hospital for Children
Wilmington, Delaware

Jamie Gasco, MD
Department of Neurological Surgery
University of Virginia
Charlottesville, Virginia

Nicole Glover, BA
Durango Orthopedic Associates/Spine Colorado
Durango, Colorado

Pankaj A. Gore, MD
Division of Neurological Surgery
Barrow Neurological Institute
St. Joseph's Hospital and Medical Center
Phoenix, Arizona

Carl N. Graf, MD
Department of Spine Surgery
Illinois Spine Institute
Schaumburg, Illinois

Jonathan N. Grauer, MD
Associate Professor
Department of Orthopaedics and Rehabilitation
Yale University School of Medicine
New Haven, Connecticut

Tooraj Gravori, MD
Fellow
Cedars Sinai Spine Center
Institute for Spinal Disorders
Los Angeles, California

Zbigniew Gugala, MD, PhD
Assistant Professor
Department of Orthopaedic Surgery and Rehabilitation
University of Texas Medical Branch
Galveston, Texas

Troy D. Gust, MD
Resident
Department of Neurosurgery
University of Kansas
Kansas City, Kansas

Regis W. Haid Jr., MD
Medical Director
Piedmont Spine Center and Neuroscience Service Line
Piedmont Hospital
Atlanta Brain and Spine Care
Atlanta, Georgia

Mitchel Harris, MD
Associate Professor
Chief of Orthopaedic Trauma
Department of Orthopaedic Surgery
Brigham and Women's Hospital
Boston, Massachusetts

James S. Harrop, MD
Associate Professor of Neurological and Orthopedic Surgery
Thomas Jefferson University
Philadelphia, Pennsylvania

Neal G. Haynes, MD
Chief Resident
Department of Neurosurgery
University of Kansas
Kansas City, Kansas

Robert Heary, MD
Professor of Neurological Surgery
UMDNJ—New Jersey Medical School
Newark, New Jersey

John Heller, MD
Professor of Orthopaedic Surgery
Spine Fellowship Director
The Emory Spine Center
Emory University School of Medicine
Atlanta, Georgia

Alan Hilibrand, MD
Professor of Orthopaedic Surgery and Neurosurgery
Thomas Jefferson University Hospital
Jefferson Medical College/The Rothman Institute
Philadelphia, Pennsylvania

Langston T. Holly, MD
Assistant Professor of Neurosurgery
David Geffen UCLA School of Medicine
Los Angeles, California

R. John Hurlbert, MD, PhD, FRCSC, FACS
Associate Professor, Faculty of Medicine
Department of Clinical Neurosciences
University of Calgary
Foothills Hospital
Calgary, Canada

Manabu Ito, MD
Associate Professor of Medicine
Department of Orthopaedic Surgery
Graduate School of Medicine
Hokkaido University
Sapporo, Japan

Vivek Joseph, MBBS, FRCSI, MCh
Professor of Neurosurgery
Department of Neurological Science
Christian Medical College
Vellore, Tamil Nadu, India

Iain H. Kalfas, MD
Department of Neurosurgery
Cleveland Clinic
Cleveland, Ohio

Paul K. Kim, MD
Department of Neurosurgery
Wake Forest University
Winston-Salem, North Carolina

Yoshihisa Kotani, MD
Associate Professor of Medicine
Department of Orthopaedic Surgery
Graduate School of Medicine
Hokkaido University
Sapporo, Japan

Ajit A. Krishnaney, MD
Staff
Department of Neurosurgery
Cleveland Clinic
Cleveland, Ohio

Timothy R. Kuklo, MD, JD
Associate Professor of Orthopaedic and Neurological Surgery
Washington University
St. Louis, Missouri

Brian K. Kwon, MD, PhD, FRCSC
Assistant Professor
Department of Orthopaedics
University of British Columbia
Vancouver, British Columbia, Canada

Merrill Landers, DPT, OCS
Associate Professor
Department of Physical Therapy
University of Nevada, Las Vegas
Las Vegas, Nevada

Allan D. Levi, MD, PhD
Professor of Neurosurgery
University of Miami
Jackson Memorial Hospital
Miami, Florida

Ronald W. Lindsey, MD
Professor and Chair
Department of Orthopaedic Surgery and Rehabilitation
University of Texas Medical Branch
Galveston, Texas

Jason G. Lowenstein, MD
Orthopaedic Surgeon
SpineAustin
Austin, Texas

Steven Ludwig, MD
Associate Professor of Orthopaedics
Chief of Spine Surgery
Department of Orthopaedics
University of Maryland
Baltimore, Maryland

Ignacio N. Madrazo, MD, DSc, FACS
Professor of Neurosurgery
Neuroscience Center
Research Unit on Neurological Diseases
Centro Médico Siglo XXI, IMSS
Hospital Ángeles del Pedregal, México
CAMINA Research Laboratory
Mexico City, Mexico

Eduardo Magallón, MD
Hospital Ángeles del Pedregal
Mexico City, Mexico

David Magit, MD
Clinical Instructor
Department of Orthopaedics
Yale University/Yale New Haven Hospital
New Haven, Connecticut
Greenwich Hospital
Greenwich, Connecticut

Glen Manzano, MD
Resident
Department of Neurosurgery
University of Miami
Jackson Memorial Hospital
Miami, Florida

Robert W. Molinari, MD
Associate Professor
Department of Orthopaedics
University of Rochester
Rochester, New York

Praveen V. Mummaneni, MD
Associate Professor
Department of Neurosurgery
University of California San Francisco
San Francisco, California

Michael Nikolakis, MD
Spine Fellow
Department of Orthopaedics
University of British Columbia
Vancouver, British Columbia, Canada

Russ P. Nockels, MD
Professor
Department of Neurosurgery
Loyola University
Chicago, Illinois

John E. O'Toole, MD
Assistant Professor
Department of Neurosurgery
Rush University Medical School
Chicago, Illinois

David O. Okonkwo, MD, PhD
Assistant Professor
Department of Neurological Surgery
University of Pittsburgh Medical Center
Pittsburgh, Pennsylvania

F. Cumhur Öner, MD, PhD
Professor of Spinal Surgery
Department of Orthopedics
University Medical School Utrecht
Utrecht, The Netherlands

Rod J. Oskouian Jr., MD
Attending Neurosurgeon
Swedish Neuroscience Specialists
Swedish Medical Center
Seattle, Washington

Jeff Pan, MD
Department of Neurosurgery
Emory University School of Medicine
Atlanta, Georgia

Aditya Pandey, MD
Assistant Professor of Neurosurgery
University of Michigan
Ann Arbor, Michigan

Stephen M. Papadopoulos, MD
Barrow Neurological Institute
Phoenix, Arizona

Scott Paquette, MD, FRCSC
Clinical Assistant Professor
Department of Surgery
Division of Neurosurgery
University of British Columbia
Vancouver, British Columbia, Canada

Alpesh A. Patel, MD
Assistant Professor of Orthopaedic Surgery and Neurosurgery
University of Utah
Salt Lake City, Utah

Andrew J. Paterson, MD
Assistant Professor
Department of Orthopaedics
University of New Mexico, School of Medicine
Albuquerque, New Mexico

Stephen M. Quinnan, MD
Assistant Professor of Orthopaedic Surgery
University of Miami
Jackson Memorial Hospital
Ryder Trauma Center
Miami, Florida

Sharad Rajpal, BA, MD
Chief Resident
Department of Neurosurgery
University of Wisconsin Hospitals & Clinics
Madison, Wisconsin

Y. Raja Rampersaud, MD
Associate Professor of Surgery
Division of Orthopaedic Surgery and Neurosurgery
University of Toronto
Toronto Western Hospital
Toronto, Ontario, Canada

Wolfgang Rauschning, MD, PhD
Professor Emeritus
Department of Orthopaedic Surgery
Academis University Hospital
Uppsala, Sweden

Daniel K. Resnick, MD
Associate Professor and Vice Chairman
Department of Neurological Surgery
University of Wisconsin
Madison, Wisconsin

Gerald E. Rodts, MD
Department of Neurosurgery
Emory University School of Medicine
Atlanta, Georgia

Michael K. Rosner, MD
Associate Professor or Surgery
Uniformed Services University of the Health Sciences
Walter Reed Army Medical Center
Washington, District of Columbia

Rick C. Sasso, MD
Assistant Professor
Clinical Orthopaedic Surgery
Indiana University School of Medicine
Indianapolis, Indiana

David Schwartz, MD
Assistant Clinical Professor
Director, OrthoIndy Pine Fellowship
Department of Orthopaedic Surgery
Indiana University School of Medicine
Indiana Orthopaedic Hospital
Indianapolis, Indiana

Karl M. Schweitzer Jr., MD
Orthopaedic Surgery Resident
Duke University Medical Center
Durham, North Carolina

Nouzhan Sehati, MD
Department of Neurosurgery
University of California at Los Angeles Medical Center
Los Angeles, California

Lali H.S. Sekhon, MB, BS (Hons.I), PhD, FRACS, FACS
Adjunct Associate Professor
Spine Nevada
University of Nevada, Reno, School of Medicine
Reno, Nevada

Rajiv K. Sethi, MD
Department of Orthopaedic Surgery
Brigham and Women's Hospital
Boston, Massachusetts

Christopher I. Shaffrey, MD
Professor
Department of Neurological Surgery
University of Virginia
Charlottesville, Virginia

Rishi N. Sheth, MD
Chief Resident
Department of Neurosurgery
University of Miami
Jackson Memorial Hospital
Miami, Florida

Joseph Silvaggio, MD, BSc, FRCSC
Assistant Professor
Department of Neurosurgery and Radiology
Health Sciences Centre
University of Manitoba
Winnipeg, Manitoba, Canada

Harvey E. Smith, MD
Spine Surgery Fellow
The Rothman Institute
Philadelphia, Pennsylvania

Laura A. Snyder, MD
Medical Student
Thomas Jefferson University
Philadelphia, Pennsylvania

Volker K. H. Sonntag, MD
Barrow Neurological Institute
Vice Chairman, Division of Neurological Surgery
Chief, Spine Section, Division of Neurological Surgery
Professor of Clinical Surgery
University of Arizona
Phoenix, Arizona

Michael P. Steinmetz, MD
Assistant Professor
Center for Spine Health
Lerner College of Medicine
Cleveland Clinic
Cleveland, Ohio

Chadi Tannoury, MD
Orthopaedic Resident
The Rothman Institute
Thomas Jefferson University Hospital
Philadelphia, Pennsylvania

Nicholas Theodore, MD, FACS
Director, Neurotrauma Program
Barrow Neurological Institute
Phoenix, Arizona

Pradeep Thumbikat, MS, FRCS(Glasg)
Consultant in Spinal Injuries
Princess Royal Spinal Injuries Centre
Northern General Hospital
Sheffield, United Kingdom

Jared Toman, MD
Resident
Department of Orthopedic Surgery
Boston Medical Center
Boston, Massachusetts

Vincent Traynelis, MD
Professor of Neurosurgery
Rush University Medical Center
Chicago, Illinois

Gregory R. Trost, BS, MD
Associate Professor
Department of Neurosurgery
University of Wisconsin Hospitals & Clinics
Madison, Wisconsin

Luis M. Tumialán, MD
Department of Neurosurgery
Emory University School of Medicine
Atlanta, Georgia

Alexander R. Vaccaro, MD, PhD
The Rothman Institute at Jefferson University Hospital
Philadelphia, Pennsylvania

Brian Walsh, MD
Dean and St. Mary's Outpatient Center
Madison, Wisconsin

K. Michael Webb, MD
Division of Neurological Surgery
Barrow Neurological Institute
St. Joseph's Hospital and Medical Center
Phoenix, Arizona

Kirkham B. Wood, MD
Associate Professor
Harvard Medical School
Department of Orthopaedic Surgery
Massachusetts General Hospital
Boston, Massachusetts

Howard Yeon, MD
Department of Orthopaedic Surgery
Brigham and Women's Hospital
Boston, Massachusetts

Jim A. Youssef, MD
Durango Orthopedic Associates/Spine Colorado
Durango, Colorado

Carlos Zamorano, MD
Neurosciences Center
Hospital Ángeles de Pedregal
Mexico City, Mexico

SECTION I

Introduction

CHAPTER 1

The Changing Face of Spinal Trauma in Modern Society

Paul A. Anderson and Alexander R. Vaccaro

INTRODUCTION

Many advances have occurred in the management of spinal trauma and spinal cord injuries over the last decade. Despite much basic research in neuroprotection and spinal cord regeneration, no clinically positive benefits have occurred in humans. Multiple clinical trials are now ongoing with the hope of limiting spinal cord damage and producing reversal of established injuries in these unfortunate individuals. Improvements in general medical care, diagnostic imaging, and surgical techniques have reduced morbidity and mortality as well as the incidence of neurologic deterioration. Patients are now treated rapidly with interventions that allow mobilization and early transfer to rehabilitation centers. This chapter will review some of the salient changes that are occurring in spinal trauma and spinal cord injury research.

EPIDEMIOLOGY

The incidence of spinal cord injury in the United States is approximately 15–40 cases per million, or about 11,000 per year. This has been relatively constant over the last several decades. The male to female ratio is 4:1; although recently, more females are sustaining spinal injuries. The mean age at time of injury has increased from 28.7 years in the 1970s to 37.6 years since the year 2000. This increase is caused by general aging of the population and by an increase in the percentage of geriatric patients which has increased to approximately 5% to 10% of all spinal injured patients.

The most common etiology remains vehicular trauma in 47.5% of spinal cord injuries; falls, acts of violence (gunshot wounds), and sports are the next most common causes. Falls are increasing, especially in geriatric patients. Hopefully, fall prevention programs and treatment of osteoporosis will reduce these trends.

Dramatic increases in life span have been observed in spinal cord injury patients. However, deaths after admission still range from 4.4% to 16.7%. Causes of death include pneumonia, pulmonary embolism, and infection. Higher-level quadriplegics have an increased risk of death compared to paraplegic patients. Urinary sepsis and renal failure as a cause of mortality have significantly decreased due to improved management of patients with neurogenic bladder and bowel.

Over the last four decades, a change in severity of injuries of patients admitted to rehabilitation centers has occurred. Admissions for complete spinal cord injury have decreased from 67% to 45% over this time period. This reduction is felt to be because of improved prehospital and early hospital care (thereby preventing neurologic deterioration) and by the avoidance of laminectomy. Survivors of injuries to the occipitocervical junction are being seen with increasing frequency and range from

2.3% to 6.8% of spinal cord injury admissions. This introduces special burdens and costs to the medical trauma system, as many patients are respiratory dependent.

DIAGNOSTIC TESTING

Imaging of the spine has become an important aspect of trauma care. Protocols are now established with a goal to identify all patients with significant and unstable cervical injuries. The standard 3-view cervical spine series has been replaced in many centers by helical computed tomography (CT) with reformations. CT has increased sensitivity from 85% to 99% and is cost-effective over plain radiographs in patients who are already undergoing CT for other causes. Magnetic resonance imaging (MRI) may identify occult ligamentous injuries or cord compressive pathology. However, MRI also identifies insignificant lesions and leads, perhaps, to unnecessary or overtreatment. The use of MRI has not been proven to be a positive benefit relative to outcomes at this time.

Ideally, classification systems allow communication between practitioners, confer an impression of injury severity and instability, predict prognosis, and help to direct treatment. No classification system of cervical spine injuries has gained acceptance or has proven to be reliable. A new system has been proposed and is based on morphologic descriptions and a quantitative scale of stability. This has been shown to have excellent reliability and may improve research in the future.

EMERGENT MANAGEMENT OF SPINAL CORD INJURY

The immediate management of patients with spinal trauma remains unchanged: protect the spinal cord from further trauma, reduce fractures and dislocations, and provide long-term stability. In most cases, this is best accomplished by cranial tong traction. Additionally, the maintenance of maximum oxygen saturation and a mean arterial blood pressure of greater than 80 are important to adequately perfuse the acutely injured central nervous system tissue.

The concept of neuroprotection is to limit the secondary injuries that occur following spinal cord injuries. These injuries are caused by a variety of vascular, biochemical, cellular, and molecular events. The use of methylprednisolone as a neuroprotective agent is now controversial. Further analysis of the original clinical investigations and the addition of two randomized controlled studies have shown that any effect is, at most, modest and that significant complications can occur with its use. Currently the use of methylprednisolone is only recommended as an option in select patients. Other neuroprotective agents such as minocycline are being tested in pilot human studies.

The timing of surgery remains enigmatic. Most animal studies clearly show a time-dependent inverse relation between the duration from injury to surgical decompression and neurologic recovery. However, this has not been established in any Level I study in humans. A prospective investigation to evaluate the effect of early intervention is being performed by the Spine Trauma Study Group.

Spinal cord regeneration offers the only hope for most patients with established spinal cord injury. A number of techniques are being evaluated in animal models, but effective application in humans is most likely years away. Transplantation of embryonic stem cells, activated macrophages, and olfactory ensheathing cells show great promise. Activated macrophages transplantation is currently in Phase II investigations in the United States. Other human trials include direct spinal cord repair.

SURGICAL TECHNIQUES

Surgical techniques to manage spinal trauma are now well accepted. The majority of patients with unstable fractures are treated surgically either from an anterior or posterior approach. Decompression is now accepted as important in patients with ongoing neural compression and spinal cord injury. The technique of instrumentation, including rigid screw with plate or rod fixation, can now be applied posteriorly along the lateral masses, across the cervicothoracic and occipitocervical junction, and at

C1–C2. These modern techniques, although they increase the risk of neurovascular injury, can rigidly stabilize the spine, allow early mobilization, and minimize postoperative bracing.

COSTS

The costs of spinal cord injuries are staggering and place an enormous burden on government and families. The yearly costs of a quadriplegic are $450,000 for the first year and are approximately $52,000 per year thereafter. The estimated lifetime costs of a patient injured at age 25 with quadriplegia is $1.5 million and does not include indirect costs such as lost wages. From a cost perspective, prevention programs such as Think First appear effective.

CONCLUSION

Although no major breakthrough has occurred in regeneration or neuroprotection, measurable improvements have occurred in patients with spinal trauma. The patient survival rate is increasing, and fewer patients are deteriorating neurologically. Better diagnostic tests and surgical techniques reduce complications and allow earlier transfer to rehabilitation which facilitates and shortens overall stays and, presumably, costs. Efforts to translate basic research to human clinical trials are now ongoing with the hope of reducing morbidity and improving neurologic recovery.

SECTION II

Cervical Anatomy

CHAPTER 2

Anatomy and Development of the Immature Cervical Spine

Peter G. Gabos and Stephen M. Quinnan

PRE-EMBRYONIC PERIOD (WEEKS 0–3)

The pre-embryonic period begins with fertilization and proceeds with rapid cellular division and formation of a solid ball of cells called the morula. This cell mass cavitates at day 4 to form the blastocyst, which progressively develops as it travels to the uterus and becomes embedded during week 2. A concentration of cells forms within one end of the blastocyst cavity called the inner cell mass, or embryoblast, which will give rise to all tissues of the future embryo. The embryoblast then cavitates to form the amniotic cavity, and the embryoblast cells become a bilaminar disc with the epiblast layer dorsally adjacent to the amniotic cavity and the hypoblast layer ventrally adjacent to the yolk sac (Fig. 2.1).

EMBRYONIC PERIOD (WEEKS 3–8)

GASTRULATION

The onset and major formative events of human spine development occur during the embryonic period of gestation beginning with the formation of the trilaminar disc during gastrulation. Gastrulation is the process of formation of the three embryonic germ cell layers: ectoderm, mesoderm, and endoderm. Gastrulation is initiated with the formation of the primitive streak, which is a linear proliferation of epiblast cells that establishes the embryonic axis. At the cephalic end of the primitive streak is a slightly elevated area called the primitive node. In the center of the primitive node is a depression called the primitive pit. Along the midline is a depression called the primitive groove (Fig. 2.2). Epiblast cells migrate toward the primitive streak and invaginate underneath it at the primitive groove to displace the hypoblast cells and form the definitive endoderm. Cells that come to lie between the endoderm and epiblast form the mesoderm, and the cells that remain as the superficial epiblast form the ectoderm (see Fig. 2.2).

The mesodermal cells that migrate through the primitive pit and come to rest on the midline form the prechordal plate, a compact mass of mesoderm cranial to the primitive pit, and a dense midline tube called the notochordal process. The notochordal process grows in length as cells proliferating in the region of the primitive node add on to its proximal end and as the primitive streak regresses. The tube then fuses with the endoderm ventrally and unzips to form a midventral bar of mesoderm called the notochordal plate. The origin of the notochordal process at the primitive node becomes a patent structure called the neurenteric canal, which allows for temporary communication between the embryonic and yolk sac cavities. The notochordal plate completely detaches from the endoderm and retreats into the mesoderm-containing space by day 22–24, changing as it does so

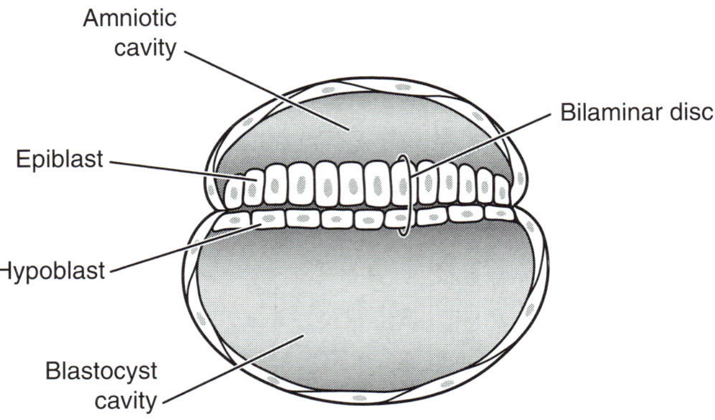

FIGURE 2.1. Bilaminar germ disc formed from the embryoblast with epiblastic cells adjacent to the amniotic cavity and hypoblastic cells bordering the blastocyst cavity.

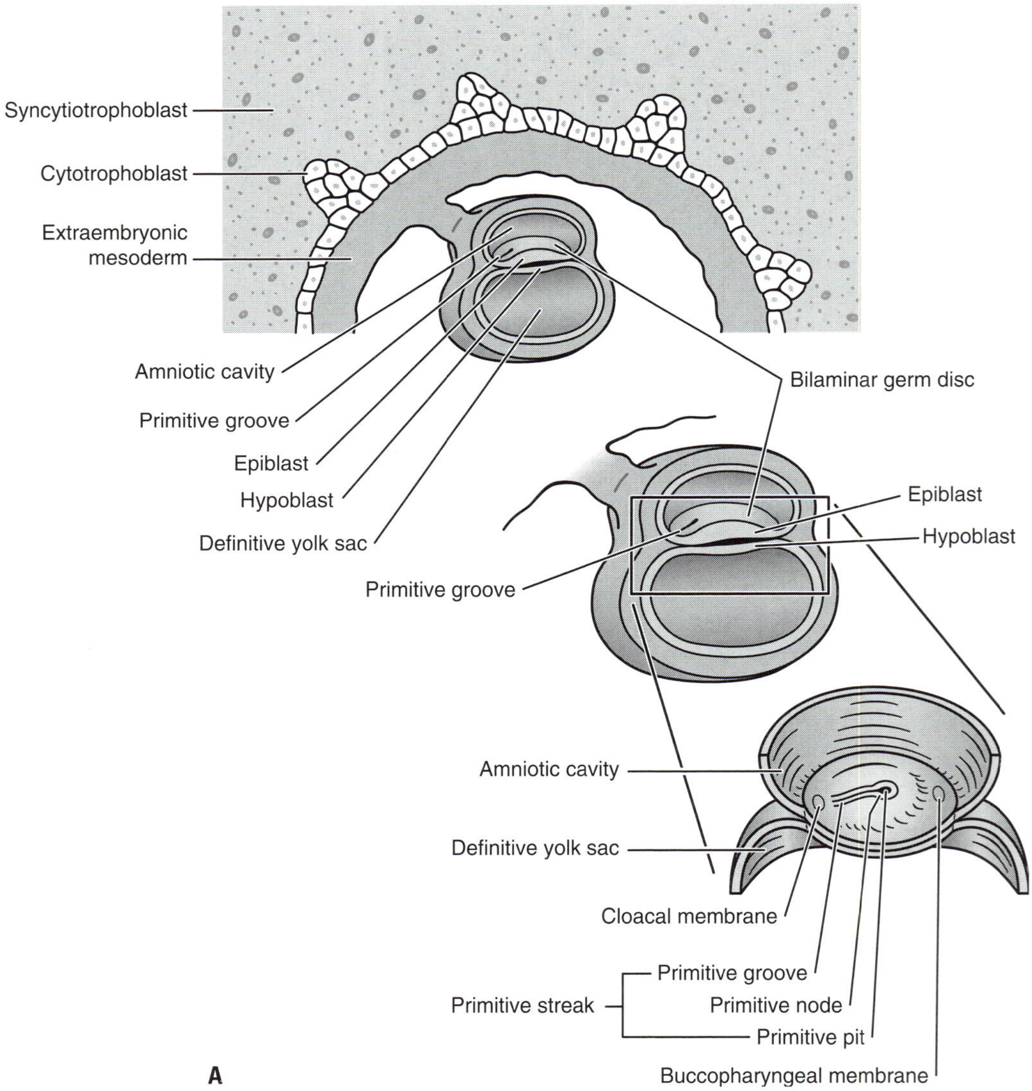

Syncytiotrophoblast
Cytotrophoblast
Extraembryonic
mesoderm
Amniotic cavity
Primitive groove
Epiblast
Hypoblast
Definitive yolk sac
Bilaminar germ disc
Epiblast
Hypoblast
Primitive groove
Amniotic cavity
Definitive yolk sac
Cloacal membrane
Primitive groove
Primitive streak
Primitive node
Primitive pit
Buccopharyngeal membrane
A

FIGURE 2.2. **A.** View of the dorsal surface of the bilaminar germ disc through the sectioned amnion at day 15 showing epiblast cells forming the primitive streak. *(continued)*

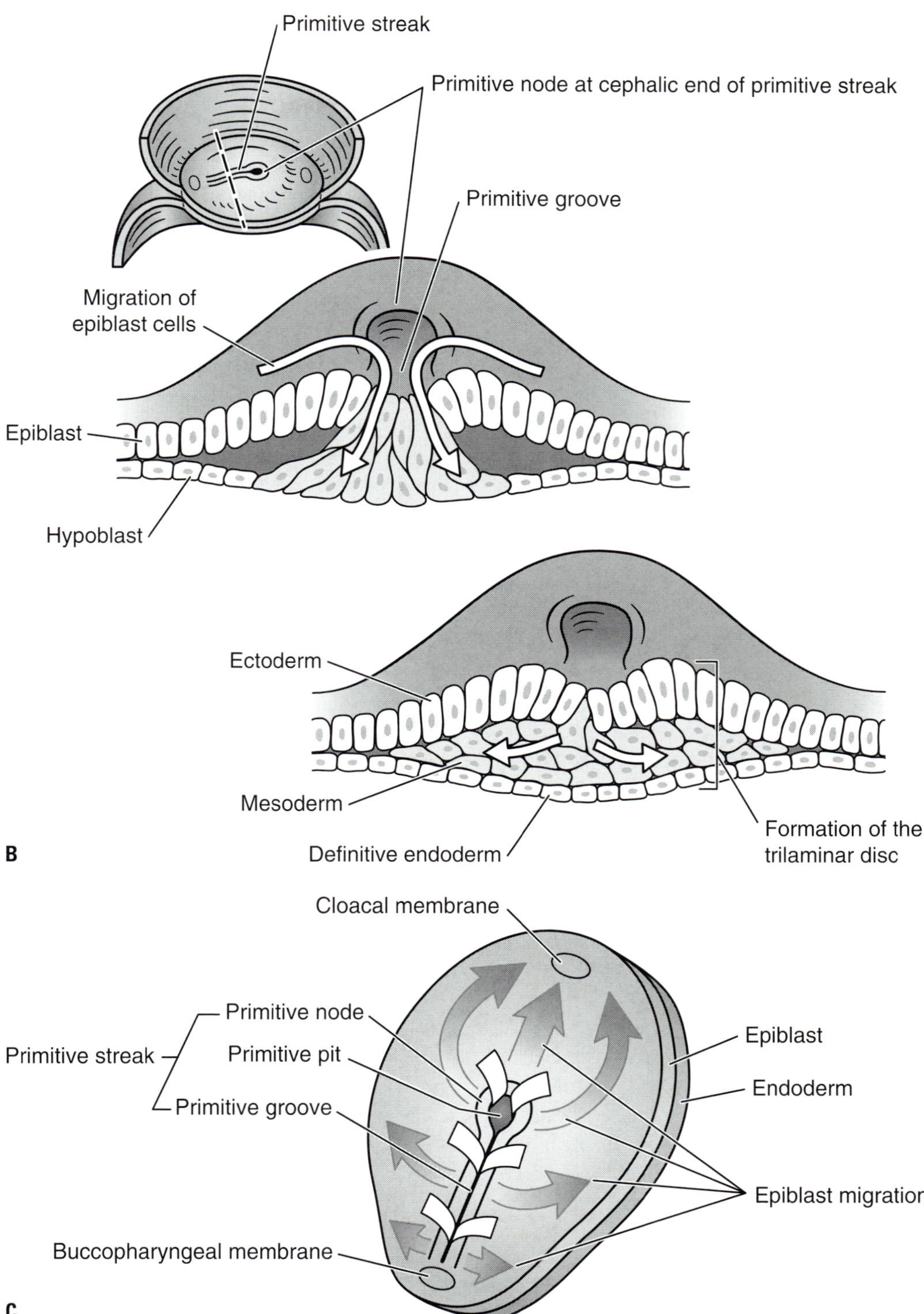

FIGURE 2.2. *(Continued)* **B.** Illustrates the movement of epiblast cells into the primitive streak to form the three layered gastrula. The cells that migrate on day 14–15 displace the hypoblast to form the endoderm. The epiblast cells that migrate on day 16 form the intraembryonic endoderm. **C.** Movement of mesoderm from specific locations within the primitive streak to well-defined destinations within the gastrula.

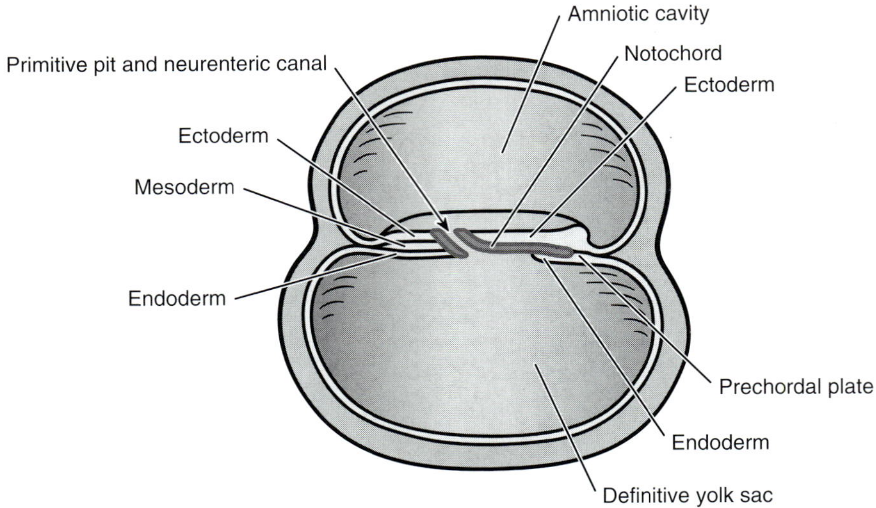

FIGURE 2.3. Sagittal section through a gastrula showing a cannulated notochordal process fusing with the endoderm to form the notochordal plate, which will become the notochord. The neurenteric canal is apparent allowing temporary communication between the amnion and yolk sac.

into a solid cellular rod called the notochord (Fig. 2.3). On either side of the midline notochord, the mesoderm cells spread out to form a loose network or sheet of mesenchyme that becomes organized into three zones that are apparent by day 19: paraxial, intermediate, and lateral plate mesoderm. The cells that migrate from the cranial end of the primitive streak form the paraxial mesoderm, the cells that migrate from the midregion of the streak form the intermediate mesoderm, and the cells that migrate from the caudal part form the lateral plate mesoderm. The paraxial mesoderm is directly adjacent to the notochord and develops into the axial skeleton, voluntary musculature, and part of the dermis of the skin. The narrower intermediate mesoderm develops into the urinary and genital systems. The flattened lateral plate mesoderm splits into two layers, ventrally forming the mesothelial covering of visceral organs and dorsally forming the inner lining of the body wall, parts of the limbs, and most of the dermis.

NEURULATION

Neurulation is the process of folding that creates the neural tube. Initiation of neurulation begins in the later half of the third week as the notochord and prechordal mesoderm signal the overlying ectoderm to thicken and form the neural plate. The neural plate elongates gradually toward the primitive streak and, by the eighteenth day, the lateral edges of the plate become elevated to form the neural folds which surround the neural groove. Fusion of the neural folds begins in the midline in the region of the neck and gradually proceeds cephalad and caudad, thereby forming the neural tube. The two ends of the neural tube communicate with the amniotic cavity through openings called neuropores. The cranial neuropore closes by approximately day 25, and the caudal neuropore closes by approximately day 27 marking the end of neurulation (Fig. 2.4).

SOMITE FORMATION

The paraxial mesoderm is organized into rounded whorl-like structures called somitomeres by the end of the third week. Somitomeres just caudal to the rostral end of the notochord develop further to form discreet blocks of segmental mesoderm called somites by day 20. Additional somites form at a rate of three to four pairs per day in a cephalocaudal direction for the next 10 days. By the end of

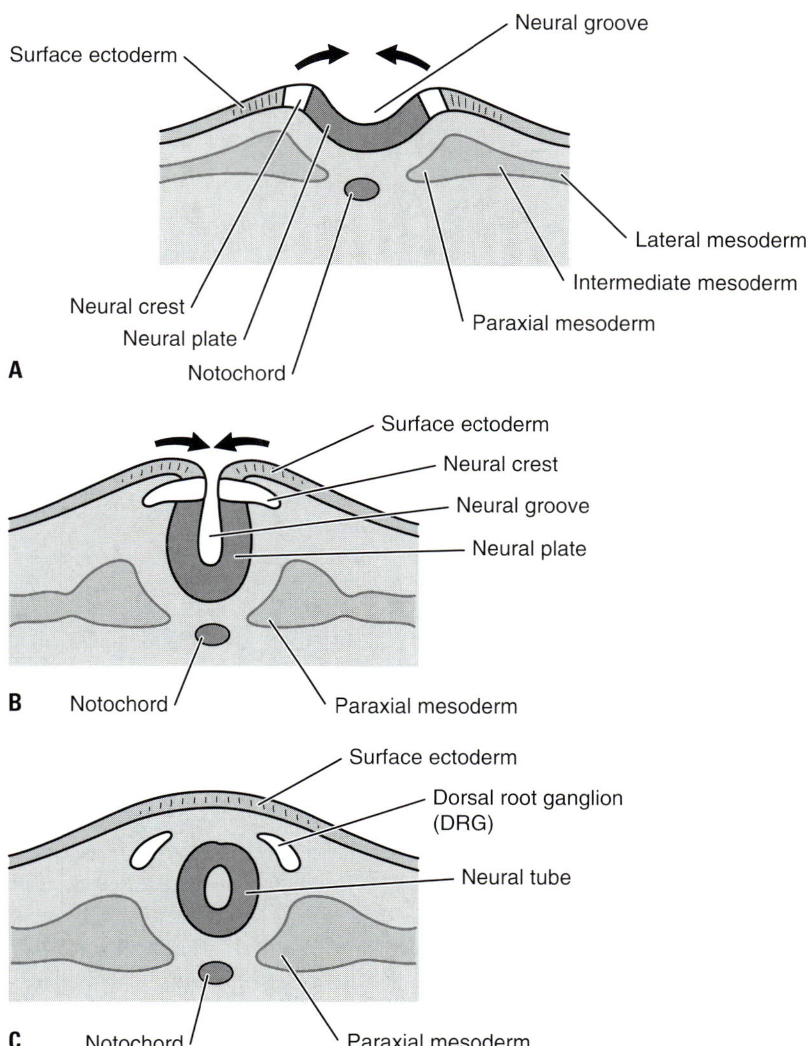

FIGURE 2.4. Axial view illustrating the formation of the neural tube and dorsal root ganglia. **A.** Neural folds form as neural ectoderm thickens laterally. **B.** Neural folds fuse to form the neural tube, and neural crest cells migrate into the underlying mesoderm to form a multitude of structures including the dorsal root ganglia **(C)**.

week 5, there are 42 to 44 pairs of somites: 4 occipital, 8 cervical, 12 thoracic, 5 lumbar, 5 sacral, and 8 to 10 coccygeal. The first occipital and last 5 to 7 coccygeal somites disappear, and the remaining final 37 pairs of somites form the axial skeleton and establish the segmental organization of the body (Fig. 2.5).

By the beginning of week 4, shortly after forming, each somite shows further differentiation into a sclerotome, myotome, and dermatome. Sclerotomes, which will develop into the vertebrae, are the first subdivision to appear as a ventromedial cell mass. The next most medial group becomes the myotome and the most lateral the dermatome. The dermomyotome is displaced laterally by expansion of the dorsolateral body wall as the sclerotomal cells proliferate. Sclerotomal cells proliferate rapidly and migrate to form the ventral portion of the sclerotome that surrounds the notochord and that forms the rudiment of the vertebral body, disks, and costal processes and to form the more dorsolateral portion that forms the rudiment of the neural arches that eventually surround the spinal canal as pedicles and laminae.

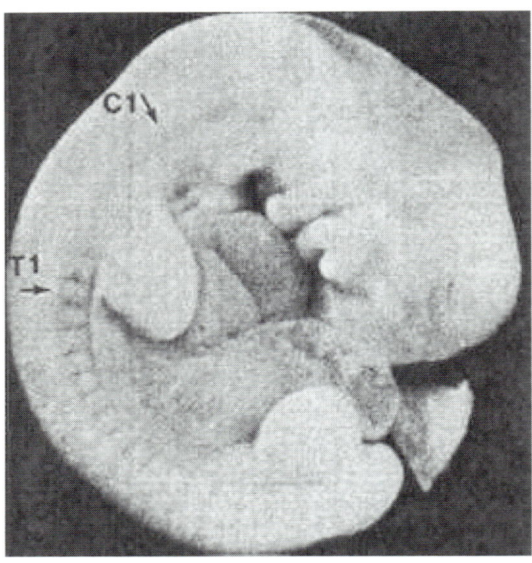

FIGURE 2.5. A 5.5-mm human embryo showing the external manifestations of the somites. The relations of the cervical somites to the limb bud presage that the nerves will be involved in the brachial plexus. The black dots rostral to the cervical somites indicate the position of the precervical somites that will form the basiocciput.

DEVELOPMENT AND OSSIFICATION OF TYPICAL VERTEBRAE

The ventral cells of the sclerotomes form a cylindrical column of loose mesenchymal tissue called the perichordal tube that surrounds the notochord. During week 6 of embryonic development, the sclerotomes undergo a metamorphosis that has traditionally been termed *resegmentation*. According to this theory, each sclerotome is divided into a cranial and a caudal part by a sclerotomic fissure (Fig. 2.6). The mesenchyme adjoining the fissure undergoes rapid cell proliferation to form cell aggregates called dense perichordal disks. Each sclerotome, therefore, contains a dense perichordal disk flanked cranially and caudally by less dense cell aggregates. The cranial half of one somite then fuses with the caudal half of the adjoining segment to form a fused loose perichordal disk, which gives rise to the primordium of the vertebral body. Intervertebral disks form from the dense perichordal disks at segmental levels with the original core of each somite. The nucleus pulposus is thought to be composed of cells of notochordal origin, whereas the surrounding anulus fibrosus develops from remaining sclerotomal cells. Meanwhile, the cells of the caudal part of the caudal hemisclerotome form the membranous precursor of the neural arch elements.[1,2]

Resegmentation was considered an ideal explanation of how muscles of separate myodermatomes could cross intervertebral disk levels to provide for voluntary motion. However, recent studies challenge the theory of resegmentation and provide an alternative explanation.[3,4,5] These studies indicate that the ventral perichordal sclerotomal cells, termed axial mesenchyme, establish a more defined perichordal tube that is a fairly homogenous cylindrical column. Areas of the perichordal tube adjacent to each somite then undergo more rapid proliferation to form the dense perichordal disks which form the intervertebral disks. In addition, the sclerotomal mesenchymal cells that have migrated more dorsolaterally form a continuous lateral column from which the neurocostal elements will be derived. The intersclerotomic cleft is obliterated, but the junctions of the myotomic arcs and the intersegmental vessels continue to mark the relative position of the now vanished cleft. The lateral column initially displays a longitudinally uniform cell density, but the cells lying medial to the cranial half of the myotome soon show a marked diminution in number, while the cells of the caudal hemisclerotome proliferate to develop an increased cell density that will form the membranous precursor of the neural arch. The intersegmental vessels remain at the superior boundary of this light region, while the associated intersegmental nerve courses within the loose cell mass. In the rostromedial part of the caudal hemisclerotome, just lateral to the dense perichordal disk of the axial mesenchyme, a rapid increase in cell concentration signals the formation of the costal process (Fig. 2.7).

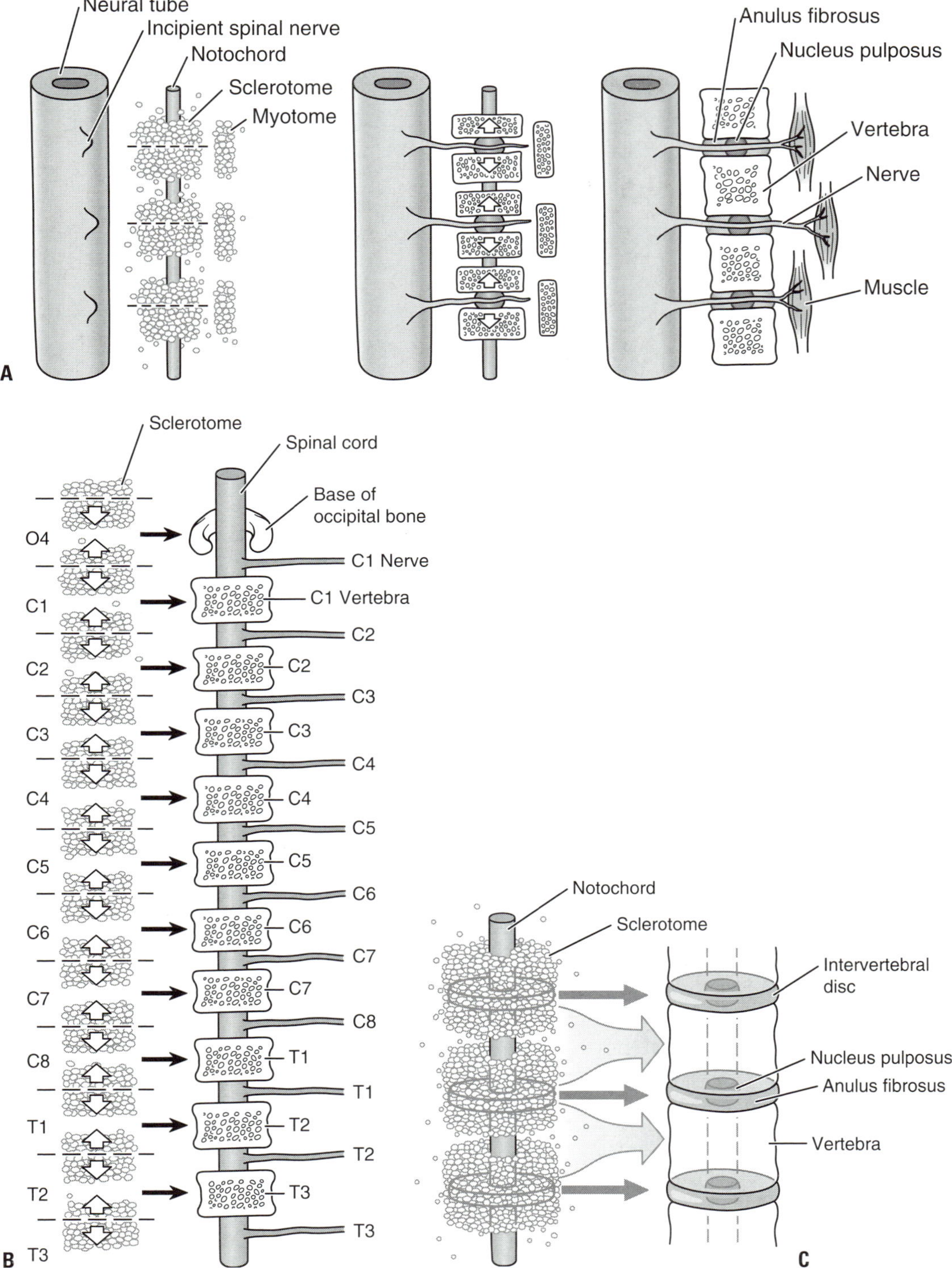

FIGURE 2.6. **A.** Represents resegmentation theory where sclerotomes split into caudal and cranial halves which recombine to form rudimentary vertebrae. **B.** Illustrates division of sclerotomes to form seven cervical vertebrae and eight cervical nerves. **C.** Relative contribution of sclerotome and notochord to vertebra and intervertebral disc.

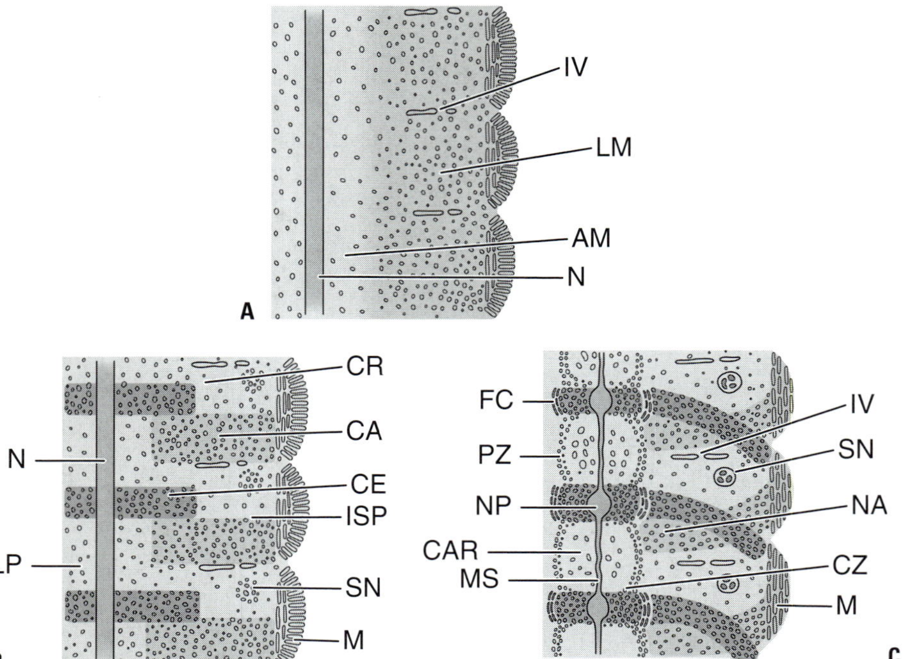

FIGURE 2.7. Illustration of early development of the mammalian vertebrae derived from information provided by Verbout and Dalgleish. **A.** Early organization of mesenchyme into columns. The notochord (N) is of uniform diameter and surrounded by loose unsegmented axial mesenchyme (AM) from which vertebral centra and discs will be derived. Lateral sclerotomic mesenchyme (LM) also lacks segmentation initially. The dermomyotome (DM) retains the original segmentation throughout this metamorphosis, and the intersegmental vessels (IV) mark the intersclerotomic boundaries. **B.** Axial mesenchyme differentiates into dense perichordal disc (DP) and loose perichordal disc (LP) that become the intervertebral disc and centrum, respectively. The lateral mesenchyme separates into loose tissue in the cranial sclerotomic region (CR), which accommodates the intervertebral vessels (IV) and the developing spinal nerves (SN), and a dense caudal sclerotomic region (CA) that is the precursor to the neural arches. A costal element (CE) organizes lateral to the incipient disc. The intersclerotomic plane (ISP) is the abrupt demarcation of cell differentiation that may produce spurious "intrasegmental clefts" in histologic preparation. **C.** The notochord has differentiated into mucoid streak (MS) within the vertebrae and the cell concentration that contributes to the nucleus pulposus (NP). The disc now shows the development of fibrocartilage (FC), and additional growth is now provided by the perichondral and chondrogenous zones (PZ, CZ). The "crossing" of the membranous precursors of the costal element (CE) and the neural arch element (NA) illustrates that the costal elements grow ventrolaterally while the neural arch grows dorsolaterally. The staggered position of the myotomes (M) relative to the neural arch elements indicates why resegmentation is not required to explain the definitive muscle–bone overlapping.

The medial and lateral sclerotomal columns appear to commingle, but as chondrification proceeds, the neurocentral synchondrosis eventually develops as an obvious demarcation between these two regions. The neural arch primordium contributes substantially to the formation of the vertebral body, especially in the cervical region where it may contribute as much as half the body mass. The costal process becomes a rib in the thoracic spine, but in the cervical and lumbar spine, it forms part of the transverse process. The costal process component of the sclerotome also gives rise to the hypochordal bow. In the neck, this structure becomes the anterior arch of the atlas, but more distally, it forms the thick portion of the anterior longitudinal ligament at each level. The costal process and hypochordal bow are the vestiges of the hemal or ventral arch in other vertebrate species such as birds and reptiles. The sclerotomes thus metamorphose to form the definitive structure of the membranous vertebral column.

CHONDRIFICATION

Chondrification begins rapidly after the mesenchymal spine is established, beginning in the upper level occipital somites and proceeding distally. Each centrum is chondrified from a pair of centers, which appear at the sixth week and coalesce shortly thereafter. Each half of the neural arch is chondrified from a center at its base, which extends ventrally to the pedicles and dorsally to the laminae. The laminar centers meet in the midline by the fourth month. The costal processes chondrify separately. As chondrification and subsequent ossification proceed, a cartilaginous connection, known as the neurocentral synchondrosis, demarcates the ossified neural arch from the ossified centra. The neurocentral synchondrosis is situated anterior to the pedicles and lies within the vertebral body, being medially located in the cervical and sacral regions. This may on occasion lead to difficulty in differentiating from a traumatic defect of the axis in early childhood (Fig. 2.8).

OSSIFICATION

Vertebral ossification involves both primary and secondary centers of ossification, similar to other bones in the body. Ossification in utero takes place in five centers, replacing the cartilage of the chondrified vertebral anlagen. These five centers are the centrum of the vertebral body, the two neural arches, and the two costal processes. At approximately the ninth week, the chondrous centrum is invaded by pericostal vessels, which produce ventral and dorsal vascular lacunae that support ossification. For this reason, the single ossification center for the centrum initially shows dorsal and ventral components, which later unify into a single ossification center. Ossification of the centrum usually begins in the lower thoracic and upper lumbar regions and develops more rapidly in the caudal than the cranial vertebrae. The centrum occasionally ossifies from two centers and if one is suppressed, a wedge-shaped hemivertebra may develop.

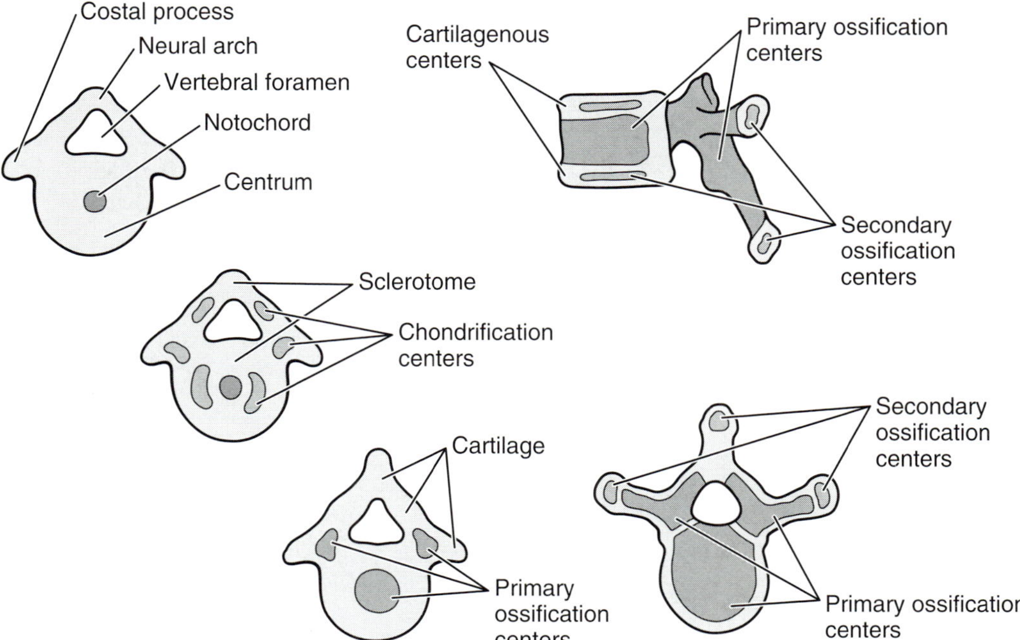

FIGURE 2.8. Four cross-sectional and one lateral view of a vertebra showing the transition from mesenchyme to cartilage through formation of primary and secondary ossification centers.

Ossification is observed in the neural arch centers by approximately the eighth week. The two neural arch centers, one for each half of the arch, appear first in the cervical region before centrum ossification is seen. At birth, the centrum, neural arches, and the costal processes at each level of the cervical spine have ossified, but these structures have not fused. The laminae of the arches first unite in the lumbar region in the first year of life, and subsequently union occurs at progressively cranial levels. The arch segments and the centra fuse at the site of the neurocentral synchondrosis, anterior to the pedicles. In the upper cervical region, the centra unites with the arches by the third year, whereas in the lower lumbar region, union is not completed until the sixth year (see Figs. 2.8 and 2.9).

Secondary centers of ossification appear at the tips of the transverse processes and within the spinous process around age 10 years in girls and 12 years in boys. The secondary centers progressively ossify these cartilaginous segments until fusing with the primarily ossified elements at age 13 years in girls and 17 years in boys. Two secondary ossification centers also appear as annular vertebral ring epiphyses on the cranial and caudal surfaces of each vertebra from the caudal surface of C2 to the cranial surface of S1. The vertebral ring epiphyses ossify initially anteriorly and progress posteriorly to form a complete disc. The ring epiphyses fuse with the rest of the vertebra by age 13 years in girls and age 17 years in boys marking the end of spinal growth. Thoracic vertebrae have additional secondary centers of ossification at the costal articular facets, which are extensions of the annular epiphyseal discs. The seventh cervical vertebra has the typical ossification centers with addition of separate secondary ossification centers for the costal processes. These appear at approximately the sixth month of fetal life and unite with the rest of the vertebra at age 6 years. If these ossification centers remain separate from

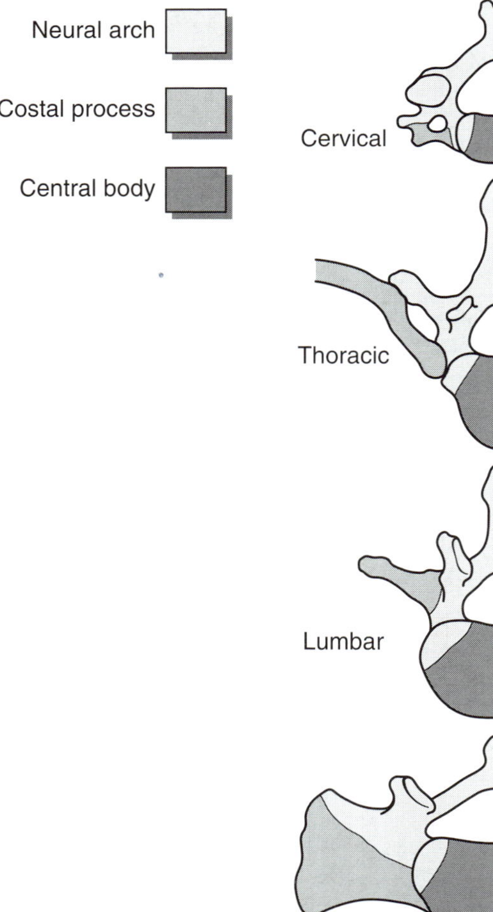

FIGURE 2.9. Comparison of relative contributions from the three primary ossific centers to the typical vertebra in each of the four major spinal areas. The neural arch ossific center contributes the most in the cervical spine.

the rest of the vertebra, they may form cervical ribs. Less commonly, separate ossification centers such as this can be seen at the sixth, fifth, and even the fourth cervical vertebrae. If cervical rib formation occurs, these ossification centers do not fuse until the end of the third decade (see Fig. 2.8).

ATYPICAL VERTEBRAL DEVELOPMENT AND THE ATLANTOAXIAL COMPLEX

The occipital region, the atlantoaxial complex, the sacrum, and the coccyx are the exceptions to the above description. The atlantoaxial complex has a complex multisegmental origin. The basiocciput arises from the fusion of the proximal occipital sclerotomes, which are perforated by cranial nerve XII (hypoglossal nerve). The C0 sclerotome, or proatlas, gives rise to the tip of the odontoid process, the anterior arch of the atlas, the dorsal part of the superior atlas facets, the upper half of the transverse ligament, the apical odontoid ligament, and the retroarticular ligaments. The anterior arch of the atlas is the enlarged hypochordal bow of the C0 sclerotome with the anterior part of the lateral mass of the atlas from the C1 sclerotome. The C1 sclerotome, or atlas, gives rise to the remainder of the atlas and the inferior major part of the odontoid process, which is considered to represent the body or centrum of the atlas (Fig. 2.10). The atlas shows an ossification center in

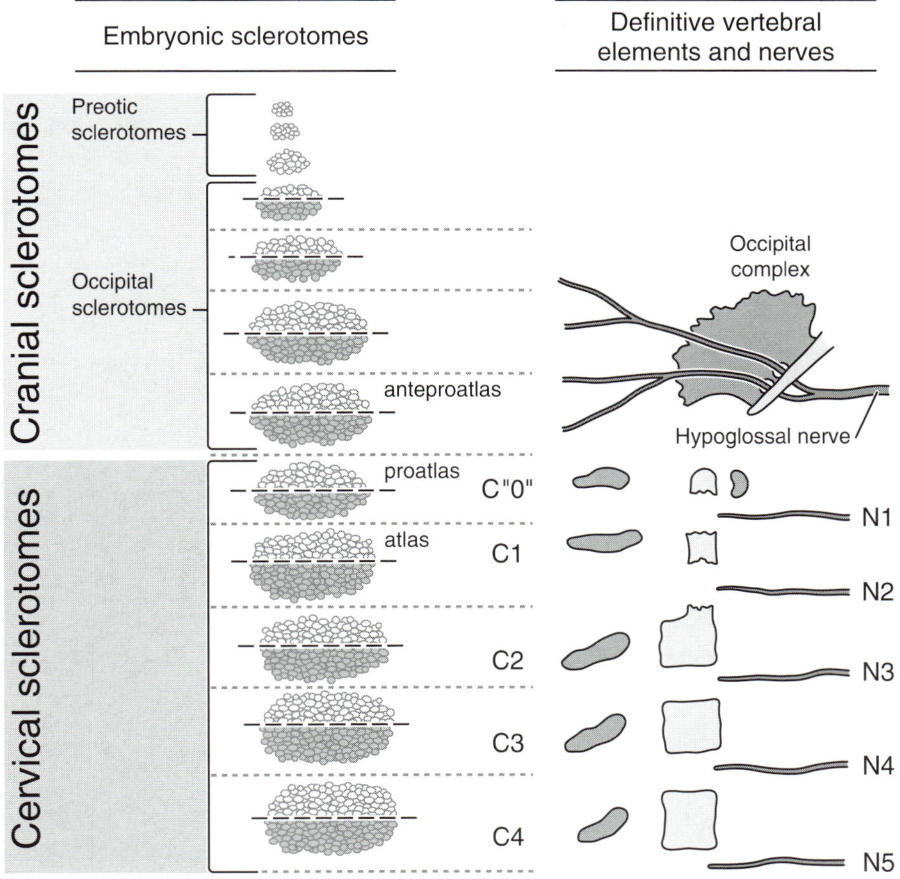

FIGURE 2.10. Illustration of the craniocervical sclerotomes and their definitive segmentally related cranial and vertebral elements and nerves. The sclerotomes of the cranial and cervical region initially form a continuum. The axis incorporates elements from three sclerotomes (C0, C1, C2), and the ring of the atlas includes neural arch components of both atlas and proatlas in addition to the hypochondral bow of the proatlas that forms the anterior arch. The caudal four cranial sclerotomes contribute to formation of the occiput, and the hypoglossal nerves form as the various occipital nerves coalesce.

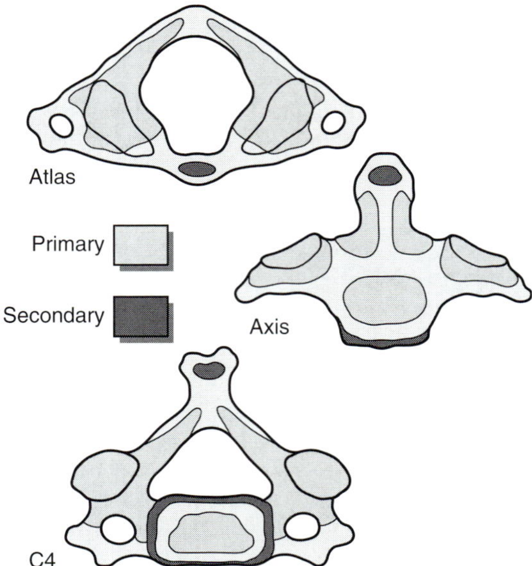

FIGURE 2.11. Schematic illustration of the ossification centers in the cervical vertebrae. The atlas contains only two primary centers at the neural arches. The secondary center that forms in the anterior arch is a derivative of the otherwise vestigial vertebral hypochondral bar found in lower vertebrates. The axis has five primary and two secondary centers of ossification. The dens ossifies from bilobed lateral centers representing what would have been the centra of C1. The apical secondary center of the dens arises within material from the proatlas. The inferior secondary center of the axis forms the ring apophysis, as in other vertebrae. The rest of the cervical vertebrae, as represented by C4, arise from three primary and two secondary centers for the ring apophysis. The secondary center at the tip of the spinous processes that is seen consistently in more caudal vertebrae are less constant in the cervical region, being most frequent in the more inferior elements (C6, C7).

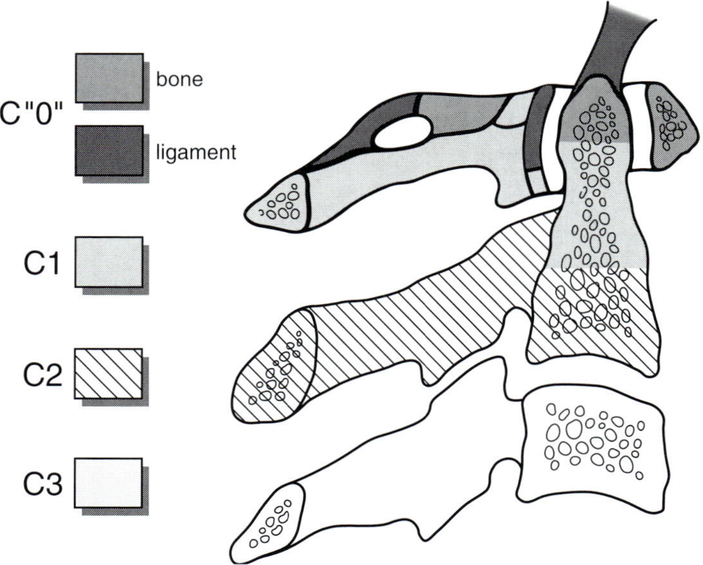

FIGURE 2.12. This illustration defines the contributions of the first three sclerotomes to the atlantoaxial complex and its syndesmotic relationships. The proatlas provides the tip of the odontoid, the anterior arch of C1, and the dorsal component of the superior atlas facet in addition to the upper half of the transverse ligament and the apical odontoid and retroarticular ligaments, which are indicated in black. The C1 sclerotome forms the rest of the posterior arch and the inferior major part of the odontoid process.

each lateral mass at about the seventh week that gradually extends into the posterior arch, where they unite between the third and fourth years. A separate center appears in the anterior arch toward the end of the first year of life, which unites with lateral masses between the sixth and eighth years (Fig. 2.11).

The central portion of the dens represents the fusion of the C0 and C1 sclerotomes. The remainder of the body of the axis and its vertebral arches are formed from C2 and C3 sclerotome components. The vertebral arch of the axis is ossified from two primary centers appearing at the seventh or eighth week and the centrum from a center appearing at the fourth or fifth month of gestation. The dens is ossified from two laterally placed centers appearing at the sixth month of gestation and uniting just before birth. At the tip of the odontoid process, a center appears at the second year of life and unites with the main mass by the twelfth year (Fig. 2.12). The base of the odontoid is separated from the body of the axis by a cartilaginous disc. The circumference of this disc is ossified, although the center remains cartilaginous until advanced age. The proximal aspect of the odontoid occasionally fails to unite with the rest of the axis and may persist as an "os odontoideum." The most caudal occipital somite, the ante-proatlas, occasionally forms a basilar tubercle or even a third condyle at the basion or anterior midline point of the foramen magnum that articulates with the tip of the odontoid. A more frank separation of this ante-proatlas segment may result in the formation of a true occipital vertebra proximal to the C1 segment.

REFERENCES

1. Bagnali KM, Harris PF, Jones PR. A radiographic study of the human fetal spine. 2. The sequence of development of ossification centres in the vertebral column. *J Anat* 1977;124:791–802.
2. Sensenig EC. The early development of the human vertebral column. *Contrib Embryol* 1949;33:21–42.
3. Dalgleish AE. A study of the development of thoracic vertebrae in the mouse assisted by autoradiography. *Acta Anat* 1985;122(2):91–98.
4. Verbout AJ. The development of the vertebral column. *Adv Anat Embryol Cell Biol* 1985;90:1–122.
5. Verbout AJ, Hudson A. The resegmentation of the embryonic vertebral column. *Proc 3rd Europ Anat Congress*, Manchester, England; 1973:215–217.

CHAPTER 3

Occiput and Upper Cervical Spine Anatomy

Christian Fras and Wolfgang Rauschning

INTRODUCTION

The cervical spine, made up of seven cervical vertebrae and their associated muscular, ligamentous, neural, and vascular tissues, serves to support the skull, allow for stable motion, and protect vital neural and vascular structures. Of the seven vertebrae, four are considered typical (C3 through C6) because of their comparatively similar structure, and three are considered atypical (C1, C2, and C7) because of their unique morphology.

This chapter will focus on the anatomy of the upper portion of the cervical spine: the caudal aspect of the occiput, C1, and C2. Although pathologic conditions in this area are less common than in other areas of the cervical spine, an understanding of the related anatomy can aid in identifying potentially catastrophic injuries. Furthermore, given the atypical nature of the vertebrae involved, a thorough understanding of their anatomy is helpful in allowing the surgeon to safely pursue operative intervention for a variety of pathologic conditions.

OSSEOUS ANATOMY

The occiput is the bony posterior covering of the cerebellum and borders the foramen magnum, where the spinal cord leaves the cranium. A useful palpable landmark in the midline of the squamous portion of the occiput is the external occipital protuberance (inion); this is the thickest portion of the occipital bone (Fig. 3.1). Other landmarks include the supreme nuchal line, the superior nuchal line, and the inferior nuchal line. Occipital bone thickness decreases significantly from the superior to the inferior nuchal line.

The foramen magnum is defined by the following borders: the posterior border is known as the opisthion; the anterior border is known as the clivus, or basion, and is formed by the basilar portion of the sphenoid and occipital bones; the lateral borders are formed in large part by the occipital condyles (Fig. 3.2). The occipital condyles are convex paired lateral prominences, typically oval or bean-shaped, and slope inferiorly from lateral to medial in the coronal plane; they make an angle of 25 to 28 degrees with the midsagittal plane. When viewed from anterior, they are wedge-shaped, extending farther medially than laterally.[1–3]

The occipital condyles articulate with the relatively shallow, cup-shaped superior articular facets of C1, forming the paired atlanto-occipital joints (Fig. 3.3). These joints are enclosed in loose joint capsules; the contribution of the atlanto-occipital joint complex to overall craniocervical stability is relatively modest, with the exception of mild restriction of anteroposterior translation.[2,4] The atlanto-occipital joint allows for approximately 20 to 30 degrees of flexion-extension and 5 to 10 degrees of lateral bending; it does not contribute significantly to rotational motion.[5,6]

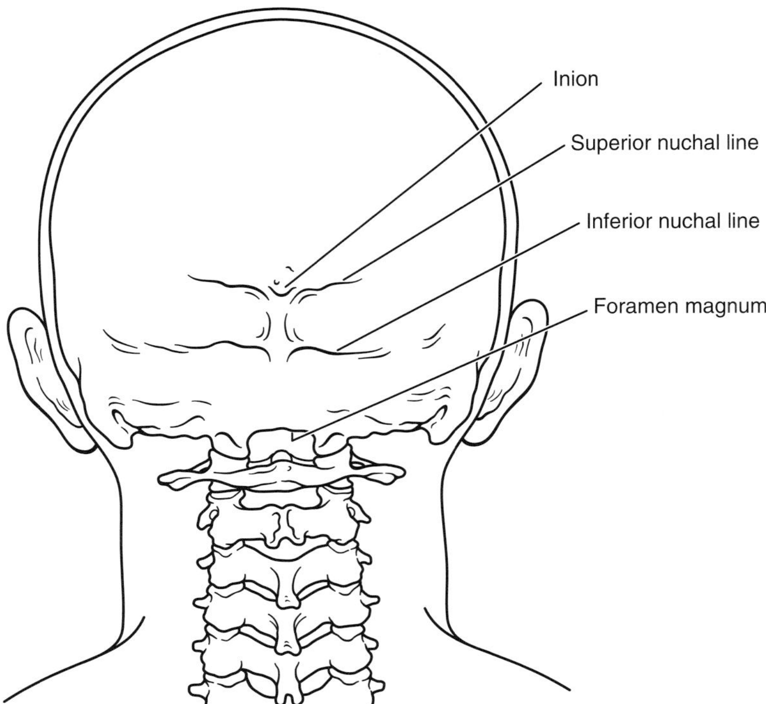

FIGURE 3.1. Upper cervical anatomy landmarks: external occipital protuberance (inion), foramen magnum, superior nuchal line, inferior nuchal line.

The first and second cervical vertebrae (or atlas and axis, respectively) are considered to be "atypical" vertebrae because of their unique structure. C1 lacks a body and a spinous process. It consists of a ringlike structure through which the spinal cord passes (the spinal canal, or vertebral foramen). The atlas is the widest cervical vertebra. The ring of C1 is composed of two lateral masses connected by a short anterior arch and a longer posterior arch; thus, it is not a symmetric ring because the anterior arch is approximately half as long as the posterior arch. At C1, the spinal canal is conveniently divided into three regions in its ventral-dorsal dimension (Steel's rule of thirds): the ventral third is occupied by the C2 odontoid process; the middle third by the spinal cord; and the dorsal third by epidural fat, meninges, and epidural vessels. Located on the ventral midline of the anterior arch is the anterior tubercle, which serves as the attachment for the anterior longitudinal ligament and longus colli muscles. On the upper dorsal surface of the posterior arch (which corresponds to the lamina of the other vertebrae) is a wide groove for the vertebral artery and first cervical nerve. In up to 15% of the population, a true arch of bone may form (the ponticulus posticus), converting this groove into the arcuate foramen.[7,8] Within each transverse process is an opening for the passage of the vertebral artery (foramen transversarium, or transverse foramen); those of the atlas are the largest in the cervical spine. Mirroring the anterior arch, on the dorsal surface of the posterior arch is the posterior tubercle, where the ligamentum nuchae attaches. The inferior surface of the posterior arch is notched, contributing to the formation of the C1-C2 intervertebral foramen.

The atlas possesses both superior and inferior articular facets, which develop from the lateral masses. The paired superior facets, articulating with the occipital condyles, are kidney shaped, elongated, and tilted medially and superiorly. The inferior facets, articulating with the axis, are more circular, are flatter, and tilt medially and inferiorly.

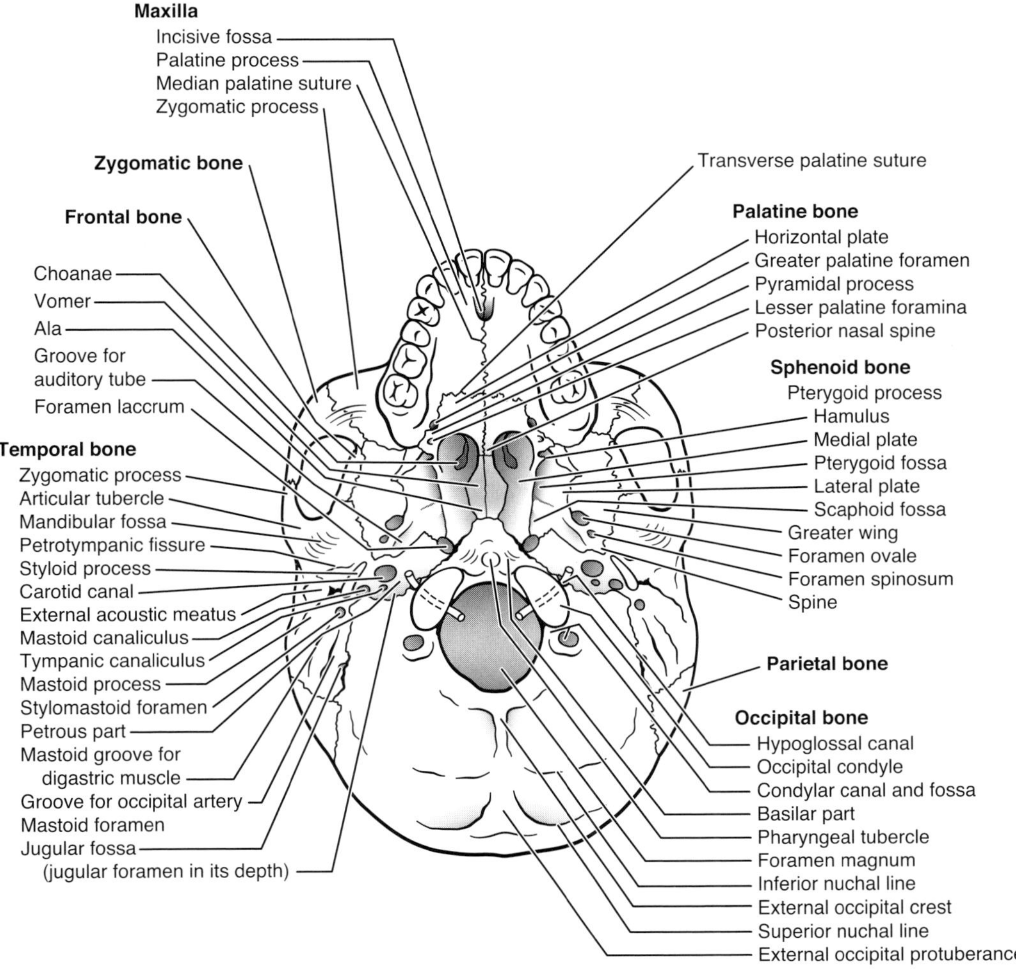

FIGURE 3.2. Foramen magnum anatomy: opisthion, clivus (or basion), basilar portion of the sphenoid and occipital bones, occipital condyles.

The predental space describes the area between the anterior arch of the atlas and the odontoid process of the axis. A diarthrodial articulation exists between the dorsal surface of the anterior ring of C1 and the ventral surface of the odontoid process.

The second cervical vertebra is the axis (also known as the epitrophysis). Its most striking feature is the dens, or odontoid process, which projects up from the body of C2 to articulate with the anterior ring of C1 and provides a pivot point for rotation of the atlas and consequently the head (Fig. 3.4). The mean height of the dens is 37.8 mm, but this and its other dimensions are highly variable.[9,10] Just lateral to the base of the dens, the body of the axis has paired facets for articulation with the inferior facets of the atlas. These are not true superior articular processes because they arise from the body and pedicle rather from the lateral masses. These facets face upward and outward. The area between the lamina and the lateral mass is ill-defined and contains a large pedicle projecting ventrally, superiorly, and medially.[11] The inferior surface of the C2 lateral mass possesses facets that face anteriorly, with very little medial or lateral angulation, to articulate with the superior facets of C3. These inferior facets of the axis are positioned more dorsal than those that articulate superiorly with the atlas. The laminae of C2 are thick and meet to form a large, bifid spinous process, which is palpable on physical examination. The transverse processes end in a single tubercle and also have a transverse foramen through which the vertebral artery passes.

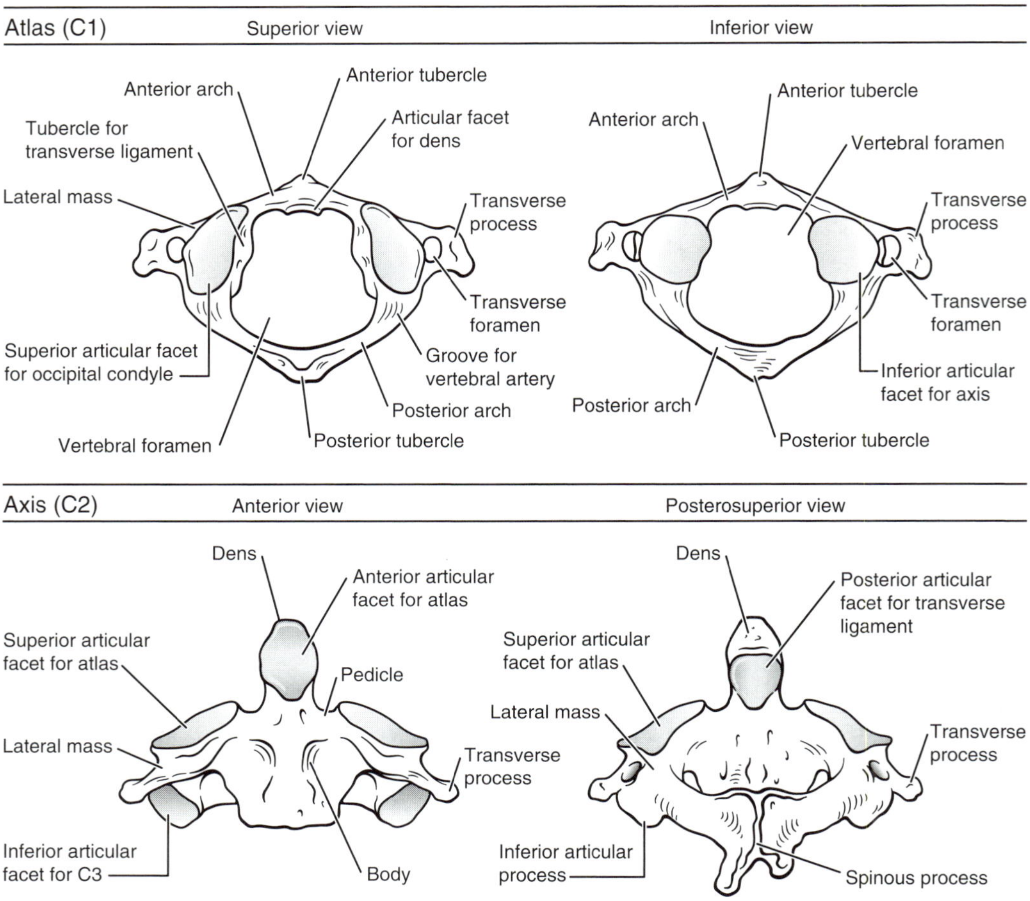

Atlas (C1)
Superior view
Inferior view
Anterior arch
Anterior tubercle
Articular facet for dens
Tubercle for transverse ligament
Lateral mass
Transverse process
Transverse foramen
Groove for vertebral artery
Superior articular facet for occipital condyle
Posterior arch
Vertebral foramen
Posterior tubercle
Anterior arch
Anterior tubercle
Vertebral foramen
Transverse process
Transverse foramen
Inferior articular facet for axis
Posterior arch
Posterior tubercle
Axis (C2)
Anterior view
Posterosuperior view
Dens
Anterior articular facet for atlas
Superior articular facet for atlas
Pedicle
Lateral mass
Transverse process
Inferior articular facet for C3
Body
Dens
Posterior articular facet for transverse ligament
Superior articular facet for atlas
Lateral mass
Transverse process
Inferior articular process
Spinous process

FIGURE 3.3. Anatomy of C1 (A,B) and C2 (C,D).

Axis (C2)
Superior view
Anterior view
Superior articular surfaces
Dens
Transverse foramen
Transverse process
Inferior articular process
Lamina
Spinous process
Dens
Anterior articular surface
Superior articular surfaces
Transverse process
Inferior articular process
Body

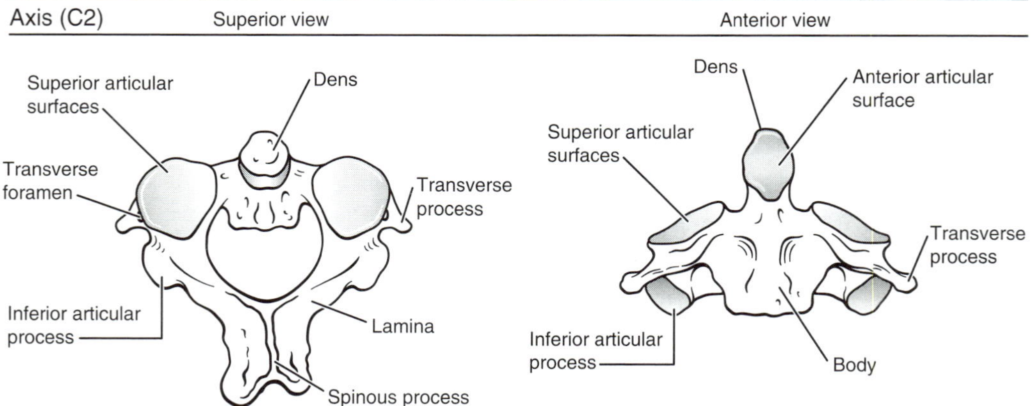

FIGURE 3.4. Anatomy of C2: dens (or odontoid process), superior articular processes, inferior articular processes.

NEURAL ELEMENTS

The spinal cord begins in the foramen magnum, at which point it is continuous with the medulla oblongata; after leaving the foramen magnum, it lies within the spinal (or vertebral) canal (Fig. 3.5). The anterior border of the spinal canal is the posterior border of the vertebral body or intervertebral disk (at C1, it is the posterior border of the dens); the lateral borders are the lateral masses and articular facets at C1 and the pedicles and inferior articular facets at C2; the posterior border is formed by the posterior arch of C1 and the lamina of C2. The cross-sectional area of the spinal canal is greatest at C2 and progressively decreases throughout the subaxial spine, being smallest at C7.[12]

On the spinal cord's dorsal surface lie the posterior and posterolateral spinal artery and vein, as well as various other small arteries and veins; on the ventral surface, within the ventral fissure (anterior median fissure), lies the anterior spinal artery and various small veins. The anterior spinal artery is formed from direct branches off the vertebral arteries that join together; the two posterior arteries arise from either the vertebral artery or the posterior inferior cerebellar arteries. In the upper cervical spine, the anterior spinal artery supplies most of the spinal cord; the remainder is largely supplied by the two posterior arteries (Fig. 3.6).[13]

The internal structure of the spinal cord can be briefly described as containing an inner, butterfly-shaped core of gray matter composed of nerve cell bodies and a surrounding outer white matter layer of nerve fibers (Fig. 3.7). The posterior horn of gray matter contains somatosensory neurons; the anterior gray matter horn contains motor neurons. The white matter of nerve fibers that surrounds the gray matter is organized into posterior, lateral, and anterior columns. The posterior

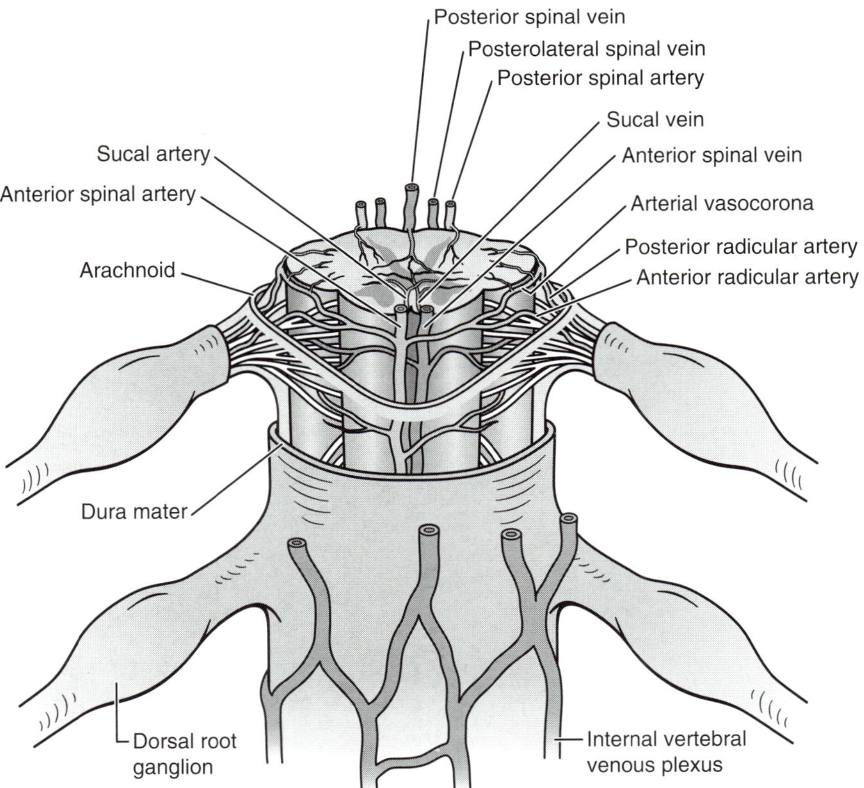

FIGURE 3.5. Spinal cord anatomy: posterior and posterolateral spinal artery and vein, ventral fissure, anterior spinal artery.

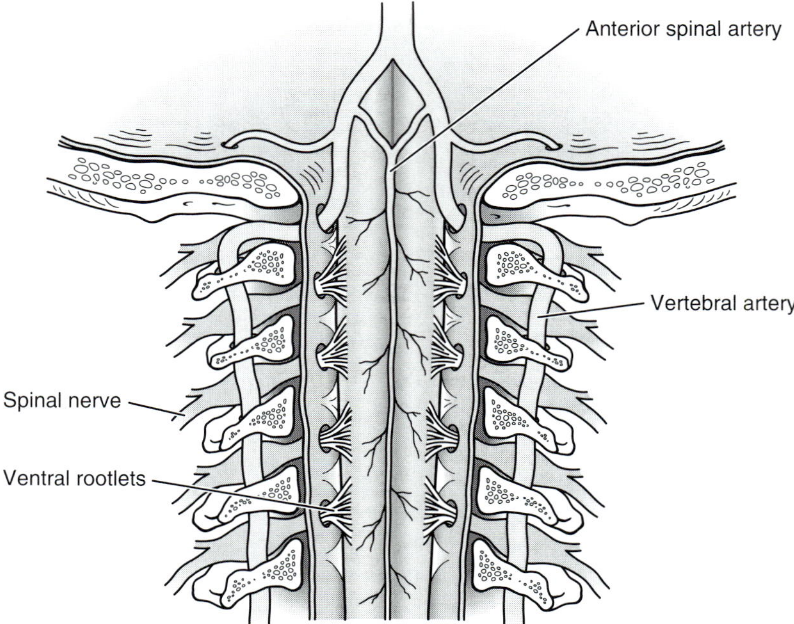

FIGURE 3.6. Anterior spinal artery.

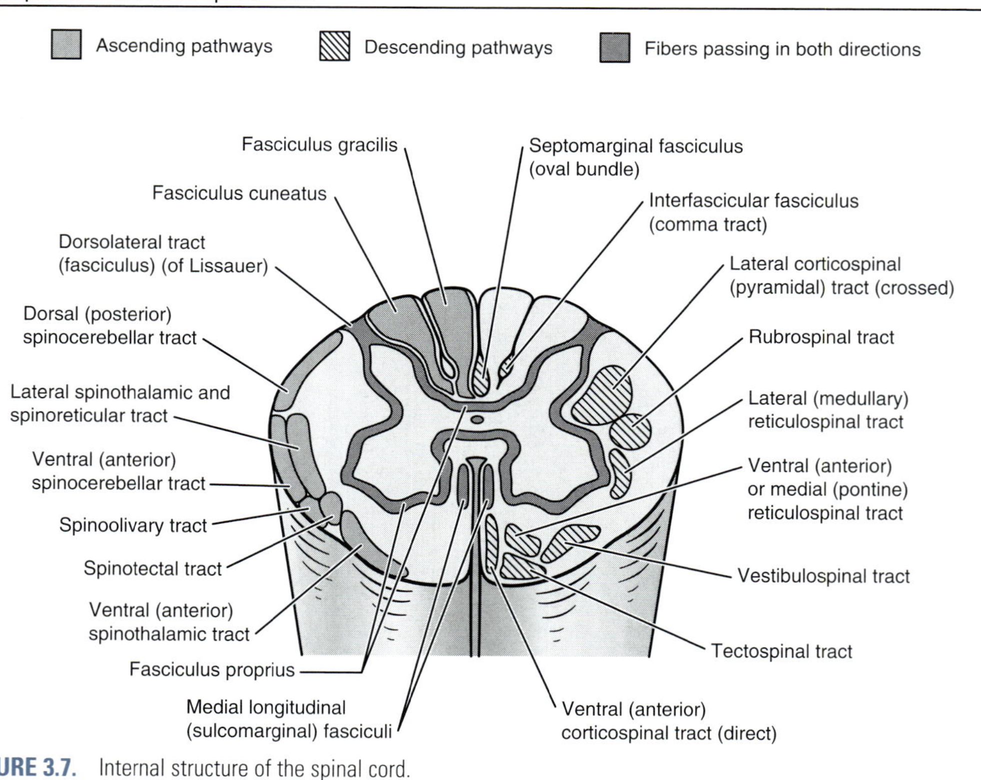

FIGURE 3.7. Internal structure of the spinal cord.

column is an ascending group of fibers relating to proprioception, vibration, and light touch sensation. The lateral column contains the lateral corticospinal and lateral spinothalamic tracts. The former is a descending pathway contributing to voluntary discrete and skillful motor function; the latter is an ascending pathway relaying pain and temperature sense. The anterior column contains several different tracts within it, including the anterior corticospinal tract (descending fibers associated with motor function) and the anterior spinothalamic tract (ascending fibers associated with light touch).

At each level of the spinal cord, a left and right spinal nerve exit; there are eight paired cervical spinal nerves. Shortly after leaving the spinal cord, the dorsal root ganglion forms (Fig. 3.8). Just beyond the dorsal root ganglion, and usually just at or outside the intervertebral foramen, the cervical spinal nerves divide into dorsal and ventral primary rami. As a general rule, the dorsal roots supply only incoming sensory information, whereas the ventral roots contain both motor and sensory fibers. The first cervical nerve exits between the occiput and C1; nerves C2 to C7 exit above the correspondingly numbered vertebrae (e.g., the C2 nerve exits just superior to the C2 vertebra, between C1 and C2; C8 exits above T1) (Fig. 3.9). The first cervical nerve exits just above the posterior arch of the atlas and posteromedial to the atlas' lateral mass. Its ventral primary ramus unites with that of the second cervical nerve, contributing fibers to the hypoglossal nerve (superior root of the ansa cervicalis); its dorsal primary ramus (also known as the suboccipital nerve) enters the suboccipital triangle, innervating the muscles of this region. There is no cutaneous branch of the C1 dorsal primary ramus.

The second cervical nerve exits between the posterior arch of C1 and the lamina of C2, just lateral to the C2 lateral mass (Fig. 3.10). Unlike other spinal nerves, the C2 nerve exits posterior

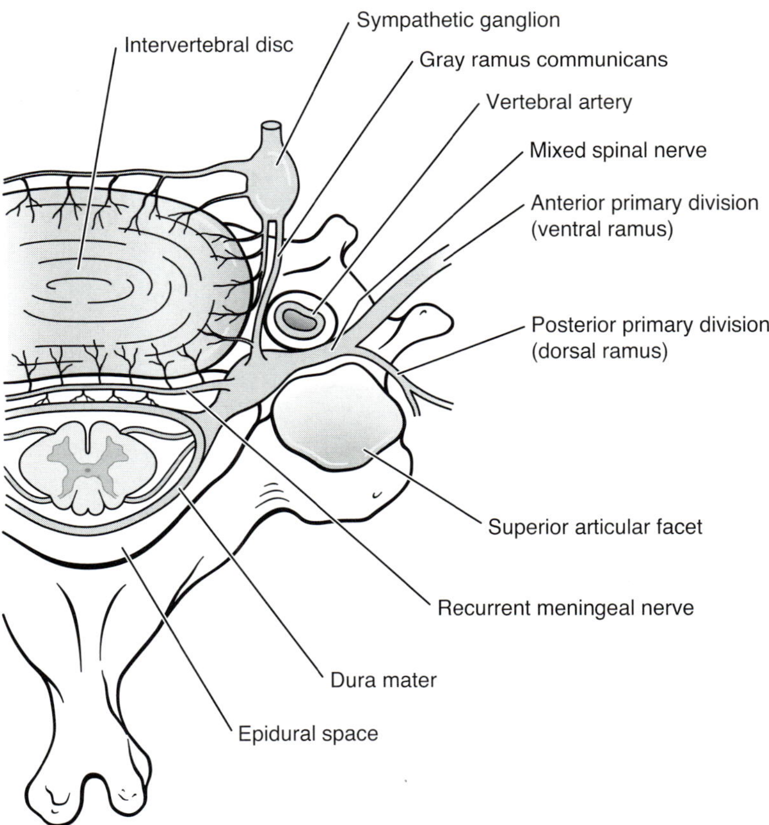

FIGURE 3.8. Cervical dorsal root ganglion.

Schematic Rendering of Cervical Plexus

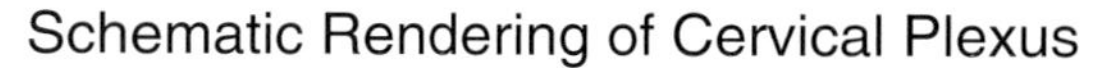

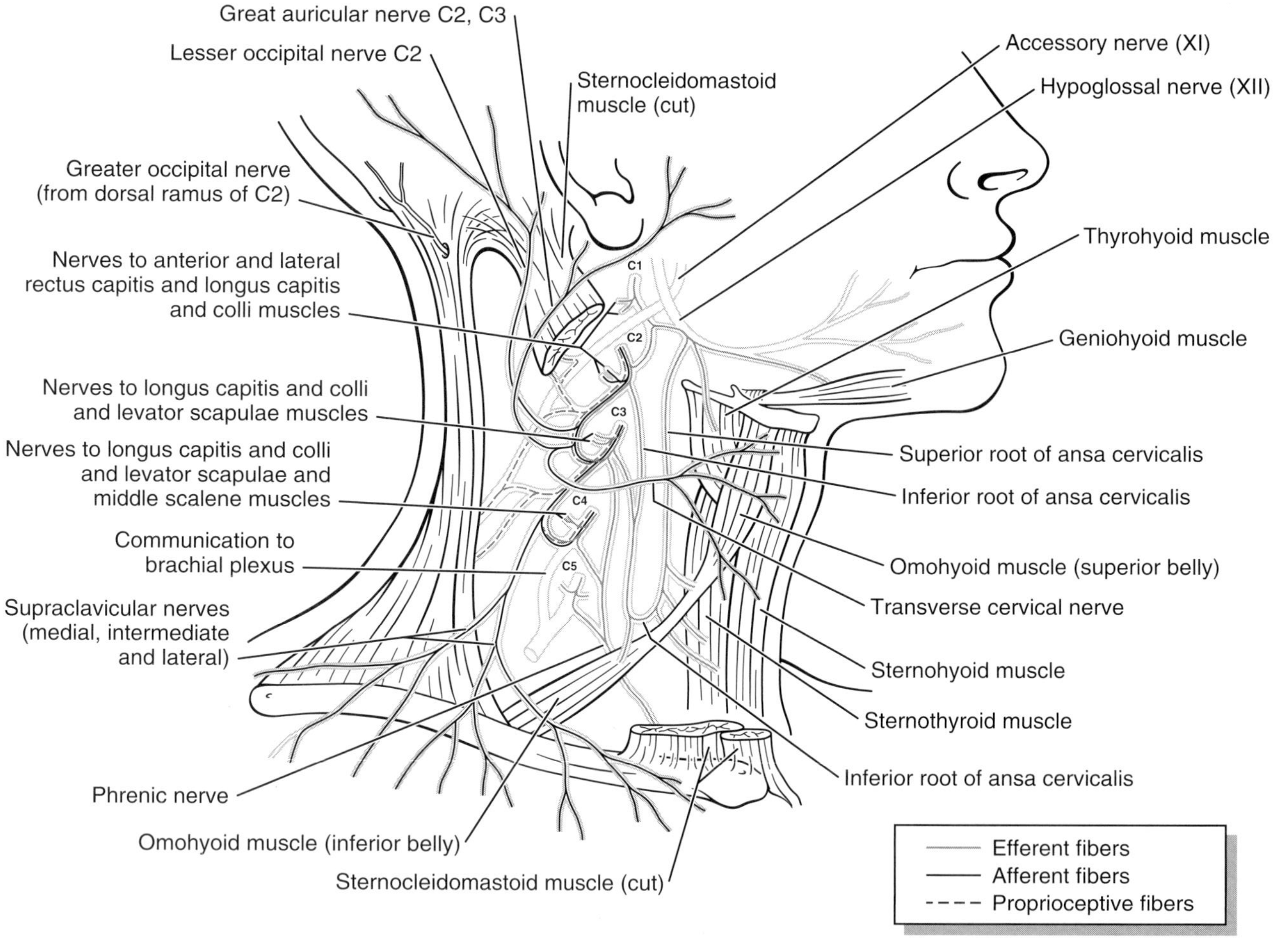

FIGURE 3.9. Cervical nerves.

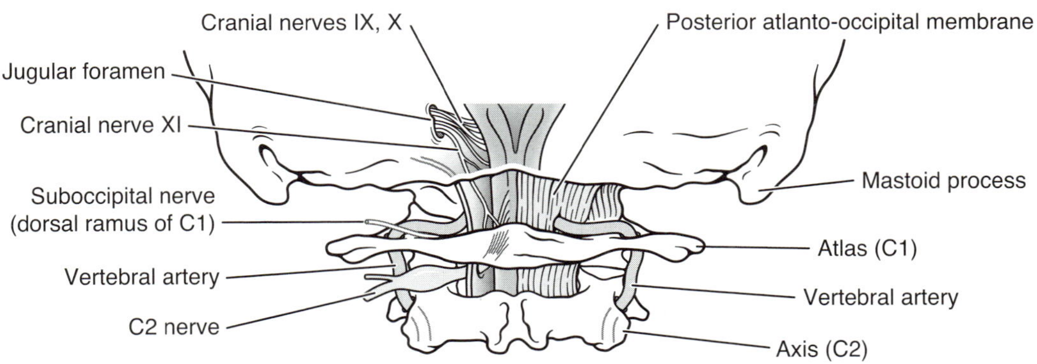

FIGURE 3.10. The C2 nerve exits posterior (rather than anterior) to the C2 superior articular surface.

(rather than anterior) to the C2 superior articular surface. The C2 dorsal rami are much larger than the ventral rami and are the largest of all the cervical dorsal rami.[14] The medial branch of the C2 dorsal rami (greater occipital nerve) runs transversely and then, in a submuscular position, superiorly to the scalp.

The third cervical nerve runs in a course similar to the remainder of the cervical nerves, exiting the vertebral canal through intervertebral foramina with borders that are similar through the rest of the cervical spine (superiorly and inferiorly are the pedicles, each of which is scalloped superiorly and inferiorly, forming the vertebral notches; posteriorly are the facet joints; and anteriorly are the intervertebral disks, uncovertebral joints, and vertebral body). The "typical" cervical vertebrae have separate anterior and posterior tubercles of their transverse processes; these tubercles are connected laterally by a costotransverse bar, which has a groove in it for the exiting spinal nerve. The typical foramen exits at an angle of 45 degrees from the midsagittal plane.[15] The principal branch of the C3 dorsal ramus is the third occipital nerve, which curves posteromedially around the superior articular process of C3, crossing the C2-C3 joint, and innervating it; it then continues medially, dorsally, and superiorly, innervating the posterior cervical musculature and the cutaneous aspects of the occipital and mastoid regions (Fig. 3.11).

The ventral (anterior) rami of nerves C1-C4 form the cervical plexus, which is located deep to the internal jugular vein and the sternocleidomastoid muscle. It is arranged in series of loops, off of which a series of branches arise. The ansa cervicalis is a loop formed from branches of nerves C1 to C3 and supplies all the strap muscles of the neck (except the thyrohyoid). The superior root of the ansa cervicalis is formed from C1 and C2 and gives off branches to the hypoglossal nerve; the inferior root is formed from C2 and C3. The cervical plexus also gives off various superficial cutaneous branches, innervating much of the skin of the anterior and posterior neck, as well as the lateral aspect of the scalp and part of the medial shoulder region; there is considerable overlap in the sensory distribution of various nerves in these areas.

VASCULATURE

The obvious focal point of any discussion of the vasculature of the cervical spine is the paired vertebral arteries. Not only are they physically intimately associated with the spine by virtue of running within the transverse foramina, but they are also the major blood supply to the cervical vertebrae and neural elements.

The vertebral arteries come off the first part of the subclavian artery, medial to the anterior scalene muscle, and run cephalad between the anterior scalene and longus colli muscles (Fig. 3.12). In most individuals, the arteries lie ventral to the transverse process of the seventh cervical vertebra, which usually does not contain a transverse foramen; they typically first enter the transverse foramen

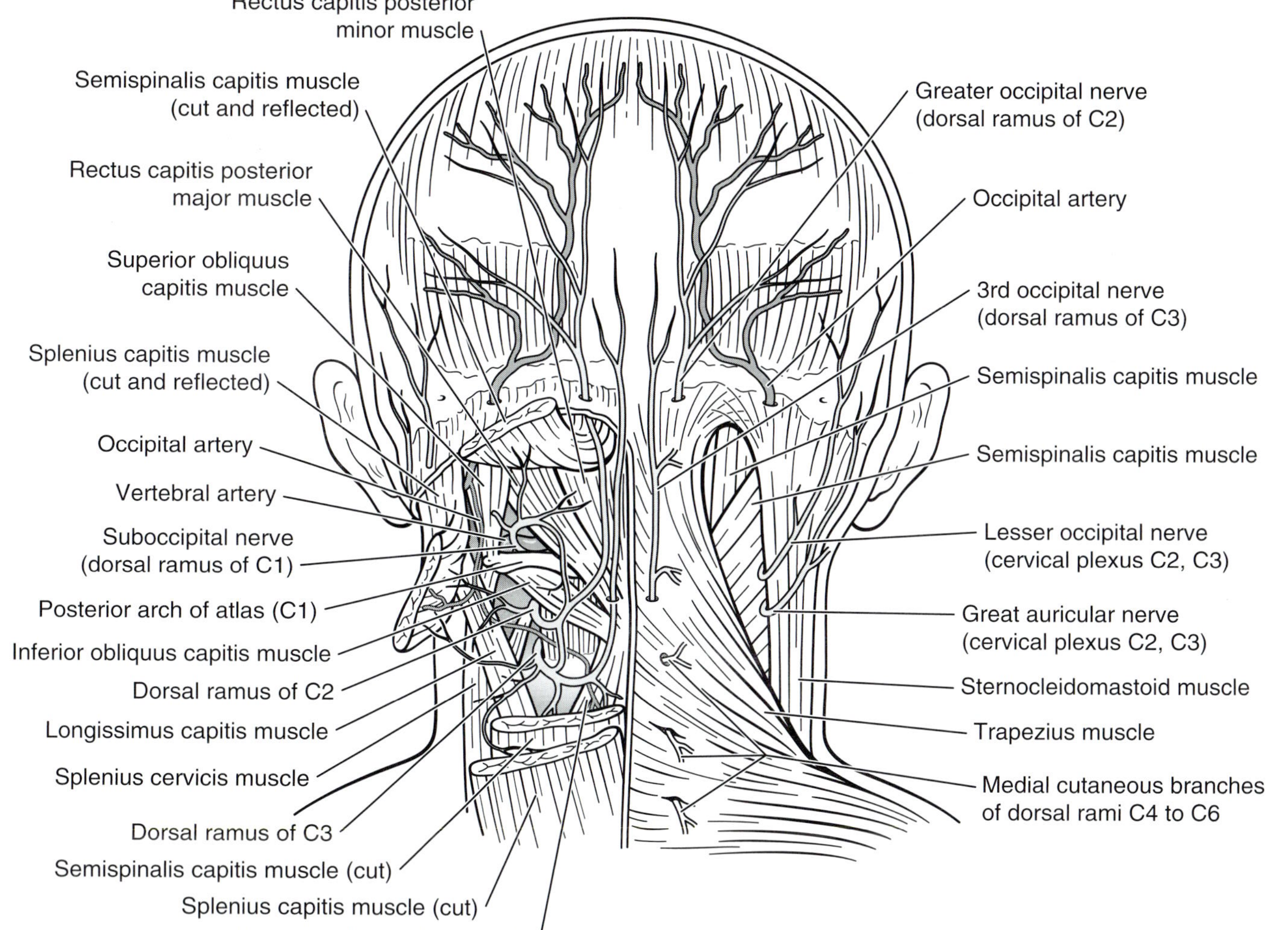

FIGURE 3.11. Innervation of the posterior cervical musculature and the cutaneous aspects of the occipital and mastoid regions.

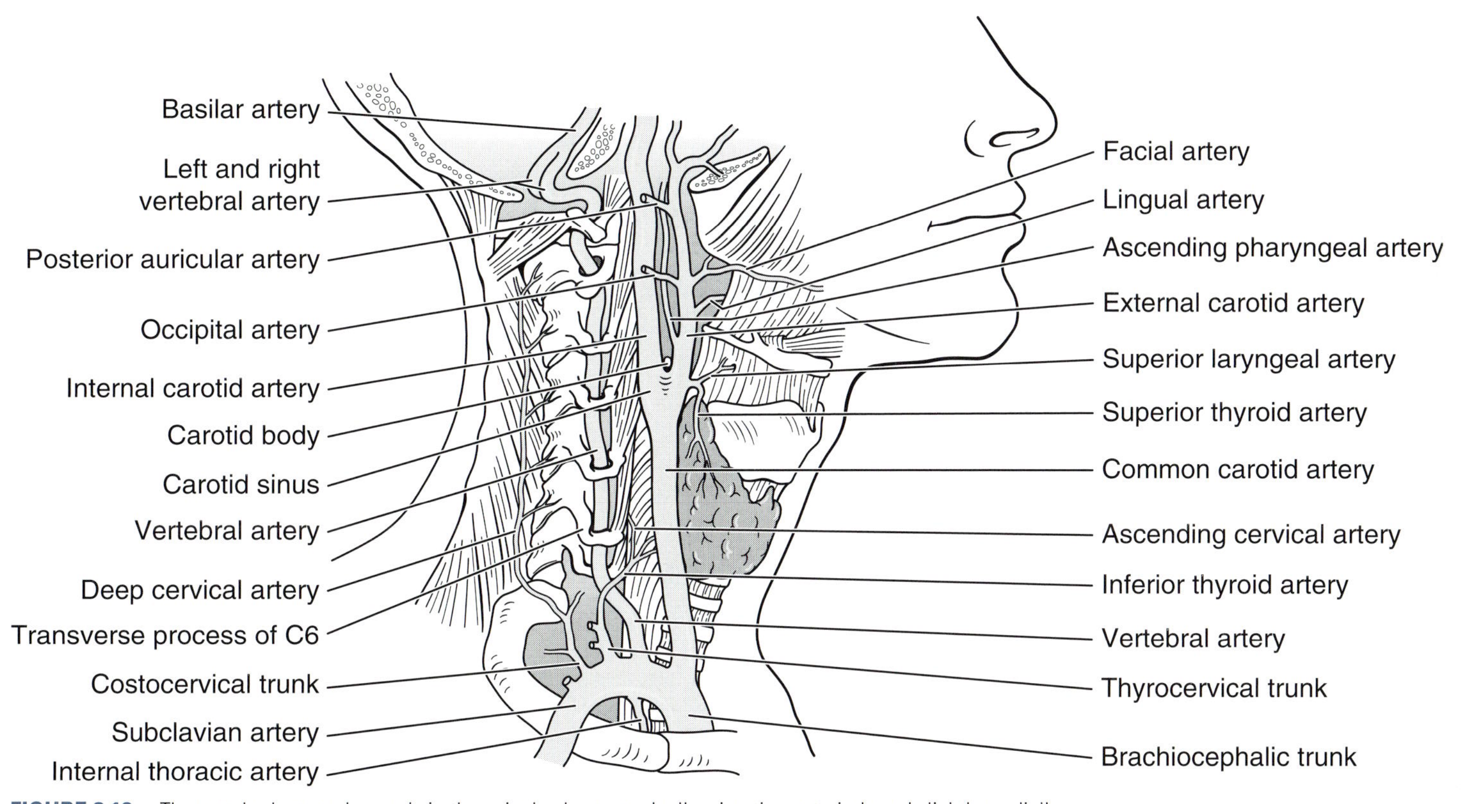

FIGURE 3.12. The vertebral artery descends in the spinal column, gradually migrating anteriorly and slightly medially.

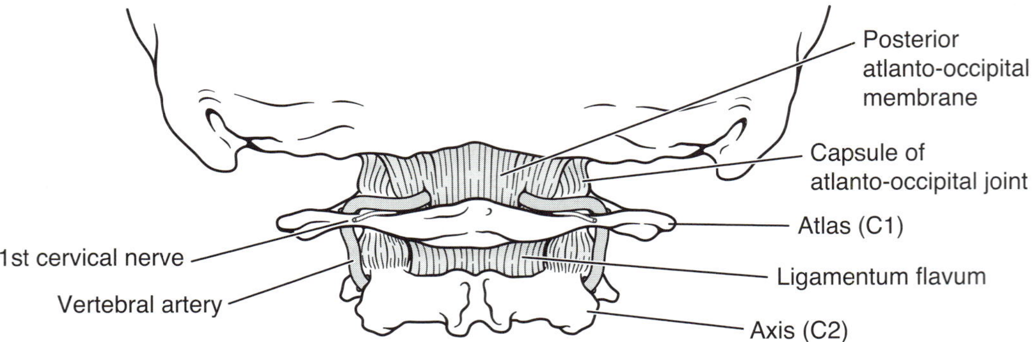

FIGURE 3.13. At C1, after passing through the transverse foramen, the arteries turn posteriorly, followed by a turn directly medial.

at the sixth cervical vertebra and thereafter run cephalad within these foramina to the level of C1. Throughout its course in the cervical spine, the vertebral artery is enclosed in a protective tunnel of fibrous tissue, bone, and muscle and is fixed to adjacent structures by connective tissue.[16] As it ascends in the spinal column, it gradually migrates anteriorly and slightly medially.[17,18] At C1, after passing through the transverse foramen, the arteries make an abrupt, almost right-angle, posterior turn, followed shortly by an equally abrupt turn directly medial, to run in a wide groove in the posterior arch of the C1 ring, passing over the ring just posterior to the superior articular facet of C1 (Fig. 3.13). Thereafter, the arteries again turn anterior and resume their cephalad progress, passing through the posterior atlanto-occipital membrane and entering the foramen magnum, where they join to form the basilar artery (Fig. 3.14). Just before forming the basilar artery, both vertebral arteries each give off a branch, which join together to form the anterior spinal artery. Vertebral artery abnormalities in the atlantoaxial region have been described in up to 2% of the population.[19]

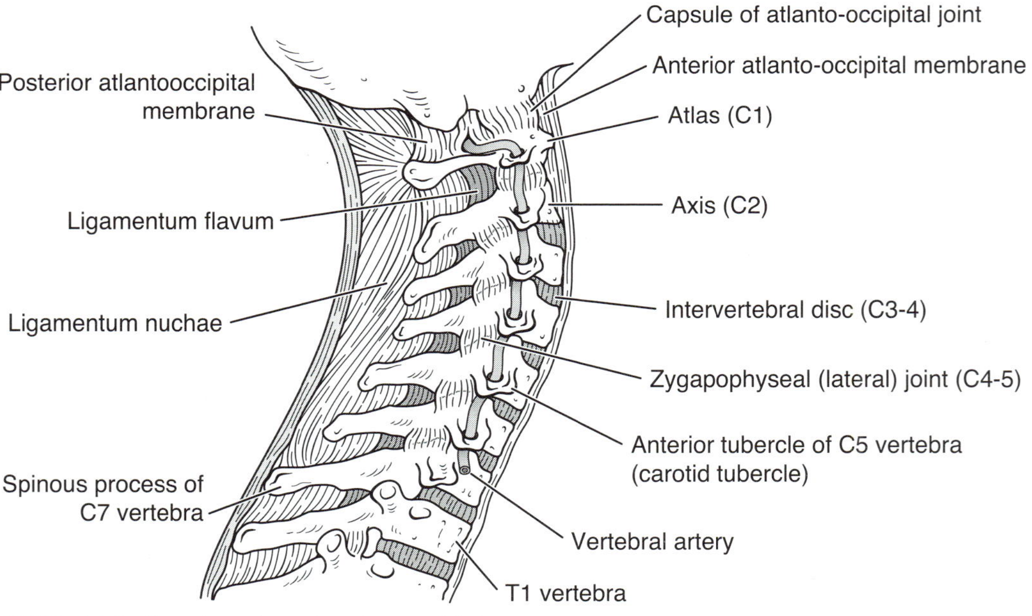

FIGURE 3.14. Posterior and anterior atlanto-occipital membranes.

Segmental vessels off the vertebral arteries provide the blood supply to the vertebrae, with separate branches supplying the anterior and posterior aspects of the vertebral bodies and the laminae. The blood supply of the dens is primarily by direct branches from the vertebral arteries, with paired anterior and posterior vessels rising along the borders of the dens, forming an "apical arcade"; anastomoses are then formed with the carotid system by horizontal arteries.[20–22] Less significant contributions to the dens blood supply also come from the alar and accessory ligaments, as well as an intraosseous supply from the C2 body.

Other vessels associated with the cervical spine include the occipital artery (a branch off the external carotid artery in the upper cervical spine), the ascending cervical artery (arising from the thyrocervical trunk or inferior thyroid artery), and the deep cervical artery (typically arising from the subclavian artery). These vessels provide blood supply to the surrounding neck muscles and soft tissues and also provide a modest blood supply to the vertebral column and neural elements.

SOFT TISSUES: JOINTS, LIGAMENTS, AND MUSCLES

The articulations between the skull, atlas, and axis have been described in some detail, particularly in regard to the morphology and orientation of the facets. The atlanto-occipital joints are synovial joints and contain synovial membranes and capsular ligaments. Contributing to the support of the atlanto-occipital complex are also the anterior and posterior atlanto-occipital membranes, which run from the anterior and posterior foramen magnum to the corresponding aspects of the ring of C1. These membranes, at their lateral extent, blend with the margins of the capsular ligaments of the atlanto-occipital joints. The posterior atlanto-occipital membrane allows the passage of the vertebral arteries and the suboccipital nerve (first cervical nerve), just above the lateral aspect of the posterior arch of C1; from the occiput to C1, the posterior atlanto-occipital membrane replaces the ligamentum flavum (a similar fibroelastic membrane also replaces the ligamentum flavum between the atlas and axis). The anterior atlanto-occipital membrane blends inferiorly at the level of the C2 body with the anterior longitudinal ligament.

The atlas articulates with the axis at three joints: the two lateral atlantoaxial synovial joints, between the C1 inferior articular facets and the C2 superior articular surfaces, and the median atlantoaxial joint, between the anterior ring of C1 and the anterior aspect of the dens. This latter joint is a pivot joint, with a synovial membrane and capsular ligaments anterior and posterior to the dens. The lateral atlanto-occipital joints are reinforced by an accessory ligament extending from the posterior aspect of C2 superiorly and laterally to the lateral mass of C1.

Multiple ligaments connect C1 and C2, as well as the occiput and C2 (Fig. 3.15). The ligamentum nuchae is located dorsally and extends from the external occipital protuberance distally, attaching to the posterior tubercle of C1 and the tips of the spinous processes of the remaining cervical vertebrae. However, the majority of the ligaments contributing to the stable relationship of the occiput, atlas, and axis are located ventral to the spinal cord. The cruciate ligament is formed by the transverse ligament of C1 (transverse atlantal ligament) and its superior and inferior ligamentous extensions that connect it to the anterior aspect of the foramen magnum and the posterior aspect of the C2 body, respectively. The inferior extension to the C2 body is further subdivided into a superior longitudinal band, which connects to the superior aspect of the dens, and an inferior longitudinal band, which connects to the base of the C2 body. The transverse ligament extends from tubercles located laterally on the dorsal surface of the anterior C1 ring, around the posterior aspect of the superior portion of the dens. The paired alar ligaments extend from the tip of the dens to each occipital condyle, also contributing, en route, a small band to the lateral masses of C1. The apical ligament runs from the superior tip of the dens to the anterior edge of the foramen magnum. In some individuals, a ligamentous connection exists between the anterior ring of C1 and the base of the dens, termed the anterior atlantodental ligament.[23] The tectorial membrane runs from the anterior aspect of the foramen magnum and basion to the posterior aspect of the base of the C2 vertebral body, at which point it merges with the posterior longitudinal ligament, which runs distally for the remainder

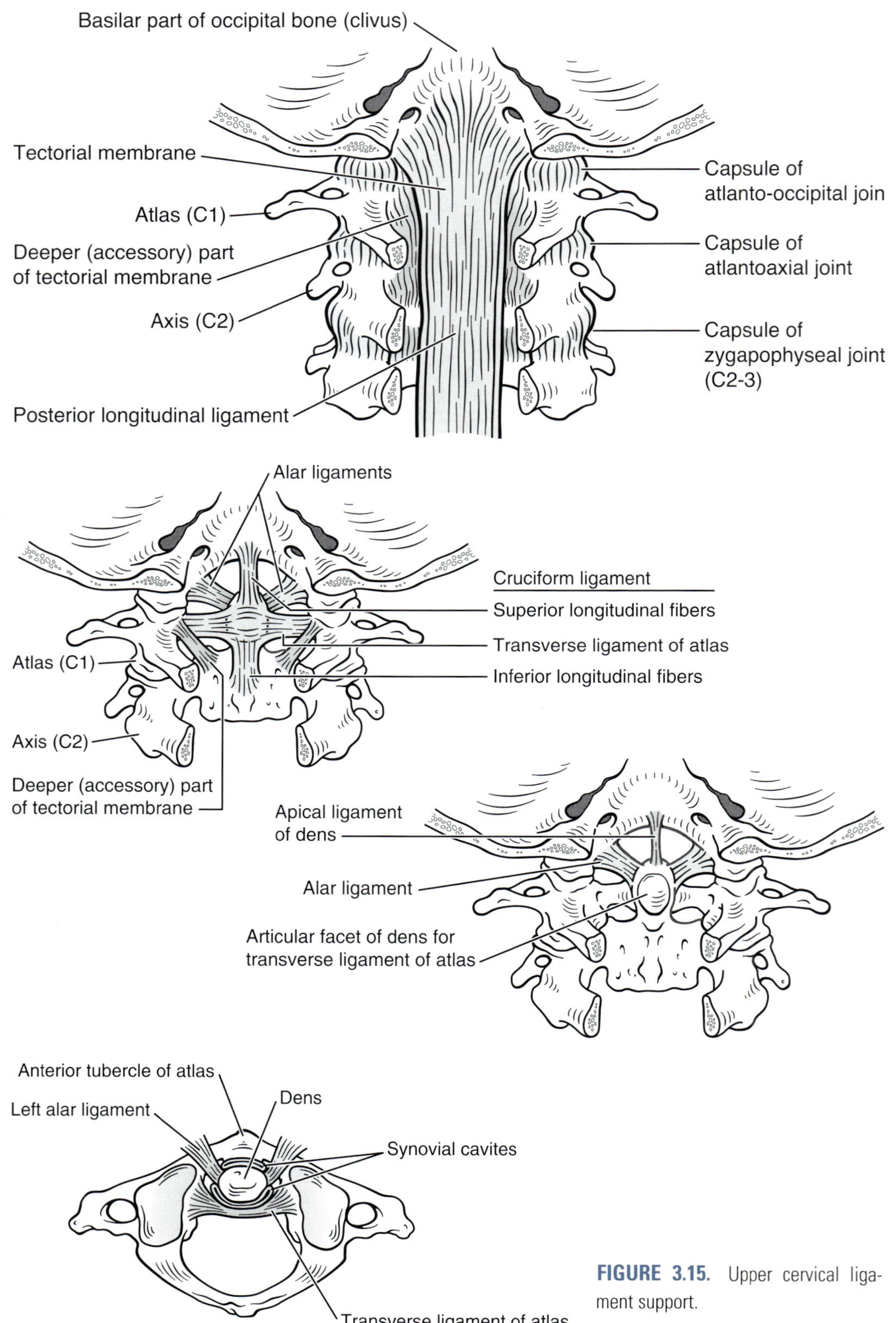

FIGURE 3.15. Upper cervical ligament support.

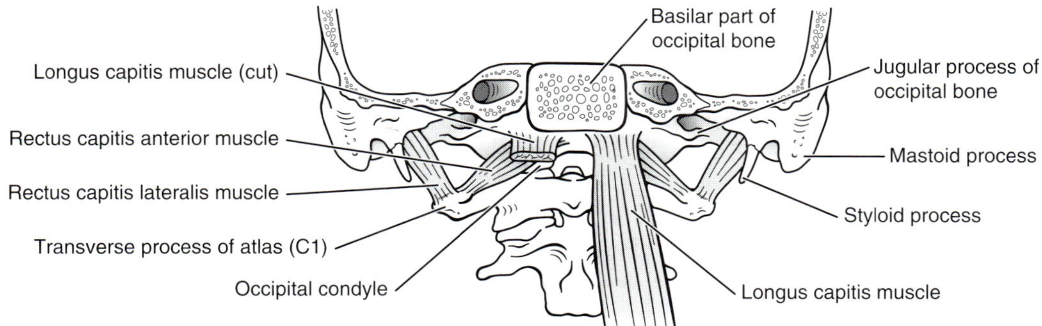

FIGURE 3.16. Upper cervical spine musculature: rectus capitis anterior, rectus capitis lateralis, suboccipital muscles.

of the spine. Both the anterior and posterior longitudinal ligaments are rather loosely adhered to the vertebral periosteum, but are closely adhered to the anulus fibrosus of the intervertebral disks.

Proceeding from dorsal to ventral, the ligaments of the anterior aspect of the proximal cervical spine and occiput are arranged in the following layers: tectorial membrane; cruciate ligaments; alar ligaments; apical ligament; and, most ventrally, the anterior atlanto-occipital membrane.

A few muscles are specifically associated with the upper cervical spine, including the rectus capitis anterior and rectus capitis lateralis anteriorly and the suboccipital muscles posteriorly (Fig. 3.16). The rectus capitis anterior originates from the anterior surface of the lateral mass and the base of the transverse process of C1; it inserts on the anterior aspect of the foramen magnum and the basilar portion of the occiput. The rectis capitus anterior flexes and stabilizes the head and provides some stability to the atlanto-occipital joint. The rectus capitis lateralis originates from the superior surface of the transverse process of C1 and inserts onto the inferior aspect of the jugular process of the occipital bone; it also stabilizes the atlanto-occipital joint and contributes to lateral side bending of the head. Both muscles are innervated by C1 and C2.

Posteriorly, the suboccipital muscles are a group of four pairs of muscles that are deep to the erector spinae; they include the obliquus capitis superior and inferior and the rectus capitis posterior major and minor (Fig. 3.17). The obliquus capitis superior is the most superior and lateral of all the

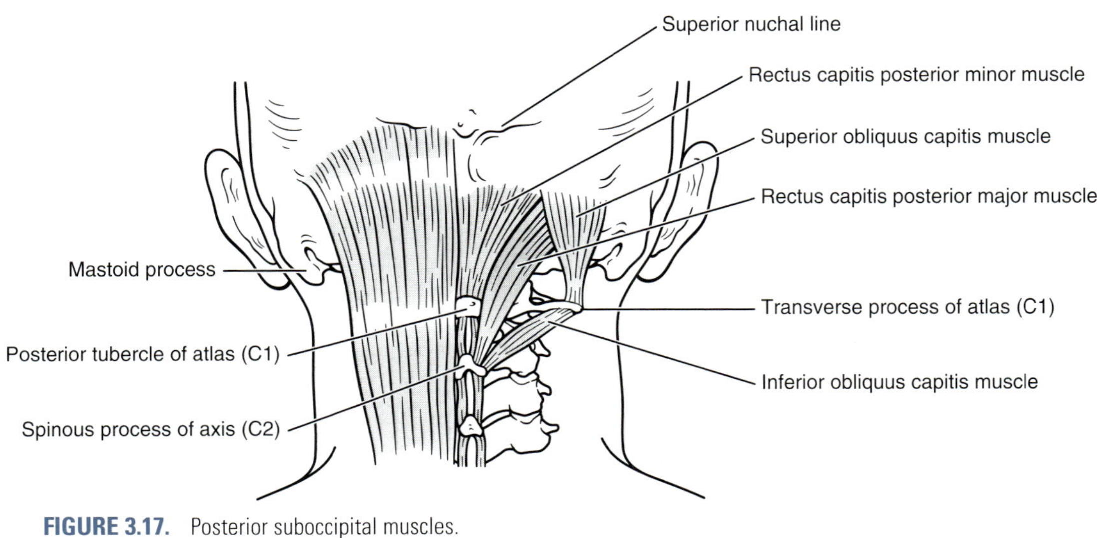

FIGURE 3.17. Posterior suboccipital muscles.

suboccipital muscles, originating from the superior aspect of the C1 transverse process and extending superior and medial to insert onto the occiput between the superior and inferior nuchal lines; it assists in head extension and ipsilateral lateral head bending. The obliquus capitis inferior and rectus capitis posterior major both originate from the spinous process of C2 and extend superiorly and laterally. The obliquus capitis inferior inserts onto the inferior aspect of the C1 transverse process and participates in ipsilateral head rotation; the rectus capitis posterior major runs medial to the obliquus capitis inferior, inserting onto the occipital bone on the lateral aspect of the inferior nuchal line, and assists with head extension and ipsilateral rotation. Finally, the rectus capitis posterior minor lies medial to the major, arising from the posterior tubercle of the C1 arch, and inserting onto the occiput's inferior nuchal line, just medial to the insertion of the rectus capitis posterior major; it assists in head extension. All of the suboccipital muscles are ultimately innervated by the suboccipital nerve.

REFERENCES

1. Gardner E, Gray D, O'Rahilly R. *Human anatomy*. Philadelphia, PA: WB Saunders, 1975.
2. Anderson PA, Montesano PX. Morphology and treatment of occipital condyle fractures. *Spine* 1988;13:731–736.
3. Pfirrmann CW, Binkert CA, Zanetti M, et al. MR morphology of alar ligaments and occipitoatlantoaxial joints: study in 50 asymptomatic subjects. *Radiology* 2001;218:133–137.
4. Avellino AM, Mann FA, Grady MS, et al. Why acute cervical spine injuries are "missed" in infants and children. *Top Spinal Cord Inj Rehabil* 2000;6(suppl):203.
5. Dvorak J, Schneider E, Saldinger P, et al. Biomechanics of the cranio-cervical region: the alar and transverse ligaments. *J Orthop Res* 1988;6:452–461.
6. Crisco JJ, Panjabi MM, Dvorak J. A model of the alar ligaments of the upper cervical spine in axial rotation. *J Biomech* 1991;24:607–614.
7. Stubbs D. The arcuate foramen: variability in distribution related to race and sex. *Spine* 1992;17:1502–1504.
8. Young JP, Young PH, Ackermann MJ, et al. The ponticulus posticus: implications for screw insertion into the first cervical lateral mass. *J Bone Joint Surg Am* 2005;87:2495–2498.
9. Heller JG, Alson MD, Schaffler MB, et al. Quantitative internal dens morphology. *Spine* 1992;17:861–866.
10. Heggeness M, Doherty B. The trabecular anatomy of the axis. *Spine* 1993;18:1945–1949.
11. An HS, Gordin R, Renner K. Anatomic considerations for plate-screw fixation of the cervical spine. *Spine* 1991;16(suppl);S548–S551.
12. Panjabi M, Duranceau J, Goel V, et al. Cervical human vertebrae: quantitative three-dimensional anatomy of the middle and lower regions. *Spine* 1993;16:861–874.
13. Dommisse GF. The blood supply of the spinal cord. *J Bone Joint Surg Br* 1974;56:225–235.
14. Bogduk N. The clinical anatomy of the cervical dorsal rami. *Spine* 1982;7:319–320.
15. Czervionke LF, Daniels DL, Ho PSP, et al. Cervical neural foramina: correlative anatomic and MR imaging study. *Neuroradiology* 1988;169:753–759.
16. Chop P, de Miranda Neto NH, Lucas, GA, et al. The vertebral artery: its relationship with adjoining tissues in its course in the intra and intertransverse processes in man. *Rev Paul Med* 1992;110:245–250.
17. Ebraheim N, Lu J, Brown J. Vulnerability of vertebral artery in anterolateral decompression for cervical spondylosis. *Clin Orthop* 1996;322:146–151.
18. Vaccaro A, Ring D, Scuderi G. Vertebral artery location in relation to the vertebral body as determined by two-dimensional computed tomography evaluation. *Spine* 1994;19:2637–2641.
19. Sato K, Watanabe T, Yoshimoto K. Magnetic resonance imaging of C2 segmental type of vertebral artery. *Surg Neurol* 1994;41:45–51.
20. Althoff B, Goldie IF. The arterial supply of the odontoid process of the axis. *Acta Orthop Scand* 1977;48: 622–629.
21. Schatzker J, Rorabeck CH, Waddell JP. Fractures of the dens (odontoid process): an analysis of thirty-seven cases. *J Bone Joint Surg Br* 1971;53:392–405.
22. Schiff DCM, Parke WW. The arterial blood supply to the odontoid process. *J Bone Joint Surg Am* 1973;55: 1450–1456.
23. Dvorak J, Panjabi M. Functional anatomy of the alar ligaments. *Spine* 1987;12:183–189.

CHAPTER 4

Subaxial Cervical Spine

Luis M. Tumialán, Wolfgang Rauschning, and Praveen V. Mummaneni

INTRODUCTION

Below the atlas and axis lie the five remaining vertebrae of the cervical spine, collectively referred to as the subaxial cervical spine. These vertebrae have subtle variations in their osseous, vascular, and neural anatomy. A thorough understanding of this complex anatomy facilitates comprehension of the mechanisms of injury and operative treatment in this region.

OSSEOUS ANATOMY

The osseous region of the spine bears less weight than the thoracolumbar spine; the vertebral bodies from C3 to C7 are small relative to their respective arches and transverse foramina. The angular dimensions of the cervical vertebral bodies are similar to the geometry of a rhombus, with differing heights anteriorly and posteriorly and varying depths superiorly and inferiorly. All of these dimensions increase with submillimeter increments when proceeding from C3 to C7.[1] The mean sagittal and parasagittal depths of the middle vertebral body in the subaxial spine have been reported to be approximately 14 mm, a useful reference point when considering instrumentation in this area of the spine.[2]

Projecting posterolaterally from the vertebral bodies are shortened pedicles that give rise to the superior articular facet. Viewed posteriorly, these structures form columns on the lateral aspect of the laminas and are therefore referred to as the articular pillars or lateral masses. Extending posteromedially from each lateral mass are the lamina of the posterior arch, which fuse at the midline to form the spinous process. The spinous processes of the third, fourth, and fifth cervical vertebrae are usually bifid, whereas the seventh is longer and tapered, making it the most prominent of the processes and typically palpable on physical examination (Fig. 4.1). Hence, the C7 vertebra is also referred to as the vertebra prominens. The C6 spinous process may be a single projection or bifid.

On the lateral-most aspects of each vertebral body are the uncinate processes (Fig. 4.2). These bony ridges project from the posterolateral aspect of each cervical vertebral body and serve as the limit of the outer border of the anulus fibrosus. These processes are a useful landmark for the relative position of the vertebral artery, which lies laterally, and the spinal nerves, which reside posterolaterally. This process articulates with the inferior aspect of the superior vertebral body, forming a posterolateral area of articulation, known as the uncovertebral joint, or Luschka's joint. The superior surface of the uncovertebral joint is transversely concave because of the uncinate process, and the inferior surface is reciprocally convex. The major role of this joint is to limit posterior translation and lateral bending while offering torsional stability in the cervical spine.[3] Ligaments extending from the posterior longitudinal ligament cover this articulation posterolaterally.

Immediately lateral to the uncinate processes are the transverse foramina (also referred to as the foramen transversaria), which serve as the conduit for the vertebral artery (Figs. 4.3 and 4.4). These

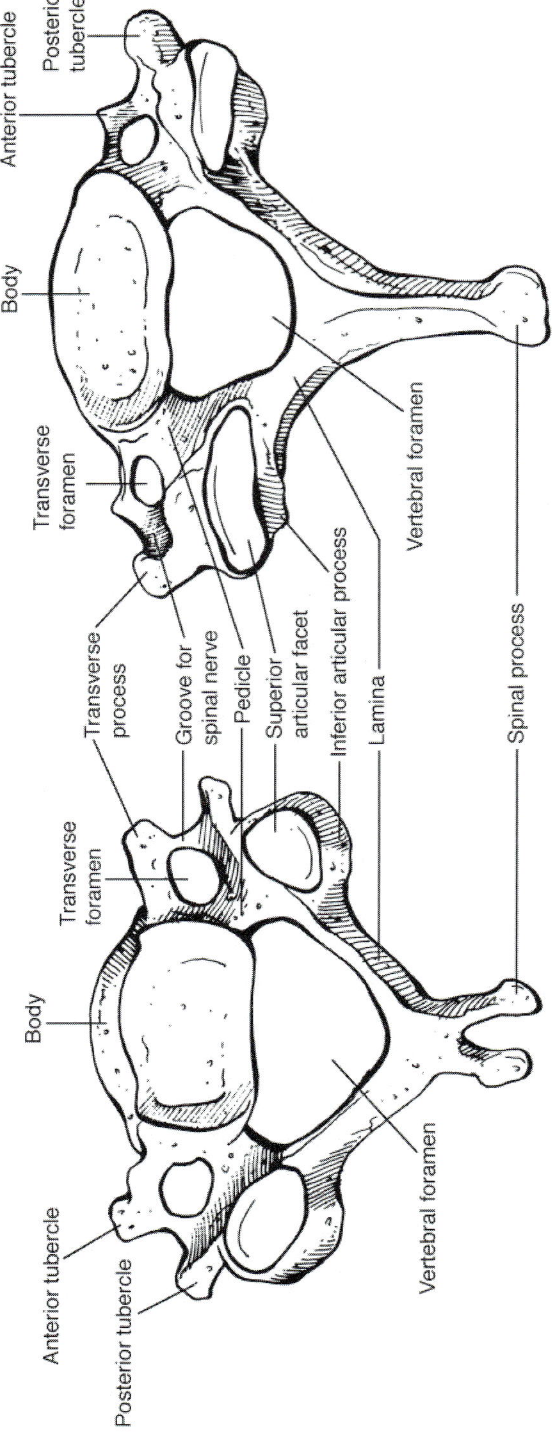

FIGURE 4.1. Fourth cervical vertebra: superior view; seventh cervical vertebra: superior view.

C3
C4
C5
Uncinate process
Zygapophyseal joint
Interarticular part
Intervertebral foramen for spinal nerve

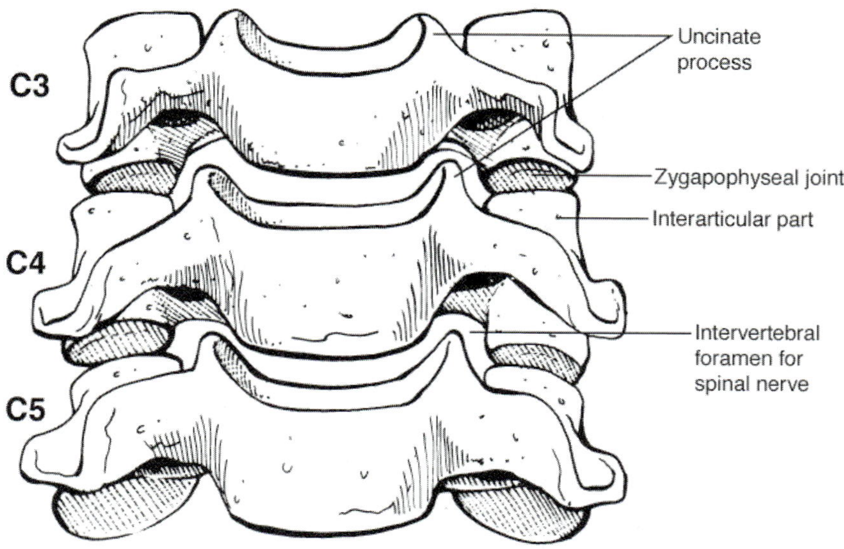

FIGURE 4.2. Third, fourth, and fifth cervical vertebrae: anterior view.

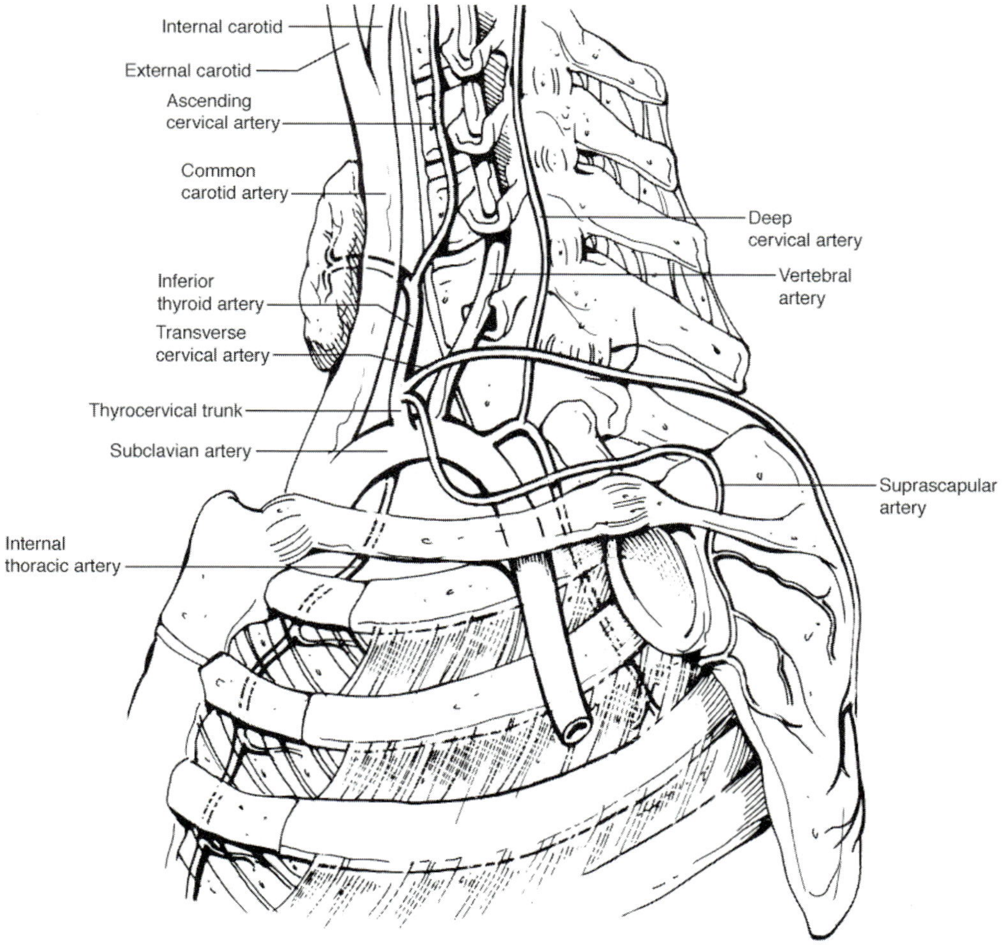

Internal carotid
External carotid
Ascending cervical artery
Common carotid artery
Inferior thyroid artery
Transverse cervical artery
Thyrocervical trunk
Subclavian artery
Internal thoracic artery
Deep cervical artery
Vertebral artery
Suprascapular artery

FIGURE 4.3. Right lateral schematic view.

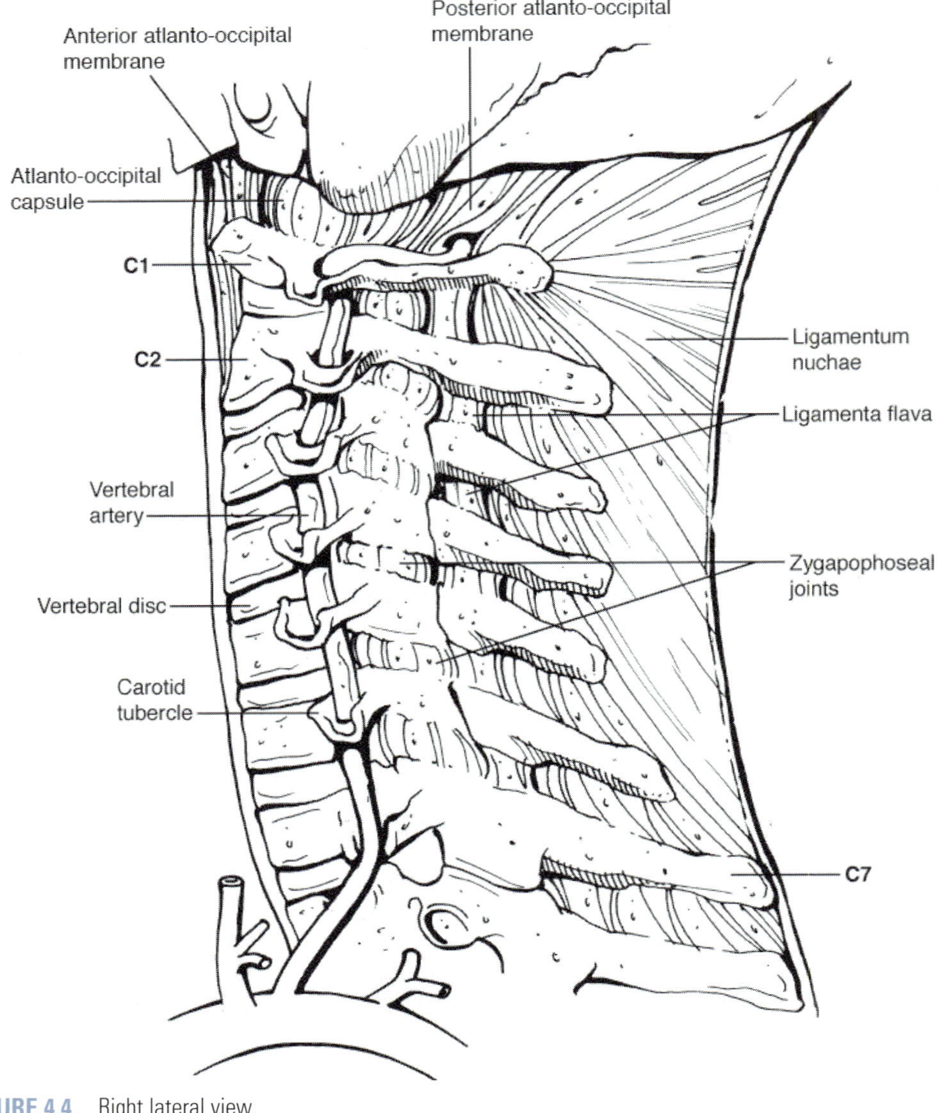

FIGURE 4.4. Right lateral view.

foramina are formed by a vestigial costal element fused to the vertebral body. In addition to the vertebral artery, multiple veins and the sympathetic nervous plexus course within these foramina. Consistent with the fact that most humans have a left dominant vertebral artery, the left foramina transversaria are generally larger than the corresponding foramina on the right. Anomalies of these foramina include their complete absence, duplication (up to 7%), or triplication (less than 1%).[4] The distance from the lateral apex of the uncinate process to the medial border of the transverse foramen gradually decreases from C6 to C4, thereby bringing the vertebral artery more medial in the upper cervical spine. Several anatomic and radiographic studies have demonstrated that the foramina transversaria of the more cephalad cervical vertebrae were more medial and more dorsal than the foramina of the lower cervical spine, thus making the vertebral artery more susceptible to injury in the midcervical area than in the lower cervical spine during anterior cervical surgery. Yet another subtlety is that the anterior-posterior diameter of these foramina gradually increases from C3 to C6.[2]

The lateral-most aspect of each vertebra ends in a transverse process posteriorly and a rudimentary rib or costal process anteriorly. The anterior tubercle of the transverse process, which represents the rib element, is most prominent at C6 and is referred to as the carotid tubercle of Chassaignac at that level. Collectively, the tubercles arise from both the anterior and posterior aspects of the transverse process and act as origin and insertion points for the anterior and posterior cervical musculature, respectively. In between the tubercles lies the costotransverse lamella, or spinal nerve sulcus. As the ventral ramus of each spinal nerve exits from the spinal column, it courses over this groove.[5]

NEURAL AND VASCULAR ANATOMY

The paired vertebral arteries arise from the subclavian or brachiocephalic artery, pass by the transverse process of C7 anteriorly and laterally, and then enter the foramen transversaria at C6 (Fig. 4.5). Anomalies of the vertebral arteries do occur; however, they are primarily limited to the origin of the vessel from the aortic arch or proximal to the arch of C1. The segment of the vertebral artery from C6 to C1 is where the artery is most vulnerable to injury during anterior cervical spine surgery. Of note, during its ascent from C7 to C3, the vertebral artery becomes slightly closer to the exiting nerve root. The lateral aspect of the vertebral artery is covered by a venous plexus.[4]

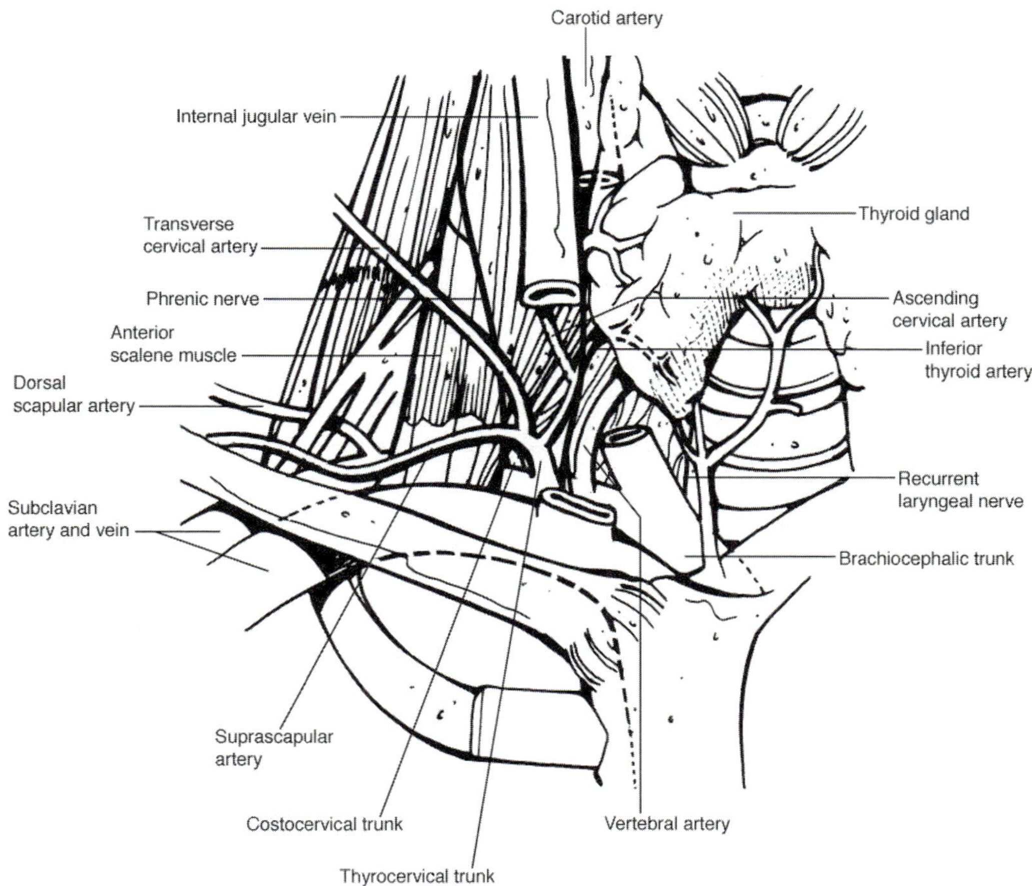

FIGURE 4.5. Right anterior dissection.

The intervertebral foramen is formed by the inferior posterior elements of the superior vertebra and the superior posterior elements of the adjacent inferior vertebra. The pedicle of the superior vertebra forms the anterior superior arch of the foramen, and the uncinate process forms the anterior inferior aspect of the arch. The posterior component of the intervertebral foramen consists of the superior and inferior facets or, collectively, the facet joint. The size of the intervertebral foramen demonstrates an increased trend of height and width from cephalad to caudad. Biomechanically, flexion of the cervical spine increases the dimensions of the intervertebral foramina and extension decreases it. At each level, the ventral root of the spinal nerve is adjacent to the uncinate process anteriorly and the pedicle inferiorly. The contribution of the uncinate process to the anterior inferior aspect of the intervertebral foramen varies depending on the level. The uncinate processes in the upper cervical spine are smaller and contribute less to the intervertebral foramen than in the lower cervical spine. This subtle anatomical variation has direct implications in the anterior decompression of a nerve root. Anterior foraminotomy may be adequately accomplished with removal of approximately the posterior third of the uncinate process in the upper cervical spine, whereas the lower levels would require removal of the posterior half of the uncinate process for adequate decompression.[3]

As the nerve root exits the intervertebral foramen, it courses along a groove within the transverse process. The spinal nerves from C3 to C7 exit the dural sac to lie in front of the superior articular process. At the anterolateral corner of the superior articular process, they divide into a larger ventral ramus and smaller dorsal ramus as they exit from the intervertebral foramina.[6] The ventral ramus of the cervical spinal nerve courses over the sulcus in between the anterior and posterior tubercles and then proceeds in an anterolateral direction to form the cervical and brachial plexus. The dorsal ramus of the spinal nerve runs posteriorly around the superior articular process supplying the facet joint, ligaments, deep muscles, and skin of the posterior neck. The dorsal ramus of the spinal nerve courses close to the base of the superior articular process.

The lateral masses also have a complex anatomic relationship with the vertebral arteries and the cervical roots, which pass in proximity to these structures. If the lateral mass is considered in quadrants, anterior to the superomedial and inferomedial quadrants courses the vertebral artery and anterior to the inferomedial and inferolateral quadrants resides the nerve root. Of note, neither of the aforementioned structures course anterior to the superolateral quadrant, thereby prompting some authors to refer to this quadrant as the "safe quadrant."[7] The anterior-posterior size of the lateral mass decreases from C3 to C7 incrementally by only several millimeters.[1]

LIGAMENTS AND INTERVERTEBRAL DISCS

Each cervical vertebra articulates with the adjacent vertebrae at the intervertebral disc space anteriorly and the facet joints posteriorly. The intervertebral disc consists of three components: the anulus fibrosus, the nucleus pulposus at the center of the disc, and the cartilaginous endplates at the vertebral body–anulus fibrosus interface superior and inferior. The anulus fibrosus and the endplates are secured both anteriorly and posteriorly by the anterior and posterior longitudinal ligaments, respectively. These ligaments extend over the entire length of the spine and are the major stabilizers of the intervertebral joints. The anterior longitudinal ligament is strongly adherent to the intervertebral discs, hyaline cartilage endplates, and margins of the vertebral bodies. It remains loosely attached to the middle aspect of the vertebral bodies, where it fills the anterior concavity of the vertebral body. The posterior longitudinal ligament extends downward from the tectorial membrane. It is widest in the upper cervical spine and tapers caudally.[8]

The posterior articulations are supported collectively by the ligamentum flavum, ligamentum nuchae, interspinal ligament, and capsule of the facet joint. The ligamentum nuchae spans from the occiput to the spinous process of C7. The deep fibers of the ligamentum nuchae attach to the spinous process of each cervical vertebra and reinforce the interspinous ligaments. There are two ligamenta flava at each level, which attach to the anterior surface of the vertebral arch above and the superior margin of the vertebral arch below. The right and left ligamenta flava fuse posteriorly and merge with the interspinous ligaments.

SUPERFICIAL VASCULAR, NEURAL, AND MUSCULAR ANATOMY

Immediately deep to the sternocleidomastoid muscle lies the carotid sheath, which contains the carotid artery, internal jugular vein, and vagus nerve. The common carotid artery lies anterior to the transverse process of C4 to C6. At the upper border of the thyroid cartilage, the common carotid artery divides into its internal and external components. The vagus nerve descends within the carotid sheath on either side and gives off the recurrent laryngeal nerves. The left recurrent laryngeal nerve first descends into the thorax, then courses around the aortic arch before it ascends in the tracheoesophageal groove. The right recurrent laryngeal nerve emerges at the level of the first part of the subclavian artery, then ascends obliquely in the tracheoesophageal groove. It next crosses midline at the level of C6 and may be found anterior or posterior to the inferior thyroid artery.[9]

On the cervical spine itself, the most adherent musculature is the longus colli muscles. This muscle group is the longest and the most medial of the prevertebral muscles. These muscles act as an invaluable marker to delineate the midline when approaching the subaxial spine anteriorly. The longus colli extends from the anterior tubercle of the atlas to the bodies of the third cervical to the third thoracic vertebra, with other attachments to the transverse processes of the third to sixth cervical vertebrae. In addition to demarcating the midline, this muscle group also is the position on which lies the sympathetic trunk below the prevertebral fascia.[10] The sympathetic ganglia may be at risk when the longus colli muscle is stripped from the vertebral bodies or transverse processes, manifesting clinically as Horner syndrome when damaged. Dissections have demonstrated the sympathetic trunk to lie on average 11 mm lateral to the medial border of the longus colli muscle. For this reason, a blunt-tip retractor should be placed securely beneath the surface of the longus colli muscle rather than on the surface, to minimize such an injury.[11]

REFERENCES

1. Francis C. Dimensions of the cervical vertebrae. *Anat Rec* 1955;122(4):603–609.
2. Panjabi MM, Duranceau J, Goel V, et al. Cervical human vertebrae: quantitative three-dimensional anatomy of the middle and lower regions. *Spine* 1991;16:861–869.
3. Kotani Y, McNulty P, Abumi K, et al. The role of anteromedial foraminotomy and the uncovertebral joints in the stability of the cervical spine: a biomechanical study. *Spine* 1998;23:1559–1565.
4. Heary R, Albert T, Ludwig S, et al. Surgical anatomy of the vertebral arteries. *Spine* 1996;21:2074–2080.
5. Ebraheim N, An H, Xu R, et al. The quantitative anatomy of the cervical nerve root groove and the intervertebral foramen. *Spine* 1996;21:1619–1623.
6. Xu R, Kang A, Ebraheim N, et al. Anatomic relation between the cervical pedicle and the adjacent neural structures. *Spine* 1999;24:451–454.
7. Pait T, McAllister P, Kaufman H. Quadrant anatomy of the articular pillars (lateral cervical mass) of the cervical spine. *J Neurosurg* 1995;82:1011–1014.
8. Yilmazlar S, Kocaeli H, Uz A, et al. Clinical importance of ligamentous and osseous structures in the cervical uncovertebral foraminal region. *Clin Anat* 2003;16:404–410.
9. Tew J, Mayfield F. Complications of surgery of the anterior cervical spine. *Clin Neurosurg* 1976;23:424–434.
10. Kiray A, Arman C, Naderi S, et al. Surgical anatomy of the cervical sympathetic trunk. *Clin Anat* 2005; 18:179–185.
11. Jónsson H, Rauschning W. Surgical anatomy of the cervical spine. *Tech Orthopaed* 1994;9(1)18–29.

SECTION III

Biomechanics of the Cervical Spine

CHAPTER

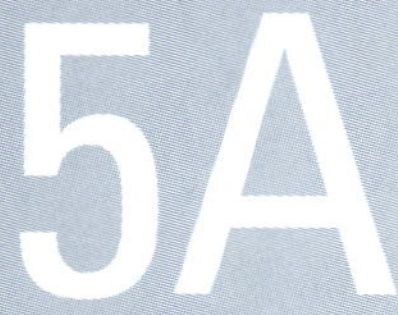

Cervical Spine Kinematics and the Biomechanics of the Injured Cervical Spine: Craniocervical Junction (Occiput-C2)

Sharad Rajpal and Gregory R. Trost

INTRODUCTION

The upper cervical spine is very complex and highly susceptible to injury. To understand why this is the case, a systematic evaluation of the morphology and biomechanics of this region is a necessary but arduous task. Although many different biomechanical models have helped elucidate the mechanisms involved in spinal trauma, their conclusions necessitate certain assumptions. Experimental studies contribute different pieces to the puzzle because of the myriad of possible modeling approaches: isolated spinal components (ligaments, etc.), functional spinal units, multisegmental spinal units, entire cervical column, entire spinal column, cadaver, autopsy, etc. The biomechanics of trauma is even more difficult, involving additional variables, such as magnitude of impact, location of impact, direction of impact, rate of impact, relative position of the spinal elements at the time of impact, and so forth. Traumatic injury to the spine occurs in a dynamic setting and may not adhere to the constraints of a given mathematical model. The goal of this chapter is to describe pertinent aspects of the kinematics of the normal upper cervical spine and the relevant biomechanics in adult spinal trauma.

UNIQUE ANATOMY

Although the anatomy of the occipital-atlantoaxial (C0-C1-C2) joint is described in a previous chapter, it is important to emphasize certain unique anatomic features composing this particular joint.

1. *Vertebral shape.* The occipital condyles (C0), the ring of C1 (atlas), and the odontoid process are all uniquely shaped, whereas the basic design of the vertebrae below C2 (axis) is similar.
2. *Angle of facet complex (joint).* The shape and position of the articulating processes, among other factors, help dictate the pattern of movement of the spine. The C0-C1 articulating joints have convex surfaces on the occiput and concave grooves on C1. Between C1-C2, the two intervertebral joints are convex on both articulating bones, whereas the two odontoid joints include one between the dens and anterior arch of atlas and one between the dens and the transverse ligament.
3. *Intervertebral disc.* The intervertebral disc supports loads, absorbs compression, and resists tension and shearing forces during physiologic movement. Although intervertebral discs play a crucial role in spine biomechanics, they are not present between C0-C1 or C1-C2.

4. *Ligaments.* Ligaments are responsible for allowing restrained movement of the spine, thereby playing a key role during spinal injury. The shape of the load-displacement curve is similar for each ligament, which carries loads most effectively in the directions of its fibers. The specific function of each ligament is dictated by its architecture, orientation, and location within the vertebral column. Several ligaments are unique to the upper cervical spine, such as the transverse and alar ligaments.
5. *Spinal muscles.* The spinal muscles are divided into two groups: the preventral and postvertebral muscles. Their overall biomechanical function includes (a) generating moment-arm and torque, (b) providing resistance to external loads, and (c) providing stability. The spinal muscles of the upper cervical spine are responsible for the unique motions involving the calvarium, atlas, and axis.
6. *Spinal canal.* The spinal canal is larger at C1-C2 than anywhere else in the axial skeleton. This has implications for the presence of any associated neurologic injury during spinal trauma.

BIOMECHANICS OF THE NORMAL UPPER CERVICAL SPINE

The occipital-atlantoaxial joint complex is designed for moving the head smoothly through all axes of motion while protecting vital neural elements. To effectively discuss abnormal behaviors of the spine, such as in trauma, one must first discuss normal behaviors of the spine. Based on numerous biomechanical studies, average ranges of three-dimensional movement have been established for the occipital-atlantoaxial complex (Table 5A.1).

Local anatomic elements are responsible for physiologic limitations in various axes of motion. The C0-C1 junction contributes combined capital flexion-extension of 25 degrees, with approximately 20 degrees occurring at the C1-C2 joint. Flexion at C0-C1 is restricted by the osseous tip of the dens making contact with the anterior edge of the foramen magnum. The tectorial membrane is responsible for limiting several motions in the upper cervical spine: (a) C0-C1 extension, (b) C1-C2 forward flexion beyond neutral flexion of C0-C1, and (c) C1-C2 extension. If the tectorial membrane is incompetent, hyperextension at C0-C1 is limited by contact between the posterior arch of C1 and the occiput. Sixty percent of axial rotation of the entire cervical spine occurs within the upper cervical spine alone, with the remaining 40% occurring in the subaxial cervical spine. The majority of this axial rotation occurs around C1-C2 (40 degrees unilateral axial rotation) because of the unique articulating surface between the C1-C2 lateral masses and decreased presence of ligamentum flavum. Each alar ligament is the main restraint for contralateral axial rotation: with slight rotation, the ipsilateral alar ligament tightens first; with extreme rotation, the ipsilateral alar ligament shortens by winding around the dens, whereas the contralateral alar ligament tightens to limit any further

TABLE 5A.1 Average Range-of-Motion Values for Individual Joints of the Upper Cervical Spine

Joint	Motion	Range of Motion (degrees)
Occipital-atlantal (C0-C1)	Combined flexion/extension	25
	Unilateral axial rotation	5
	Unilateral lateral bending	5
Atlantoaxial (C1-C2)	Combined flexion/extension	20
	Unilateral axial rotation	40
	Unilateral lateral bending	5

Source: White AA, Panjabi MM. *Clinical Biomechanics of the Spine.* 2nd ed. Philadelphia: Lippincott, 1990:92.

TABLE 5A.2 Failure Strengths for Ligaments of the Upper Cervical Spine

Spinal Level	Ligament Type	Average Force (N)	Average Deformation (mm)
C0-C1			
	Anterior atlanto-occipital membrane	233	18.9
	Posterior atlanto-occipital membrane	83	18.1
C1-C2			
	Anterior longitudinal ligament	281	12.3
	Atlantoaxial membrane	113	8.7
	Capsular ligament	157	11.4
	Transverse ligament	354	
C0-C2			
	Apical ligament	214	11.5
	Alar ligament	286	14.1
	Vertical cruciate ligament	436	25.2
	Tectorial membrane	76	11.9

Source: White AA, Panjabi MM. *Clinical Biomechanics of the Spine.* 2nd ed. Philadelphia: Lippincott, 1990:22.

rotation. It is important to note that the instantaneous axis of rotation (IAR) at C1-C2 is around the spinal cord, which helps minimize any distortion of this structure during rotation. Axial rotation at C0-C1 is considered insignificant. One-side (unilateral) lateral bending is minimal at both the C0-C1 and C1-C2 articulations (5 degrees each). On lateral flexion to one side, the contralateral alar ligament tightens and limits further flexion. Translation within the upper cervical spine is also minimal, especially at C0-C1. At C1-C2, anteroposterior translation is limited to approximately 2 to 3 mm as a result of the strong transverse ligament holding the dens to the anterior ring of C1. The ligaments of the upper cervical spine are quite strong, which explains why ligament failure in the upper cervical spine occurs uncommonly. Table 5A.2 provides the average failure strengths for various upper cervical spine ligaments.

Although physiologic motions of the spine are sometimes studied and described individually for simplicity reasons, they are inherently connected. This phenomenon of *coupling* is defined as movement of the spine in one axis that obligates movement along another axis. An example of coupling is when lateral bending results in rotation. Coupling is most apparent in the upper cervical spine and varies with motion type and spine location. To help further examine the motions of the cervical spine in three dimensions, Panjabi et al.[1] studied the effect of posture (full flexion, neutral, and full extension) on the kinematics of the upper cervical spine (axial torque and lateral bending). They found that the posture of the head in the sagittal plane alone affects the three-dimensional motions of the upper cervical spine in a complex manner: while certain movements remain unaffected, others either increase or decrease with changes in posture. These effects were also found to be different between C0-C1 and C1-C2.[1]

BIOMECHANICS OF THE INJURED UPPER CERVICAL SPINE

Different parts of the spine respond differently to similar external forces. The upper cervical spine has unique and complex anatomy that makes it vulnerable to traumatic injury. During injury, the normal physiologic parameters of the spinal elements (bones, ligaments, muscles, etc.) are exaggerated, often to the point of failure. The most instructive method to discuss the biomechanics of trauma of the upper cervical spine is to describe specific injury patterns. It is important to remember that many classification schemes exist for specific injury patterns, only some of which have gained recognition. Diagnosis and treatment of individual upper cervical spine injuries, however, is beyond the scope of this chapter.

OCCIPITAL CONDYLE FRACTURE

Occipital condyle fractures (OCFs) are frequently found in association with C1 fractures and are often difficult to diagnose. OCFs are grouped into three types according to the Anderson and Montesano classification system (Fig. 5A.1).[2] Type I fractures are typically the result of an impaction-type injury from asymmetric axial forces applied to the head. The result is a comminuted fracture of the occipital condyle at the insertion of the ipsilateral alar and apical ligament complex with minimal or no displacement of fragments into the foramen magnum. Spinal stability is due to the intact tectorial membrane and contralateral alar ligament. Type I fractures are sometimes seen with other lateral mass fractures in the upper cervical spine (most commonly the C1 ring). Type II fractures are often the result of distraction-type forces applied through the alar and apical ligament complex. The result is a basilar skull fracture extending to, and involving, the occipital condyle, with an intact alar and apical ligament complex. Type III fractures represent avulsion-type fractures of the occipital condyle by the alar ligament. This appears as a fracture of the distal tip of the occipital condyle, resulting in a free condylar fragment that may become displaced into the foramen magnum toward the odontoid process. There may also be disruption of the contralateral alar ligament and tectorial membrane. Type III OCFs occur from excessive loading in rotation, lateral bending, or a combination of the two.

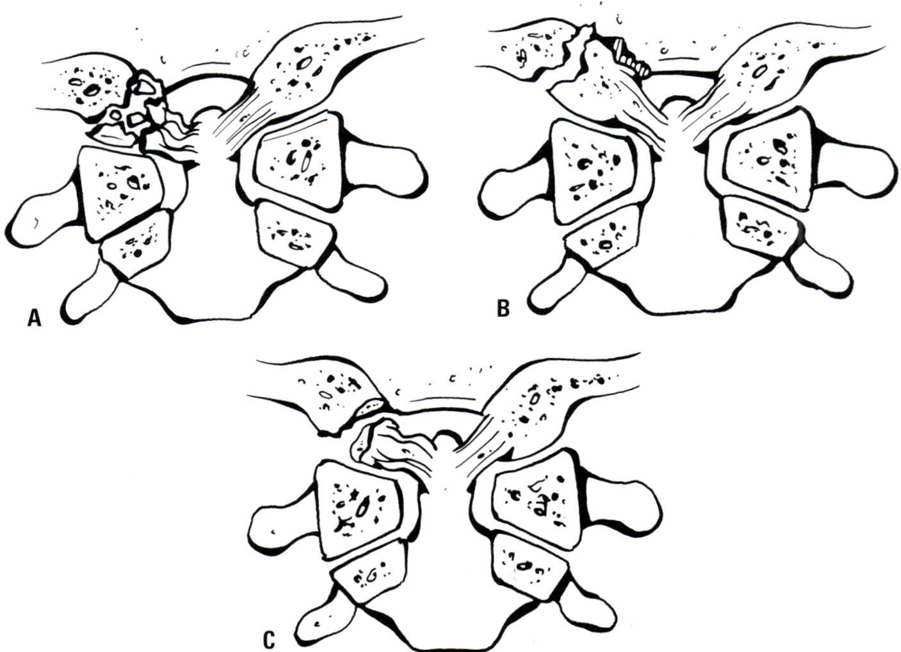

FIGURE 5A.1. Classification of occipital condyle fractures as proposed by Anderson and Montesano. **A.** Type I: impacted type. **B.** Type II: basilar skull type. **C.** Type III: avulsion type. (Source: Anderson PA, Montesano PX. Morphology and treatment of occipital condyle fractures. *Spine* 1988;13:732, Figure 1A,B,C, with permission.)

ATLAS (C1) FRACTURE

The C1 ring is responsible for regulating movement between the occiput and C2, as well as transferring the weight of the cranium from the occipital condyles to the lateral masses of C2 through its own lateral masses. This relationship is responsible for the various fracture patterns seen in the atlas, which can be divided into multiple groups: isolated anterior or posterior arch fractures, combined anterior and posterior arch fractures (burst or Jefferson fracture), lateral mass fractures, and transverse process fractures. Comminuted C1 ring fractures are most often caused by axial loading (typically a direct blow to the vertex of the calvarium), with subsequent compression of the atlas by the occipital condyles. Depending on the location of the head in relation to the upper cervical spine, this may produce unilateral, bilateral, or rotatory fracture patterns. The anterior arch is weakest in the axial plane, and the posterior arch is weakest in the sagittal plane. Fracture sites for the atlas ring occur at the thinnest portions, which include the transitional regions from the posterior and anterior arches to the lateral masses. In the posterior arch, this includes the vertebral artery groove (an important clinical consideration). In the Jefferson fracture, there is bilateral spreading of the lateral masses, with failure in both the posterior and anterior arches. Lateral displacement of the lateral masses greater than 7 mm indicates risk for tearing of the insertions of the transverse atlantal ligament. Lateral mass fractures of C1 are typically due to axial loading coupled with lateral bending. This particular fracture may be seen in combination with either an OCF or C2 lateral mass fracture. Posterior arch fractures are typically produced by compression-hyperextension. This results in contact between the posterior arch of C1 and the occiput or C2 spinous process, causing a C1 posterior arch or C2 spinous process fracture. Isolated anterior arch fractures are uncommon and believed to occur from avulsion of the superior attachment of the longus colli muscle.

Landells and Van Peteghem[3] proposed a classification system based on atlas fracture patterns (Fig. 5A.2). Type I fractures are confined to either the anterior or posterior arch. Type II fractures involve

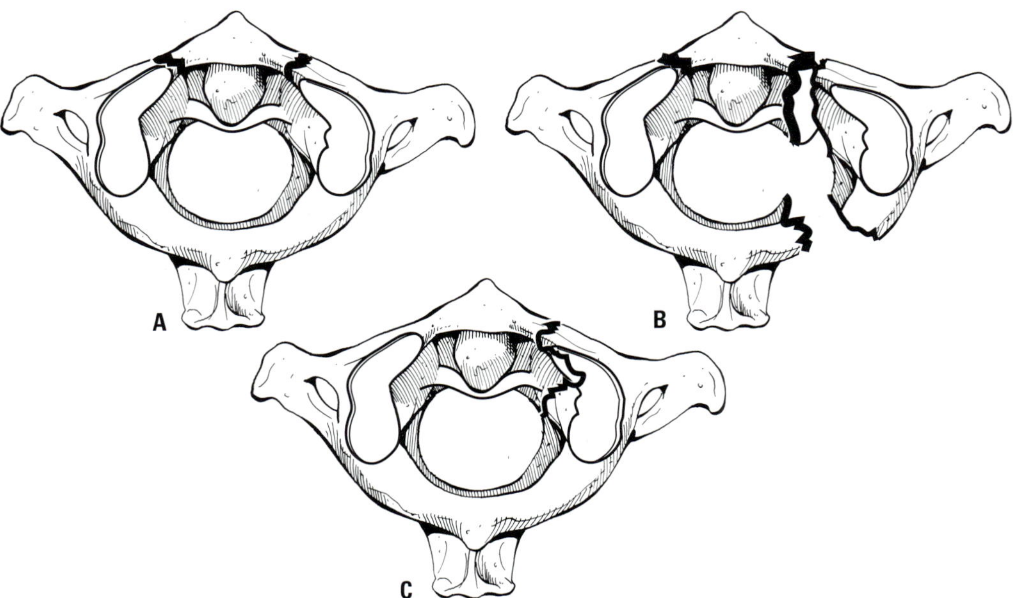

FIGURE 5A.2. Classification of atlas fractures as proposed by Landells and Van Peteghem. **A.** Type I fractures are confined to a single arch (anterior or posterior). **B.** Type II fractures involve both arches and include the classic Jefferson's fracture. **C.** Type III fractures involve the lateral mass, with or without a fracture of an arch. (Source: Landells CD, Van Peteghem K. Fractures of the atlas: classification, treatment, and morbidity. *Spine* 1988;13:451, Figures 1,2,3, with permission.)

both anterior and posterior arch fractures (akin to the Jefferson fracture), with possible lateral displacement of the lateral masses. Type III fractures primarily involve the lateral masses, although there may also be extension into either the anterior or posterior arch.[3]

AXIS (C2) FRACTURE

The unique anatomy of C2 leads to distinct fracture patterns. In general, the axis is subject to similar axial loading forces on the spine as the atlas but is less prone to burst fracturing because of the thickness of its lamina. Axis fractures typically occur in flexion and extension and usually do not produce neurologic symptoms. Three of the more common axis fracture patterns include traumatic spondylolisthesis (hangman fracture), odontoid process fractures, and vertical dorsal C2 body fractures.

Traumatic Spondylolisthesis

Traumatic spondylolisthesis was originally attributed to the mechanism of hyperextension-distraction injuries characterized by victims of judicial hangings. Traumatic spondylolisthesis is thus often referred to as the hangman fracture. Today, fractures within the C2 pedicles are seen in diving and automobile accidents. The typical scenario is that of an unrestrained passenger in a motor vehicle being thrown forward and suffering hyperextension-compression from striking the windshield. The C2 vertebra is, in essence, compressed by the opposing forces of C1 and C3. With sudden hyperextension and axial loading, the weight of the cranium is transmitted to the C1-C2 lateral masses through the occipital condyles and into the base of the axis. The anterior structures are initially stressed, with ensuing compression of the posterior facets that ultimately causes failure at the weakest portions of the axis at the pedicles (isthmus) of C2 (Fig. 5A.3).[4] This fracture pattern therefore typically involves bilateral fractures through the pars interarticularis or pedicles, with separation of the anterior vertebral elements

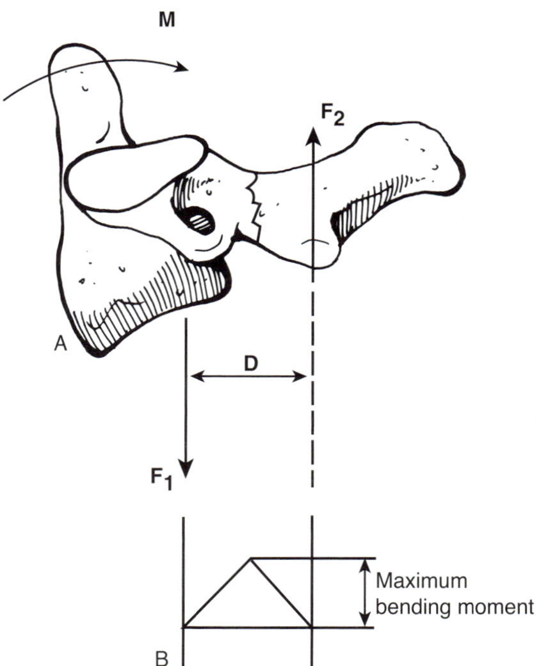

FIGURE 5A.3. Mechanical vulnerability of the C2 vertebra is presented with the multiple forces that act on the C2 vertebrae by the ring of C1 and C3. (Source: White AA, Panjabi MM. *Clinical Biomechanics of the Spine.* 2nd ed. Philadelphia: Lippincott, 1990:212, Figure 4-30.)

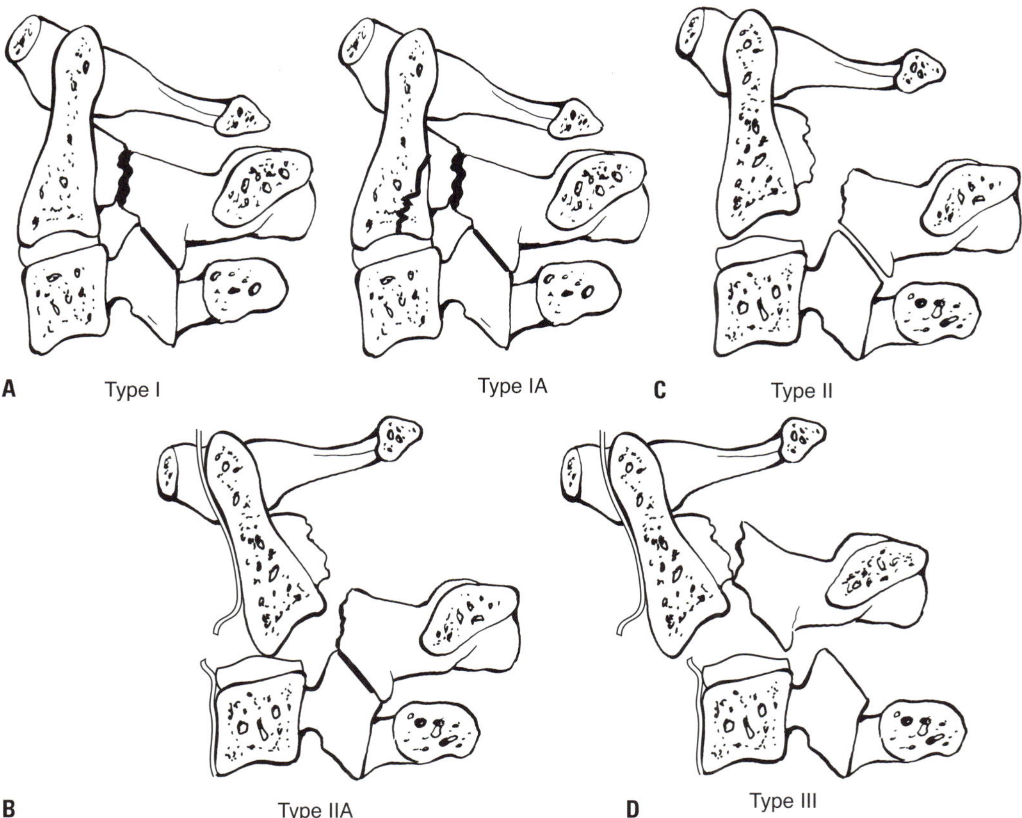

FIGURE 5A.4. Classification of traumatic spondylolisthesis as proposed by Levine and Edwards. **A.** Type I. **B.** Type II. **C.** Type IIa. **D.** Type III. (Source: Winn HR ed. *Youmans Neurological Surgery.* 5th ed. Philadelphia: Saunders, 2003:4905, Figure 315-8, with permission.)

from the posterior vertebral elements. The fracture line may travel into the C2 body or cross the superior articular surface. Although posterior ligamentous structures usually remain intact, the C2-C3 intervertebral structures become largely distracted from the combination of extension and distraction of the upper cervical spine. In contrast to hanging, in which the bending moment creates extension with tensile forces on the cervical spine, automobile accidents produce compressive forces on the cervical spine with a similar bending moment.

There are four patterns of traumatic spondylolisthesis classically described by Levine and Edwards[5] based on the degree of angulation and displacement (Fig. 5A.4). Type I fractures are often due to hyperextension with axial loading and include bilateral pars fracture, no angulation, less than 3 mm of translation, an intact C2-C3 disc, and typically intact anterior longitudinal (ALL) or posterior longitudinal ligaments (PLL). Type II fractures (most common fracture subtype) are often due to rebound hyperflexion and compression after initial hyperextension-axial loading. This fracture subtype often includes bilateral pars fracture, disruption of the PLL, C2-C3 disc rupture, possible ALL disruption, greater than 3 mm of translation, and greater than 10 degrees of angulation. Type IIa fractures are a type II variant and include a fracture line that is more oblique than vertical and located just anterior to the facet joints; type IIa fractures are thus similar to type II except for the presence of greater angulation and less displacement. Type IIa fractures result from greater force in flexion than extension, with possible posterior distraction. Type III fractures are the most severe and are due to either a submental traction injury or flexion followed by compression and include all the characteristics of a type II fracture as well as bilateral C2-C3 facet capsule dislocations.

Odontoid Process (Dens) Fracture

The most common type of axis fracture is the odontoid process fracture. Anderson and D'Alonzo[6] classified dens fractures into three types (Fig. 5A.5). Type I fractures (rare) are through the tip of the odontoid process, likely as a result of avulsion of the alar ligament from its attachment to the tip of

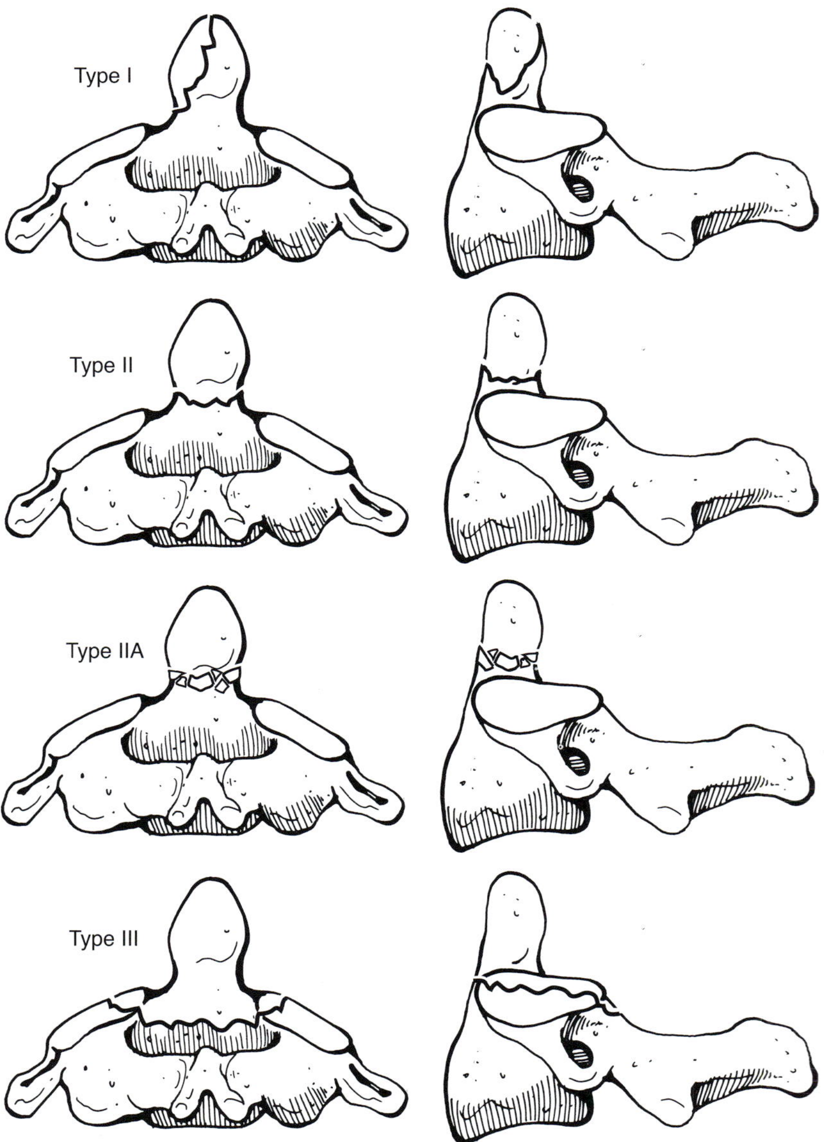

FIGURE 5A.5. Classification of odontoid process fractures as proposed by Anderson and D'Alonzo. Type I fracture is through the tip of the odontoid process. Type II is fracture at the base of the odontoid process. If there are comminuted bone fragments at the fracture site, the fracture classification is modified to Type IIA. Type III fracture is through the C2 body and may involve the superior articulating surface. (Source: Anderson LD, D'Alonzo RT. Fractures of the odontoid process. *J Bone Joint Surg Am* 1974;56:1664, Figure 1. Reprinted with permission from the Journal of Bone and Joint Surgery, Inc.)

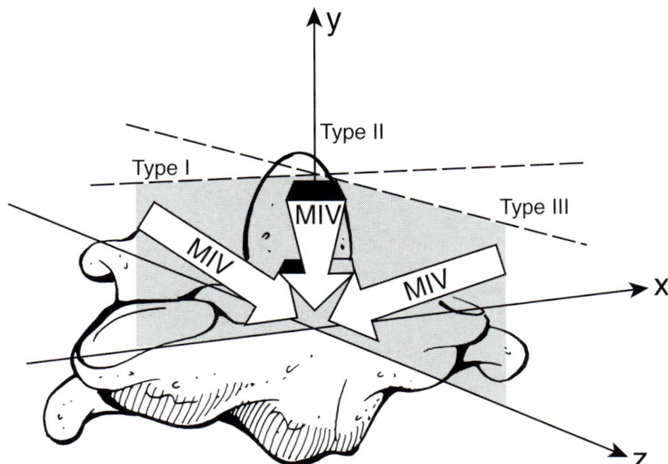

FIGURE 5A.6. Vector of injury producing various subtypes of dens fractures. Type III fractures occurred from a combination of horizontal shear and vertical compression directed in the sagittal plane (anterior or posterior impact). Type II fractures occurred with a similar type of impact except directed 45 degrees to the sagittal plane. Type I fractures were produced when the same combined impact was directed 90 degrees lateral to the sagittal plane. (Source: White AA, Panjabi MM. *Clinical Biomechanics of the Spine.* 2nd ed. Philadelphia: Lippincott, 1990:200, Figure 4-19.)

the dens. Type II fractures are the most common and occur at the base of the odontoid process. If there are comminuted bone fragments at the fracture site, the fracture classification is modified to type IIA. Type III dens fractures occur through the C2 body and may involve the superior articulating surface. The mechanism of injury required to produce various dens fracture patterns was studied by Althoff[7] (Fig. 5A.6). Althoff's experimental studies revealed that fractures of the odontoid process did not occur simply from hyperextension, hyperflexion, or horizontal shear (anterior or posterior), but instead from varying *combinations* of vertical compression and horizontal shear. To fracture the odontoid process, the direction of the impact needed to be directed in such a way that only minimal movement occurred at the C0-C1 joint or subaxial cervical spine. As the compression and shear vectors were directed more laterally and out of the sagittal plane, the more cephalad was the fracture of the dens. In experimental studies, type III fractures occurred from a combination of horizontal shear and vertical compression directed in the sagittal plane (anterior or posterior impact). Type II fractures occurred with a similar type of impact except directed 45 degrees to the sagittal plane. Type I fractures were produced when the same combined impact was directed 90 degrees lateral to the sagittal plane. Other authors have found type I fractures to occur with lateral flexion and rotation, producing tension on the alar ligaments. The degree of displacement of the odontoid usually reflects the degree of associated ligamentous injury and angle of the fracture. Benzel et al.[8] believe the Anderson and D'Alonzo type III dens fracture does not anatomically involve the odontoid process and therefore should be reclassified with C2 body fractures (see following discussion).

Vertical Axis Vertebral Body Fractures

Benzel et al.[8] described *vertical* fracture patterns of the C2 vertebral body that were not addressed by Anderson and D'Alonzo (Fig. 5A.7). These vertical fractures are grouped into two major types based on their fracture orientation: coronal (type I) versus sagittal (type II). Type I fractures have four possible mechanisms of injury: (a) extension with axial loading, (b) hyperextension with axial loading, (c) flexion-axial load, and (d) flexion-distraction. Type II fractures are due to axial loading until C2 body failure (assuming the C1 ring and the occipital condyles remain strong and resist fracturing). If the vector of the axial load is oriented slightly lateral, a variant of the type II fracture is produced,

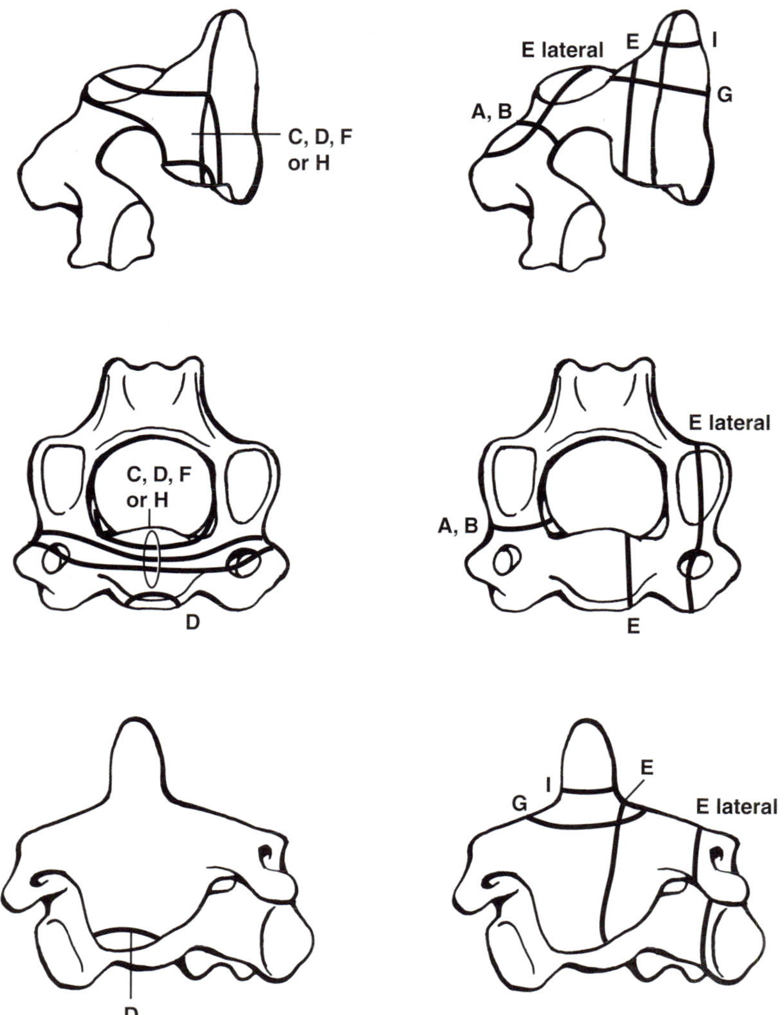

FIGURE 5A.7. Classification of vertical C2 vertebral body fractures as proposed by Benzel et al. (Source: Benzel ED, Hart BL, Ball PA, et al. Fractures of the C2 vertebral body. *J Neurosurg* 1994;81:212, Figure 7, with permission.)

with the fracture line oriented vertically through the foramina transversarium and along the pars interarticularis. The type III fracture of Anderson and D'Alonzo is the same pattern and mechanism of injury as a type III horizontal rostral fracture in the classification of Benzel et al.[8]

COMBINATION FRACTURES, DISLOCATIONS, AND SUBLUXATIONS

The constant physiologic interaction and dependence of individual spinal segments within the upper cervical spine naturally translates into occasional contiguous injuries. Two of the more common injuries include atlanto-occipital dislocation and atlantoaxial subluxation and dislocation.

Atlanto-occipital (C0-C1) Dislocation

Atlanto-occipital dislocation (AOD) can produce devastating neurologic deficits and mortality. In traumatic AOD, the patient may suffer an associated injury to the brainstem at the spinal-medullary junction, resulting in respiratory arrest. With improved prehospital spine immobilization management, the number of patients arriving at emergency departments alive has increased over the years.

The most important structures in maintaining C0-C1 stability are the tectorial membrane and the alar ligaments. Tremendous forces in hyperflexion, hyperextension, lateral flexion, or varying combination can cause this injury pattern, which results in either complete or almost-complete disruption of ligamentous structures between the occiput and the remainder of the upper cervical spine. The most common mechanism for AOD is thought to be a shear-type load on the C0-C1 joint from lateral translation of the skull in relation to the atlas, with subsequent rotation and distraction causing tectorial membrane rupture.

Atlantoaxial (C1-C2) Subluxation and Dislocation

The stability of the atlantoaxial joint rests on an intact transverse ligament. This ligament is mostly responsible for preventing abnormal translation of C1 on C2, even in the face of intact alar ligaments.[9] White and Panjabi,[10] after reviewing the literature, have tried to group abnormal patterns of subluxation and dislocation of this joint into two major types: (1) translatory and (2) rotatory. Within these major groups are further defined subgroups: (1.A) bilateral anterior translation, (1.B) bilateral posterior translation, (2.A) unilateral anterior rotation, (2.B) unilateral posterior rotation, and (2.C) unilateral combined anterior and posterior rotation. Although not all of these conditions occur secondary to trauma, descriptions of all are provided for completeness. Biomechanical studies to confirm the information provided in the following section are still being evaluated and clarified.

Bilateral Anterior and Bilateral Posterior Displacement. Bilateral anterior displacement (BAD) of C1 on C2 is more common than bilateral posterior displacement (BPD) of C1 on C2 (Fig. 5A.8). In BAD, the magnitude of force is so tremendous that it often produces either a fracture of the dens or rupture of the transverse ligament. Typically the direction of force is anteriorly in the sagittal plane, with the neck in slight flexion. Similarly, a BPD of C1 on C2 is secondary to forces directed in the sagittal plane from anterior to posterior, though most descriptions of this injury are in patients with an abnormal dens (i.e., infected, congenitally defective, absent, etc.). In posteriorly directed forces accompanied by slight distraction, the dens remains intact as the anterior arch of C1 "rides" over the odontoid process and becomes locked behind the dens.

Unilateral Anterior and Unilateral Posterior Displacement. With unilateral anterior displacement (UAD), one of the two articular masses shifts anteriorly, creating an abnormally large interval between the dens and the ring of C1 (see Fig. 5A.8). Regardless of left-sided or right-sided UAD, the IAR occurs laterally through the facet joint, which remains dorsal. Unilateral posterior displacement (UPD) is the least common type of rotary injury (see Fig. 5A.8). Although UPD is similar to UAD in that the IAR occurs around the contralateral facet joint, the interval between the dens and the ring of C1 in this type of injury remains somewhat normal.

Unilateral Combined Anterior and Posterior Displacement. In this type of injury, there is essentially a combination of UAD and UPD, producing abnormal rotatory displacement of C2 in relation to C1, with one lateral mass dislocating posteriorly and one lateral mass dislocating anteriorly. The IAR in this injury is centered abnormally over the region of the odontoid process (see Fig. 5A.8).

CONCLUSION

Upper cervical spine biomechanics in trauma is quite complex and governed by many interdependent factors. In principle, the direction of force applied to the cervical spine and the strength of both immediate and adjacent spinal elements will dictate the type and location of injury. Although experimental models provide invaluable information for understanding the pathology of cervical spine trauma, additional patient variables must be considered in the clinical setting (degenerative diseases, arthritis, age, gender, etc.). Increasing clinical awareness and more sophisticated biomechanical spine models are continuing to enhance our understanding of traumatic upper cervical spine injuries.

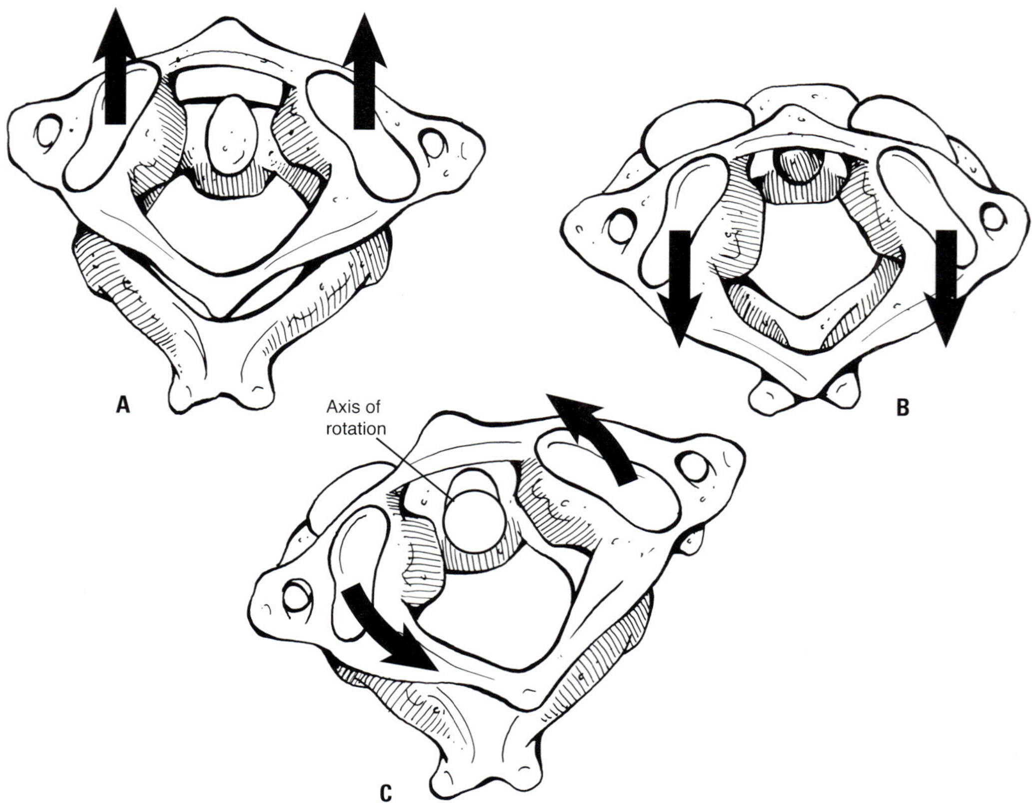

FIGURE 5A.8. **A.** Pattern of bilateral anterior and posterior translation of C1 on C2. (Source: White AA, Panjabi MM. *Clinical Biomechanics of the Spine.* 2nd ed. Philadelphia: Lippincott, 1990:295, Figure 5-19, and 296, Figure 5-21.) **B.** Pattern of unilateral anterior and posterior rotatory displacement of C1 on C2 with their instantaneous axes of rotation (IAR). (Source: White AA, Panjabi MM. *Clinical Biomechanics of the Spine.* 2nd ed. Philadelphia: Lippincott, 1990:297, Figure 5-23, and 299, Figure 5-25.) **C.** Pattern of unilateral combined anterior and posterior rotatory displacement of C1 on C2 with its instantaneous axis of rotation (IAR). (Source: White AA, Panjabi MM. *Clinical Biomechanics of the Spine.* 2nd ed. Philadelphia: Lippincott, 1990:299, Figure 5-26.)

REFERENCES

1. Panjabi MM, Oda T, Criso JJ, et al. Posture affects motion coupling patterns of the upper cervical spine. *J Orthop Res* 1993;11:525–536.
2. Anderson PA, Montesano PX. Morphology and treatment of occipital condyle fractures. *Spine* 1988;13:731–736.
3. Landells CD, Van Peteghem K. Fractures of the atlas: classification, treatment, and morbidity. *Spine* 1988;13:450–452.
4. Schneider RC, Livingson KE, Cave AJE, et al. "Hangman's fracture" of the cervical spine. *J Neurosurg* 1965;22:141–154.
5. Levine AM, Edwards CC. The management of traumatic spondylolisthesis of the axis. *J Bone Joint Surg Am* 1985;67:217–226.
6. Anderson LD, D'Alonzo RT. Fractures of the odontoid process. *J Bone Joint Surg Am* 1974;56:1663–1674.
7. Althoff B. Fractures of the odontoid process: an experimental study. *Acta Orthop Scand Suppl* 1979;177:1–95.
8. Benzel ED, Hart BL, Ball PA, et al. Fractures of the C2 vertebral body. *J Neurosurg* 1994l;81:206–212.
9. Fielding W, Cochran GB, Lawsing JF 3rd, et al. Tears of the transverse ligament of the atlas: a clinical and biomechanical study. *J Bone Joint Surg* 1974;56:1683–1691.
10. White AA, Panjabi MM. *Clinical Biomechanics of the Spine.* 2nd ed. Philadelphia: Lippincott, 1990:1–125, 169–378.

CHAPTER 5B

Cervical Spine Kinematics and the Biomechanics of the Injured Cervical Spine: Subaxial Cervical Junction (C3-C7)

David O. Okonkwo, Jamie Gasco, Christopher I. Shaffrey, Harvey E. Smith, and Alexander R. Vaccaro

INTRODUCTION

The motions (kinematics) of the subaxial cervical spine are dictated by the unique anatomic relationships of the bony and soft tissue structures of the C3-C7 vertebral segments. Biomechanical properties of the subaxial cervical spine responsible for stability are dictated by the force tolerances of these components. As a result of the nonlinear biomechanical properties of the subaxial cervical spine, the design of effective in vivo models that mimic the human spine with fidelity is still under constant development. The determinants of injury are the point of application; the force vector, including magnitude and direction; and the rate of loading.[1–3] Under load the cervical spine can buckle, creating moments in one direction at one level and the opposite at another.

SUBAXIAL CERVICAL SPINE

ANATOMIC COMPONENTS OF THE SUBAXIAL CERVICAL SPINE

Vertebrae

Unique anatomic characteristics differentiate the cervical vertebral bodies from other segments of the spine. In the coronal plane, the interbody junction (uncovertebral joint) has a saddlelike or ellipsoid appearance, with anterior-posterior and medial-lateral concavities.[4] The inferior endplates form a curved lip in the sagittal plane designed to prevent anterior displacement of the caudal vertebral body. The superior endplates have a craniocaudal anteroposterior orientation that enables the movement of flexion-extension with the cephalad vertebral level. The particular disposition of the articulating facets enables flexion-extension and rotation around an axis perpendicular to the facet joint, rather than around an axis perpendicular to the endplate (Fig. 5B.1).[5] The 45-degree upward orientation of the facet surfaces also precludes motion in the anterior plane.

Facet Joints

Understanding the orientation of the facets, or zygapophyseal joints, is critical to understanding the biomechanics of injury affecting the subaxial cervical spine. The facet joint, composed of a fibrous capsular membrane, a synovial membrane and fluid, articular cartilage, and superior and inferior articular

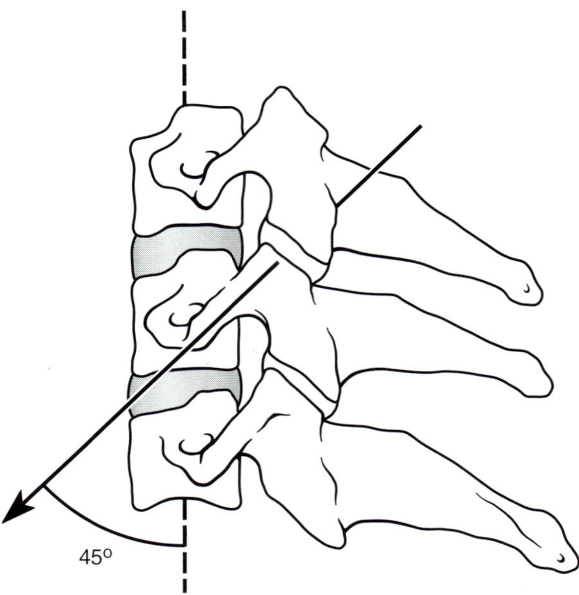

FIGURE 5B.1. Flexion-extension and rotation in the subaxial cervical spine occur around the axis perpendicular to the facet joint (*solid arrow*), and not around the axis perpendicular to the endplate (*dotted line*). The facet joints are oriented at an upward angle of 45 degrees.

processes, acts as a pillar that absorbs one-fifth of axial compressive loads and half of extension and rotational loads.[6–8] The superior articular processes have a variable orientation that determines the limits of motion of the cervical spine segments. The spatial orientation of the superior articular process from C3 downward varies from posteromedial to posterolateral. In general, above the C5-C6 level, the superior articular facets are oriented posteromedially and below C5-C6, its orientation is posterolateral. This transition in orientation may be gradual (over two to five successive vertebrae) or sudden (adjacent vertebrae). However, individual anatomic variations are the norm, and fixed patterns of change in orientation should not be inferred.[9,10] The posteromedial orientation of the superior articular processes of C3 facilitates head rotation by fixing the C2 vertebra; posterolateral orientation of the lower cervical levels facilitates flexion, extension, rotation, and lateral bending.

In addition to the stability afforded by the zygapophyseal joints, there are prominent anatomic articulations on the lateral borders of the superior and inferior surfaces of the bodies of C3 through C7. These lips fit together to form what are called the Luschka joints, uncovertebral joints, or lateral interbody joints. Whether these structures represent "true" joints is controversial, and the role of uncovertebral joints in the biomechanics of cervical spine injuries is not clearly known.

Spinal Ligaments

The ligaments are a major stabilizing component of the cervical spine and are critical for both intrinsic spinal stability and surgical stabilization techniques. The spinal ligaments serve to facilitate smooth spinal motions and maintain the articulated alignment of the spine. During supraphysiologic loads, the ligaments are a key source of protection against dislocation and neural element injury.

The anterior longitudinal ligament (ALL), at the anterior and anterolateral surfaces of the vertebral bodies, serves to limit extension and prevents excessive distraction. The ALL in the cervical spine is substantially weaker than that in lower parts of the spine. The posterior longitudinal ligament (PLL), which is narrow over the bodies and widens as it attaches to the discs, limits flexion and reinforces the central portion of the discs. The PLL is broad and strong in the cervical spine and is the key ligament resisting injury from flexion, extension, and distraction injury vectors (see later discussion).

The ligamentum flava are paired ligaments that attach laminae of contiguous vertebrae. The ligamentum flava prevent excessive flexion and act to buffer extension. The capsular ligaments serve to limit facet dislocation. The interspinous ligaments and supraspinous ligaments (the "posterior ligament complex") resist flexion and are an important, often overlooked, contributor to cervical spinal stability. These ligaments are key resistors of cervical facet dislocation. With aging, the elastin component of spinal ligaments fibroses and the risk for ligamentous injury increases.[11]

Ligaments are uniaxial structures that resist tensile or distractive forces.[8,12] Their viscoelastic properties determine a rate-dependent internal response (including injury) to external loading: if gradual reorientation of fibers is allowed (slow-rate mechanism), avulsion of the ligament may occur; with high rates of loading, disruption of fibers is more likely.[3] The integrity and function of the spinal ligaments is also critical in stabilization surgeries, and it is clear that common spinal surgical procedures induce significant changes in the biomechanical properties of the spinal ligaments.[13]

Intervertebral Discs

The anulus of the intervertebral disc is thick anteriorly and tapers laterally and posteriorly, with the nucleus of the disc residing in an eccentric location. This wedge shape of the disc contributes to the lordosis (anterior convexity) of the cervical spine and dictates an asymmetric internal load share. Yoganandan et al.,[8] in finite element analysis of combined loading, demonstrated that the ventral region of the disc experiences higher axial forces under all loading models, whereas shear forces primarily affect the dorsal anulus.

In contrast to the ligaments, which are arranged in a uniaxial manner to resist tension, the intervertebral discs are designed to sustain compression primarily through the nucleus pulposus (proteoglycan). Tension, shear, bending, and torsion force vectors are distributed mainly to the anulus fibrosus (collagen).

Spinal Cord

Although the spinal cord and its coverings do not contribute significantly to force tolerances in the subaxial cervical spine, the tolerances of these structures should be considered when viewing risk for neurologic deficit from specific injury vectors such as distraction. For example, denticulate ligaments are strongest in the cervical region and limit cranial-caudal motion of the spinal cord.[14] Numerous investigators have demonstrated a tethering effect of the denticulate ligaments on the spinal cord. Thus, the denticulate ligaments may exacerbate spinal cord damage during distraction injuries. The present understanding of the contribution of viscoelastic properties of the spinal cord and its coverings and attachments in pathologic states is limited at best.

NORMAL SUBAXIAL CERVICAL SPINE KINEMATICS

Table 5B.1 lists the normal degrees of motion in the adult subaxial cervical spine.[15–18] Figure 5B.2 illustrates the three-dimensional coordinate axes, corresponding positive moments, and injury force vectors of the cervical spine.

Flexion-extension is the principal motion of the subaxial cervical spine. Initially it was thought that flexion of the cervical spine began in the upper cervical region, with the spinous processes fanning out in stepwise progression through the lower cervical segments.[19] This has been challenged by contemporary studies incorporating dynamic, high-speed cineradiography. Flexion-extension is, in fact, a multistep process that begins in stepwise progression from C6-C7 through C4-C5.[20] The initial phase is followed next by craniocervical junction flexion, followed by flexion at C2-C4, during which time slight extension occurs at C6-C7. The final phase of flexion occurs again at C4-C7. Extension occurs essentially in the reverse order of the phases of flexion and, again, is initiated and terminated at C6-C7. The highest degrees of flexion occur at C5-C6, likely accounting for both the high rate of degenerative changes and the high rate of flexion-compression injury at this level. The most common level fractured is C5.

TABLE 5B.1 Degrees of Motion in the Subaxial Cervical Spine

LEVEL	Motion Flexion-Extension[15,18]	Axial Rotation*[16]	Lateral Bending[17]	Translation†[16]
C3-4	15.2 ± 3.8	4.5 ± 1.1	3.5 ± 1.4	0.6 ± 0.2
C4-5	17.1 ± 4.5	4.6 ± 1.1	3.3 ± 1.0	0.9 ± 0.3
C5-6	17.1 ± 3.9	4.0 ± 1.1	4.3 ± 1.4	0.9 ± 0.2
C6-7	18.1 ± 6.1	1.6 ± 1.8	5.7 ± 1.9	0.6 ± 0.3

*Recall that 50% of axial rotation occurs at C1-C2.
†Translation does not occur in the absence of axial rotation.

Axial rotation in the cervical spine, on the other hand, is rather limited in the subaxial cervical spine because of facet joint orientation, as illustrated previously. Lateral bending is, in part, enabled by the vertebral body–disc–vertebral body Luschka joints, which forms in the anulus fibrosus during childhood and is fully developed by the third decade of life. Higher degrees of lateral bending occur above C5 (see Table 5B.1).

Translation in the subaxial cervical spine is limited by the orientation of the facets, by the spinal ligaments, and by the anulus. The most common mechanism of shear strain is whiplash injury (flexion-extension).[21]

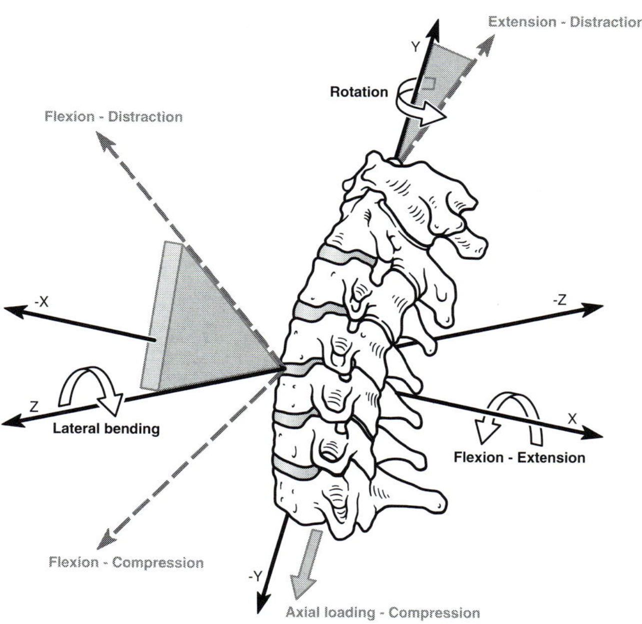

FIGURE 5B.2. The three-dimensional coordinate axes, positive moments, and injury force vectors around the motion segments of the cervical spine. Rotation, lateral bending, and flexion-extension are the corresponding positive moments around each of the three coordinate axes (*X, Y, Z*). Injury force vectors of flexion-distraction, extension-distraction, flexion-compression, and axial loading are illustrated in gray.

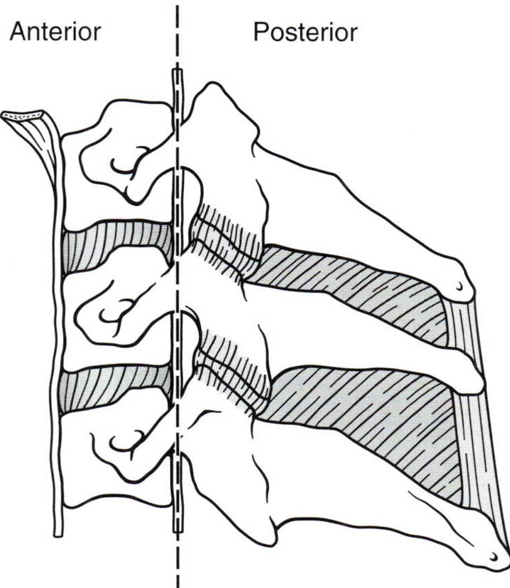

FIGURE 5B.3. The two-column concept of the subaxial cervical spine. In Holdsworth's two-column concept, the anterior column consists of the anterior longitudinal ligament, the vertebral bodies, intervertebral discs, and posterior longitudinal ligament. The posterior column includes the laminae, spinous process, ligamentum flavum, and posterior ligamentous complex (interspinous and supraspinous ligaments).

BIOMECHANICS OF SUBAXIAL CERVICAL SPINE INJURIES

Two-Column Concept of Spinal Stability

The two-column concept of the cervical spine was proposed in Holdsworth's landmark paper[22] in 1963. The anterior column consists of the vertebral body, anterior and posterior longitudinal ligaments, and intervertebral discs; the posterior column consists of the facet joints, capsular ligaments, spinous processes, laminas, and interspinous ligaments (Fig. 5B.3). Denis' three-column concept of spinal stability[23] is fashioned for injuries involving the thoracic and lumbar spine. At present, the majority of biomechanistic theories have used the two-column theory to evaluate injury mechanisms of the subaxial cervical spine.

Holdsworth[22] contended that instability occurs with injury to the posterior ligamentous complex in association with an anterior column injury. As mentioned previously, the determinants of cervical spinal column injury are the magnitude, vector, and rate of force application sustained by the cervical spine.[1–3] White and Panjabi[12] defined instability as "loss of the ability of the spine under physiologic loads to maintain its pattern of displacement so that there is no initial or additional neurologic deficit, no major deformity, and no incapacitating pain." It may result from ligamentous injury with or without an associated bony injury.

The most common level injured is C5-C6, believed to be due to the higher degree of flexion-extension motion (see Table 5B.1) at this level compared to the rest of the cervical spine.

Compression Injuries

Argenson et al.[24] built on the schemata of Allen et al.[1] and Harris et al.[25] to classify subaxial cervical spine injuries on the principal force vectors producing specific patterns of injury (Table 5B.2). The first of these force vectors is compression injury, which may occur in association with flexion or extension.

TABLE 5B.2 Argenson Classification of Subaxial Cervical Spine Injuries[24]

Type	Injury Mechanism (%)	Injury Pattern (%)	Characteristics
A	Compression injuries (33)	I: Anterior compression (wedge) fracture (3) II: Comminuted fracture (7) III: Teardrop fracture (23)	Principally bony damage; often associated with flexion forces
B	Flexion/extension/ distraction injuries (28)	I: Moderate whiplash with neurologic injury (5) II: Severe whiplash (sprain) (14) III: Bilateral facet fracture-dislocation (9)	Principally disc and ligamentous damage
C	Rotation injuries (39)	I: Unilateral facet fracture (20) II: Fracture separation of the articular pillar (10) III: Unilateral dislocation (9)	Asymmetric lesions; rotation is always associated with lateral flexion

Pure axial loading as a cause of cervical spine injury is relatively rare below C2, described in only 7% of subaxial injuries in the series by Argenson et al.[24] (Axial loading in atlantoaxial injuries was discussed previously.) Pure axial compression often results in a comminuted fracture, which may or may not result in bone retropulsed into the spinal canal endangering the neural elements (Fig. 5B.4).

The most common force resulting in traumatic spinal cord injuries or unstable cervical spinal fractures is compression with flexion (see Table 5B.2). Force vectors directed in flexion may result in distraction of the posterior elements and compression of anterior elements. Clinically, axial loading with a flexion vector directs force through the anterior column (anterior aspect of the vertebral body and the intervertebral disc). Less severe degrees of force result in a compression or wedge fracture, whereas a severe force may result in an unstable teardrop (flexion-compression) fracture (Fig. 5B.4).

Flexion-Extension-Distraction Injuries

A second group of injury force vectors are flexion-extension-distraction injuries, commonly known as whiplash injuries. These injuries are characterized by disproportionate injury to the spinal ligaments and intervertebral disc compared to the bony elements.

The physiologic movements of flexion and extension are, as mentioned earlier, modulated by the PLL, which is strong in the cervical spine. Thus, when the PLL remains intact after a whiplash injury (with moderate force magnitude), the transverse axis of the spine remains intact and neurologic injury is rare. However, when the PLL is disrupted in more severe injuries, often in association with failure of the posterior anulus, unstable spinal lesions are produced. Unstable lesions happen when failure of the PLL and posterior anulus occurs in combination with anterolisthesis, endplate angulation greater than 10 degrees, facet malalignment, or distracted vertebral segments resulting from posterior ligamentous complex injury.[26]

Bilateral fracture-dislocation (or jumped facets; Fig. 5B.5) results in PLL failure and disruption of the posterior ligamentous complex (supraspinous or interspinous ligaments). This ligamentous injury has important implications for clinical management of flexion-compression injuries: traction with larger weights may result in significant distraction; halo fixation is more likely to fail with ligamentous injury; and an anterior procedure jeopardizes the remaining intact anterior longitudinal ligament, worsening stability and increasing the likelihood of pseudarthrosis.

Extension-distraction injuries are far less common than flexion-distraction injuries, but their consequences tend to be more severe in terms of spinal instability and neurologic compromise.[27]

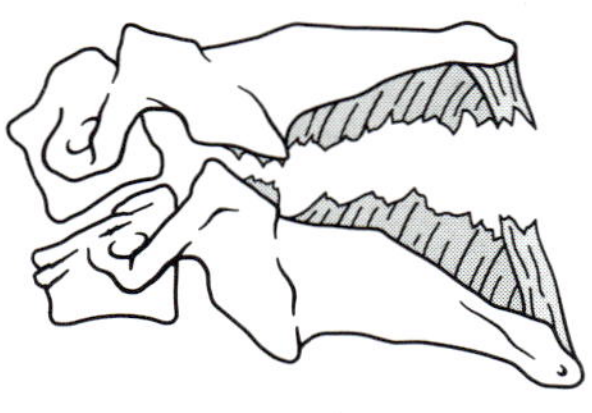

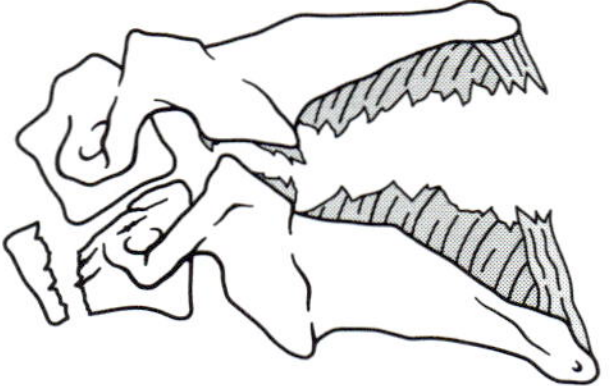

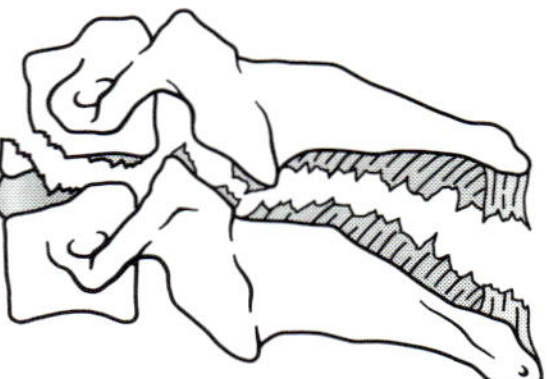

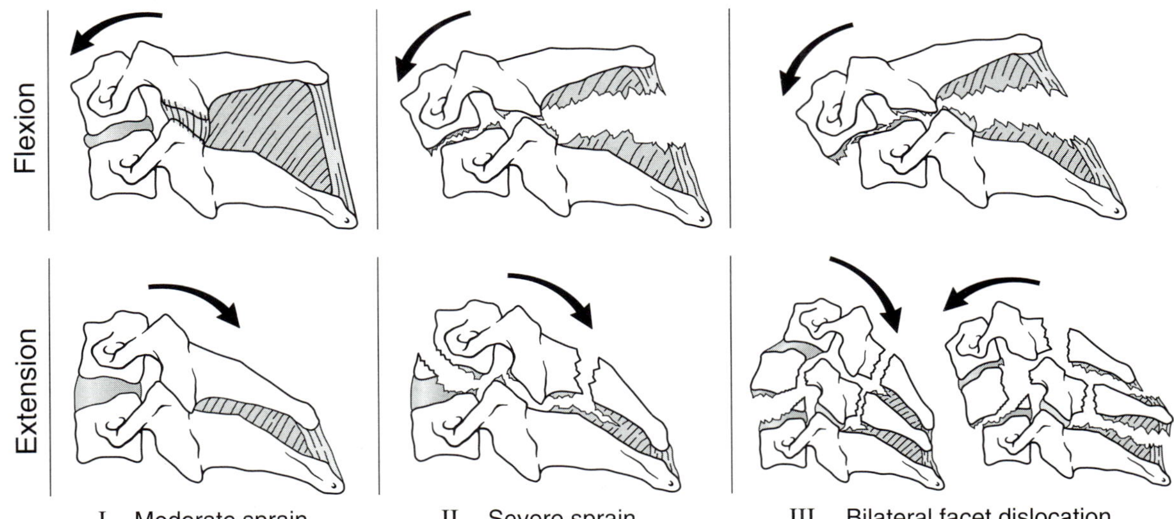

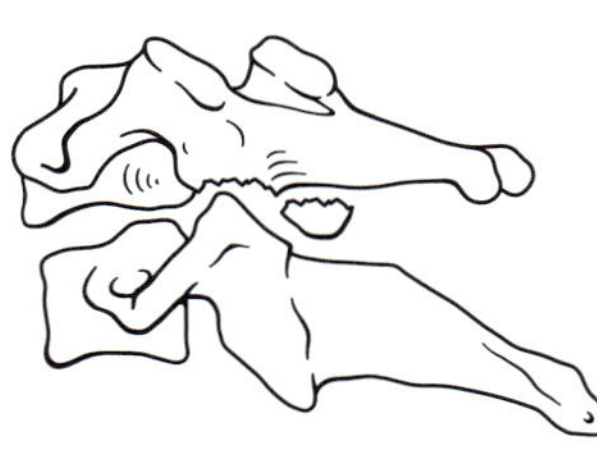

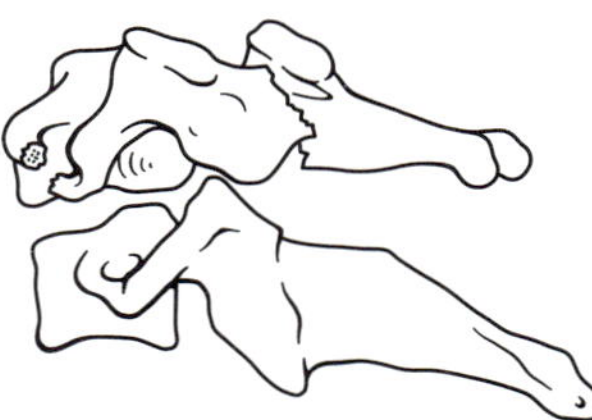

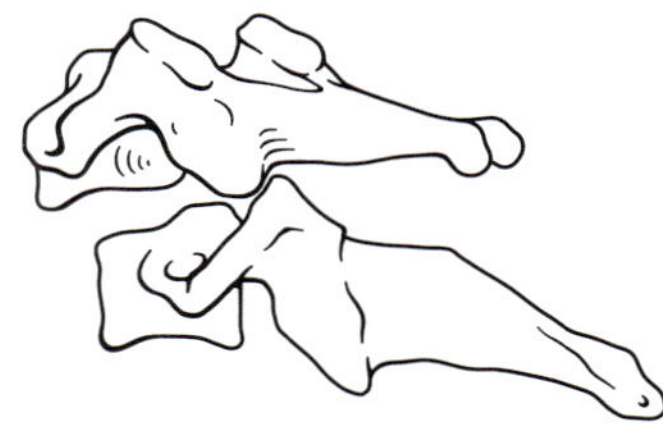

FIGURE 5B.4. Mechanistic classification of subaxial cervical spine injuries. The classification schema of Argenson et al groups cervical spine traumatic injuries by injury force vector. (Modified from Argenson C, De Peretti F, Ghabris A, et al. A scheme for the classification of lower cervical spine injuries. *Maîtrise Orthopédique* 2006, with permission.)

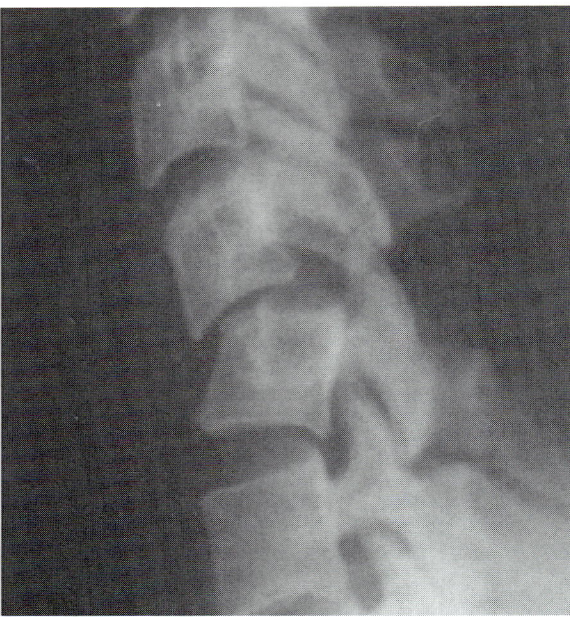

FIGURE 5B.5. Severe flexion-distraction injury force vectors may produce bilateral fracture-dislocation, or jumped facets. Bilateral jumped facets, as seen here, occur when the traumatizing injury force persists in the setting of posterior longitudinal ligament failure and disruption of the supraspinous and interspinous ligaments. The radiographic hallmark of bilateral jumped facet is more than half forward displacement of one vertebral body over the next.

In mild and moderate whiplash injuries, static and dynamic radiographs may be normal, but subclinical ligamentous injury and delayed deformity may arise. This is supported experimentally by microscopic histologic analysis demonstrating multilevel disc and ALL injury in spines that appeared radiographically normal. These spines may demonstrate exaggerated but subpathologic motion at multiple levels on motion segment analysis following sagittal extension vector injury forces.[28]

Rotational Injury

Rotational injury manifests clinically in the form of asymmetric lesions such as a unilateral dislocation and/or fractured facets or fractures of the articular pillar (the facets absorb half of the load resulting from rotational forces applied to the cervical spine). Rotational injuries are designated type C injuries in the classification of Argenson et al.[24] (see Table 5B.2 and Fig. 5B.4). Rotational injury always occurs with lateral flexion vectors superimposed on rotation. Spinal column alignment is, in general, maintained following rotational injuries. Rotational injuries are typically stable, with the possible exception of certain unilateral facet dislocations in which there may be injury to the PLL (often intact in a unilateral facet dislocation).

Burst Fractures

Prior experimental models suggested that burst fractures begin at the endplates as a result of increased pressure and superoinferior bulging of the nucleus pulposus[29,30]; however, more recent finite element data indicate that bulging or expansion of the disc results in higher degrees of downward force being distributed to the facets, initiating the following sequence[31]:

1. An axial load at a high rate forces the inferior articular facet in a caudal and anterior direction into the superior articular facet causing a rotational deformity to the transverse process.

2. The rotational deformity of the facets transmits a tensile force to the second column through the pedicle that ultimately extends into the center of the body.
3. Fracture occurs in the posterior region of the vertebral body, producing a wedge-shaped fragment of bone.
4. The fragment is projected in the spinal canal, stretching the PLL and compressing the cord. The bone fragment is subsequently forced back anteriorly by the action of both the cord/dura and the PLL after maximum level of deformity is reached.

SUBAXIAL CERVICAL SPINE INJURY CLASSIFICATION SYSTEM

A subcommittee of the Spine Trauma Study Group reviewed the literature pertaining to the classification techniques for subaxial cervical trauma and developed the Subaxial Cervical Spine Injury Classification (SLIC) system,[32] building on the concepts developed in creating the Thoracolumbar Injury Classification and Scoring (TLICS) system,[33,34] classifying injuries according to their morphology, integrity of the posterior ligamentous complex, and neurologic status of the patient. The goal of the SLIC system and methodology is to address concerns regarding other classification systems (limited intraobserver and interobserver reproducibility, too cumbersome for clinical use, and a need to directly translate the information provided by classification to clinical decision making in a facile manner.) The SLIC scale assigns points to the injury based on morphology, integrity of the discoligamentous complex, and neurologic status of the patient (Table 5B.3). The clinical decision for surgical versus nonsurgical management is based on the

TABLE 5B.3 SLIC System

Component	Points
Morphology	
No abnormality	0
Compression	1
Burst	+1 = 2
Distraction	3
Rotation/translation	4
Discoligamentous complex	
Intact	0
Indeterminate	1
Disrupted	2
Neurologic Status	
Intact	0
Root injury	1
Complete cord injury	2
Incomplete cord injury	3
Continuous cord compression with neurologic deficit (modifier)	+1

SLIC score, with injuries scoring 1 to 3 managed nonoperatively and injuries scoring 5 or more likely necessitating surgical management. The SLIC scoring system is designed to facilitate consideration of the key injury components that should be considered in clinical decision making; individual patient considerations and confounding variables should be assessed when appropriate, and the SLIC score should be considered a guideline to facilitate clinical decision making. The SLIC system has demonstrated good initial reliability and validity data, but the system remains to be clinically validated.

CONCLUSION

Understanding the unique anatomy shared by all segments from C3 to T1 allows recognition of common injury patterns. The important components to stability are the bodies and lateral masses with accompanying ligaments, including ALL, PLL, discs, and nuchal ligaments. The force vector, location of application, and rate of loading will ultimately determine the injury and its severity. Once an injury is identified, reversing the force vector can usually be used to correct malalignment.

REFERENCES

1. Allen BL Jr, Ferguson RL, Lehmann TR, et al. A mechanistic classification of closed, indirect fractures and dislocations of the lower cervical spine. *Spine* 1982;7:1–27.
2. Pintar FA, Yoganandan N, Voo L. Effect of age and loading rate on human cervical spine injury threshold. *Spine* 1998;23:1957–1962.
3. Yoganandan N, Pintar F, Butler J, et al. Dynamic response of human cervical spine ligaments. *Spine* 1989;14:1102–1110.
4. Penning L, Wilmink JT. Rotation of the cervical spine: a CT study in normal subjects. *Spine* 1987;12:732–738.
5. Bogduk N, Mercer S. Biomechanics of the cervical spine. I: Normal kinematics. *Clin Biomech (Bristol, Avon)* 2000;15:633–648.
6. Mercer S, Bogduk N. Intra-articular inclusions of the cervical synovial joints. *Br J Rheumatol* 1993;32:705–710.
7. Tonetti J, Peoc'h M, Merloz P, et al. Elastic reinforcement and thickness of the joint capsules of the lower cervical spine. *Surg Radiol Anat* 1999;21:35–39.
8. Yoganandan N, Kumaresan S, Pintar FA. Biomechanics of the cervical spine. II: Cervical spine soft tissue responses and biomechanical modeling. *Clin Biomech (Bristol, Avon)* 2001;16:1–27.
9. Milne N. The role of zygapophysial joint orientation and uncinate processes in controlling motion in the cervical spine. *J Anat* 1991;178:189–201.
10. Pal GP, Routal RV, Saggu SK. The orientation of the articular facets of the zygapophyseal joints at the cervical and upper thoracic region. *J Anat* 2001;198:431–441.
11. Iida T, Abumi K, Kotani Y, et al. Effects of aging and spinal degeneration on mechanical properties of lumbar supraspinous and interspinous ligaments. *Spine J* 2002;2:95–100.
12. White A III, Panjabi M. *Clinical Biomechanics of Spine*. 2nd ed. Philadelphia: JB Lippincott, 1990.
13. Kotani Y, Cunningham BW, Cappuccino A, et al. The effects of spinal fixation and destabilization on the biomechanical and histologic properties of spinal ligaments: an in vivo study. *Spine* 1998;23:672–682.
14. Tubbs RS, Salter G, Grabb PA, et al. The denticulate ligament: anatomy and functional significance. *J Neurosurg* 2001;94:271–275.
15. Maiman D, Millington P, Novak S, et al. The effect of the thermoplastic Minerva body jacket on cervical spine motion. *Neurosurgery* 1989;25:363–367.
16. Ishii T, Mukai Y, Hosono N, et al. Kinematics of the subaxial cervical spine in rotation in vivo three-dimensional analysis. *Spine* 2004;29:2826–2831.
17. Ishii T, Mukai Y, Hosono N, et al. Kinematics of the cervical spine in lateral bending: in vivo three-dimensional analysis. *Spine* 2006;31:155–160.
18. Maiman DJ, Pintar FA, Groff MW, et al. Concepts and mechanisms of biomechanics. In: Winn HR, ed. *Youmans Neurological Surgery*. 5th ed. Philadelphia: WB Saunders, 2004:4181–4201.
19. Buonocore E, Hartman JT, Nelson CL. Cineradiograms of cervical spine in diagnosis of soft-tissue injuries. *JAMA* 1966;198:143–147.
20. Van MH, Drukker J, Sanches H, et al. Cervical spine motion in the sagittal plane (I) range of motion of actually performed movements, an x-ray cinematographic study. *Eur J Morphol* 1990;28:47–68.

21. Reitman CA, Mauro KM, Nguyen L, et al. Intervertebral motion between flexion and extension in asymptomatic individuals. *Spine* 2004;29:2832–2843.
22. Holdsworth H. Fractures, dislocations, and fracture-dislocations of the spine. *J Bone Joint Surg* 1963;45:6–20.
23. Denis F. The three column spine and its significance in the classification of acute thoracolumbar spinal injuries. *Spine* 1983;8:817–831.
24. Argenson C, De Peretti F, Ghabris A, et al. A scheme for the classification of lower cervical spine injuries. *Maîtrise Orthopédique* 2006.
25. Harris JH Jr, Edeiken-Monroe B, Kopaniky DR. A practical classification of acute cervical spine injuries. *Orthop Clin North Am* 1986;17:15–30.
26. Louis R. [Cervical sprains and cervical herniated discs (author's transl)]. *Nouv Presse Med* 1979;8:1843–1849.
27. Cusick JF, Yoganandan N, Pintar F, et al. Cervical spine injuries from high-velocity forces: a pathoanatomic and radiologic study. *J Spinal Disord* 1996;9:1–7.
28. Stemper BD, Yoganandan N, Pintar FA, et al. Anterior longitudinal ligament injuries in whiplash may lead to cervical instability. *Med Eng Phys* 2005;28:515–524.
29. Roaf R. A study of the mechanics of spinal injuries. *J Bone Joint Surg Br* 1960;42:810–823.
30. Tran NT, Watson NA, Tencer AF, et al. Mechanism of the burst fracture in the thoracolumbar spine: the effect of loading rate. *Spine* 1995;20:1984–1988.
31. Wilcox RK, Allen DJ, Hall RM, et al. A dynamic investigation of the burst fracture process using a combined experimental and finite element approach. *Eur Spine J* 2004;13:481–488.
32. Vaccaro AR, Hulbert RJ, Patel AA, et al. The Subaxial Cervical Spine Injury Classification System. *Spine* 2007;32:2365–2374.
33. Vaccaro AR, Zeiller SC, Hulbert RJ, et al. The thoracolumbar injury severity score: a proposed treatment algorithm. *J Spinal Disord Tech* 2005;18:209–215.
34. Vaccaro AR, Lehman RA Jr, Hurlbert RJ, et al. A new classification of thoracolumbar injuries: the importance of injury morphology, the integrity of the posterior ligamentous complex, and neurologic status. *Spine* 2005;30:2325–2333.

CHAPTER 5C

Cervical Spine Kinematics and the Biomechanics of the Injured Cervical Spine: Cervicothoracic Junction (C7-T1)

Daniel R. Fassett and Darrel S. Brodke

INTRODUCTION

The cervicothoracic junction is a specialized transition zone within the spine. It is prone to injury and can be difficult to stabilize. The vertebrae are slightly different from those above and below, and the associated stress concentration should be considered when surgical treatment is considered.

The incidence of traumatic injuries at the cervicothoracic junction (Fig. 5C.1) has been reported to be as high as 9% of all cervical injuries.[1] The transitional anatomy and complex biomechanics of this region can make conservative and operative treatment of fractures in this area challenging.[2,3] Two main factors place the cervicothoracic junction at risk. The first is the transition between the highly mobile cervical spine and the rigid thoracic spine. The second is the change in sagittal alignment that naturally occurs, with the lordotic cervical spine meeting the kyphotic thoracic spine. These factors both result in considerable energy concentration directly at the cervicothoracic junction, a factor that should be strongly considered when treating traumatic injuries in this area.

The cervicothoracic junction osteology reveals changes in the vertebrae consistent with the increased forces seen in this region. The vertebral body of C7 is larger than the other cervical vertebral bodies and able to withstand greater compressive loads.[4,5] The pedicles of C7 and T1 are also larger than the pedicles of the vertebra discussed previously and below the cervicothoracic junction, which provides more structural stability.[6] In addition, the C7-T1 facet articulation, which more closely resembles a thoracic facet, is more vertically inclined (approximately 65 degrees) than the other cervical facets (approximately 45 degrees) in the sagittal plane.[4,7,8] This greater inclination serves to resist translation forces, which may be great on this transitional segment and also reduce the amount of axial rotation.[7] The length of the spinous processes of C7 and T1 also act to provide more stability. Although the intraspinous, supraspinous, and nuchal ligaments tend to be weak compared to other ligamentous structures, the long spinous processes of C7 and T1 act as a lever arm around the flexion-extension axis of rotation and increase the contribution of these ligaments to stability in limiting flexion.[9]

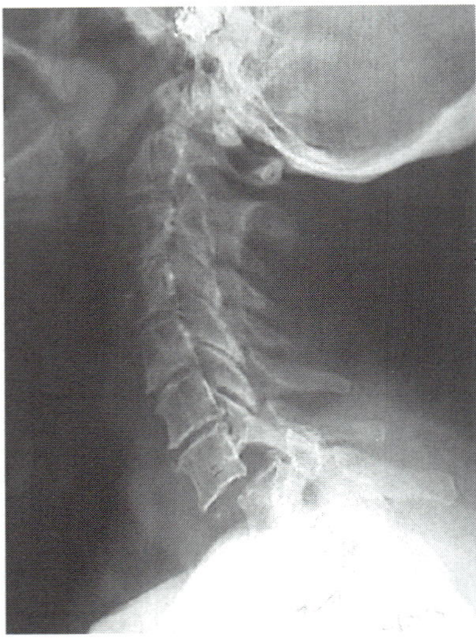

FIGURE 5C.1. Bilateral facet fracture dislocation at C7-T1.

The C7-T1 articulation is the least mobile articulation in the cervical spine. This articulation allows mostly flexion-extension motion, with approximately 5 to 9 degrees of physiologic motion in this plane. With the steep angulation of the facets, lateral bending and axial rotation are limited at C7-T1, with only 2 to 4 degrees of lateral bending and 2 to 5 degrees of axial rotation.[10,11]

A limited number of biomechanical studies have specifically addressed the complexity of forces and instrumentation at the cervicothoracic junction. These have tended to support posterior constructs for stabilization over anterior and longer constructs over those that end at the C7-T1 location. Bueff et al.[12] reported that posterior stabilization of the cervicothoracic junction with hooks and rods had statistically more stiffness compared to that with anterior cervical plates. Kreshak et al.[13] studied the kinematics of posterior stabilization of two-column and three-column traumatic injuries at the cervicothoracic junction. They found that posterior stabilization was sufficient for two-column injuries with greater stiffness than intact specimens. In three-column injuries, the stiffness with posterior instrumentation decreased, especially in extension.

CONCLUSION

The authors recommend posterior stabilization for two-column injuries at the cervicothoracic junction and combined anterior-posterior instrumentation for three-column injuries in this area.

Ames et al.[14] also compared anterior and posterior stabilization techniques at the cervicothoracic junction in destabilized cervical spines. They found that posterior pedicle screw instrumentation reduced motion better than anterior plating, especially in lateral bending and axial rotation. They also noted that stability of posterior instrumentation improved when the pedicle screw instrumentation was extended from T1 to T2 and the combination of anterior and posterior instrumentation produced significantly more stability than either anterior or posterior instrumentation alone.

The biomechanics of the cervicothoracic junction are unique because of the transition from mobile cervical spine to rigid thoracic spine and the transition from lordotic to kyphotic segments. Close examination of the osteology reveals changes consistent with the special needs of this region. Treatment of the unstable cervicothoracic junction must take into account this biomechanical environment.

REFERENCES

1. Nichols CG, Young DH, Schiller WR. Evaluation of cervicothoracic junction injury. *Ann Emerg Med* 1987; 16:640–642.
2. Chapman JR, Anderson PA, Pepin C, et al. Posterior instrumentation of the unstable cervicothoracic spine. *J Neurosurg* 1996;84:552–558.
3. An HS, Vaccaro A, Cotler JM, et al. Spinal disorders at the cervicothoracic junction. *Spine* 1994;19:2557–2564.
4. Milne N. The role of zygapophysial joint orientation and uncinate processes in controlling motion in the cervical spine. *J Anat* 1991;178:189–201.
5. Panjabi MM, Duranceau J, Goel V, et al. Cervical human vertebrae: quantitative three-dimensional anatomy of the middle and lower regions. *Spine* 1991;16:861–869.
6. Bailey AS, Stanescu S, Yeasting RS, et al. Anatomic relationships of the cervicothoracic junction. *Spine* 1995;20:1431–1439.
7. Ghanayem AJ, Zdeblick TA, Dvorak J. Functional anatomy of joints, ligaments, and discs. In: Clark CR, ed. *The Cervical Spine.* Philadelphia: Lippincott-Raven, 1998:45–52.
8. Panjabi MM, Oxland T, Takata K, et al. Articular facets of the human spine: quantitative three-dimensional anatomy. *Spine* 1993;18:1298–310.
9. Takeshita K, Peterson ETK, Bylski-Austrow D, et al. The nuchal ligament restrains cervical spine flexion. *Spine* 2004;29:E388–E393.
10. White AA, Panjabi MM. *Clinical Biomechanics of the Spine.* 2nd ed. Philadelphia: JB Lippincott, 1990.
11. Miura T, Panjabi MM, Cripton PA. A method to simulate in vivo cervical spine kinematics using in vitro compressive preload. *Spine* 2002;27:43–48.
12. Bueff HU, Lotz JC, Colliou OK, et al. Instrumentation of the cervicothoracic junction after destabilization. *Spine* 1995;20:1789–1792.
13. Kreshak JL, Kim DH, Lindsey DP, et al. Posterior stabilization at the cervicothoracic junction: a biomechanical study. *Spine* 2002;27:2763–2770.
14. Ames CP, Bozkus MH, Chamberlain RH, et al. Biomechanics of stabilization after cervicothoracic compression-flexion injury. *Spine* 2005;30:1505–1512.

SECTION IV

Evaluation of the Cervical Spine Injured Patient

CHAPTER 6

Prehospital Management

Christopher M. Bono

INTRODUCTION

Care for a patient with a potential cervical spine injury begins before the patient arrives at the hospital. This first includes general considerations such as assessing airway, air exchange, and hemodynamic stability (the often cited A, B, C, or airway, breathing, circulation). Although primarily geared toward saving the patient's life, they are also critical to maintaining adequate perfusion of an injured spinal cord to maximize neurologic recovery. Following in temporal sequence, but more important for avoiding secondary neurologic injury, immobilization of the spine includes application of a cervical collar, in-line traction during head and neck maneuvers, and transfers using a rigid backboard. This chapter will review the current data and recommendations concerning these issues.

SECURING AN AIRWAY

Airway security is crucial to the overall survival of the patient. In the unconscious or obtunded patient, an adequate airway is the most imminent priority. First, it must be determined if the traumatized victim is able to breathe spontaneously. This is determined by listening for breath sounds at the mouth and auscultation of the lungs.

If spontaneous breathing is not present, the next step must be to inspect the oral and nasal cavities and upper airway. Any gross obstruction, such as blood, secretions, or tissues, should be cleared before attempting forced respirations, because they can become pushed distally and obstruct the passage of air. Next, bag-mask ventilation ("bagging") should be attempted.[1] A conforming mask should cover the nose and mouth. This is connected to a bag-valve resuscitator that is manually squeezed to infuse air into the patient's lungs.

Air should flow easily, with little resistance. Keeping the patient's head in a neutral position with the mouth open maximizes patency of the upper airway and is important in avoiding displacement of a potential spine injury. If the mouth cannot be maintained open, the jaw might be dislocated anteroinferiorly at the temporomandibular joint (the so-called jaw thrust) (Fig. 6.1). This is the airway maneuver of choice for those with suspected cervical spine fractures or dislocations.[2]

In the minority of cases, bag-mask ventilation is not successful. Persistent bleeding, laryngeal swelling, or anatomic variants can sometimes inhibit air exchange. In these cases, endotracheal intubation might be performed in the field on an emergent basis. With intubation, manipulation of the neck can potentially displace unstable cervical fractures or dislocations. Manual in-line stabilization should be maintained throughout the intubation process. This is achieved by a dedicated person (other that performing the intubation) firmly supporting the head on either side with his or her hands.

In-field intubation should be reserved as a last resort. It is best to proceed with intubation in the more controlled setting of a hospital emergency room, where other options, such as fiberop-

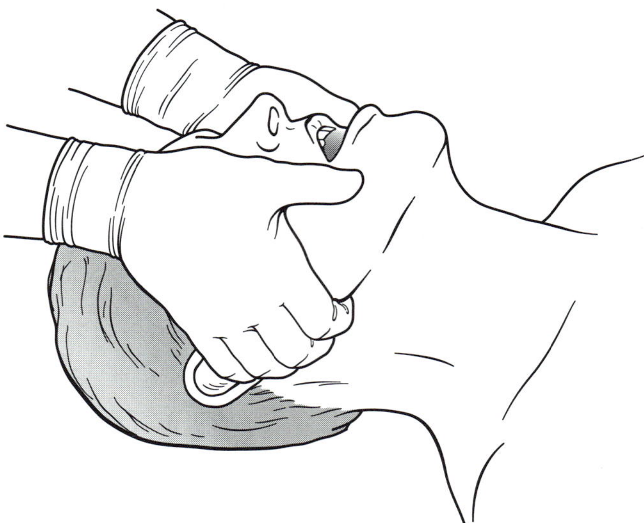

FIGURE 6.1. To maintain airflow, place the patient's head in a neutral position with the mouth open. If the mouth cannot be maintained open, dislocate the jaw anteroinferiorly at the temporomandibular joint (the "jaw thrust").

tic[3] or nasotracheal[4] intubation can be safely performed if needed. In the field, a cricothyroidotomy might be the safest alternative for difficult airway control in a patient with a potentially unstable spine.[4]

Helmets, as used for sports or motorcycling, are often in place at the time of initial evaluation. They should be kept in place during in-field evaluation and medical stabilization.[5] Optimally, a helmet should be maintained until radiographic evaluation of the cervical spine has been performed.[5] Safe removal of a helmet in a patient with a potential cervical spine injury requires a team of coordinated individuals. Of importance, the face mask or visor can and should be removed. This enables access to the eyes, nose, and mouth for inspection and airway management.

HEMODYNAMIC RESUSCITATION

Hemodynamic assessment and resuscitation should begin in the field. Maintaining hemodynamic stability is crucial to patient survival. In addition, it may also be important in minimizing further ischemia to a compromised spinal cord.[6] Vale et al.[7] prospectively examined a cohort of 64 patients with acute spinal cord injury in whom the mean arterial blood pressure was maintained above 85 mm Hg. At 1-year follow-up, 60% of patients with a complete spinal cord injury improved at least one Frankel (American Spinal Injury Association) grade, 30% regained the ability to walk, and 20% had some bladder function. Notwithstanding the multitude of other covariables, the authors concluded that acute and emergent maintenance of blood pressure is a critical component to optimizing neurologic recovery. Based on less objective data, others have recommended maintaining an arterial oxygen partial pressure of at least 100 mm Hg (torr).[6]

Although pressure is best monitored by an intra-arterial manometer, this is not feasible in the prehospital scenario, leaving the examiner to rely on cuff measurements alone. In-field cuff pressure measurements combined with pulse assessment is critical to initial resuscitation of spine-injured victims. Patients with spinal cord injury often present with neurogenic shock. In distinction from hemorrhagic shock, in which compensatory tachycardia is usually present, neurogenic shock results in hypotension accompanied by bradycardia. This results from loss of the normal sympathetic response to low blood pressure. Pressure should be restored by a combination of postural maneuvers (Trendelenburg position), judicious fluid infusion, and vasopressor administration. If neurogenic shock is treated as purely hypovolemic shock, fluid overload can quickly ensue, leading to pulmonary edema or other systemic medical complications.

Large-bore intravenous access should be obtained in a patient requiring fluid resuscitation. In most patients, a peripheral intravenous catheter can be easily placed. A 14- or 16-gauge catheter is preferred for rapid infusion of fluid. Patients who have lost a large portion of their blood volume (either from hemorrhage or pooling) can present a challenge. Collapse of the peripheral venous complex may make it nearly impossible to locate an adequate vein for access. In these cases, the on-scene practitioner can place a femoral (groin) line. The location of the vein is distal to the inguinal ligament and just medial to the femoral artery, which is usually palpable even in severely hypovolemic patients.

Central line placement is usually not performed in the field. In the rare circumstance that a femoral line cannot be placed, the next best option may be a subclavian line. This is more risky than a femoral line because misplacement of the needle can lead to a pneumothorax, with potentially devastating consequences in a compromised patient. An internal jugular line should not be attempted in the field. It requires removal of the cervical collar, as well as some rotation of the head or neck to the contralateral side. This can potentially lead to displacement of an unrecognized cervical fracture.

The goal of venous access is to replace fluids in a volume-depleted patient. In spine-injury patients, hypotension can be related to bleeding (volume loss) or peripheral vasodilation from loss of sympathetic tone (neurogenic shock). Thus, pressure resuscitation and maintenance should be achieved with a combination of fluid replacement and administration of vasopressors (vasoconstrictors). Care must be taken to recognize the coexistence of both of these entities. Overly aggressive fluid replacement in a patient with neurogenic shock can lead to pulmonary edema; vasopressors without fluid replacement in a patient with hypovolemic shock can lead to organ ischemia.

IN-FIELD IMMOBILIZATION

Manual immobilization of the head and neck should be maintained until a hard cervical collar can be applied. A hard collar should be applied as soon as possible after initial inspection of the patient. The patient should not be moved before placement of a collar. Various types of cervical orthoses are available, all of which contain an anterior window to accommodate a tracheostomy tube or facilitate an emergency cricothyrotomy. Less motion is allowed by the NecLoc (Ossur Americas Trauma and Spine, Paulsboro, NJ) collar compared to the Miami J (Jeroma Medical, Moorestown, NJ), Philadelphia (Ossur Americas Trauma and Spine, Paulsboro, NJ), Aspen (Aspen Medical Productions, Irvine, CA), and Stifneck (Laerdal Inc., Wappingers Falls, New York, NY) devices[8]; however, a clinical difference has yet to be demonstrated. In-field application of Gardner-Wells tongs and traction appears to be the most effective means of immobilizing the cervical spine.[9] However, this can potentially distract an underlying and unrecognized occipitocervical dissociation. In addition, it is not routinely available to most emergency medical technicians.

The neck should be immobilized by supplemental manual in-line stabilization during transfers even with the collar in place. Likewise, in-line stabilization should be used whenever the cervical collar has been temporarily removed. The patient should be moved from the field to the stretcher with the use of a rigid backboard to minimize displacement of thoracic or lumbar injuries. A slider board can facilitate these transfers. Log-roll technique and spinal precautions should be observed at all times. Alternatively, a lift-and-slide maneuver can be used with equivalent motion prevention of a potentially unstable spine injury.[10]

IMMOBILIZATION AFTER GUNSHOT WOUNDS TO THE HEAD AND NECK

Gunshot wounds to the head and neck frequently involve the cervical spine.[11–13] Despite their relative frequency, there remains a paucity of evidence-based data concerning management of these serious injuries. Particularly, the role of routine cervical immobilization after gunshot wounds to the head and neck remains unclear. Most agree that low-velocity gunshot wounds to the spine are usually inherently mechanically stable.[14–17] Despite this, routine cervical immobilization after neck and head gunshot wounds in the form of a hard cervical collar is usually recommended until radiographic evaluation of the spine can be performed. In cases in which airway and respiration are not compromised and the patients are easily hemodynamically resuscitated, it seems prudent to postpone removal of the collar until spinal imaging has been performed. However, in cases with concomitant injuries such as hemorrhage or laryngeal edema, a cervical collar can impede life-saving procedures, such as cricothyrotomy or neck exploration.

To better understand this issue, one must first examine the likelihood of cervical fracture after a gunshot wound. Previous authors have stratified the risk for fracture after gunshot wounds to the head.[14–16] Studies have demonstrated a 0% incidence of cervical fractures after isolated gunshot wounds to the calvaria.[16,18] With wounds extending outside the calvaria, a 10% incidence of cervical spine fracture has been found.[16] With gunshot wounds involving the maxillary and orbital regions, a 10% and 20% rate of cervical fracture, respectively, has been reported.[14] The rate of cervical fracture after gunshot wounds to the neck has varied from 22% to 25%.[19,20] Glaringly absent from these studies, however, is distinction between stable and unstable fractures.

In a recent analysis of the stability of fractures after gunshot wounds, Medzon et al.[21] found that the overall rate of cervical spine fracture was 23% after gunshot wounds to the head or neck. Of these fractures, 16% were unstable, making the overall incidence of unstable spine fractures only 3.7% of cases. None occurred in patients who were examinable and neurologically intact. Although these data suggest that the cervical collar can be removed and spinal precautions discontinued in alert and awake patients without spinal cord injury, it must be acknowledged that the numbers were too low to actually consider whether the risk for unstable fracture truly approaches zero. To further limit such conclusions, one must consider that an unstable spine fracture is possible in a neurologically intact patient after a gunshot wound.[22]

REFERENCES

1. Smith CE, Fallon WF. Sevoflurane mask anesthesia for urgent tracheostomy in an uncooperative trauma patient with a difficult airway. *Can J Anaesth* 2000;47:242–245.
2. ILCOR. Adult basic life support. *Circulation* 2000;102:22–59.
3. Mulder DS, Wallace DH, Woolhouse FM. The use of fiberoptic bronchoscope to facilitate endotracheal intubation following head and neck trauma. *J Trauma* 1975;15:638–640.
4. Bivins HG, Ford S, Bezmalinovic Z, et al. The effect of axial traction during orotracheal intubation of the trauma victim with an unstable cervical spine. *Ann Emerg Med* 1989;17:25–29.
5. Swenson TM, Lauerman WC, Blanc RO, et al. Cervical alignment in the immobilized football player: radiographic analysis before and after helmet removal. *Am J Sports Med* 1997;25:226–230.
6. Vaccaro AR, An HS, Betz RR, et al. The management of acute spinal trauma: prehospital and in-hospital emergency care. *Instr Course Lect* 1997;46:113–125.
7. Vale FL, Burns J, Jackson AB, et al. Combined medical and surgical treatment after acute spinal cord injury: results of a prospective pilot study to assess the merits of aggressive medical resuscitation and blood pressure management. *J Neurosurg* 1997;87:239–246.
8. Askins V, Eismont FJ. Efficacy of five cervical orthoses in restricting cervical motion: a comparison study. *Spine* 1997;22:1193–1198.
9. Neville S, Watts C, Loos L, et al. Use of traction in cervical spine fractures during interhospital tranfer by aircraft. *J Spinal Disord* 1990;3:67–76.
10. DelRossi G, Horodyski M, Heffernan TP, et al. Spine-board transfer techniques and the unstable cervical spine. *Spine* 2004;29:E134–E44.
11. Farmer J, Vaccaro A, Balderston R, et al. The changing nature of admission to a spinal cord injury center: violence on the rise. *J Spinal Disord* 1998;11:400–403.
12. Roye W, Dunn E, Moody J. Cervical spinal cord injury: a public catastrophe. *J Trauma* 1988;28:1260–1264.
13. Lin S, Vaccaro A, Reich S, et al. Low-velocity gunshot wounds to the spine with an associated transperitoneal injury. *J Spinal Disord* 1995;8:136–144.
14. Kihtir T, Ivatury R, Simon R, et al. Early management of civilian gunshot wounds to the face. *J Trauma* 1993;35:569–575.

15. Kupcha P, An H, Cotler J. Gunshot wounds to the cervical spine. *Spine* 1990;15:1058–1063.
16. Kennedy F, Gonzalez P, Beitler A, et al. Incidence of cervical spine injury in patients with gunshot wounds to the head. *South Med J* 1994;87:621–623.
17. Cornwall EE, Chang DC, Bonar JP, et al. Thoracolumbar immobilization for trauma patients with torso gunshot wounds: is it necessary? *Arch Surg* 2001;136:324–327.
18. Chong C, Ware D, Harris J. Is cervical spine imaging indicated in gunshot wounds to the cranium? *J Trauma* 1998;44:501–502.
19. Ordog GJ, Albin D, Wasserberger J, et al. 110 bullet wounds to the neck. *J Trauma* 1985;25:238–246.
20. Isiklar Z, Lindsey R. Low-velocity civilian gunshot wounds of the spine. *Orthopedics* 1997;20:967–972.
21. Medzon R, Rothenhaus T, Bono CM, et al. Stability of cervical spine fractures after gunshot wounds to the head and neck. *Spine* 2005;30:2274–2279.
22. Apfelbaum JD, Cantrill SV, Waldman N. Unstable cervical spine without spinal cord injury in penetrating neck trauma. *Am J Emerg Med* 2000;18:55–57.

CHAPTER 7A

Physical Evaluation: American Spinal Injury Association Classification

Bizhan N.M.N. Aarabi

INTRODUCTION

Over the past three decades, there has been significant progress in the management of spinal cord injury.[1–7] The arrival time for an injured patient to a trauma center today in many instances remains under 60 minutes. Trauma centers equipped with spiral computed tomography (CT) and 24-hour magnetic resonance imaging (MRI) have been able to define injury profile within a few hours, and intensive care units have been able to prevent secondary systemic insults more efficiently.[8–14] Animal experimentation has clearly shown that injury-induced secondary insult to the spinal cord parenchyma starts within minutes and continues for hours to weeks.[15–28] Stem-cell technology, novel pharmaceutical agents, and earlier decompression may offer new hope for better functional recovery.[29–40] Standardizing neurologic and functional classification of spinal cord injury and increasing interrater reliability of assessment tools may help tailor future interventions that may be predictive in improving long-term outcomes.[41–48]

ASSESSMENT TOOLS

In his 1992 Heiner Sell lecture of the American Spinal Injury Association (ASIA), Dr. Ditunno[49] finished his sentence with the phrase "we have began." His statement referred to our chronic difficulties with introduction of an assessment tool capable of measuring severity of spinal cord injury, being predictive of outcome and prognosis while possessing a high degree of interrater reliability. Historically, this work began in 1912 when Lovett[50] attempted grading muscle strength in patients with poliomyelitis descriptively into normal, good, fair, poor, and zero. It took 30 years before the British Medical Research Council, in 1943, replaced these descriptors with numerical values from 0 to 5. From 1969 to 1979, Frankel et al.,[51] Bracken et al.,[52] and Lucas and Ducker[53] introduced their versions of descriptive and numerical classifications of spinal cord injury, which were influential in methylprednisolone trial outcome studies. Others have introduced complementary classifications, each adding a small step in describing indices of change, being recovery or neurologic worsening.[54–56] Over the years, we have learned better predictors of outcome, such as superficial nociception, and less benefit from splitting dorsal column function into position, vibration, and light and crude touch sensations as reliable instruments of change.[57,58]

S.L. Stover, during his presidency of ASIA from 1980 to 1982, suggested the need for a work group introducing a system of neurologic classification following spinal cord injury.[49] In 1982,

ASIA described severity of injury as categories of paraplegia, complete injury, incomplete injury, and neurologic levels. It provided key sensory dermatomes and key muscles for sensory and motor classification and defined zone of injury and Frankel classification.[59] The 1982, 1988, and 1990 modifications of ASIA Standards for Neurological and Functional Classification of Spinal Cord Injury were followed by a major step in an attempt to develop the International Standards for Neurological and Functional Classification of Spinal Cord Injury. ASIA brought together a multidisciplinary group of investigators from different specialties and continents to put together the International Standards for Neurological and Functional Classification of Spinal Cord Injury (ISCSCI).[59–61] This classification introduced a universally accepted numerical scale of measurement of the severity of spinal cord injury, to make possible communication across a variety of independent variables such as outcome, intervention, endpoints, prognosis, and rehabilitation.[62–76] The validity of the 1992 version of ISCSCI and its interrater reliability are still being intensely evaluated until we see a universally accepted tool with high degree of predictability of injury, prognosis, outcome, and efficacy of intervention.[49,62,64–66,73,77–81]

MODIFIED STANDARD NEUROLOGIC CLASSIFICATION OF SPINAL CORD INJURY/AMERICAN SPINAL INJURY ASSOCIATION IMPAIRMENT SCALE

The following items are checked in Modified Standard ASIA classification:

Motor Scale

The Motor Scale is divided into six grades:

0 Total paralysis
1 Palpable or visible contractions
2 Active movement, gravity eliminated
3 Active movement, against gravity
4 Active movement, against some resistance
5 Active movement, against full resistance
NT Not able to test

Motor and sensory scales for each segment is determined according to the following charts (Tables 7A.1 and 7A.2).

TABLE 7A.1 ASIA Motor Strength Examination of 10 Muscles in the Upper and Lower Extremities

Cord Segment	Tested Muscle	Left							Right						
		0	1	2	3	4	5	NT	0	1	2	3	4	5	NT
C5	Elbow flexors														
C6	Wrist extensors														
C7	Elbow extensors														
C8	Finger flexors														
T1	Finger abductors														
L2	Hip flexors														
L3	Knee extensors														
L4	Ankle dorsiflexors														
L5	Long toe extensors														
S1	Ankle plantar flexors														

TABLE 7A.2 Light Touch and Pin Prick Sensory Examination Considering 28 Dermatomes

	Light Touch								Pin Prick							
	Left				Right				Left				Right			
Dermatome	0	1	2	NT	0	1	2	NT	0	1	2	NT	0	1	2	NT
C2																
C3																
C4																
C5																
C6																
C7																
C8																
T1																
T2																
T3																
T4																
T5																
T6																
T7																
T8																
T9																
T10																
T11																
T12																
L1																
L2																
L3																
L4																
L5																
S1																
S2																
S3																
S4-5																

The sum total of each side is determined and recorded.

Light touch and pin-prick sensation are graded according to the key points on sensory dermatomes, as shown in Figure 7A.1.

Numerical values of sum total of pin-prick and light touch sensation are recorded separately.

The following items are also checked in Modified Standard Neurological Classification of Spinal Cord Injury/ASIA Impairment Scale:

1 Voluntary anal contraction at S4-S5.
2 Voluntary anal sensation at S4-S5.

3 Complete and incomplete status of spinal cord injury.
4 Neurologic level.
5 Motor and sensory levels of spinal cord injury.
6 Zones of partial preservation: motor and sensory.
7 ASIA Impairment Scale: Frankel A, B, C, D, E.
8 Status of bulbocavernosus reflex.

Definitions

Neurologic level: The most caudal segment of spinal cord with normal sensory and motor function on both sides

Sensory level: The most caudal injury segment with intact sensation bilaterally

Motor level: The most caudal injury segment with at least a strength equal to 3 out of 5 bilaterally

Sensory score: Sum total of pin-prick and light touch scores reflecting the degree of spinal cord injury

Motor score: Sum total of motor score (0–5) of the 10 myotomes reflecting the degree of segmental injury of the spinal cord

Zone of partial preservation: Sensory and motor function reflecting segments with partial preservation of function caudal to the neurologic level of injury; term used in patients with complete spinal cord

Tetraplegia: Functional loss resulting from complete spinal cord injury at the level of cervical spine

Paraplegia: Functional loss resulting from complete spinal cord or cauda equina injury caudal to cervical segments

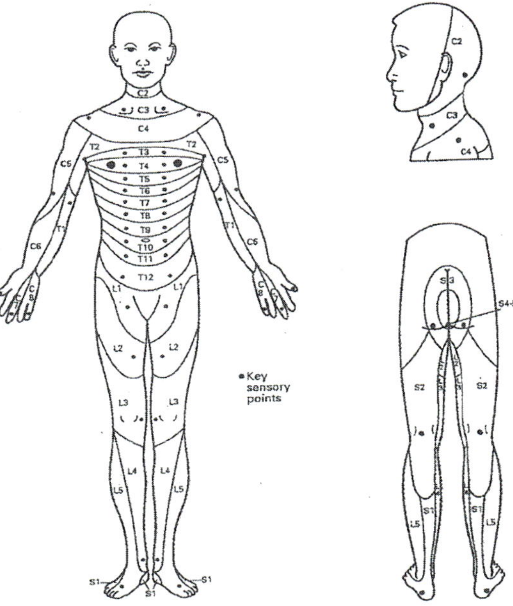

0-Absent Sensation
1-Impaired Sensation
2-Normal Sensation
NT-Not able to test

FIGURE 7A.1. Light touch and pin-prick sensation is evaluated in each dermatome demonstrated. (Adapted from American Spinal Injury Association. *International Standards for Neurological Classification of Spinal Cord Injury.* Chicago: American Spine Injury Association, reprint 2008.)

Quadriparesis: Incomplete loss of function (sensory, motor, autonomic) as a consequence of cervical spinal cord injury
Paraparesis: Incomplete loss of function (sensory, motor, autonomic) caudal to cervical spinal cord segments
Dermatome: Sensory supply of skin confined to a single sensory nerve root
Myotome: Specified number of muscle fibers supplied by a single motor segment
Skeletal level: Spinal level with the most severe bony structural damage after trauma
Incomplete: Partially preserved function caudal to the neurologic level of spinal cord injury
Complete: Total loss of function below a spinal injury segment

CLINICAL RECORD FOR A PATIENT WITH SPINAL CORD INJURY

A 51-year-old man fell and was transferred to a level I trauma center with an incomplete spinal cord injury (Frankel C). His examination was recorded using the following Modified Standard ASIA Classification of Neurological Injury (Tables 7A.3, 7A.4, and 7A.5). CT and MRI of the cervical spine revealed a flexion-compression teardrop fracture of C3 with a herniated disc at C3-C4 and evidence of spinal cord injury (MR type 3).[13] The patient underwent an urgent C3-C4 discectomy with partial corpectomy followed by an arthrodesis and internal fixation of the vertebral bodies of C3 and C4. Preoperative and postoperative studies are shown in Figures 7A.2 and 7A.3. At 18 days after admission, the patient's ASIA motor score was 72, ASIA impairment D, with intact light touch. Pin-prick sensation was present throughout, with half in the right L4, L5, and S1 dermatomes. There was voluntary anal sensation and contraction. There was slight hyperreflexia in all reflex groups but continued absence of the bulbocavernosus reflex.

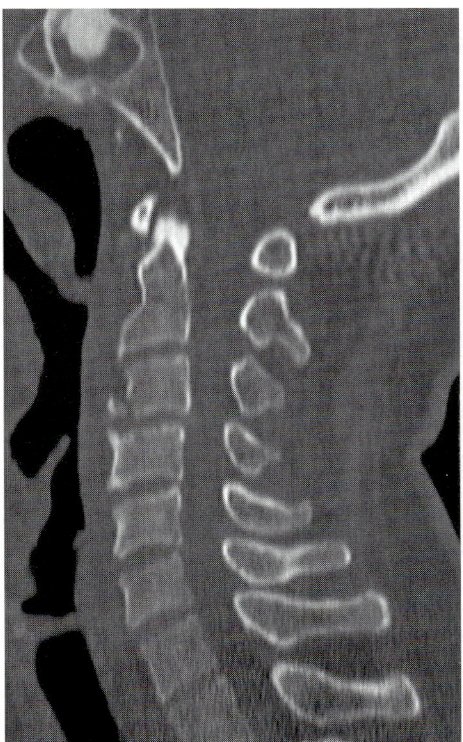
A

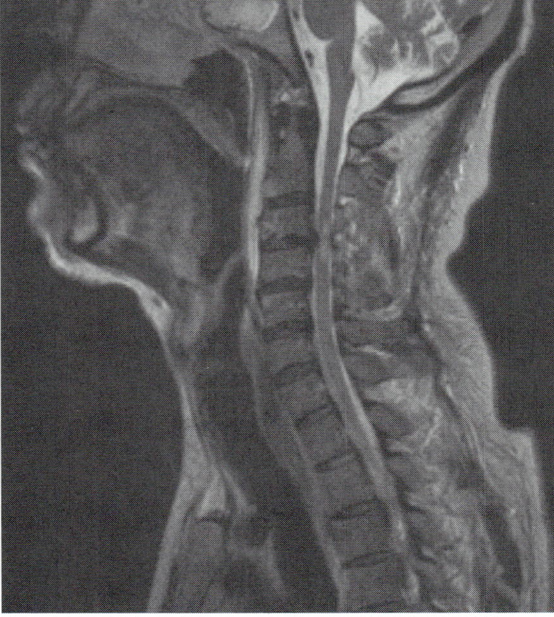
B

FIGURE 7A.2. Computed tomography and magnetic resonance imaging of the cervical spine revealed a flexion compression teardrop fracture of C3 with a herniated disc at C3-C4 and evidence of spinal cord injury.

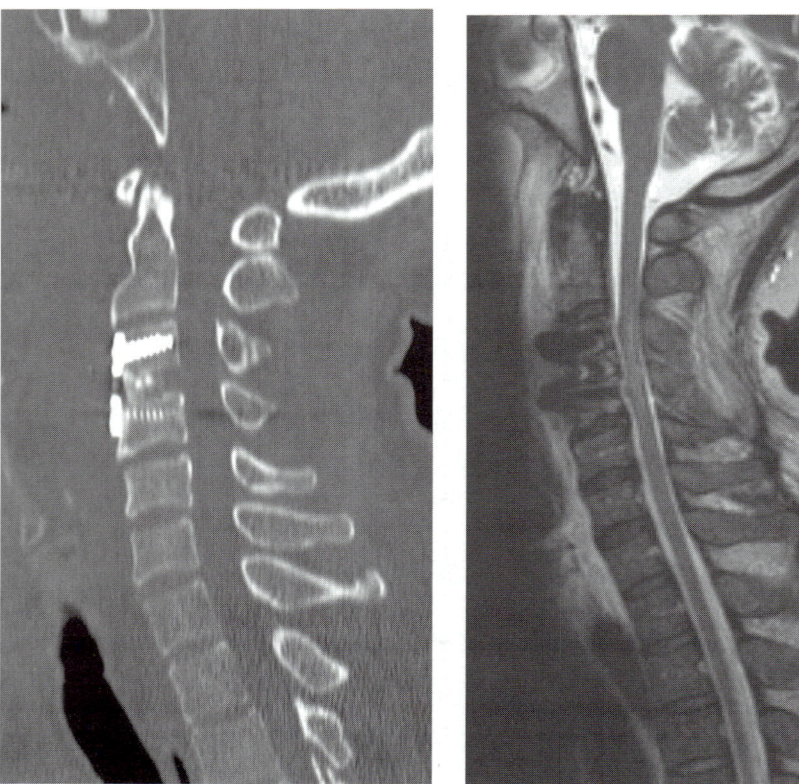

FIGURES 7A.3. The patient underwent a C3-C4 discectomy with partial corpectomy and internal fixation of C3 and C4.

NEUROLOGIC EXAMINATION

TABLE 7A.3 Motor Examination at Admission

Myotomal Muscle Group	Right Muscle Strength						Left Muscle Strength					
	0	1	2	3	4	5	0	1	2	3	4	5
Elbow flexors					✓						✓	
Wrist extensors	✓						✓					
Elbow extensors		✓						✓				
Finger flexors	✓						✓					
Finger abductors	✓						✓					
Hip flexors	✓						✓					
Knee extensors	✓						✓					
Ankle dorsiflexors			✓						✓			
Long toe extensors			✓						✓			
Ankle plantar flexors			✓						✓			

0 = Total paralysis; 1 = palpable or visible contraction; 2 = active movement, gravity eliminated; 3 = active movement, against gravity; 4 = active movement, against some resistance; 5 = active movement, against fall resistance; NT = not able to test.

TABLE 7A.4 Sensory Examination at Admission

	Pin-prick									Light touch							
	Right				Left					Right				Left			
	0	1	2	NT	0	1	2	NT		0	1	2	NT	0	1	2	NT
C2			✓				✓		C2			✓				✓	
C3			✓				✓		C3			✓				✓	
C4			✓				✓		C4			✓				✓	
C5			✓				✓		C5			✓				✓	
C6		✓					✓		C6			✓				✓	
C7		✓					✓		C7			✓				✓	
C8		✓					✓		C8			✓				✓	
T1		✓					✓		T1			✓				✓	
T2		✓					✓		T2			✓				✓	
T3		✓					✓		T3			✓				✓	
T4		✓					✓		T4			✓				✓	
T5		✓					✓		T5			✓				✓	
T6		✓					✓		T6			✓				✓	
T7		✓					✓		T7			✓				✓	
T8		✓					✓		T8			✓				✓	
T9		✓					✓		T9			✓				✓	
T10		✓					✓		T10			✓				✓	
T11		✓					✓		T11			✓				✓	
T12		✓					✓		T12			✓				✓	
L1		✓					✓		L1			✓				✓	
L2		✓					✓		L2			✓				✓	
L3		✓					✓		L3			✓				✓	
L4		✓					✓		L4			✓				✓	
L5		✓					✓		L5			✓				✓	
S1		✓					✓		S1			✓				✓	
S2			✓				✓		S2			✓				✓	
S3			✓				✓		S3			✓				✓	
S4/S5			✓				✓		S4/S5			✓				✓	

Sensory scale: 0 = absent, 1 = impaired, 2 = normal, NT = not able to test.

TABLE 7A.5 Functional Impairment Scale

			1/30/06	Total	2/16/06	Total
Sensory score	Pin-prick	Right	36	92	53	109
		Left	56		56	
	Light touch	Right	56	112	56	112
		Left	56		56	
Motor score	Right	11	22	36	72	
	Left	11		36		
Voluntary anal sensation		Present		Present		
Voluntary anal contraction		Present		Present		
Bulbocavernosus reflex		Present		Absent		
Abnormal reflexes		Absent		Absent		
ASIA impairment scale					C	
Spinal cord injury					Incomplete	
Zones of partial preservation					Not applicable	
Neurologic level					C4	
Motor level					C5	
Sensory level					C5	
Skeletal level					C3/C4	

REFERENCES

1. Ball PA. Critical care of spinal cord injury. *Spine* 2001;26:S27–S30.
2. Benzel EC, Doezema D. Prehospital management of the spinally injured patient. In: Narayan RK, Wilberger JE Jr, Povlishock JT, eds. *Neurotrauma*. New York: McGraw-Hill Health Professions Division, 1996:1113–11120.
3. Hadley MN, Walters BC, Grabb PA, et al. Clinical assessment after acute cervical spinal cord injury: guidelines for the management of acute cervical spine and spinal cord injuries. *Neurosurgery* 2002;50:S21–S29.
4. Tator CH, Benzel EC, eds. *Contemporary Management of Spinal Cord Injury: From Impact to Rehabilitation*. Park Ridge, IL: American Association of Neurological Surgeons, 2000:91–98.
5. McAfee PC. Cervical spine trauma. In: Frymoyer JW, ed. *The Adult Spine: Principles and Practice*. New York: Raven Press, 1991:1063–1106.
6. Pasquale M, Fabian TC. Practice management guidelines for trauma from the Eastern Association for the Surgery of Trauma. *J Trauma* 1998;44:941–956.
7. Tator CH, Rowed DW, Schwartz ML, et al. Management of acute spinal cord injuries. *Can J Surg* 1984;27:289–293.
8. Banit DM, Grau G, Fisher JR. Evaluation of the acute cervical spine: a management algorithm. *J Trauma* 2000;49:450–456.
9. Benzel EC, Hart BL, Ball PA, et al. Magnetic resonance imaging for the evaluation of patients with occult cervical spine injury. *J Neurosurg* 1996;85:824–829.
10. Chee SG. Review of the role of magnetic resonance imaging in acute cervical spine injuries. *Ann Acad Med Singapore* 1993;22:757–761.
11. Chiu WC, Haan JM, Cushing BM, et al. Ligamentous injuries of the cervical spine in unreliable blunt trauma patients: incidence, evaluation, and outcome. *J Trauma* 2001;50:457–463.
12. Schaefer DM, Flanders A, Northrup BE, et al. Magnetic resonance imaging of acute cervical spine trauma. *Spine* 1989;14:1090–1095.
13. Schaefer DM, Flanders AE, Osterholm JL, et al. Prognostic significance of magnetic resonance imaging in the acute phase of cervical spine injury. *J Neurosurg* 1992;76:218–223.
14. Sees DW, Rodriguez Cruz LR, Flaherty SF, et al. The use of bedside fluoroscopy to evaluate the cervical spine in obtunded trauma patients. *J Trauma* 1998;45:768–771.

15. Anderson DK. Chemical and cellular mediators in spinal cord injury. *J Neurotrauma* 1991;9:143–145.
16. Anderson DK, Means ED, Waters TR, et al. Spinal cord energy metabolism following compression trauma to the feline spinal cord. *J Neurosurg* 1980;53:375–380.
17. Anderson TE, Stokes BT. Experimental models for spinal cord injury research: physical and physiological considerations. *J Neurotrauma* 1992;9(suppl 1):S135–S142.
18. Balentine JD, Greene WB. Ultrastructural pathology of nerve fibers in calcium-induced myelopathy. *J Neuropathol Exp Neurol* 1984;43:500–510.
19. Banik NL, Shields DC, Ray S, et al. Role of calpain in spinal cord injury: effects of calpain and free radical inhibitors. *Ann New York Acad Sci* 1998;844:131–137.
20. Blight AR. Delayed demyelination and macrophage invasion: a candidate for secondary cell damage in spinal cord injury. *CNS Trauma* 1985:2:299–315.
21. Carlson G, Gordon C, Wada E, et al. Vascular re-perfusion and neural preservation after spinal cord injury. *J Neurotrauma* 1998;15:860.
22. Carlson GD, Gorden CD, Nakazowa S, et al. Perfusion-limited recovery of evoked potential function after spinal cord injury. *Spine* 2000;25:1218–1226.
23. Carlson SL, Parrish ME, Springer JE, et al. Acute inflammatory response in spinal cord following impact injury. *Exp Neurol* 1998;151:77–88.
24. de la Torre JC. Spinal cord injury: review of basic and applied research. *Spine* 1981;6:315–335.
25. Edwards L, Nashmi R, Jones O, et al. Upregulation of Kv 1.4 protein and gene expression after chronic spinal cord injury. *J Comp Neurol* 2002;443:154–167.
26. Stokes BT. Experimental spinal cord injury: a dynamic and verifiable injury device. *J Neurotrauma* 1992;9:129–131.
27. Tarlov IM. Spinal cord compression studies. III: Time limits for recovery after gradual compression in dogs. *Arch Neurol Psychiatry* 1954;71:588–597.
28. Yanase M, Sakou T, Fukuda T. Role of N-methyl-D-aspartate receptor in acute spinal cord injury. *J Neurosurg* 1995;83:884–888.
29. Albert TJ, Kim DH. Timing of surgical stabilization after cervical and thoracic trauma. Invited submission from the Joint Section Meeting on Disorders of the Spine and Peripheral Nerves, March 2004. *J Neurosurg Spine* 2005;3:182–190.
30. Bakshi A, Barshinger AL, Swanger SA, et al. Lumbar puncture delivery of bone marrow stromal cells in spinal cord contusion: a novel method for minimally invasive cell transplantation. *J Neurotrauma* 2006;23:55–65.
31. Brustle O, Jones KN, Learish RD, et al. Embryonic stem cell-derived glial precursors: a source of myelinating transplants. *Science* 1999;285:754–756.
32. Duh MS, Shepard MJ, Wilberger JE, et al. The effectiveness of surgery on the treatment of acute spinal cord injury and its relation to pharmacological treatment. *Neurosurgery* 1994;35:240–248.
33. Fehlings MG, Perrin RG. The role and timing of early decompression for cervical spinal cord injury: update with a review of recent clinical evidence. *Injury* 2005;36:B13–B26.
34. Fehlings MG, Sekhon LH, Tator C. The role and timing of decompression in acute spinal cord injury: what do we know? What should we do? *Spine* 26(suppl 24):S101–S110.
35. Hakalo J, Wronski J. Importance of early operative decompression of spinal cord after cervical spine injuries. *Neurol Neurochir Pol* 2004;38:183–188.
36. Kishan S, Vives MJ, Reiter MF. Timing of surgery following spinal cord injury. *J Spinal Cord Med* 2005;28:11–19.
37. La Rosa G, Conti A, Cardali S, et al. Does early decompression improve neurological outcome of spinal cord injured patients? Appraisal of the literature using a meta-analytical approach. *Spinal Cord* 2004;42:503–512.
38. Nakamura M, Toyama Y, Okano H. [Transplantation of neural stem cells for spinal cord injury]. *Rinsho Shinkeigaku* 2005;45:874–876.
39. Tator CH, Fehlings MG, Thorpe K, et al. Current use and timing of spinal surgery for management of acute spinal surgery for management of acute spinal cord injury in North America: results of a retrospective multicenter study. *J Neurosurg* 1999;91(suppl 1):12–18.
40. Yamazaki T, Yanaka K, Fujita K, et al. Traumatic central cord syndrome: analysis of factors affecting the outcome. *Surg Neurol* 2005;63:95–99.
41. Bracken MB, Collins WF, Freeman DF, et al. Efficacy of methylprednisolone in acute spinal cord injury. *JAMA* 1984;251:45–52.
42. Fehlings MG, Baptiste DC. Current status of clinical trials for acute spinal cord injury. *Injury* 2005;36(suppl 2): B113–B122.
43. Hadley MN, Walters BC, Grabb PA, et al. Guidelines for the management of acute cervical spine and spinal cord injuries. *Neurosurgery* 2002;50:S1–S199.
44. Hall ED, Springer JE. Neuroprotection and acute spinal cord injury: a reappraisal. *NeuroRx* 2004;1:80–100.
45. Hurlbert RJ, Moulton R. Why do you prescribe methylprednisolone for acute spinal cord injury? A Canadian perspective and a position statement. *Can J Neurol Sci* 2002;29:236–239.

46. Hurlbert RJ. The role of steroids in acute spinal cord injury: an evidence-based analysis. *Spine* 2001;26(suppl 24):S39–S46.
47. O'Connor PA, McCormack O, Gavin C, et al. Methylprednisolone in acute spinal cord injuries. *Ir J Med Sci* 2003;172:24–26.
48. Short D. Is the role of steroids in acute spinal cord injury now resolved? *Curr Opin Neurol* 2001;14:759–763.
49. Ditunno JF Jr. American spinal injury standards for neurological and functional classification of spinal cord injury: past, present and future. 1992 Heiner Sell Lecture of the American Spinal Injury Association. *J Am Paraplegia Soc* 1994;17:7–11.
50. Lovett RW. *Treatments of Infantile Paralysis.* Philadelphia: P. Blakiston's Son & Company, 1917.
51. Frankel HL, Hancock DO, Hyslop G, et al. The value of postural reduction in the initial management of closed injuries of the spine with paraplegia and tetraplegia. I. *Paraplegia* 1969;7:179–192.
52. Bracken MB, Webb SB Jr, Wagner FC. Classification of the severity of acute spinal cord injury: implications for management. *Paraplegia* 1978;15:319–326.
53. Lucas JT, Ducker TB. Motor classification of spinal cord injuries with mobility, morbidity and recovery indices. *Am Surg* 1979;45:151–158.
54. Botsford DJ, Esses SI. A new scale for the clinical assessment of spinal cord function. *Orthopedics* 1996; 15:1309–1313.
55. Chehrazi B, Wagner FC Jr, Collins WF Jr, et al. A scale for evaluation of spinal cord injury. *J Neurosurg* 1981; 54:310–315.
56. Tator CH, Rowed DW, Schwartz ML. Sunnybrook Cord Injury Scales for Assessing Neurological Injury and Neurological Recovery. In: Tator CH, ed. *Early Management of Acute Spinal Cord Injury.* New York: Raven Press, 1982:7–24.
57. Bedbrook GM, Prince HG. A study of the influence of posterior column sensory sparing on initial presentation of cervical injuries on the ultimate prognosis. *Paraplegia* 1987;25:441–445.
58. Crozier KS, Graziani V, Ditunno JF Jr, et al. Spinal cord injury: prognosis for ambulation based on sensory examination in patients who are initially motor complete. *Arch Phys Med Rehab* 1991;72:119–121.
59. American Spinal Injury Association. *Standards for Neurological Classification of Spinal Injury Patients.* Chicago: ASIA, 1982.
60. American Spinal Injury Association. *Standards for Neurological Classification of Spinal Injury Patients.* Chicago: ASIA, 1989.
61. American Spinal Injury Association. *International Standards for Neurological and Functional Classification of Spinal Cord Injury.* Chicago: ASIA/IMSOP, 1992.
62. Bednarczyk JH, Sanderson DJ. Comparison of functional and medical assessment in the classification of persons with spinal cord injury. *J Rehabil Res Dev* 1993;30:405–411.
63. Cohen ME, Ditunno JF Jr, Donovan WH, et al. A test of the 1992 International Standards for Neurological and Functional Classification of Spinal Cord Injury. *Spinal Cord* 1998;36:554–560.
64. Coleman WP, Geisler FH. Injury severity as primary predictor of outcome in acute spinal cord injury: retrospective results from a large multicenter clinical trial. *Spine J* 2004;4:373–378.
65. Ditunno JF Jr, Young W, Donovan WH, et al. The international standards booklet for neurological and functional classification of spinal cord injury. American Spinal Injury Association. *Paraplegia* 1994;32:70–80.
66. El Masry WS, Tsubo M, Katoh S, et al. Validation of the American Spinal Injury Association (ASIA) motor score and the National Acute Spinal Cord Injury Study (NASCIS) motor score. *Spine* 1996;21:614–619.
67. Geisler FH, Coleman WP, Grieco G, et al. Measurements and recovery patterns in a multicenter study of acute spinal cord injury. *Spine* 2001;26:S68–S86.
68. Ishida Y, Tominaga T. Predictors of neurologic recovery in acute central cervical cord injury with only upper extremity impairment. *Spine* 2006;27:1652–1658.
69. Marino RJ, Ditunno JF Jr, Donovan WH, et al. Neurologic recovery after traumatic spinal cord injury: data from the Model Spinal Cord Injury Systems. *Arch Phys Med Rehab* 1999;80:1391–1396.
70. Middleton JW, Truman G, Geraghty TJ. Neurological level effect on the discharge functional status of spinal cord injured persons after rehabilitation. *Arch Phys Med Rehab* 1998;79:1428–1432.
71. Oleson CV, Burns AS, Ditunno JF, et al. Prognostic value of pinprick preservation in motor complete, sensory incomplete spinal cord injury. *Arch Phys Med Rehab* 2005;86:988–992.
72. Ota T, Akaboshi K, Nagata M, et al. Functional assessment of patients with spinal cord injury: measured by the motor score and the Functional Independence Measure. *Spinal Cord* 1996;34:531–535.
73. Priebe MM, Waring WP. The interobserver reliability of the revised American Spinal Injury Association standards for neurological classification of spinal injury patients. *Am J Phys Med Rehabil* 1991;70:268–270.
74. Schurch B, Schmid DM, Kaegi K. Value of sensory examination in predicting bladder function in patients with T12-L1 fractures and spinal cord injury. *Arch Phys Med Rehab* 2003;84:83–89.
75. Toh E, Arima T, Mochida J, et al. Functional evaluation using motor scores after cervical spinal cord injuries. *Spinal Cord* 1998;36:491–496.

76. Waters RL, Adkins R, Yakura J, et al. Prediction of ambulatory performance based on motor scores derived from standards of the American Spinal Injury Association. *Arch Phys Med Rehab* 1994;75:756–760.
77. Ditunno JF Jr, Burns AS, Marino RJ. Neurological and functional capacity outcome measures: essential to spinal cord injury clinical trials. *J Rehabil Res Dev* 2005;42:35–41.
78. Ditunno JF Jr, Graziani V, Tessler A. Neurological assessment in spinal cord injury. *Adv Neurol* 1997;72:325–333.
79. Ditunno JF Jr. New spinal cord injury standards, 1992. *Paraplegia* 1992;30:90–91.
80. Donovan WH, Kopaniky D, Stolzmann E, et al. The neurological and skeletal outcome in patients with closed cervical spinal cord injury. *J Neurosurg* 1987;66:690–694.
81. Jonsson M, Tollback A, Gonzales H, et al. Inter-rater reliability of the 1992 international standards for neurological and functional classification of incomplete spinal cord injury. *Spinal Cord* 2000;38:675–679.

CHAPTER 7B

Physical Examination: Classification of Cervical Spine Injuries

Paul A. Anderson and Alexander R. Vaccaro

INTRODUCTION

Trauma to the spine results in many injury patterns as a result of its unique anatomy and the variable direction and magnitude of forces causing injury. As a result, no classification system of subaxial cervical spine injuries is accepted as a standard, despite the primary importance of classification in determining prognosis and treatment. Newer imaging modalities with increased sensitivities further divide injury patterns into more groups at the expense of less specificity.

The purpose of a classification system is to allow communication between practitioners, assess severity of injury, determine prognosis, direct treatment, and provide quantitative data for research. Currently used systems do not fulfill these objectives. Sensitivity and specificity rarely have been evaluated and when tested on classification systems show poor correlations.[1,2] In most systems only descriptions or mechanisms are given without a judgment of severity of injury. Even in a given fracture type, a range of injury is often present. Finally, the lack of reliability and validity limits research methods to accurately assess pathologic biomechanics and clinical outcomes.

The important principles of a classification system are reliability and validity. Reliability is the reproducibility of the system by the same or other observers and at different time periods. This is often measured by kappa (κ) coefficients or interclass correlation coefficients (ICC). These values range from 0 to 1, with values greater than 0.75 representing excellent reliability.[3] Validity is the ability to accurately measure the condition under consideration. Furthermore, classification systems must be easy to learn, applicable under a variety of conditions, and adaptable as new information or new assessment tools become available. Classifications often represent a simplification or idealized model because, in reality, biologic systems represent variability rather than an arbitrary line of demarcation. Mirza et al.[4] identified six expectations for an ideal classification system: identification and terminology, injury and treatment, characteristics, neurologic factors, grading, and prognostic factors. They noted that none of the currently available spine classification systems (for subaxial cervical classification) fulfill all of these expectations.

This chapter will review historically the most accepted classification systems, propose a new method of a quantifiable system, and assess its reliability.

CLASSIFICATION SYSTEMS

Classification systems are most commonly based on a description of morphology, hypothesized mechanisms of injury, and stability. Another important component is severity of neurologic injury.

MORPHOLOGIC DESCRIPTION

Morphologic systems use plain radiographic images and computed tomography (CT) (or rarely magnetic resonance imaging [MRI]) to describe injury pathoanatomy (Table 7B.1). Examples are

TABLE 7B.1 Morphologic Description of Subaxial Cervical Fracture

Anterior column injuries
Isolated
Compression fractures
Transverse process fractures
Traumatic disc herniations
Complex
Burst fractures
Disc distraction with or without avulsion fractures
Flexion axial loading fractures
Compression fracture with posterior ligamentous disruption
Lateral column injuries
Isolated
Superior facet fractures
Inferior facet fractures
Lateral mass pedicle fractures
Complex
Fractures with separation of lateral mass
Unilateral facet dislocations with or without fractures
Bilateral facet dislocations with or without fractures
Posterior column injuries
Isolated
Spinous process fractures
Lamina fractures
Complex
Posterior ligamentous injuries with or without fractures
Special cases
Bilateral pedicle fractures with traumatic spondylolisthesis
Spinal cord injury without radiographic abnormality
Fractures in ankylosed spine

bursting fractures, isolated lamina fractures, and facet dislocations. Limitations of morphologic descriptions are that these are broad groupings with no assessment of severity of injury. Also, terms describing mechanism of injuries are now associated with specific morphologic patterns, thus blending the two systems.

MECHANISTIC SYSTEMS

Evaluation of the mechanism of injury is important to predict severity of injury and behavior. It may also indicate specific methods for treatment. For example, a hyperextension injury resulting in disc distraction may be best treated with an anterior fusion. Alternatively, a hyperflexion injury with resulting posterior ligamentous disruption would be treated with posterior fusion. An important concept to consider is the primary injury vector. This has been described by White and Panjabi[5] as the major force vector resulting in injury. From this, one can infer which structures are likely to be incompetent.

However, judging the specific mechanism from radiographs is not precise. Many confounding variables occur during injury that may affect injury patterns. These include the exact direction of forces, site of impact (if any), attitude or head position, magnitudes of acceleration and deceleration forces, restraints, preexisting disease, and countercoup, or rebound, forces. For example, Shono[6] applied impact loads to the vertex of the cranium, creating both axial loading–type fractures and facet fracture-dislocations. Similarly, patients involved in the same traumatic events may have differing patterns of spinal injuries.

STABILITY

Stability is paramount to prognosis and planning the treatment of spinal injuries, second in importance only to neurologic injury. Nicoll[7] first described the stability concept when determining which injury pattern allowed return to work in Welsh miners who had thoracolumbar fractures. Those with fracture dislocations and posterior ligamentous injuries, in general, could not return to work and thus were defined as having unstable injuries. More recently, White and Panjabi[8] provided the best definition of stability: "ability of the spine under physiologic loads to maintain a relationship between vertebral segments in such a way that there is neither damage nor subsequent irritation of the spinal cord or nerve roots, and, in addition, there is no development of incapacitating deformity or pain due to structural changes."

In clinical practice, physicians must assess each patient and judge stability at the time of initial evaluation and during the course of treatment. This concept is, however, difficult from a practical standpoint. Even if one judges the spine stable, it is important to serially reevaluate patients given the frequency of occult instability.

DETERMINANTS OF STABILITY

The determinant of stability is the integrity of osseous and ligamentous structures. In the subaxial cervical spine, the osseous structures are the vertebral bodies, the lateral columns or pillars with articulations connected to the bodies by pedicles, the lamina, and the spinous processes. Important ligamentous structures from anterior to posterior are the anterior longitudinal ligament, disc-anulus complex, posterior longitudinal ligament, facet capsules, ligamentum flavum, and nuchal ligaments, including the interspinous, supraspinous, and ligamentum nuchae. Of equal or greater importance to stability are the neurologic elements.

Humans have many congenital variations and disease states that alter the risk for neurologic injury and thus spinal stability. Most notable is the spinal canal size and spinal ankylosis. Congenitally small spinal canals (<13 mm midsagittal diameter) predispose to greater neurologic injury from displacement of fractures or even no apparent skeletal injury.[9] Spinal ankylosis from fusion, ankylosing spondylitis, and diffuse idiopathic skeletal hyperostosis (DISH) are increasingly being recognized as predisposing to significant instability, even in seemingly innocuous nondisplaced fractures.

As described by White and Panjabi,[8] stability is dichotomous: stable or unstable. However, in reality, there is a spectrum of variability. To address this limitation, they developed a checklist for clinical instability. This analytical tool was based on cadaveric biomechanical experiments but has never been validated or tested for reliability. In their system, one or two points are assigned for presence of injuries to various components of the spine, degree of neurologic injury, residual deformation, canal size, and other patient factors. A score of 5 indicates instability but does not indicate treatment methods, such as surgery. Although it is useful as a framework to evaluate patients, the lack of validation and inconsistencies in the descriptions limit its usefulness. However, a high score such as 5 or greater usually indicates, in the authors' experience, a minimum requirement of a halo vest or surgical stabilization.

PATIENT ASSESSMENT

Accurate classification of cervical spine injuries requires clinical and radiographic examination. A patient history, if possible, should be obtained, determining modes of injury, direction and magnitude of force factors, associated injuries, and preexisting disease. Transient neurologic symptoms imply significant cervical displacement and potential instability.

The physical examination consists of log-rolling and spinal inspection from occiput to the sacrum. The spine is palpated and tenderness elicited. Reproducible focal tenderness is highly sensitive in greater than 98% of patients but not specific in awake, alert patients without distracting injuries.[10] Palpable gaps between spinous processes are pathognomonic for disruption of the posterior ligamentous complex. Disruptions of the posterior ligamentous complex are the most significant signs of instability.[11] Severe pain and difficulty in log-rolling patients indicates a potentially unstable fracture. The examination is completed by critical neurologic and perineal examination.

In most cases, the classification can be based on plain radiographs and at least one cross-sectional imaging modality. Standard radiographic views are the three-view series: anteroposterior (AP), open-mouth, and lateral. This should include the cervicothoracic junction. In a trauma setting, these studies have been largely replaced by CT with reconstructions. CT has significantly higher sensitivity and is cost-effective in patients who are already undergoing CT for other purposes.[12]

MRI has increased sensitivity over CT, especially for subtle or nondisplaced fractures and for identification of ligamentous disruptions, disc disruptions, and herniations and for assessment of canal and cord integrity.[13] In the author's opinion, it is not routinely needed to determine the classification; however, it is helpful in some cases, especially when evaluating suspicious ligamentous injuries.

HISTORICAL SYSTEMS

Over the past century, researchers have attempted to categorize and develop treatment algorithms for cervical spine injuries.

WATSON-JONES

Watson-Jones[14] identified three basic fracture types and emphasized developing specific treatment algorithms for each injury type. These injury patterns include crush (wedge) fractures, comminuted (burst) fractures, and fracture dislocations. He recommended specific reduction maneuvers emphasizing complete realignment for each different fracture type. The system formed an excellent basis for most remaining systems.

BOHLER

Bohler,[15] concurrent with Watson-Jones, critically analyzed 1200 patients with spinal injuries. He reviewed radiographs and had artistic drawings created for each one. In more than 50 cases, he dissected and autopsied the spine, determining the effect of reduction maneuvers. Similar to

Watson-Jones, he described specific closed techniques for the various injury types. Based on this experience, he proposed a mechanistic classification system with seven fracture types. Many of the terms he proposed such as flexion-distraction and shear fractures are used today.

HOLDSWORTH

Holdsworth[11] expanded Nicoll's concept of stability and applied it to subaxial cervical spine injuries. He included all basic concepts of classification, including fracture types, mechanism, and stability. He noted that the spine consists of two columns, anterior and posterior. Of special importance to stability was the posterior osteoligamentous complex. Disruption of this was a strong predictor of treatment failure and sign of instability. He also correctly noted that fracture dislocations, especially rotational fractures, had the greatest instability.

BOHLMAN

Bohlman reviewed 300 patients with cervical spine injuries, of which 186 had subaxial trauma.[16] He categorized those into morphologic patterns based on spinal region. These broad groups included injuries involving the articular processes such as unilateral and bilateral facet dislocations, injuries of the vertebral body without subluxation, and posterior element fractures. He used common descriptive terminology. He noted that many injuries occur across all levels and correlated the type of injury to risk of neurologic dysfunction.

FERGUSON AND ALLEN

Ferguson and Allen proposed a mechanistic classification based on a review of 165 patients.[17] They divided cases into six large groups of phylogenies. Based on presumed mechanism, each phylogeny was divided into two to five patterns based on increasingly severe injury. This system is based on a critical analysis of injury force vectors or factors and is logically formulated along an increasing instability scale. It has been used reliably for many biomechanical experiments and occasionally in human investigations. Their basic hypotheses are well worth considering, as follows:

1. The forces producing injury can be divided into major and minor force vectors or factors.
2. They can be deduced from radiographic evaluation.

Increasing-severity injuries are related to increasing magnitude of force. In different patients, similar injuries will result from application of similar force vectors or factors. Last, there is a spectrum of injury ranging from trivial to severe in each basic phylogeny.

Limitations of this system are the large number of fracture types, which reduces reliability, and injuries are assumed to occur primarily in a sagittal plane, which does not account for coupled vectors and does not logically account for rotational injuries, such as unilateral and bilateral facet dislocations.

LOUIS

Louis developed a different model in which the spine is considered as a tripod with three legs or columns.[18] The vertebral body anteriorly and each pillar or lateral mass forms the three columns. The posterior osteoligamentous complex acts as a spring or tensioning band. Louis attempted to quantify injury severity by assigning grades for each of the three columns, from 0 to 2 points for progressive amounts of injury. An unstable injury was present when the score was greater than 2. This classification system, however, has not been used widely to date.

AO

The AO group has an established model for classification of skeletal injury using three broad groups (A to C) with many subdivisions. Magerl used similar principles in devising a system for the spine.[19] A-type fractures result from failure in compression, B-type fractures result from distraction, and C-type fractures result from failure that occurs because of rotation or translation. For the subdivisions, each group is based on increasing severity of injury. Ultimately more than 57 cases have been described. This system has many of the tenets of a good classification system, especially for progression of injury severity increasing with higher grades. Unfortunately, this system is clinically difficult to use and has poor reliability. Oner et al.[1] compared the AO system to the Dennis system for thoracolumbar fractures. Correlation coefficients were poor. In general, these were less than 0.25 for the AO system and only slightly better for the Dennis system. Similarly, Wood et al.[2] demonstrated that the interobserver agreement between the AO and Dennis systems was only fair, although intraobserver agreement was satisfactory. Validation in the cervical spine has not occurred.

ADVANCES IN CLASSIFICATION OF SPINAL INJURIES

Much research has focused on injury biomechanics in hope of developing strategies to prevent or lessen injury. This, unfortunately, has not aided in the development of a universally accepted classification system. Imaging, especially cross-sectional CT, has increased sensitivities to detect injuries and allow a more comprehensive determination of severity of injury. Few of these advances have been used in fracture classifications. MRI can identify occult injuries and especially ligamentous disruptions. However, increased sensitivity is offset by decreased specificity because many findings (such as trivial fractures and soft tissue edema) have unknown or little significance but now require further evaluation and perhaps unnecessary treatment. Research methods evaluating reliability of schemes are now more frequently performed. Thus far, current classification systems are disappointingly poor, with only fair interobserver and intraobserver reliability.[1,2] Clearly, development of a reliable system based on new technology of assessment and known biomechanical studies is needed.

A major focus of the Spine Trauma Study Group is to develop a valid reliable classification system. Three components are needed to adequately describe lower cervical spine injuries: a morphologic description, quantification of stability, and a measurement of neurologic injury. The latter was described in a previous section.

MORPHOLOGIC DESCRIPTION

The morphologic description is based on identification of the major spinal injury region. Although a simplification, this approach allows the use of commonly recognized terminology. The descriptions avoid use of eponyms and mechanisms whenever possible. Groups of injuries are placed together. Division is not needed because this will be further assessed by the quantification of stability. Isolated injuries are those limited to one bony or ligamentous structure. Complex injuries are those associated with bone and ligamentous disruption or that extend over more than one region of the spine. The spine is broadly divided, similar to Bohlman's system, into the anterior column, lateral column, and posterior column.[20]

ANTERIOR COLUMN INJURY

Isolated Injuries

Isolated anterior column injuries include fractures of the transverse process, compression fractures, and disc distraction without subluxation.

Complex Injuries

Complex anterior column injuries result from significant forces, especially axial loading with either flexion or extension. Bony injuries include burst fractures in which the weight-bearing vertebral body is split into many fragments and a segment is retropulsed into the spinal canal. A varying degree of posterior ligamentous injury is present, including laminar fractures and posterior ligamentous complex disruption. The coronally split vertebral body fracture, also called the flexion-axial loading, or teardrop fracture, results from high-energy forces. The vertebral body is split coronally from the anterior cortex through to the inferior endplate, and the vertebral body is rotated posteriorly into the spinal canal. A small triangular piece of the anterior-inferior vertebral body is created, the so-called teardrop. As in the burst fracture, the posterior ligamentous complex may be disrupted.

Disc distraction injuries are being increasingly recognized, perhaps as a result of the increased use of MRI. In these, there is failure of the anterior longitudinal ligament and disc anulus, which creates opening, or diastasis, across the disc space. Small avulsions may be present and were previously called the extension teardrop, most commonly at C2. In more severe cases, disc distraction occurs with retrolisthesis or posterior vertebral subluxation and spinal cord injury. These injuries are continuums from the isolated injuries described earlier.

LATERAL COLUMN INJURY

Isolated Injuries

Isolated lateral column injuries include nondisplaced inferior and superior articular facet fractures, as well as lateral mass fractures without vertebral subluxation.

Complex injuries

Complex lateral column injuries are frequent but, in general, are mistaken for a benign-appearing pattern that can develop progressive subluxation. These injuries may occur unilaterally or bilaterally. Examples include unilateral facet dislocation with or without fracture, fracture separations of the lateral mass, and bilateral facet dislocations with or without fracture.

The unilateral facet dislocation is caused by axial rotation and is associated with approximately 25% anterior translation of the vertebral body. In the majority of cases there will be associated facet fracture. Another associated injury is disruption of the posterior longitudinal ligament complex. Fracture separation of the lateral mass is often mistaken for unilateral facet dislocation because the amount of vertebral body translation also ranges from 0% to 25%.[21] In this case, there is fracture of the pedicle at its base and through the lamina where it connects to the lateral mass. This creates a free-floating lateral mass that will rotate forward, thereby no longer creating a stop to anterior rotation. Also, unlike the unilateral facet dislocation, subluxation of both the cranial and caudal levels may occur.

Bilateral facet dislocations are usually associated with facet fracture and bilateral lamina and always with posterior ligamentous complex disruption. Vertebral body subluxation ranges from 25% to 50% or even greater. In rare cases, total ligamentous disruption occurs and distraction between vertebral bodies is present or created during traction. Traumatic injury to the disc with herniation in the spinal canal occurs in up to 50% of cases, but its significance is highly controversial.

POSTERIOR COLUMN INJURIES

Isolated Injuries

Isolated injuries of the posterior column include injury to spinous process and lamina fractures.

Complex Injuries

Complex injuries are posterior ligamentous complex injuries. These injuries are commonly seen with other fracture patterns but also may be seen as an isolated pattern. They may initially be difficult to diagnose because minimal radiographic changes may be present. Often the hallmark of the posterior ligamentous complex disruption is focal kyphosis and mild widening between the spinous processes. With increasing kyphosis, facet subluxation or a perched position or facet diastasis is observed.

SPECIAL CASES

Several injury patterns do not fit the groupings described in the previous sections. These include fractures in patients with ankylosed spines, traumatic spondylolisthesis, and spinal cord injury without radiographic abnormality (SCIWORA). Patients with injuries who have an ankylosed spine from ankylosing spondylitis, DISH, or surgery or congenitally have alterations in mechanics and stability. The injuries usually consist of transverse fracture planes that may occur through the disc or body, exiting in the pedicle and facet joints. In such patients the spine should be considered unstable even when injuries appear as nondisplaced. Traumatic spondylolisthesis is a unique fracture thought to be from hyperextension, similar to a hangman fractures and traumatic spondylolisthesis of the lumbar spine.[16] The forced hyperextension causes bilateral pedicle fracture. Continuation of forces occurs through the disc, resulting in discoligamentous injury and anterior vertebral body translation. The spinal canal is often enlarged so that neurologic deficits are not as great as might be expected. SCIWORA indicates patients with spinal cord injuries without observable radiographic cause. Although no skeletal injury is observed, the spine should be considered unstable because sufficient deformation occurs to result in spinal cord injury. This syndrome is classically seen in children, in whom the spinal column deforms elastically to a greater degree than the neural elements. Consequently, with deformation, the spinal cord fails under tension and no observable skeletal injury occurs. In some cases, injuries are through the cartilaginous endplate, which are difficult, if not impossible, to diagnose. Elderly patients also sustain spinal injury without radiographic abnormalities. In these cases, patients usually have preexisting small spinal canals (<13 mm) with spondylotic changes. During hyperextension or axial loading transiently, the spinal cord is pinched between an infolding ligament and a bulging disc or osteophyte, causing a spinal cord injury.

CERVICAL SPINE INJURY SEVERITY SCORE

The purpose of the Cervical Spine Injury Severity Score is to quantitatively measure the degree of instability. We had hypothesized that injury patterns with high scores indicate the need for surgery, whereas lower ones would be treated nonoperatively. A middle, or gray, zone will be present in which either treatment may be appropriate. The score, when added to morphologic descriptions, can give an exact summary of the type and severity of injury, allowing better comparison between treatment methods and assessment of prognosis. The Cervical Spine Injury Severity Score is based on grading the four different spinal regions using a visual analog scale (VAS).

FOUR COLUMNS

The spine is divided into four columns or zones: anterior, posterior, right lateral mass (pillar), and left lateral mass (pillar) (Fig. 7B.1A). The anterior column includes the anterior longitudinal ligament, vertebral body, disc anulus, and posterior vertebral body. The posterior column includes the posterior ligamentous complex, including the nuchal ligament, interspinous and supraspinous ligaments, the spinous process, lamina, and ligamentum flavum. Each lateral column includes the pedicle, lateral mass, superior and inferior facet to the junction of the lamina, and lateral mass and facet capsules.

ANALOG SCORE

Each of the four zones is scored independently using a VAS ranging from 0 to 5 (see Fig. 7B.1B). The scores are summed, giving a total from 0 to 20, with 0 being no injury and 20 the most unstable condition.

The VAS is graded based on fracture displacement and severity of ligamentous disruption. Scores can be fractional, and the VAS is used similar to a pain VAS (see Fig. 7B.1B). Generally a score of 1 indicates a nondisplaced fracture and a score of 5 is the worst injury for that zone. For

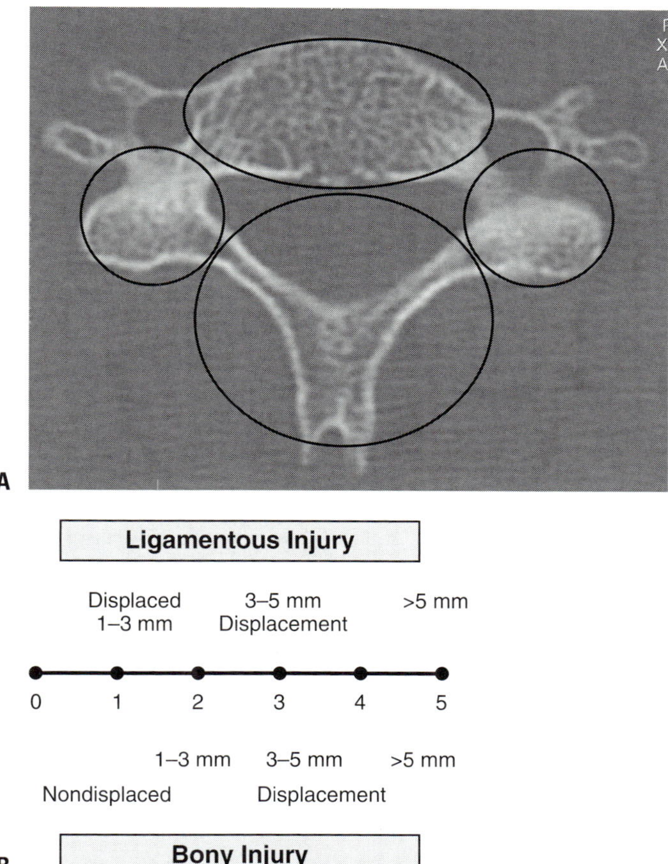

FIGURE 7B.1. **A.** The cervical spine is divided into four columns: anterior, right pillar, left pillar, and posterior. **B.** Analog scores (0–5) are used to score each column independently. A nondisplaced fracture is given a score of 1, and increasing scores are given for increasing displacement. A 5 is assigned for the worst injury that can occur to that column.

instance, a complete facet fracture dislocation is given a score of 5, and a facet fracture with subluxation of 3 to 4 mm is assigned a value of 3. Similarly, a subtle increase in spreading between spinous processes may be a 2.5, and a complete separation is a 5.

RELIABILITY

The Cervical Spine Injury Severity Score was tested for reliability. Thirty-five consecutive patients with cervical trauma were identified. Radiographs and CT images were downloaded as Digital Imaging and Communications in Medicine (DICOM) images and stored on CD. They were then read using eFilm Lite (MERGE Healthcare, Milwaukee, WI) by 10 observers who, after being given instructions, randomly graded the cases. Five additional cases were repeated to establish intraobserver reliability. Reliability was assessed using ICCs. A score greater than 0.75 was considered excellent, 0.4 to 0.75 was considered fair or moderate, and less than 0.4 was considered to be poor.[3]

The injury patterns were well distributed from minor and less severe to severe instabilities. The mean score was 8.2 with a standard deviation of 6.6. Intraobserver ICC showed excellent agreement at 0.97 to 0.99. Similarly the intraobserver ICC again showed excellent agreement, ranging from 0.75 to 0.98. These results indicate that the Cervical Spine Injury Severity Score is highly reliable in qualification of severity of injury.

CASE EXAMPLES

CASE 1

A 45-year-old man fell, striking his head (Fig. 7B.2). He presented with bilateral weakness in the C7 distribution but otherwise had a normal neurologic examination. He had a disc distraction injury, with comminuted fractures of both lateral masses. His injury is scored as anterior, 3.5; right pillar, 4.5; left pillar, 2; posterior, 1; with a total of 11.

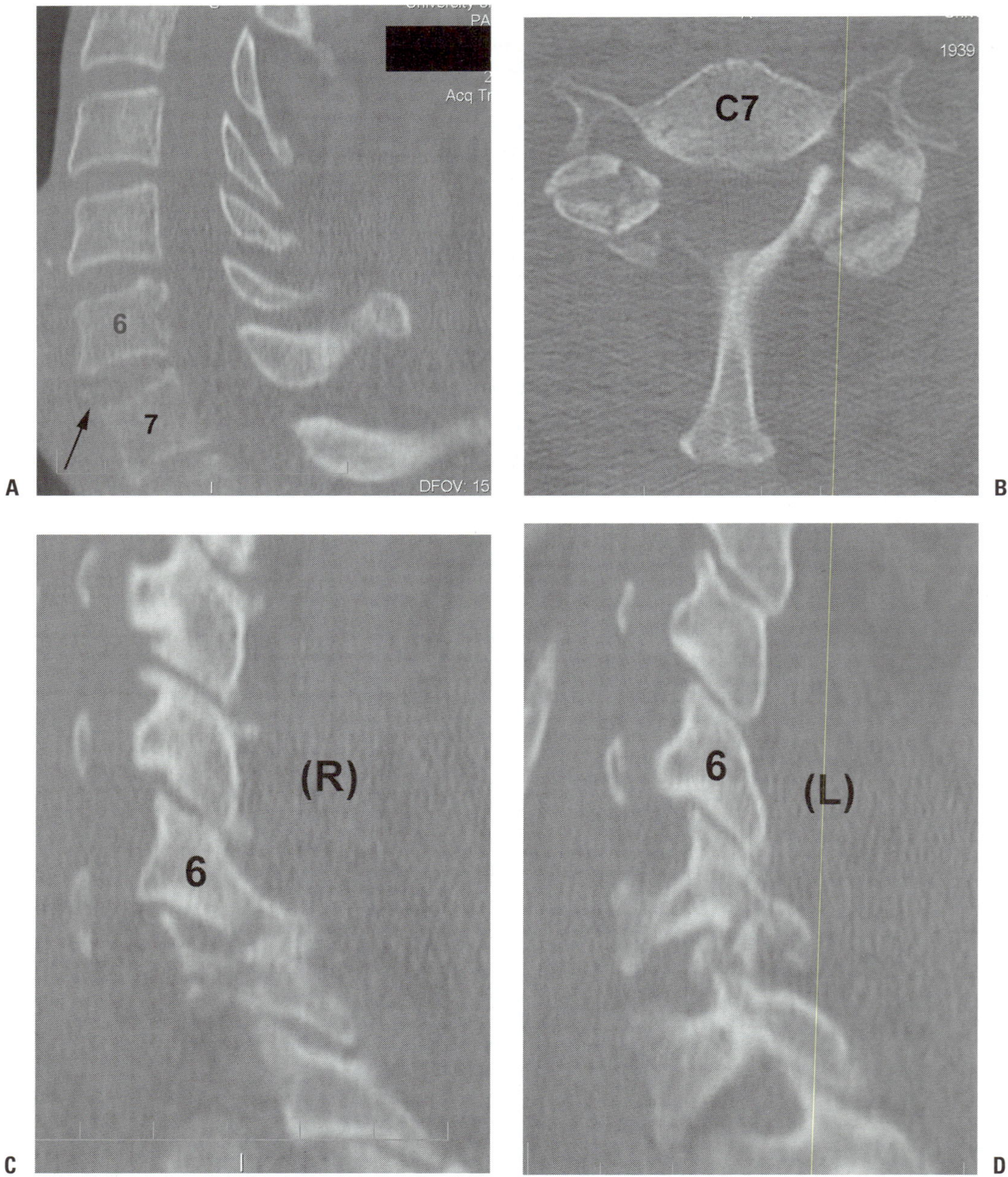

FIGURE 7B.2. **A.** Sagittal computed tomography (CT) image of patient with disc distraction injury. A small avulsion is seen with widened disc space. The anterior score is a 3.5, and posterior score is 1.0. **B.** Axial CT showing bilateral comminution of lateral masses. **C.** Right sagittal CT image. A fracture dislocation of the facet is present. The right pillar score is 4.5. **D.** Left sagittal CT. Fracture of facet without dislocation and a score of 2 is assigned. The total score is equal to 11.

CASE 2

A 22-year-old man incurred a diving injury sustaining a flexion–axial loading injury and complete C4 quadriplegia (Fig. 7B.3). His injury score is scored as anterior, 5; right pillar, 4.5; left pillar, 1; posterior, 5; with a total of 15.5.

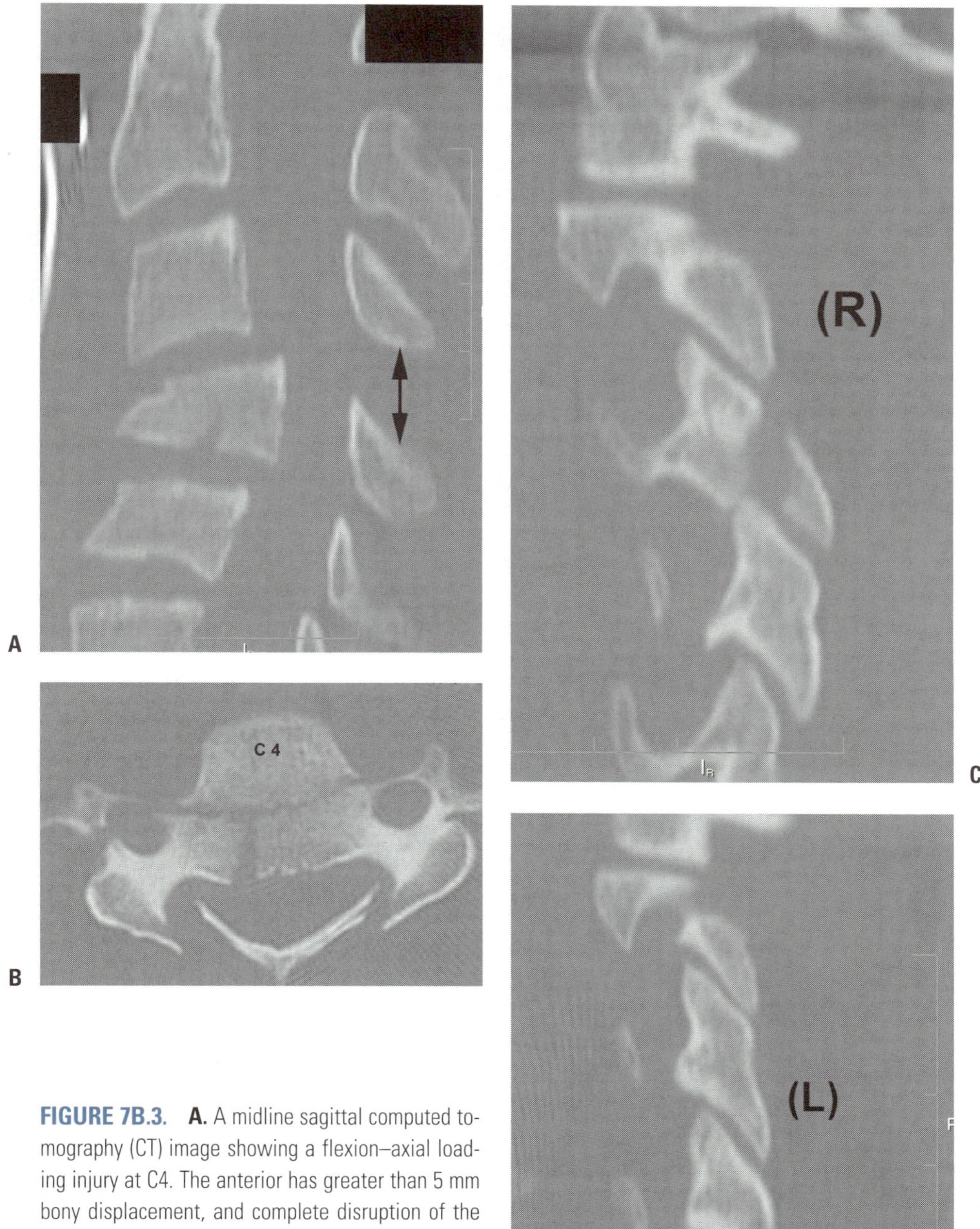

FIGURE 7B.3. **A.** A midline sagittal computed tomography (CT) image showing a flexion–axial loading injury at C4. The anterior has greater than 5 mm bony displacement, and complete disruption of the posterior osteoligamentous complex is present. Both columns are scored a 5. **B.** Axial CT image. **C.** Right sagittal CT image. A fracture subluxation of the right facet is present. A score of 4.5 is given. **D.** Left sagittal CT image. Minimal diastasis of C6-C7 facet with a score of 1. The total score is equal to 15.5.

CASE 3

A 16-year-old male patient involved in a motor vehicle crash had transient quadriparesis and a compression fracture of C7, with posterior ligamentous disruption (Fig. 7B.4). His injury score is scored as anterior, 3; right pillar, 1; left pillar, 3; posterior, 5; with a total of 12.

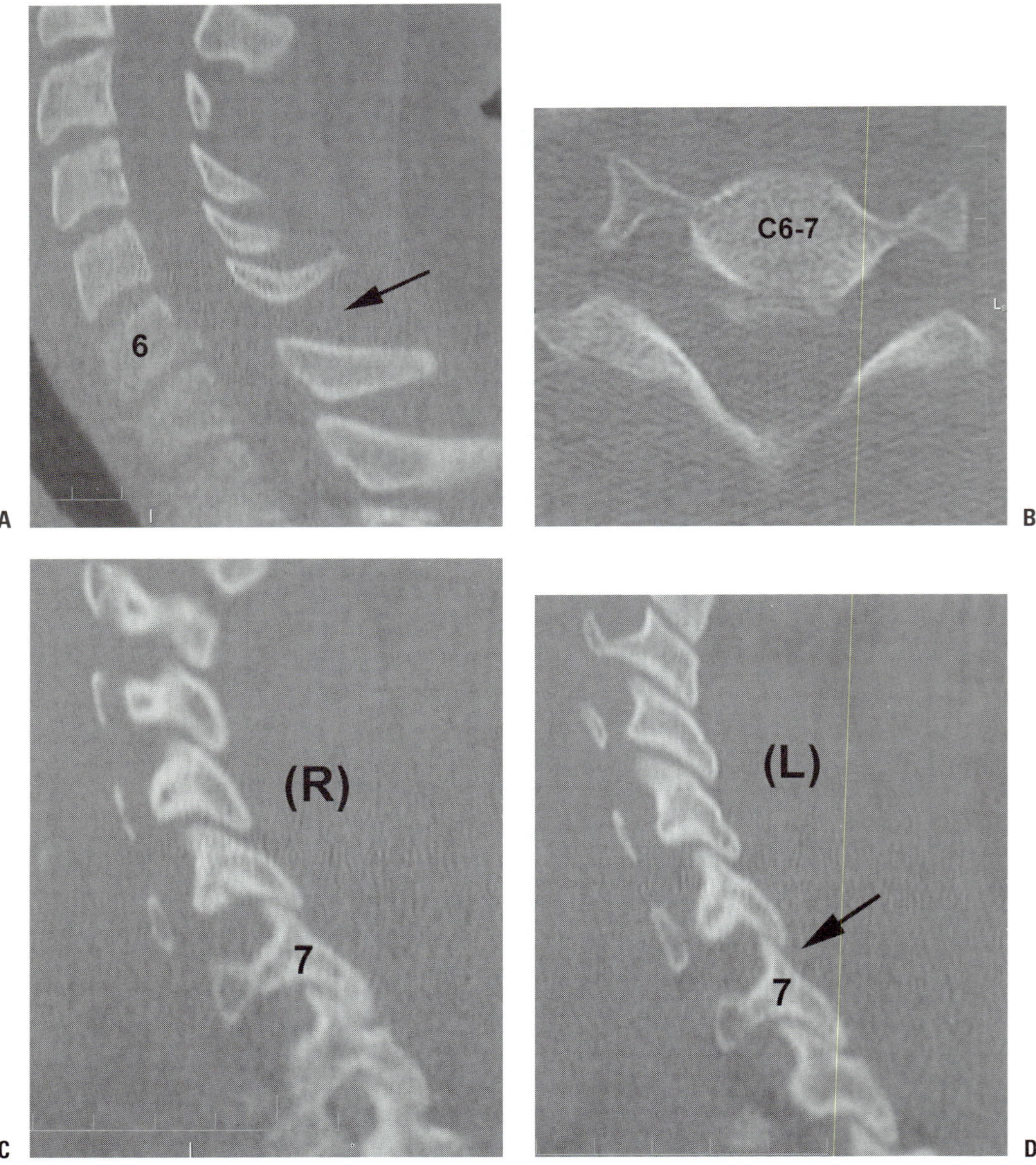

FIGURE 7B.4. **A.** A 16-year-old male patient with compression fracture at C7 and posterior ligamentous injury at C6-C7. A small avulsion of ring apophysis at C6 is present. The anterior score is 3 and posterior 5. **B.** Axial CT image. **C.** Right pillar sagittal CT image showing a nondisplaced fracture of the facet, scored as 1. **D.** Left pillar sagittal CT image. A perched facet at C6-C7 is present; score equals 3. Total injury severity score is 12.

CASE 4

A 23-year-old man sustained a burst fracture of C7 and incomplete quadriplegia (Fig. 7B.5). His injury score is scored as anterior, 5; right pillar, 2.5; left pillar, 1; posterior, 5; with a total of 13.5.

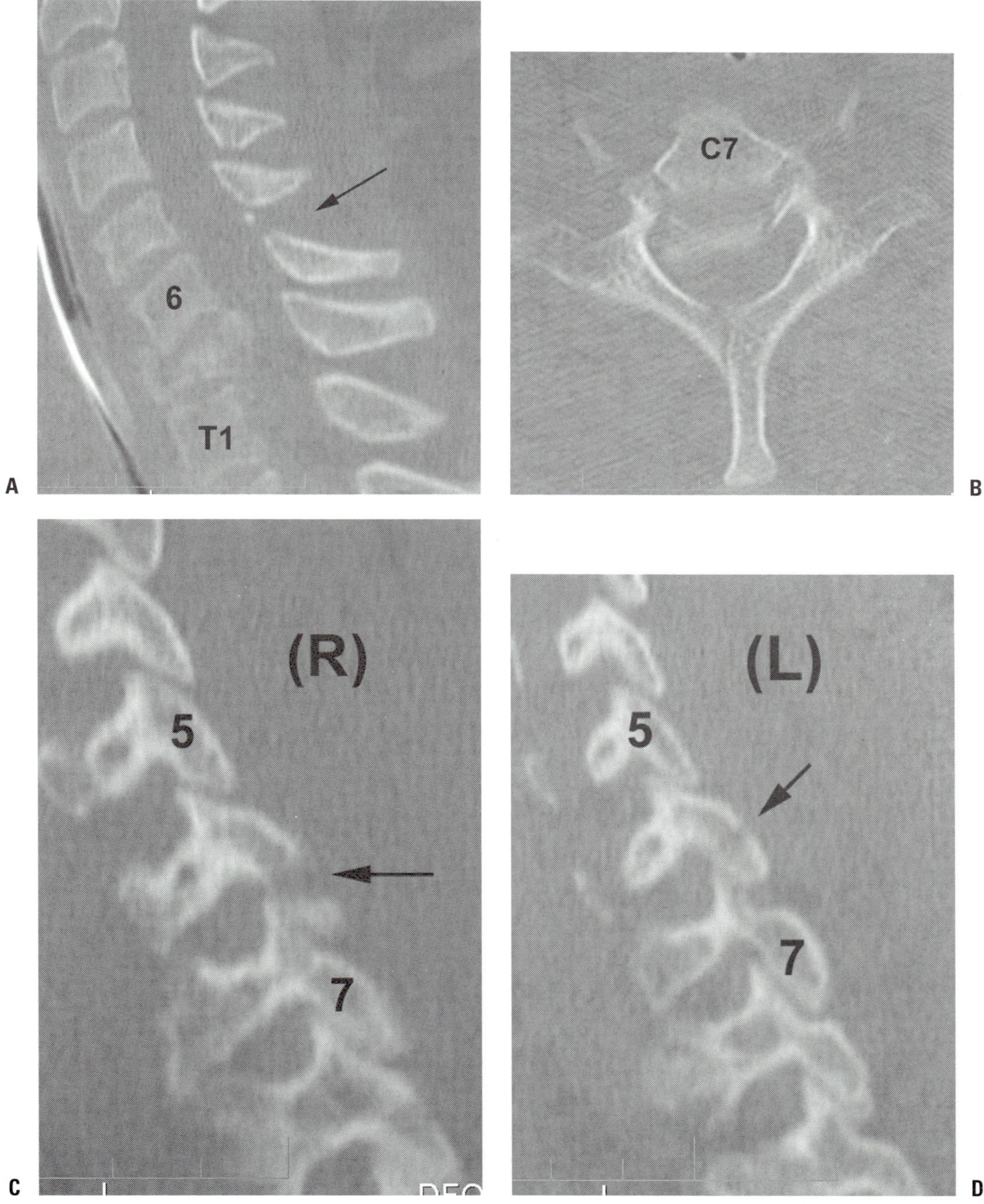

FIGURE 7B.5. **A.** A burst fracture with posterior ligamentous injury of C7 is seen on sagittal CT image. Posterior ligaments appear completely disrupted at C5-C6. Bony retropulsion of greater than 5 mm is present, and both the anterior and posterior columns are assigned a 5. **B.** Axial CT image shows burst components and a minimally displaced spinous process fracture. **C.** Right sagittal CT image demonstrates a displaced inferior facet fracture with a score of 2.5. **D.** Left sagittal CT image shows nondisplaced inferior facet fracture with a score of 1. Total injury severity score is 13.5.

CONCLUSION

The classification of spinal injuries is important because there are a large number of injury patterns that need to be efficiently communicated between spinal care physicians. An effective classification system allows communication among practitioners, is reliable, correlates to severity of injury or instability, predicts prognosis, and, of importance, helps direct treatment. No current system fulfills these attributes. We propose combining a morphologic description with a quantitative score, the Cervical Spine Injury Severity Score. The morphologic descriptions are based on commonly used terms and avoid eponyms and mechanism of injury. The Cervical Spine Injury Severity Score is based on independent scoring of the four spinal columns and ranges from 0 to 20. This system was highly reliable, with an interclass correlation score greater than 0.88. Further research is ongoing relative to using the system with MRI and validation of the system biomechanically and clinically.

REFERENCES

1. Oner FC, Ramos LM, Simmermacher, RK et al. Classification of thoracic and lumbar spine fractures: problems of reproducibility—a study of 53 patients using CT and MRI. *Eur Spine J* 2002;11:235–245.
2. Wood KB, Khanna G, Vaccaro AR, et al. Assessment of two thoracolumbar fracture classification systems as used by multiple surgeons. *J Bone Joint Surg Am* 2005;87:1423–1429.
3. Shrout PE, Fleiss JL. Intraclass correlations: uses in assessing rater reliability. *Psychol Bull* 1979;86:420–428.
4. Mirza SK, Mirza AJ, Chapman JR, et al. Classifications of thoracic and lumbar fractures: rationale and supporting data. *J Am Acad Orthop Surg* 2002;10:364–377.
5. White AA, Panjabi MM. *Clinical Biomechanics of the Spine.* 2nd ed. Philadelphia: Lippincott Williams & Wilkins, 1990.
6. Shono Y, McAfee PG, Cunningham BW. The pathomechanics of compression injuries in the cervical spine. Nondestructive and destructive investigative methods. *Spine* 1993;18(14): 2009–2019.
7. Nicoll EA. Fractures of the dorsolumbar spine. *J Bone Joint Surg Br* 1949;31:376–394.
8. White AA, Panjabi M. Kinematics. In: White AA, Panjabi M, eds. *Clinical Biomechanics of the Spine.* 2nd ed. Philadelphia: Lippincott, 1990:92–102.
9. Eismont FJ, Clifford S, Goldberg M, et al. Cervical sagittal spinal canal size in spine injury. *Spine* 1984;9:663–666.
10. Gonzalez RP, Fried PO, Bukhalo M, et al. Role of clinical examination in screening for blunt cervical spine injury. *J Am Coll Surgeons* 1999;189:152–157.
11. Holdsworth F. Fractures, dislocations, and fracture-dislocations of the spine. *J Bone Joint Surg Am* 1970; 52:1534–15551.
12. Wintermark M, Mouhsine E, Theumann N, et al. Thoracolumbar spine fractures in patients who have sustained severe trauma: depiction with multi-detector row CT. *Radiology* 2003;227:681–689.
13. Emery SE, Pathria MN, Wilber RG, et al. Magnetic resonance imaging of posttraumatic spinal ligament injury. *J Spinal Disord* 1989;2:229–233.
14. Watson-Jones R. The results of postural reduction of fractures of the spine. *J Bone Joint Surg Br* 1938; 20:567–586.
15. Bohler L. *Die techniek de knochenbruchbehandlung imgrieden und im kriege.* Vienna: Verlag von Wilhelm Maudrich, 1930.
16. Anderson PA, Bohlman HH. Anterior decompression and arthrodesis of the cervical spine: long-term motor improvement. II: Improvement in complete traumatic quadriplegia. *J Bone Joint Surg Am* 1992;74:683–692.
17. Ferguson RL, Allen BL Jr. A mechanistic classification of thoracolumbar spine fractures. *Clin Orthop Relat Res* 1984;189:77–88.
18. Louis R. Spinal stability as defined by the three-column spine concept. *Anat Clin* 1985;7:33–42.
19. Magerl F, Aebi M, Gertzbein SD, et al. A comprehensive classification of thoracic and lumbar injuries. *Eur Spine J* 1994;3:184–201.
20. Bohlman HH. Acute fractures and dislocations of the cervical spine: an analysis of three hundred hospitalized patients and review of the literature. *J Bone Joint Surg Am* 1979;61:1119–1142.
21. Levine AM, Mazel C, Roy-Camille R. Management of fracture separations of the articular mass using posterior cervical plating. *Spine* 1992;17:S447–S454.

CHAPTER 8

Preimaging Cervical Spine Clearance Guidelines for Trauma Patients

Ronald W. Lindsey and Zbigniew Gugala

INTRODUCTION

Emergency department clearance of the cervical spine is one of the highest priorities in early assessment and treatment of trauma patients. Annually, more than 10 million patients present for trauma care in the United States, and the risk for cervical spine injury must be considered.[1–3] Actual cervical spine injury occurs in only approximately 1% to 3% of blunt trauma patients, although these projections may vary depending on the injury mechanism.[4–8] A multitude of confounding, distracting, and potentially devastating issues make the cervical spine clearing process particularly challenging in this setting. Therefore, the need for a concise, yet thorough, approach to cervical spine clearance mandates that efficacious clearance guidelines are established and adhered to.

Traditionally, most physicians have considered imaging the principal, if not the sole, method by which the cervical spine should be cleared.[9] This opinion resulted in the tendency for many physicians to ignore the merits of the history and physical examination and impeded the development of dependable clinical indicators of cervical injury. Unfortunately, most of the initial cervical spine clearance protocols depended almost entirely on indiscriminate imaging.[10] The problems with this approach have become well known and include (a) a large number of inadequate radiographs, (b) an even larger number of normal radiographs, (c) delay of the trauma patient's workup and treatment, (d) compromise of medical personnel time and attention, (e) inefficient use of institutional resources, (f) increased patient and staff radiation exposure, and (g) increased medical costs.

Twenty years ago, Jacobs and Schwartz[11] reported a study in which they analyzed the emergency physician's ability to clinically predict the presence of cervical spine injury in trauma patients and noted that only 50% of the injuries were appropriately predicted. However, when the same physicians were asked to predict which patients did not have an injury, they were 94% successful. Inadvertently, this study not only emphasized the true focus of cervical spine clearing (i.e., accurately determining the absence of cervical spine injury), but affirmed that clinical clearing of a cervical injury was more feasible than clinical injury detection. Furthermore, the same authors were able to identify clinical variables that correlated positively with cervical injury.

Until recently, significant physician support for clinical assessment as the exclusive modality to affect cervical spine clearing in the emergency department did not exist. In a retrospective series of 1686 consecutive trauma patients subjected to cervical spine clearing, Lindsey et al.[12] questioned the efficacy of routine cervical spine imaging. These authors demonstrated cervical spine injury in less than 2% of patients, and most of these injuries were not threatening to the spine's stability or the patient's neurologic status. The same study also analyzed a prospective group of 600 patients; of the 1% of patients with cervical spine injury, all presented with neck pain, demonstrated neurologic deficit, or were obtunded. The authors suggested that the cervical spine of many trauma patients could be effectively cleared by clinical assessment alone, and this opinion supported the conclusion of others. A study by Bachulis et al.[13] emphasized the predictive power of neck pain in the alert patient; all alert patients in their series with cervical injury had neck pain. Fischer,[14] in another study, corroborated these findings, but also identified neurologic deficit as an important clinical predictor of cervical injury. Although these concepts were initially considered controversial, they have proven to be prophetic. Recently, as a result of several prospective randomized clinical trials, all modern cervical clearing guidelines actively seek to identify trauma patients in whom the cervical spine can be successfully cleared by clinical assessment modalities alone.

Therefore, the objective of this chapter is to discuss the present guidelines for clinical clearing of the cervical spine in trauma patients before imaging. This includes (a) defining the concept of trauma clearing and its principal objective, (b) identifying the three basic trauma patient groups that determine the most appropriate clearing process, (c) establishing the basic clinical clearing (history and physical examination) components, (d) the Advanced Trauma Life Support (ATLS) guidelines for clearing, (e) the most popular clinically based clearing instrument, and (f) the authors' proposed algorithm for clinical clearance of the cervical spine.

CERVICAL SPINE CLEARANCE: DEFINITION AND OBJECTIVES

Cervical spine clearance in the trauma setting is defined as reliably ruling out the presence of cervical injury in a patient when cervical injury does not exist. Contrary to the common misconception, cervical clearance is not intended to classify an injury or determine its most appropriate treatment. Clearance simply declares that an injury is not present. The clearing process always requires a complete clinical evaluation, but only occasionally warrants adjunctive imaging. Ideally, clearing should occur at the earliest point in the trauma assessment process that it can be accomplished reliably. However, the clearance process does not place its major emphasis on the haste with which it is accomplished, but rather on its accuracy.

The fundamental objective of cervical spine clearance is to improve the efficiency and accuracy of the entire trauma assessment process. When cervical spine injury can reliably be ruled out, neck immobilization precautions can be discontinued, additional neck diagnostic or therapeutic modalities are not warranted, and the trauma evaluation can focus on the other areas of the patient's assessment. Considerable pressure may be placed on the emergency clinician to expeditiously clear, especially when the index of suspicion for injury is low. However, one should accept that some patients simply cannot be cleared in the acute setting. If cervical spine injury cannot be reliably excluded, vigilant cervical spine precautions are maintained, and efforts to establish a definitive position on the status of the cervical spine must continue.

BASIC CERVICAL TRAUMA PATIENT CLEARANCE GROUPS

A comprehensive clinical examination is imperative before cervical spine clearance can even be considered. A reliable clinical examination requires that the patient is alert, oriented, and cooperative. The clinician's initial objective should be to establish the patient's level of consciousness. The level of patient consciousness has been classified using the Ransohoff Scale,[15] which consists of six levels of alertness ranging from full orientation through deep coma (Table 8.1). In the criteria, a patient with Class 1 level of consciousness should be alert, respond immediately to questions, and follow complex commands. More commonly, the Glasgow Coma Scale (which consists

TABLE 8.1 Ransohoff Classification of Consciousness Levels

Class	Description
1	Alert; responds immediately to questions; may be disoriented and confused; follows complex commands
2	Drowsy, confused, uninterested; does not lapse into sleep when undisturbed; follows only simple commands
3	Stuporous; sleeps when not disturbed; responds briskly and appropriately to noxious stimuli
4	Deep stupor; responds defensively to prolonged noxious stimuli
5	Coma; no appropriate response to any stimuli; includes decorticate and decerebrate responses
6	Deep coma; flaccidity; no response to any stimuli

Adapted from: Ransohoff J, Fleischer A. Head injuries. *JAMA* 1975;234:861–864, with permission.

of six levels of alertness ranging from full orientation to deep coma) (Table 8.2) has been used to determine a patient's level of alertness. By these criteria, alertness is defined by spontaneous eye opening, oriented verbal response, and the ability to obey commands. Only a fully alert patient (Ransohoff Class 1 or Glasgow Coma Scale >14) is capable of undergoing a dependable physical examination and is the only type of patient in which cervical injury can be reliably excluded, with or without supplemental imaging.[16]

An alert patient can provide a valid history and enable a creditable physical examination and corroborate the data obtained from all other diagnostic modalities. Even when cervical imaging appears unremarkable, injury cannot be conclusively excluded unless the patient is able to contribute to the

TABLE 8.2 Glasgow Coma Scale

Feature	Response	Score
Eye opening	Spontaneous	4
	To speech	3
	To pain	2
	None	1
Verbal response	Oriented	5
	Confused conversation	4
	Words inappropriate	3
	Sounds incomprehensible	2
	None	1
Motor response	Obeys commands	6
	Localizes pain	5
	Flexion normal	4
	Flexion abnormal	3
	Extended	2
	None	1
Total Coma Score		**3–15**

process. The clinician's ability to perform a reliable clinical examination is essential in the clearance process and constitutes the principal basis by which patients can be divided into one of the following three groups[16]:

Group I: Patients for whom clinical examination alone can rule out presence of cervical spine injury without the need for diagnostic imaging

Group II: Patients who can be cleared only when clinical examination is supplemented with diagnostic imaging

Group III: Patients who cannot be clinically examined at the time of emergency department presentation and consequently are not candidates for cervical spine clearance, even if adjunctive imaging is negative

GROUP I

Group I includes patients who meet all of the five following criteria[17]: (a) full alertness, (b) no intoxication, (c) no midline tenderness, (d) no focal neurologic deficit, and (e) no distracting painful injury (Table 8.3).

A randomized, prospective study by the NEXUS group of 34,069 patients demonstrated that significant cervical spine injury could be reliably excluded by physical examination alone.[18] Among the patients who met these clinical criteria, only two demonstrated significant cervical spine injury.[1] One patient had a clavicle fracture that was not considered to be a disqualifying distracting injury. Another patient was an asymptomatic man with a history of multiple motorcycle accidents, and it was unclear whether a cervical spine fracture was an acute or chronic injury. The reliability of cervical spine clearance by physical examination of the alert patient has been corroborated by other studies.[12–14] These studies demonstrated that many trauma patients are alert on presentation to a medical facility and, therefore, can potentially be clinically cleared. Successfully cleared patients do not require further diagnostic measures, and cervical spine precautions can be discontinued.

TABLE 8.3 Clinical Cervical Spine Clearance Criteria as Defined by the NEXUS Group

1. Altered neurologic function is present if any of the following is present: (a) Glasgow Coma Scale score of 14 or less; (b) disorientation to person, place, time, or events; (c) inability to remember 3 objects at 5 minutes; (d) delayed or inappropriate response to external stimuli; or (e) any focal deficit on motor or sensory examination. Patients with none of these individual findings should be classified as having normal neurologic function.
2. Patients should be considered intoxicated if they have either of the following: (a) a recent history of intoxication or intoxicating ingestion or (b) evidence of intoxication on physical examination. Patients may also be considered to be intoxicated if tests of bodily secretions are positive for drugs that affect level of alertness, including a blood alcohol level greater than 0.08 mg/dL.
3. Midline posterior bony cervical spine tenderness is present if the patient complains of pain on palpation of the posterior midline neck from the nuchal ridge to the prominence of the first thoracic vertebra or if the patient evinces pain with direct palpation of any cervical spinous process.
4. Patients should be considered to have a distracting painful injury if they have any of the following: (a) a long bone fracture; (b) a visceral injury requiring surgical consultation; (c) a large laceration, degloving injury, or crush injury; (d) large burns; or (e) any other injury producing acute functional impairment. Physicians may also classify any injury as distracting if it is thought to have the potential to impair the patient's ability to appreciate other injuries.

Adapted from: Hoffman JR, Wolfson AB, Todd K, et al. Selective cervical spine radiography in blunt trauma: methodology of the National Emergency X-Radiography Utilization Study (NEXUS). *Ann Emerg Med* 1998;32:461–469, with permission.

GROUP II

Fully oriented and alert patients who demonstrate symptoms of neck pain, tenderness, neurologic deficit, or decreased mobility on physical examination require additional diagnostic assessment to effectively clear the cervical spine.

This group also includes patients with a distracting injury or past history of cervical spine pathology. Additional diagnostic studies typically consist of three-view radiography (anteroposterior [AP], lateral, open-mouth odontoid) and may include adjunctive computed tomography (CT) or magnetic resonance imaging (MRI).[16] Voluntary lateral flexion-extension radiography is indicated only after symptomatic treatment has failed over a brief period (typically 2 weeks) and is not generally recommended in the acute setting.

An alert patient who presents with partial or complete neurologic deficit is assumed to have a spine injury and therefore requires imaging. Whether the deficit is due to spinal cord, spinal root, or peripheral nerve injury, an exhaustive diagnostic effort must be made to rule out spine instability and injury. Throughout this process, the physician must strictly adhere to all precautionary spine immobilization techniques, even if the initial examination suggests a complete neurologic deficit. Plain radiography and/or sophisticated imaging are always indicated to diagnose and categorized the injury. Prophylactic modalities such as high-dose steroid administration, when indicated, may be instituted emergently. Serial examinations, ideally by the same physician(s), is recommended whether the patient's neurologic deficit is partial or complete to document neurologic progression or improvement during the workup.

GROUP III

In obtunded trauma patients, strict adherence to basic principles of cervical spine external support and stabilizing precautions is recommended.

Imaging to detect but not to definitively exclude injury is always required in these patients. Imaging should begin with the standard three-view plain radiographic series, followed by CT or MRI as indicated. If patients are undergoing CT for other reasons, the plain radiographs may be eliminated and routine cervical spine CT performed. This can be a cost-saving and time-saving method. If cervical spine imaging is positive, this should be addressed in accordance with the standard of care for that particular injury. If cervical spine imaging findings are negative, the prudent physician is obliged to maintain all neck precautions until the patient becomes more alert and receptive to supplemental clinical assessment. In some cases this may not be feasible because the presence of a closed head injury and subsequent spine precaution modalities may be lessened or eliminated as determined by the treating physician.[19–22]

The efficiency of cervical spine clearance can be greatly enhanced by the assignment of patients to one of these three groups. Although one of the primary clinical objectives will always be to increase the sensitivity of cervical injury detection, the emergency clinician must be cognizant that the greater challenge is to be proficient in cervical injury exclusion. Cervical spine imaging alone, which is more sensitive for injury detection than it is specific for injury exclusion, cannot substitute for a thorough clinical evaluation in establishing clearance. Moreover, the effectiveness of cervical spine imaging in clearance of the cervical spine can be enhanced when it is combined with a valid clinical assessment.

MANAGEMENT OF PATIENTS DURING CERVICAL CLEARANCE

In the prehospital phase of trauma management, one should assume cervical spine injury to be present in all patients. Cervical spine immobilization is uniformly applied and can consist of a cervical collar and/or securing the head to the backboard with tape.[23,24] Although neck immobilization in trauma patients has recently been questioned because of reported elevations in intracranial pressure and an increased risk for respiratory problems,[25] routine rigid neck immobilization is still recommended as the standard for all trauma patients.[26]

After arrival to the hospital, all external neck support should be maintained. These principles apply even during the assessment of the airway; the head and neck should not be excessively flexed, extended, or rotated at this juncture. If external neck support must be temporarily removed (e.g., to inspect a neck wound), a member of the trauma team should manually maintain control of the head and neck using in-line immobilization techniques.[23] The physician's adherence to these precautions cannot be overstated; one publication has noted the potential for progression of neurologic worsening after the arrival to a hospital setting.[27] Subsequently, the first premise in clearing trauma patients for neck injury is the assumption that all patients may have a cervical spine injury, and they should be managed accordingly until cervical pathology can be definitely excluded.[28]

If other injuries warrant initial or greater attention, the cervical spine evaluation can be safely deferred as long as neck immobilization is diligently maintained. The only aspects of the initial assessment of the trauma patient that are of greater priority than the cervical spine are the patient's airway, breathing, circulation, and head and brain. A patent airway should be expeditiously identified or established immediately after the trauma patient's arrival to the hospital. Breathing must then be documented or external ventilation initiated. Hemorrhage, the most prevalent cause of preventable deaths after trauma, must be quickly controlled to ensure hemodynamic stability.[23] Finally, a neurologic evaluation is performed to establish the patient's level of consciousness, and, if a brain injury exists, it must also be managed emergently. Cervical spine clearance becomes the focus of the evaluation only after these "ABCs" have been addressed.

THE COMPONENTS OF CLINICAL CLEARANCE OF THE CERVICAL SPINE

HISTORY

A detailed history is essential in the cervical spine assessment of trauma patients. The initial priority in obtaining a valid history is an early, accurate determination of the patient's level of alertness. Although the ideal history is one obtained from an alert, oriented trauma victim, significant information is also available from a host of other individuals who may have experienced the same mishap or are simply familiar with the scene of the accident (e.g., police, emergency medical technicians, other passengers, witnesses). In addition to documenting the mechanism of injury, the history should provide a detailed account of the events and the patient's condition immediately after injury up to the time of presentation to a medical facility.[29] Information regarding the victim's past medical history, especially as it pertains to previous cervical spine conditions, is helpful. Special attention should be given to elderly patients who have sustained a fall or minor trauma; these individuals are particularly susceptible to a cervical spine injury.[30,31]

The risk for cervical spine injury and its severity can be directly correlated with the energy associated with the traumatic insult.[11,13,32] Therefore, the level of energy (high versus low) and the manner by which the trauma is sustained (direct versus indirect) are crucial information. The clinician should determine if the accident is the result of a high-speed motor vehicular accident (MVA) or a fall from a considerable height versus an altercation. If due to a fall, the approximate height of the fall should be calculated; if due to an MVA, the record should reflect whether the patient was restrained (wearing a seatbelt) or ejected from the vehicle. Furthermore, was direct injury sustained to the occiput or was there an indirect whiplash injury?

The previously noted study by Jacobs and Schwartz[11] not only established the feasibility of clinical clearance of the cervical spine but also identified variables that seemed to correlate with an increased risk for cervical spine injury (Table 8.4). In a recent study by Stiell et al,[33] the authors calculated the odds ratios for several clinical variables that could predict a significant cervical spine injury (Table 8.5). Although these variables may serve to heighten one's awareness of the risk for cervical spine injury, ruling out the presence of these variables alone does not establish cervical clearance.

TABLE 8.4 Variables Positively Correlating with Cervical Spine Injury

Variable	*p* value
Motor vehicle accident	0.052
Fall >10 feet	0.007
Neck tenderness	0.002
Numbness	0.001
Loss of sensation	0.001
Weakness	0.001
Neck spasm	0.001
Loss of muscle power (0–5)	0.001
Decreased sensation	0.001
Loss of anal tone/wink	0.001
Fall <10 feet	0.083
Low-energy injury	0.700
Drug/alcohol intoxication	0.400
Flexion/extension	0.400
Compression/torsion	0.960
Head trauma	0.370
Neck pain	0.140
Headache	0.140
Loss of consciousness	0.382
Bradycardic hypotension	0.760

Adapted from: Jacobs LM, Schwartz R. Prospective analysis of acute cervical spine injury: a methodology to predict injury. *Ann Emerg Med* 1986;15:44–49, with permission.

PHYSICAL EXAMINATION

The physical examination, albeit challenging in the acute posttraumatic environment, is essential for valid clearance of the cervical spine. This principle exists regardless of whether adjunctive imaging is also deemed necessary to complete the process. The physical examination can be accomplished accurately only in patients who demonstrate a Glasgow Coma Scale score greater than 14, and therefore, it is feasible only for patients in groups I and II. Unlike the obtunded patients in group III, the group I and II patients are alert and oriented to participate in a physical examination that must demonstrate their ability to respond to complex commands, voluntarily mobilize their necks, indicate symptomatic anatomic regions, and undergo comprehensive neurologic evaluations. Group II patients, although suitable for physical examination, are not candidates for clinical clearance and must undergo appropriate imaging to complete a valid clearing process. In only group I patients can a physical examination be performed and the cervical spine be definitively cleared by clinical assessment alone if that examination is normal.

The initial physical examination of the trauma patient should consist of a static assessment. At this stage, the physical examination is performed while the external cervical support remains in place, the neck is not manipulated, and the patient is maintained in a supine posture. The static stage components of the physical examination that have positively correlated with cervical spine injury

TABLE 8.5 Odds Ratios of a Clinical Variable Predicting Clinically Significant Cervical Spine Injury

Variable	OR (95% CI)*
Dangerous mechanism†	5.2 (3.7–7.3)
Age ≥65 years	3.7 (2.4–5.6)
Paresthesias in extremities	2.2 (1.4–3.3)
Ambulatory at any time after injury	1.0 (0.7–1.5)
Sitting position in emergency department	0.61 (0.3–1.2)
Delayed onset of neck pain	0.4 (0.3–0.7)
Absence of midline neck tenderness	0.5 (0.3–0.8)
Able to rotate neck 45 degrees left and right	0.04 (0.01–0.3)
Simple rear-end MVA‡	0.08 (0.03-0.2)

*CI, Confidence interval; MVA, motor vehicular accident; OR, odds ratio.
† Fall from ≥1 m; axial load to the head; high-speed MVA, rollover, or ejection; bicycle collision; recreational motorized vehicular collision.
‡ Excludes vehicle pushed into oncoming traffic, hit by bus or large truck, rollover, or hit by high-speed vehicle; collision.
Adapted from: Stiell IG, Wells GA, Vandemheem KL, et al. The Canadian C-Spine Rule for radiology in alert and stable trauma patients. *JAMA* 2001;286:1841–1848, with permission.

include: the presence of neck pain, focal neck tenderness or spasm, and/or neurologic deficits.[11] Neurologic deficit of any degree precludes the ability to achieve clinical clearance, and adjunctive cervical spine imaging is mandatory.[16] Many clinicians suggest that cervical spine injury should be assumed present in the neurologically compromised patient until further workup can conclusively establish its absence. Particular attention must be given to patients who sustain direct face, head, or neck trauma.[34–37] Although neck injury usually occurs through an indirect injury mechanism (e.g., whiplash), patients who sustain direct trauma above the shoulders are particularly at significant risk for cervical spine injury.

The second phase of the physical examination of group I patients consists of a dynamic evaluation. External neck support should be removed, and, while the patient is still supine, the patient should be asked to voluntarily perform neck flexion-extension, rotation, and lateral bending. If these maneuvers are successfully performed without pain or a change in the patient's neurologic status, the examiner should apply gentle axial load to the cervical spine by compressing or distracting the skull. If the neck and patient remain asymptomatic after these maneuvers, the patient can be permitted to sit or stand upright. The components of the static assessment should be reviewed as needed to ensure that they are unchanged. At this juncture, the clinician must also determine if the patient projects any degree of apprehension related to neck or neurologic status that would warrant further evaluation. If the patient is without apprehension and has conclusively demonstrated a normal physical examination in both the static and dynamic phases of assessment, the cervical spine can be clinically cleared without adjunctive diagnostic modalities.

The physical examination alone can be unreliable in select patients even if they appear lucid. Major injuries to the chest, abdomen, pelvis, or even the extremities (e.g., open fractures) may alter the patient's perception of subtle neck or neurologic symptoms and, thereby, negate the feasibility of clinical clearance. As previously noted, a patient's history of past neck pathologic conditions would do likewise. Perhaps the most frequently encountered setting that threatens reliable clinical clearance is the unruly intoxicated or drugged patient in whom accurate imaging is not possible. These patients are often briefly admitted to the hospital for observation until they become detoxicated. Although a later physical examination may suggest that cervical spine injury is unlikely, the clinician must still consider supplemental imaging if any degree of the patient's behavior appears altered.

ADVANCED TRAUMA LIFE SUPPORT GUIDELINES FOR CERVICAL SPINE CLEARANCE

The Advanced Trauma Life Support (ATLS) guidelines for screening patients for cervical spine injury are listed in Table 8.6.[23] Their recommendations for clinical clearance are applicable only to the adult patient who is fully awake, alert, and sober. When these criteria are met, the next priority is to establish the patient's neurologic status. Any degree of neurologic deficit would suggest that clinical clearance alone is not feasible and appropriate imaging is mandatory. In the alert, neurologically intact patient, the external cervical support (collar) can be removed and the neck assessed for pain while the patient remains supine. During this assessment the clinician should determine if the neck

TABLE 8.6 ATLS Guidelines for Clearing Cervical Spine

1. **The presence of paraplegia or quadriplegia is presumptive evidence of spinal instability.**
2. **Patients who are awake, alert, sober, and neurologically intact, have no neck pain or midline tenderness:** These patients are extremely unlikely to have an acute C-spine fracture or instability. With the patient in a supine position, remove the collar. If there is no significant tenderness, ask the patient to voluntary move his neck from side to side. Never force the patient's neck. If there is no pain, have the patient voluntarily flex and extend the neck. If there is no pain, C-spine radiography is not necessary.
3. **Patients who are awake, alert, neurologically intact, cooperative, but do have neck pain or midline tenderness:** All such patients should undergo three-view radiography (lateral, AP, open-mouth odontoid) of the C-spine with axial CT images of areas of suspicion or of the lower cervical spine, if not adequately visualized on the plain films. If these films are normal, remove the collar. Under the care of a knowledgeable doctor, obtain flexion and extension, lateral cervical spine films with the patient voluntarily flexing and extending the patient's neck. If the films show no subluxation, the patient's C-spine can be cleared and the collar removed. However, if any of these films are suspicious or unclear, replace the collar and obtain consultation from a spine specialist.
4. **Patients who have an altered level of consciousness or cannot describe their symptoms:** Lateral, AP, and open-mouth odontoid films with CT supplementation through suspicious areas should be obtained on all such patients. If the entire C-spine can be visualized and is found to be normal, the collar can be removed after appropriate evaluation by a doctor skilled in the management of spine-injured patients. Clearance of the C-spine is particularly important if the pulmonary or other care of the patient is compromised by inability to mobilize the patient.
5. **When in doubt leave the collar on.**
6. **Consult:** Doctors who are skilled in the evaluation and management of the spine-injured patient should be consulted in all cases in which a spine injury is detected or suspected.
7. **Backboards:** Patients who have neurologic deficits (quadriplegia or paraplegia) should be evaluated quickly and taken off the backboard as soon as possible. A paralyzed patient who is allowed to lie on a hard board for more than 2 hours is at high risk for developing serious decubiti.
8. **Emergency situations:** Trauma patients who require emergent surgery before a complete workup of the spine can be accomplished should be transported and moved carefully with the assumption that an unstable spine injury is present. The collar should be left on and the patient log-rolled.

is symptomatic while at rest, voluntarily mobilized, or on palpation. The absence of neck pain without neurologic deficit in these alert patients achieves clinical clearance of the cervical spine, and the focus of the trauma workup can be directed elsewhere. However, if focal neck symptoms can be solicited or neurologic deficit exists, clinical assessment alone is insufficient and further diagnostic modalities are warranted before clearance can be accomplished.

The ATLS guidelines also provide recommendations on how to optimally protect the cervical spine throughout the entire trauma diagnostic and therapeutic process.[23] First, external neck support should be maintained until a conclusive position on the cervical spine has been established. Second, they suggest that the backboard, a necessity in the acute phase, should be eliminated after a couple of hours to avoid decubiti. Next, if the patient requires surgery to thwart a life-threatening condition before cervical spine clearance, the clinician should assume that an unstable neck injury exists and the entire surgical team should approach the patient accordingly. Finally, the ATLS guidelines recognize that a thorough cervical spine evaluation may occasionally exceed the capabilities of the trauma physician and suggests that a physician with spine expertise be consulted, not simply for detected injuries, but when cervical clearance cannot be decisively established.

It must be emphasized that the ATLS cervical spine guidelines were developed for the physician providing comprehensive, initial care for the traumatized patient. These guidelines provide a basic diagnostic and therapeutic algorithm designed to assist the nonspecialized physician in maintaining a rational, generalized approach to cervical spine clearance.[21,38] The guidelines are not intended to be the authoritative treatise on cervical spine injury detection or treatment; rather, the intent is to minimize the risk for overall morbidity or mortality in the trauma patient by an early inadequate suspicion of or external support for neck injuries. Furthermore, although the ATLS recommendations were compiled by knowledgeable specialists, they have been advocated without scientific validation. Recently, however, the concept of clinical clearance of the cervical spine has received considerable attention in the spine trauma literature.[1,12–14,39–43] Three clinical cervical spine clearance guidelines have gained popularity and warrant discussion.

EAST GUIDELINES FOR CERVICAL SPINE CLEARANCE

The Eastern Association for Surgery of Trauma (EAST) recognized the merits of an evidence-based protocol and endeavored to establish national consensus-based clinical guidelines that included screening recommendations for cervical clearance.[40] These clinical guidelines were formulated by a panel of trauma surgeons who were instructed to assess the scientific quality of the available evidence on the topic. The panel then defined criteria for cervical spine clearance based on the extent to which they could be supported by the evidence that existed at the time. The final recommendations were abridged after presentation to the EAST National Meeting in 1997, and these revisions were adopted. Subsequently, an update to EAST guidelines has been available for download online on the EAST website (http://www.east.org/tpg/chap3.pdf).[44]

The EAST group recognized cervical spine instability as a frequent, challenging problem confronting physicians providing acute trauma care. The complexity of this problem not only encompasses some serious medical concerns (e.g., missed or inappropriately treated cervical spine injury), but also represents major economic and legal issues. The clinical question initially addressed by this group was simply "which trauma patients require cervical spine radiography?" which suggests that there is a core group of trauma patients for whom radiographs are not warranted. Furthermore, EAST noted that although there was a plethora of literature on cervical spine instability and trauma, a Class I (prospective, randomized, and controlled) clinical trial did not exist. Therefore, their recommendations were made from Class II evidence and were deemed only reasonably justifiable.[40]

The literature at that time recognized that in the overwhelming majority of trauma patients, the assessment of the cervical spine is negative for injury.[12,18,45,46] With this understanding, the consensus EAST recommendation identified that select trauma patients could be successfully cleared for cervical spine injury without radiography. Their indications for clinical screening included patients who are awake, have no mental status changes, are without neck pain, have no distracting injuries, and have no neurologic deficit. All other patients, by their selective criteria, required imaging. Although the EAST cervical clearance recommendations for high-risk trauma patients (i.e., with neck symptoms, neurologic compromise, or an altered mental state) remain controversial,[40,44] clinician support for the feasibility of select cervical spine clearance solely by clinical evaluation has been sustained.[47]

THE NEXUS GUIDELINES

The National Emergency X-Radiography Utilization Study (NEXUS) Guidelines constitute the largest study to date designed to validate clinical criteria that could reliably clear the cervical spine in trauma patients.[18] In this multicenter, prospective, observational study, five clinical criteria were used to exclude the need for cervical spine radiography in the trauma setting. These criteria included: (a) normal alertness, (b) absence of intoxication, (c) absence of cervical tenderness, (d) absence of focal neurologic deficit, and (e) absence of a painful distracting injury (see Table 8.3).[17] Standard trauma three-view X-ray images were obtained for all patients and correlated with clinical criteria.

The NEXUS study reviewed 34,069 patients; cervical spine injury was determined in 818 patients, and the clinical criteria failed to suggest injury (false negative) in only 8 patients (Fig. 8.1).[17] Among the patients with false-negative findings, only two had injuries that were considered clinically significant. Although this decision instrument was 99.6% sensitive for the presence of injury, it was only 12.9% specific. These clinical cervical clearance criteria would have eliminated radiography in

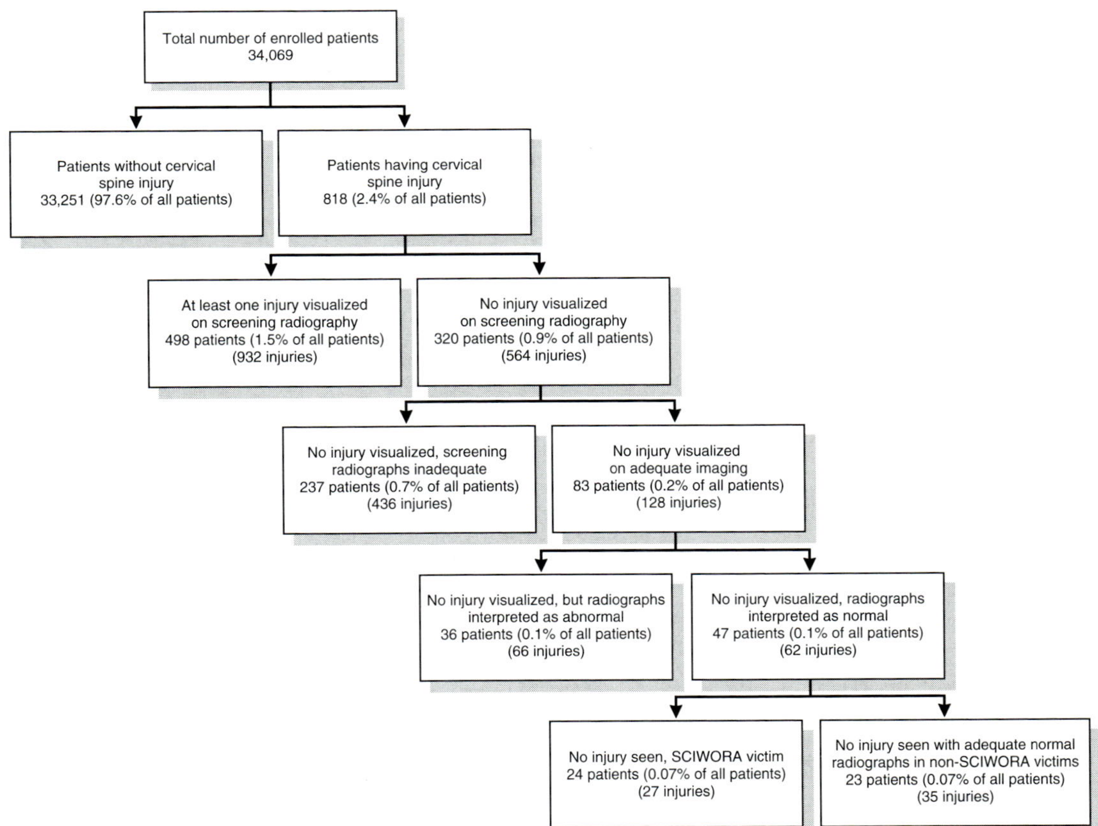

FIGURE 8.1. The distribution of the patients from the NEXUS study classified by the injury status and radiographic findings (SCIWORA, Spinal Cord Injury without Radiographic Abnormality).

4309 (12.6%) patients. The authors concluded that these clinical assessment criteria were reliable in excluding injury and effective in decreasing the need for routine cervical spine imaging.

The NEXUS study could be criticized for its low, 12.9% specificity. Furthermore, two of the clinical parameters, intoxication and painful distracting injuries, were found to be poorly reproducible.[33] In this large, well-controlled study, the low incidence of cervical spine injury further emphasized the need for a more efficient clinical instrument to clear the cervical spine without imaging.

THE CANADIAN C-SPINE RULE

Stiell et al.[33] performed a prospective cohort study of alert, stable trauma patients to determine clinical parameters that would exclude the need for imaging to clear the cervical spine (Fig. 8.2). The top priority of neck clearance was readily accepted by these authors, who also recognized that 98% of acute trauma patients present without cervical spine injury. The indiscriminate use of radiography as a screening tool was viewed as not only increasing costs, but also as precluding an expeditious acute trauma workup. The study assessed trauma patients for 20 standardized clinical parameters in a multicenter effort to determine whether cervical clearance could be reliably achieved without radiography.

The study possessed several unique features. First, its primary outcome measure was not simply the absence of injury, but the absence of clinically significant injury. Clinically significant injury was defined as a fracture, dislocation, neurologic deficit, or soft tissue injury that would require stabilization or specialized follow-up. Clinically insignificant cervical injuries include osteophyte avulsions, isolated transverse process fractures, isolated posterior spinous process fractures, and vertebral body compression fractures with less than 25% collapse. Clinically insignificant injuries were confirmed after 14 days by the following criteria: (a) no or mild neck pain, (b) no or mild restriction of neck mobility, (c) no cervical collar requirement, and (d) the patient is able to return to full or normal employment.

The Canadian C-Spine Rule study prospectively applied their clinical variable to 8424 patients.[33] The study was able to successfully exclude the necessity for cervical spine clearance radiography for patients who could satisfactorily respond to three simple questions related to the presence of (a) high-risk factors (increased age, dangerous mechanism, paresthesia), (b) low-risk factors that would prohibit the safe assessment of neck range of motion, and (c) the patient's ability to voluntarily rotate the neck (Table 8.5). The initial multicenter study using this instrument demonstrated that only 58% of trauma patients warranted radiography, with a sensitivity of 95% for cervical spine injury detection and a specificity of 42.5% for cervical spine injury exclusion. Moreover, the Canadian C-Spine Rule proved to be relatively favorable with regard to intraobserver reliability.

However, this study has several limitations. Although all patients were followed clinically, only select patients received confirmatory radiography. The distinction between important and unimportant cervical spine injury can be biased and, therefore, is controversial. Furthermore, the study's cohort did not constitute a consecutive series of patients. Despite this, the Canadian C-Spine Rule added credence to the merits of clinical cervical spine clearance criteria in select alert trauma patients.[48]

THE AUTHORS' ALGORITHM FOR CLINICAL CLEARANCE OF THE CERVICAL SPINE

The authors have developed an algorithm (Fig. 8.3) for clinical clearance of the cervical spine based on the existing literature. It begins by assuming that a cervical spine injury may be present in all trauma patients. The initial clinical examination should immediately establish the level of patient consciousness. If the patient is obtunded (group III), imaging is indicated to assess for cervical spine injury; if imaging is negative, conclusive clearance cannot be achieved until the patient becomes lucid. This management scenario typically occurs in the intoxicated patient, but should also apply to individuals with traumatic brain injury. If the patient is alert (either immediately or after detoxication), a more thorough history can be obtained and a more thorough physical examination can be performed. Alert patients with neurologic deficit, neck pain (with or without voluntary neck mobilization), or a

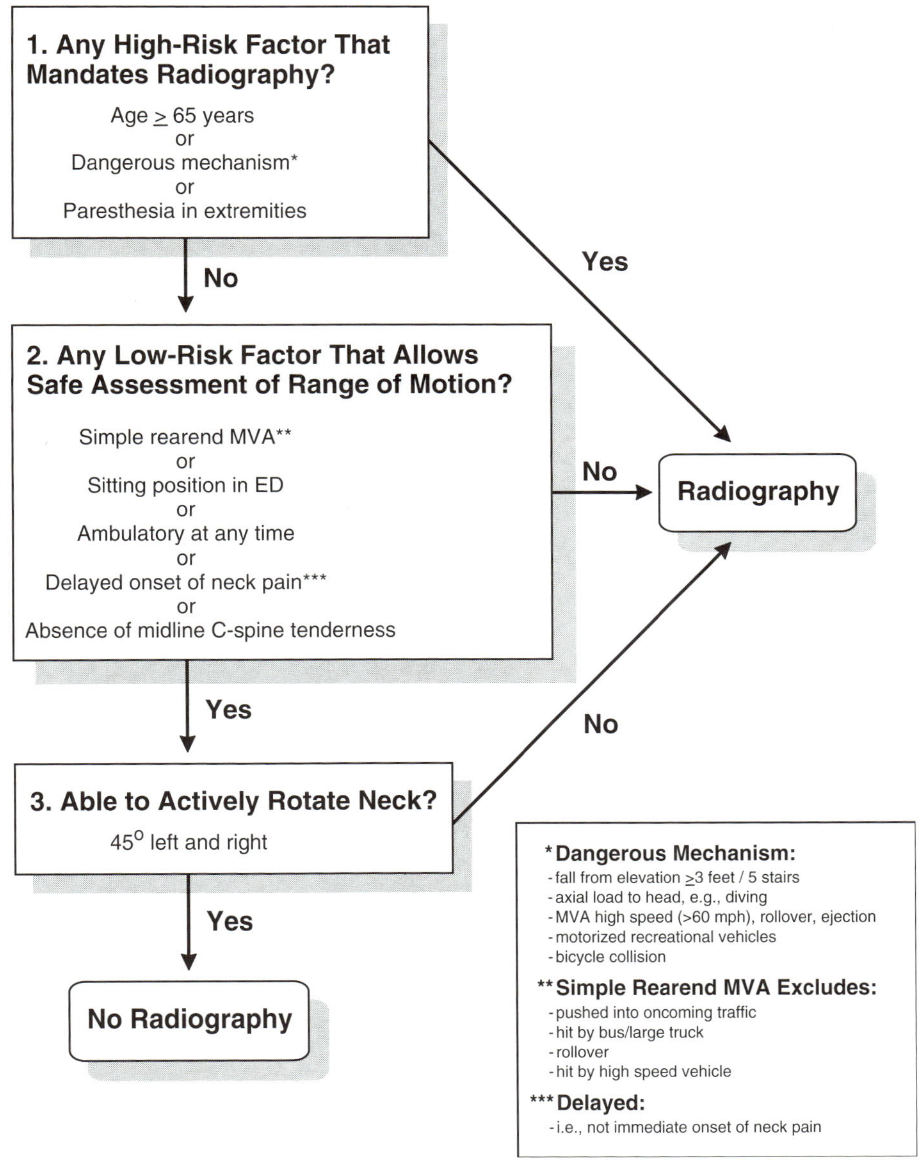

FIGURE 8.2. The Canadian C-Spine Rule Study design.

major distracting injury (group II) cannot be cleared until adjunctive imaging confirms the absence of cervical spine injury. Alert patients without neurologic deficit, neck pain, or a major distracting injury (group I) constitute the only patients in whom clinical clearance of the cervical spine is appropriate. Cervical spine imaging is not indicated in those group I patients who satisfy these clinical guidelines. In these select patients, cervical spine precautions can be discontinued, and the trauma team should direct its focus to the other aspects of the patient's care.

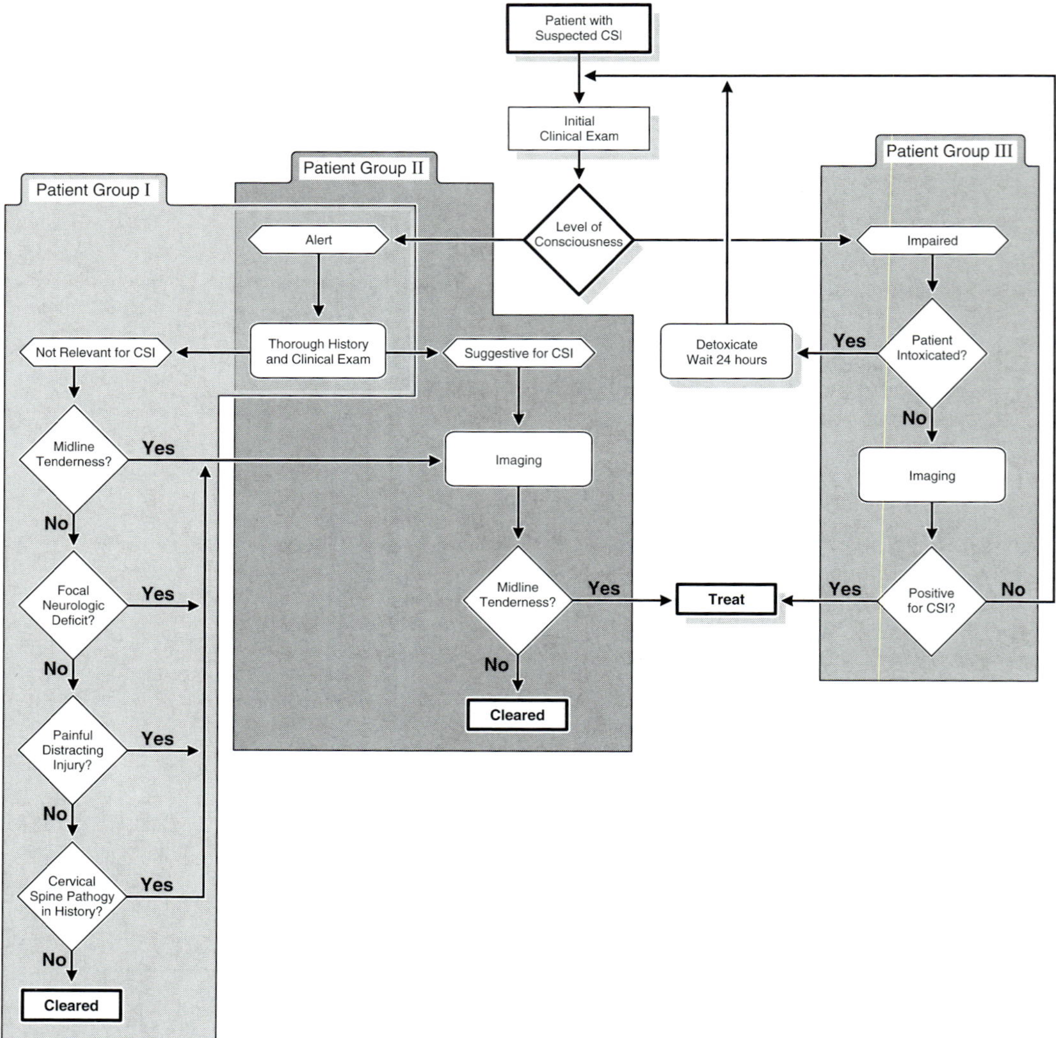

FIGURE 8.3. The authors' new algorithm of clearing the cervical spine for blunt trauma patients. Only a fully awake and alert patient (Ransohoff Class 1 or Glasgow Coma Scale >14) can reliably be cleared of a cervical spine injury with or without supplemental imaging. (CSI, cervical spine injury).

CONCLUSION

Although the modern approach to clearance of the cervical spine in the trauma patient has improved dramatically in recent years, many aspects of the existing evaluation protocols are still inadequate. The algorithms that are currently applied are not sufficiently comprehensive, forgo ease of application for improved specificity, or are often more focused on cervical injury detection than its exclusion.

The absence of penetrating trauma to the neck in existing cervical spine clearance protocols reflects their failure to be suitably comprehensive. Epidemiologic studies suggest that gunshot injury has become a leading cause for spinal cord injury in the United States, much of which is due to direct neck trauma.[49,50] The surgical literature has recognized the increased risk for patient morbidity and mortality with gunshot injury to the neck; however, current cervical spine clearance guidelines continue to neglect the problem. Clinical cervical spine clearance is not feasible in trauma patients with a

TABLE 8.7 Comparison of NEXUS and Canadian C-Rule Studies

Variable	NEXUS	C-Spine Rule
Total patients	34,069	6185*
Positive for cervical injury	818	151
Sensitivity	99.6%	100%
Specificity	12.9%	42.5%

*Patients who underwent radiographic examination of the cervical spine.

penetrating injury to the neck. All of these patients should be assessed by plain cervical spine radiography; many of these patients may warrant more sophisticated imaging (e.g., arteriography, barium swallow, computerized tomography) to rule out the presence of visceral injury.[50] If the present gunshot injury trends continue, future cervical spine clearance guidelines must include this mechanism in their evaluation algorithms.

The next major consideration for a cervical spine clearance protocol would be the ease by which it can be applied in the hectic, highly stressed emergency department environment. The Canadian C-Spine Rule has the highest reported specificity (42.5%) of currently validated clinical decision-making instruments. However, with this algorithm, the physician has to evaluate an exorbitant number of clinical variables.[33] This inherent complexity would require a clinical study to establish its interreliability and intrareliability. Conversely, the NEXUS algorithm, with its lower specificity (12.9%), consists of only five simple criteria (Table 8.7). The less complex nature of the NEXUS instrument not only ensures its timely application, but also suggests that it would be more readily accepted. Therefore, the optimal clinical cervical spine clearance protocol must not solely establish high sensitivity and specificity, but also demonstrate *sensibility* to be universally accepted.[16,42]

Finally, future cervical spine algorithms for trauma patients must address semantics. Cervical spine injury detection, clearance, screening, and evaluation are terms that are commonly confused; moreover, many trauma algorithms offer guidelines that simultaneously attempt both to clear and detect cervical spine injury. Cervical spine injury clearance and detection should form the basis for two separate algorithms because the information they seek differs. Cervical spine injury detection algorithms are in response to the inquiry: "Is a cervical spine injury present?" It is always the second question to be asked, and the answer may require complex and sophisticated diagnostic modalities. However, cervical spine clearance algorithms are in response to the inquiry: "Is a cervical spine injury absent?" This is the first question to be asked when assessing trauma patients. If it cannot be reliably answered affirmatively, the second question must be asked. The more adept future guidelines become at answering this first question, the more proficient we will become in clinically clearing the cervical spine in trauma patients.

REFERENCES

1. Hoffman JR, Schriger DL, Mower W, et al. Low-risk criteria for cervical-spine radiography in blunt trauma: a prospective study. *Ann Emerg Med* 1992;21:1454–1460.
2. Grossman MD, Reilly PM, Gillett T, et al. National survey of the incidence of cervical spine injury and approach to cervical spine clearance in US Trauma Centers. *J Trauma* 1999;47:684–690.
3. Lowery DW, Wald MM, Browne BJ, et al. NEXUS Group: epidemiology of cervical spine injury victims. *Ann Emerg Med* 2001;38:12–16.
4. Velmahos GC, Theodorou D, Tatevossian R, et al. Radiographic cervical spine evaluation in the alert asymptomatic blunt trauma victim: much ado about nothing. *J Trauma* 1996;40:768–774.
5. Ross SE, Schwab CW, David ET, et al. Clearing the cervical spine: initial radiologic evaluation. *J Trauma* 1987;27:1055–1060.

6. Shaffer MA, Doris PE. Limitation of the cross table lateral view in detecting cervical spine injuries: a retrospective analysis. *Ann Emerg Med* 1981;10:508–513.
7. Roberge RJ, Samuels JR. Cervical spine injury in low-impact blunt trauma. *Am J Emerg Med* 1999;17:125–129.
8. Ryan MD, Henderson JJ. The epidemiology of fractures and fracture-dislocations of the cervical spine. *Injury* 1992;23:38–40.
9. Spain DA, Trooskin SZ, Flancbaum L, et al. The adequacy and cost effectiveness of routine resuscitation-area cervical-spine radiographs. *Ann Emerg Med* 1990;19:276–278.
10. Petri R, Gimbel R. Evaluation of the patient with spinal trauma and back pain: an evidence based approach. *Emerg Med Clin North Am* 1999;17:25–39.
11. Jacobs LM, Schwartz R. Prospective analysis of acute cervical spine injury: a methodology to predict injury. *Ann Emerg Med* 1986;15:44–49.
12. Lindsey RW, Diliberti TC, Doherty BJ, et al. Efficacy of radiographic evaluation of the cervical spine in emergency situations. *South Med J* 1993;86:1253–1255.
13. Bachulis BL, Long WB, Hynes GD, et al. Clinical indications for cervical spine radiographs in the traumatized patient. *Am J Surg* 1987;153:473–478.
14. Fischer RP. Cervical radiographic evaluation of alert patients following blunt trauma. *Ann Emerg Med* 1984;13:905–907.
15. Ransohoff J, Fleischer A. Head injuries. *JAMA* 1975;234:861–864.
16. Lindsey RW, Gugala Z. Clearing of the cervical spine. In: The Cervical Spine Research Society Editorial Committee: Clark R, Benzel EC, Currier BL, et al., eds. *The Cervical Spine.* 4th ed. Philadelphia: Lippincott Williams & Wilkins, 2005:375–386.
17. Hoffman JR, Wolfson AB, Todd K, et al. Selective cervical spine radiography in blunt trauma: methodology of the National Emergency X-Radiography Utilization Study (NEXUS). *Ann Emerg Med* 1998;32:461–469.
18. Hoffman JR, Mower WR, Wolfson AB, et al. Validity of a set of clinical criteria to rule out injury to the cervical spine in patients with blunt trauma. National Emergency X-Radiography Utilization Study Group. *N Engl J Med* 2000;343:94–99.
19. Stassen NA, Williams VA, Gestring ML, et al. Magnetic resonance imaging in combination with helical computed tomography provides a safe and efficient method of cervical spine clearance in the obtunded trauma patient. *J Trauma* 2006;60:171–177.
20. Widder S, Doig C, Burrowes P, et al. Prospective evaluation of computed tomographic scanning for the spinal clearance of obtunded trauma patients: preliminary results. *J Trauma* 2004;56:1179–1184.
21. Harris MB, Kronlage SC, Carboni PA, et al. Evaluation of the cervical spine in the polytrauma patient. *Spine* 2000;25:2884–2891.
22. D'Alise MD, Benzel EC, Hart BL. Magnetic resonance imaging evaluation of the cervical spine in the comatose or obtunded trauma patient. *J Neurosurg* 1999;91(suppl 1):54–59.
23. American College of Surgeons Committee on Trauma. Spine and spinal cord trauma. In: *Advanced Trauma Life Support for Doctors: The Student Manual.* 7th ed. First Impression Publishing, 2004:177–189.
24. Domeier RM. Indications for prehospital spinal immobilization. National Association of EMS Physicians Standards and Clinical Practice Committee. *Prehosp Emerg Care* 1999;3:251–253.
25. Orledge JD, Pepe PE. Out-of-hospital spinal immobilization: is it really necessary? *Acad Emerg Med* 1998; 5:203–204.
26. Hadley MN, Walters BC, Grabb PA, et al. Guidelines for the management of acute cervical spine and spinal cord injuries. *Clin Neurosurg* 2002;49:407–498.
27. Bohlman HH. Acute fractures and dislocations of the cervical spine: An analysis of three hundred hospitalized patients and review of the literature. *J Bone Joint Surg Am* 1979;61:1119–1142.
28. Walter J, Doris PE, Shaffer MA. Clinical presentation of patients with acute cervical spine injury. *Ann Emerg Med* 1984;13:512–515.
29. Prasad VS, Schwartz A, Bhutani R, et al. Characteristics of injuries to the cervical spine and spinal cord in polytrauma patient population: experience from a regional trauma unit. *Spinal Cord* 1999;37:560–568.
30. Lieberman IH, Webb JK. Cervical spine injuries in the elderly. *J Bone Joint Surg Br* 1994;76:877–881.
31. Spivak JM, Weiss MA, Cotler JM, et al. Cervical spine injuries in patients 65 and older. *Spine* 1994; 19:2302–2306.
32. Huelke D, O'Day J. Mandelsohn RA. Cervical injuries suffered in automobile crashes. *J Neurosurg* 1981; 54:316–322.
33. Stiell IG, Wells GA, Vandemheen KL, et al. The Canadian C-Spine Rule for radiography in alert and stable trauma patients. *JAMA* 2001;17;286:1841–1848.
34. Beirne JC, Butler PE, Brady FA. Cervical spine injuries in patients with facial fractures: a 1-year prospective study. *Int J Oral Maxillofac Surg* 1995;24(1 Pt 1):26–29.
35. Hackl W, Hausberger K, Sailer R, et al. Prevalence of cervical spine injuries in patients with facial trauma. *Oral Surg Oral Med Oral Pathol Oral Radiol Endod* 2001;92:370–376.

36. Ardekian L, Gaspar R, Peled M, et al. Incidence and type of cervical spine injuries associated with mandibular fractures. *Craniomaxillofac Trauma* 1997;3:18–21.
37. Haug RH, Wible RT, Likavec MJ, et al. Cervical spine fractures and maxillofacial trauma. *J Oral Maxillofac Surg* 1991;49:725–729.
38. Cohn SM, Lyle WG, Linden CH, et al: Exclusion of cervical spine injury: a prospective study. *J Trauma* 1991;31:570–574.
39. McNamara RM, Heine E, Esposito B. Cervical spine injury and radiography in alert, high-risk patients. *J Emerg Med* 1990;8:177–182.
40. Pasquale M, Fabian TC. Practice management guidelines for trauma from the Eastern Association for the Surgery of Trauma. *J Trauma* 1998;44:941–957.
41. Gonzalez RP, Fried PO, Bukhalo M, et al. Role of clinical examination in screening for blunt cervical spine injury. *J Am Coll Surg* 1999;189:152–157.
42. Stiell IG, Wells GA. Methodologic standards for the development of clinical decision rules in emergency medicine. *Ann Emerg Med* 1999;33:437–447.
43. Roberge RJ, Wears RC. Evaluation of neck discomfort, neck tenderness, and neurologic deficits as indicators for radiography in blunt trauma victims. *J Emerg Med* 1992;10:539–544.
44. Marion DW, Domeier R, Dunham CM, et al. EAST practice management guidelines for identifying cervical spine injuries following trauma: 2000 update. Available at: http://www.east.org/tpg/chap3.pdf.
45. Diliberti T, Lindsey RW. Evaluation of the cervical spine in the emergency setting: who does not need an x-ray? *Orthopedics* 1992;15:179–183.
46. Vandemark RM. Radiology of the cervical spine in trauma patients: practice pitfalls and recommendations for improving efficiency and communications. *Am J Roentgenol* 1990;155:465–472.
47. Ghanta MK, Smith LM, Polin RS, et al. An analysis of Eastern Association for the Surgery of Trauma practice guidelines for cervical spine evaluation in a series of patients with multiple imaging techniques. *Am Surg* 2002; 68:563–567.
48. Kerr D, Bradshaw L, Kelly AM. Implementation of the Canadian C-Spine Rule reduces cervical spine x-ray rate for alert patients with potential neck injury. *J Emerg Med* 2005;28:127–131.
49. Isiklar ZU, Lindsey RW. Low-velocity civilian gunshot wounds of the spine. *Orthopedics* 1997;20:967–972.
50. Lindsey RW, Gugala Z. Spinal cord injury as a result of ballistic trauma. In: Chapman JR, ed. *Spine: State of the Art Reviews.* Vol. 13. Philadelphia: Hanley & Belfus, 1999:529–547.

CHAPTER 9

Spinal Imaging in Cervical Trauma: Clearing the Cervical Spine

Rajiv K. Sethi, Howard Yeon, and Mitchel Harris

INTRODUCTION

The optimal method of assessment and management of the cervical spine in the multiply injured patient requires a consistent approach. Integral to the success of this evaluation process is maintenance of stringent spinal precautions. Spinal imaging in cervical trauma plays an essential part in evaluating both the osseous and neural elements and thus guiding treatment. However, the controversy persists as to whether a cervical spine can be "cleared" without the patient's active involvement in the physical examination.

The assessment of spinal *stability* remains a universal problem. It becomes even more difficult in the setting of polytrauma, impaired mental status secondary to head injury, and drug and alcohol intoxication. There are many issues that carry medical, legal, and economic implications when discussing the initial evaluation and management of the spinal column in the polytrauma patient. How does a clinician avoid missing occult injuries when concentrating on life-threatening or limb-threatening conditions? Who needs cervical spine radiographs in the emergency department? When should flexion-extension radiographs be obtained, and what are the indications for supplemental examinations such as computed tomography (CT) scans, magnetic resonance imaging (MRI) studies, or fluoroscopic evaluations? Finally, in the setting of the absence of bony injury, how does the clinician exclude the diagnosis of a significant soft tissue injury to the cervical spine?

Trauma patients with altered mental status or distracting injuries are often maintained in a hard cervical orthosis until they can be evaluated clinically. Immobilization in a hard collar for an extended period, especially in the intensive care unit, puts patients at risk for pressure sores and increased intracranial pressures, as well as interfering with daily nursing care.[1–4] There is evidence that decubitus formation is directly related to the length of time the collar is in place.[5,6]

Approximately 30 million injuries necessitating medical care occur annually in the United States.[1,7] Cervical spine injuries occur in 2% to 4% of all trauma patients, with nearly 30,000 neck injuries documented annually.[1,7–9] The development of the Advanced Trauma Life Support (ATLS) system by the American College of Surgeons (ACS) has aided in the evaluation and overall management of the trauma patient.[9] The ATLS protocol is applicable to any trauma patient with the implicit goal of identifying limb-threatening and life-threatening injuries while eliminating the likelihood of missed injuries and delayed diagnosis.

Integral to the ATLS protocol is the issue of accurately assessing the status of the cervical spine. However, a comprehensive protocol for evaluating and deeming the cervical spine free of injury in the polytrauma patient has not been uniformly accepted by clinicians.[10,11] This is particularly relevant to the assessment of ligamentous injuries in the polytrauma patient or the patient with altered sensorium resulting from head injury or alcohol or drug intoxication. These patients are unable to provide the necessary clinical feedback and thus are at increased risk for complications as a result of missed injuries.[8,12–18]

Missed or delayed diagnosis of a cervical spine injury can lead to the onset of a neurologic injury or the progression of an incomplete lesion.[19,20] The literature is replete with articles identifying the small subset of trauma patients who do not need radiographic assessment: the sober, alert patient without neck pain, tenderness, or the presence of distracting injuries, who can demonstrate a full, active range of motion.[9,17,21–23] Conversely, there is little agreement concerning a protocol to clear the cervical spine in the intoxicated, multiply injured, or head-injured patient.[13] The ATLS guidelines state: ". . . patients who are comatose, have an altered level of consciousness, or are too young to describe their symptoms may be cleared after normal three-view cervical spine series (trauma series) and an appropriate clinical evaluation by an orthopedic surgeon or neurosurgeon."[9] Unfortunately, there are no directives or a consensus about what comprises an appropriate clinical evaluation.

Plain radiographs of the cervical spine have largely been replaced by axial CT images and their sagittal and coronal reconstructions. The advent of multidetector CT scanners has greatly increased the speed and accuracy of the reconstructions. However, the lateral view of the cervical spine is still commonly obtained in the setting of a polytrauma victim, particularly those with hemodynamic instability. A well-performed lateral cervical spine x-ray examination with visualization from the occipital-cervical junction through the cervical thoracic junction can provide enough information to the trauma surgeons to allow the trauma patient to proceed to the operating room without additional intervention aside from the maintenance of a collar.[24]

Brown et al.[25] recently demonstrated that helical CT in their institution identified 99.3% of all fractures of the cervical, thoracic, and lumbar spine, and those missed by helical CT required minimal or no treatment.[25] Newer studies are showing that helical CT scans are cost effective. A study from Vanderbilt Medical Center showed cervical spine evaluation with helical CT scan has an expected cost of U.S. $554 per patient compared with U.S. $2142 for plain films. These authors state that helical CT scan is the preferred initial screening test for detection of cervical spine fractures among moderate- to high-risk patients seen in urban trauma centers, reducing the incidence of paralysis resulting from false-negative imaging study findings and institutional costs, when settlement costs are taken into account.[26] Similarly, more recent studies confirm the benefits of whole body CT scans for detection of visceral injuries of the abdomen as well as bony injuries of the pelvis and spine.[27–30]

Once a spinal injury is suspected or localized, dedicated CT studies of that area may be beneficial for long-term management and particularly for preoperative planning. Coronal and sagittal plane reconstructions can assist the surgeon in appreciating the degree of deformity and the severity of injury. CT reconstructions can also help to identify subtle rotational or translational deformities at the fracture site.

Detecting the presence of a ligamentous injury in the trauma patient with altered mental status poses a difficult diagnostic dilemma. The use of the CT scan as the primary radiographic instrument is highly effective for occult bony injuries but is neither sensitive nor specific for detecting ligamentous injuries.[31–33] The reasons are twofold. The plane of the ligament injury often coincides with the orientation of the CT cuts, and the soft tissue windows commonly used in conjunction with the bony windows are rarely sensitive enough to identify these injuries accurately. Sagittal reconstructions reformatted from the axial cuts can also be misleading because of minor degrees of patient movement, gantry alignment not in parallel with the spine, and the fact that the study is generally performed with the patient in the supine position, thus eliminating any of the deforming forces of gravity.

Traditionally, surgeon-controlled passive flexion-extension has been viewed as potentially dangerous to the anesthetized trauma patient and to the unprotected spinal cord. In the senior author's previously published algorithm,[11] fluoroscopically visualized surgeon-controlled flexion-extension views were used to definitively eliminate the presence of an occult ligamentous injury. This maneuver was only performed once the in-line (axial) stretch test was noted to be negative; that is, there was no evidence of gross ligamentous instability. If the in-line stretch test detected instability, the neck was maintained in an orthosis and MRI imaging was ordered.

If the stretch test was negative, the fluoroscopically visualized flexion-extension maneuver was performed. This proved to be a safe, effective method to detect three purely ligamentous injuries with a series of nearly 150 patients.[11] However, despite the presence of many other studies demonstrating the utility of a physician-controlled flexion-extension evaluation, this method has too many unresolved issues to make it practical.[34,35] Should there be spinal cord monitoring performed during the maneuver? Who should actually perform the test? What happens if the entire cervical spine cannot be visualized during the maneuver? The cumulative literature on physician-directed flexion-extension has nearly 900 patients enrolled, with 10 ligamentous injuries identified.[36] There was one recorded neurologic injury, identified in a protocol violation. Eliminating the dynamic testing method leaves MRI imaging as the next most popular option.[37,38]

MRI is the most sensitive imaging method for evaluation of soft tissues. Thus MRI of the spine provides the best imaging of neurologic structures, ligaments, and the intervertebral disc. MRI is not routinely used in the evaluation of the polytrauma patient because of the time required to perform a technically adequate scan in an environment that might not allow all of the necessary monitoring equipment. MRI is most useful in patients whose plain radiographs or CT scan results fall short of explaining their full clinical picture. This is most common in the neurologically impaired victim with "normal" appearing plain films. Vaccaro et al.[39] reported that 25% of patients with cervicothoracic injuries and a neurologic deficit on presentation had their preliminary treatment plan altered after obtaining an MRI. In the same study cohort, the authors revealed that routine MRI did not alter the treatment plan in the neurologically intact patients.

MRI can provide valuable information about the status of the ligaments without risk to the spinal cord commonly associated with physician-directed flexion-extension evaluations.[40] However, there is some controversy regarding the necessity of obtaining the MRI within 48 hours of the trauma.[41] An earlier study would benefit the assessment and management of the polytrauma patient but is often impractical because of the patient's associated injuries. Additional reviews of the benefits of MRI do not support the necessity of the 48- to 72-hour recommendation.[42–44] The senior author does not limit the use of the MRI to the initial 48 hours.

Classical teaching refers to subacute flexion-extension radiographs for definitive evaluation of occult ligamentous injuries of the cervical spine. This method is commonly used with the trauma patient who can be effectively mobilized in a collar after the CT scan is noted to be "normal." However, even in this more controlled setting, flexion-extension radiographs will not be effective if on the initial lateral radiograph the cervical-thoracic junction is unable to be visualized. Acute flexion-extension radiographs have not been demonstrated to be effective in identifying occult ligamentous injuries because of underlying muscular splinting. Therefore, flexion-extension radiographs in the early evaluation of the polytrauma patient are rarely obtained.

A clear understanding of the ATLS protocol is essential for optimal care of the multiply injured patient. The cervical spine remains an area of controversy regarding early recognition of occult injuries. The results of a previous study by Harris et al.[11] highlight the fact that neither fellowship-trained traumatologists nor spinal surgeons have a uniform approach to the assessment of the cervical spine in the setting of the multiply injured patient. Further work needs to be done regarding the standardization of protocols regarding radiologic clearance of the cervical spine.

REFERENCES

1. Davis JW, Phreaner DL, Hoat DB, et al. The etiology of missed cervical spine injuries. *J Trauma* 1993;34: 342–346.
2. Fazl M, LeFebvre J, Willinsky RA, et al. Posttraumatic ligamentous disruption of the cervical spine, an easily overlooked diagnosis: presentation of three cases. *Neurosurgery* 1990;26:674–678.
3. Gerrelts BD, Petersen EU, Mabry J, et al. Delayed diagnosis of cervical spin injuries. *J Trauma* 1991;31:905–907.
4. Webb JK, Broughton RB, McSweeney, T et al. Hidden flexion injury of the cervical spine. *J Bone Joint Surg Br* 1976;58:674–678.
5. Chendrasekhar A, Moorman DW, Timberlake GA. An evaluation of the effects of semirigid cervical collars in patients with severe closed head injury. *Am Surg* 1998;67:604–606.
6. Plaisier B, Gabram SG, Schwartz RJ, et al. Prospective evaluation of craniofacial pressure in four different cervical orthoses. *J Trauma* 1994;37:714–726.
7. National Center for Health Statistics. National Hospital Ambulatory Medical Care Survey. Hyattsville, Md: National Center for Health Statistics, 1994.
8. Bachulis BL, Long WB, Hynes GD, et al. Clinical indication for cervical spine radiographs in the traumatized patient. *Am J Surg* 1987;153:473–478.
9. Committee on Trauma, American College of Surgeons. *Advanced Trauma Life Support.* Chicago: American College of Surgeons, 1997.
10. Herr CH, Ball PA, Sargent SK, et al. Sensitivity of prevertebral soft tissue measurement of C3 for detection of cervical spine fractures and dislocations. *Am J Emerg Med* 1998;16:346–349.
11. Harris MB, Kronlage SC, Carboni PA, et al. Evaluation of the cervical spine in the polytrauma patient. *Spine* 2000;25:2884–2891.
12. Davis JW, Parks SN, Detlefs CL, et al. Clearing the cervical spine in obtunded patients: the use of dynamic fluoroscopy. *J Trauma* 1995;39:435–438.
13. Harris M, Waguespack A, Kronlage S. Clearing the cervical spine in trauma patients: are we really sure its OK to remove the collar? *Orthopedics* 1997;20:903–907.
14. Lindsey RW, Diliberti TC, Doherty BJ, et al. Efficacy of radiologic evaluation of the cervical spine in emergency situations. *South Med J* 1993;86:1253–1255.
15. MacDonald RL, Schwartz ML, Mirich D, et al. Diagnosis of cervical spine injury in motor vehicle victims: how many x-rays are enough? *J Trauma* 1990;30:392–397.
16. Roberge RJ, Wears RC, Kelly M, et al. Selective application of cervical spine radiography in alert victims of blunt trauma: a prospective study. *J Trauma* 1988;28:784–788.
17. Ross S, O'Malley KF, Delong WG, et al. Clinical predictors of cervical spine injury in blunt high energy transfer injuries [abstract]. *Ann Emerg Med* 1987;165:498–499.
18. Shaffer MA, Doris PE. Limitation of the cross table lateral view in detecting cervical spine injuries: a retrospective analysis. *Ann Emerg Med* 1981;10:508–513.
19. Reid DC, Henderson R, Saboe L, et al. Etiology and clinical course of missed spine fractures. *J Trauma* 1988;28:784–788.
20. Stiell IG, Wells GA, Vandemheen K, et al. Variation in emergency department use of cervical spine radiography for alert, stable trauma patients. *Can Med Assoc J* 1997;156:1537–1544.
21. Fisher RP. Cervical radiograph evaluation of alert patients following blunt trauma. *Ann Emerg Med* 1984;13: 905–907.
22. Ringenberg BJ, Fisher AK, Urdaneta FL, et al. Rational ordering of cervical spine radiographs following trauma. *Ann Emerg Med* 1988;17:792–796.
23. Sees DN, Rodriguez-Cruz LR, Flaherty SF, et al. The use of bedside fluoroscopy to evaluate the cervical spine in obtunded trauma patients. *J Trauma* 1998;45:768–771.
24. Geusens E, Van Breuseghem I, Pans S, et al. Some tips and tricks in reading cervical spine radiographs in trauma patients. *JBR-BTR* 2005;88:87–92.
25. Brown CV, Antevil JL, Sise MJ, et al. Spiral computed tomography for the diagnosis of cervical, thoracic, and lumbar spine fractures: its time has come. *J Trauma* 2005;58:890–895, discussion 895–896.
26. Grogan EL, Morris JA Jr, Dittus RS, et al. Cervical spine evaluation in urban trauma centers: lowering institutional costs and complications through helical CT scan. *J Am Coll Surg* 2005;200:160–165.
27. Roos JE, Hilfiker P, Platz A, et al. MDCT in emergency radiology: is a standardized chest or abdominal protocol sufficient for evaluation of thoracic and lumbar spine trauma? *AJR Am J Roentgenol* 2004;183:959–968.
28. Albrecht T, von Schlippenbach J, Stahel PF, et al. The role of whole body spiral CT in the primary work-up of polytrauma patients: comparison with conventional radiography and abdominal sonography. *Rofo* 2004;176: 1142–1150.
29. Hauser CJ, Visvikis G, Hinrichs C, et al. Prospective validation of computed tomographic screening of the thoracolumbar spine in trauma. *J Trauma* 2003;55:228–234, discussion 234–235.

30. Sheridan R, Peralta R, Rhea J, et al. Reformatted visceral protocol helical computed tomographic scanning allows conventional radiographs of the thoracic and lumbar spine to be eliminated in the evaluation of blunt trauma patients. *J Trauma* 2003;55:665–669.
31. Blacksin MF, Lee HJ. Frequency and significance of fractures of the upper cervical spine detected by CT in patients with severe neck trauma. *AJR Am J Roentgenol* 1995;165:1201–1204.
32. Schleehauf K, Ross SE, Civil ID, et al. Computed tomography in the initial evaluation of the cervical spine. *Ann Emerg Med* 1989;18:815–817.
33. Tehranzadeh J, Bonk RT, Ansari A, et al. Efficacy of limited CT for nonvisualized lower cervical spine in patients with blunt trauma. *Skeletal Radiol* 1994;23:349–352.
34. Ajani AE, Cooper DJ, Scheinkestel CD, et al. Optimal assessment of cervical spine trauma in critically ill patients: a prospective evaluation. *Anaesth Intensive Care* 1998;26:487–491.
35. Davis JW, Kaups KL, Cunningham MA, et al. Routine evaluation of the cervical spine in head-injured patients with dynamic fluoroscopy: a reappraisal. *J Trauma* 2001;50:1044–1047.
36. Sliker CW, Mirvis SE, Shanmuganathan K. Assessing cervical spine stability in obtunded blunt trauma patients: review of medical literature. *Radiology* 2005;234:733–739.
37. Bolinger B, Shartz M, Marion D. Bedside fluoroscopic flexion and extension cervical spine radiographs for clearance of the cervical spine in comatose trauma patients. *J Trauma* 2004;56:132–136.
38. Griffiths HJ, Wagner J, Anglen J, et al. The use of forced flexion/extension views in the obtunded trauma patient. *Skeletal Radiol* 2002;31:587–591.
39. Vaccaro R, Kreidel KO, Pan W, et al. Usefulness of MRI in isolated upper cervical spine fractures in adults. *J Spinal Disord* 1998;11:289–294.
40. Harris MB, Shilt J. The potentially unstable cervical spine: evaluation techniques. *Tech Orthop* 2002;17:278–286.
41. D'Alise MD, Benzel EC, Hart BL. Magnetic resonance imaging evaluation of the cervical spine in the comatose or obtunded trauma patient. *J Neurosurg* 1999;91(suppl 1):54–59.
42. Morris CG, McCoy E. Clearing the cervical spine in unconscious polytrauma victims, balancing risks and effective screening. *Anaesthesia* 2004;59:464–482.
43. Hogan GJ, Mirvis SE, Shanmuganathan K, et al. Exclusion of unstable cervical spine injury in obtunded patients with blunt trauma: is MR imaging needed when multi-detector row CT findings are normal? *Radiology* 2005;237:106–113.
44. Green RA, Saifuddin A. Whole spine MRI in the assessment of acute vertebral body trauma. *Skeletal Radiol* 2004;33:129–135.

SECTION V

Principles of Nonoperative Treatment

CHAPTER 10

Cervical Orthoses

Michael K. Rosner and Timothy R. Kuklo

INTRODUCTION

Cervical orthoses have been used for almost 5000 years; however, a standardized terminology was not developed until the 1970s by the American Academy of Orthopaedic Surgeons.[1,2] This classification categorizes cervical orthoses into two distinct groups: cervical orthoses and cervicothoracic orthoses, with the main difference being that cervicothoracic orthoses extend onto the upper thorax for additional stabilization. By considering these two broad categories, some confusion may be eliminated by the numerous named devices, which appears to cause confusion for many prescribers. Because they are classified as Class I devices, there is little oversight by the Food and Drug Administration. Unfortunately, there is also little research into the actual areas of stabilization and decreased motion, increased stress, and actual biomechanical consequences of many newer orthoses.[3–17] Additionally, with the advances in internal fixation with modern instrumentation systems and the increased pressure to return the injured to work, surgical stabilization is more popular today, and cervical orthoses are less frequently used for primarily management of cervical trauma. Recent advances in three-dimensional imaging and computer modeling, however, may help improve our understanding of their effects.[18]

At the same time, braces have significantly advanced over the past several decades as a result of the engineering advances in lightweight materials, composites, and polymer resins, which are more durable and comfortable.[19] For instance, many braces are now made of durable thermoplastic, the most popular being polypropylene, without compromised cervical stabilization.[20,21] This is a great advance from the earliest braces, which were made of iron, wood, paper, and glue.[22] Some of the biomechanical principles remain the same today and can be traced back to Hippocrates.[2] These advances, along with advanced imaging such as magnetic resonance imaging (MRI), have also improved our ability to assess alignment and fracture healing. For instance, graphite and titanium are compatible with MRI and have been used in halo vest orthoses.

Regardless, it is the duty of the prescribing spine specialist to fully understand the biomechanics of the cervical spine, injury mechanisms and forces, and biomechanical principles of various cervical orthoses to optimize their use. As well, it is the duty of the patient to understand the proper wear and care of the orthosis, which takes additional time and teaching to maximize compliance.

BIOMECHANICS OF THE CERVICAL SPINE

The cervical spine is ideally designed to maximize interaction with the environment; thus, it is a highly mobile area of the spine, which is biomechanically susceptible to injury because of the large weight of the head at the cephalad end. Range of motion is determined by disc size and flexibility, facet orientation and shape, constraining anatomy such as ligamentous laxity and the integrity of the joint capsules, and the lever arm and muscle connections. Although most motion is a combination of various directions, the simplest method to understand cervical motion is to consider the motion in terms of flexion-extension, lateral bending, and rotation.

Various studies of range of motion have been performed in a normal population. These values have been reported as an average flexion of 70 ± 10 degrees, lateral bending of 45 ± 10 degrees, and axial rotation of 75 ± 10 degrees.[23] Another way of considering flexion-extension is the relative contribution of various segments to overall motion, with approximately 50% of the flexion-extension occurring at the occiput-C1 articulation, and approximately 50% spread throughout the subaxial cervical spine. It is generally thought that C5-C6 is the most mobile segment, followed by C4-C5, which was reported as the most mobile segment by other authors.[23,24] The greatest lateral bending appears to occur at C3-C4 and C4-C5, and the greatest rotation easily occurring at C1-C2. Just as important, there also appears to be a slight anterior translation of the cephalad cervical vertebral body at each motion segment with flexion and posterior translation or return with extension.[25]

Cervical motion following instrumentation and the effect on adjacent segments should also be considered. In a computer model of disc strain after anterior cervical discectomy and fusion (ACDF), Matsunaga et al.[26] found a 20% increased strain on adjacent segment discs at 1 year follow-up for both two- and three-level fusions with anterior cervical plate. As well, they found that 11 of 13 discs with a postoperative longitudinal strain had a small herniated nucleus pulposus. This effect is exaggerated, with longer level fusions and following anterior-posterior (360 degree) fusions.[27]

The cervicothoracic junction is relatively immobile and a high-stress transitional zone as well. This is an increasingly recognized compromised area, which may have been underappreciated previously. Care should be taken to fully evaluate any potential effect of cervical orthosis "immobilization" after cervical injury or surgery on this area. With rigid internal fixation, this area is also increasingly recognized as an area potentially requiring instrumentation and fusion because it carries the highest stress loads secondary to the facet orientation changes and higher adjacent level stress loads secondary to the instrumentation.

BIOMECHANICS OF ORTHOSES

An orthosis is generally defined as an external device applied to the body to restrict motion.[1] In effect, these devices control motion or position, thus providing support and prevention of deformity as well.[17] In general, approximation of the orthosis to a bony structure will increase stability. In the cervical spine, this can be difficult because the soft tissue structures of the anterior neck do not permit any direct pressure. Therefore, stability must be obtained through the mandible and/or occiput, while resting at the base of the neck on the trapezius muscles. This can be quite difficult because the spine is highly mobile.[7–9,27–30]

CERVICAL ORTHOSES

Cervical orthoses come in a variety of materials and forms. Nonetheless, they are simply a modified cylinder, which is applied as either two connected "half shells" or as a wrapped shell usually opening in the back.[31] A soft collar is the most simplified form (Fig. 10.1). It provides very limited stability, mostly by reducing flexion-extension, because it acts primarily as a proprioceptive reminder to limit neck motion. A Velcro connector is placed posteriorly, and the soft collar is placed in the neck in neutral to slight extension depending on the height of the collar. They come

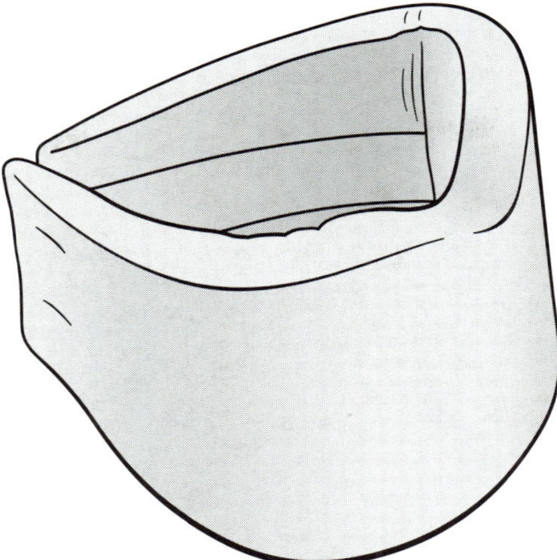

FIGURE 10.1. The soft collar has a foam insert that is designed to place the Velcro strap posteriorly.

in various sizes; however, because the collar is made of foam, a neck cutout can be easily fashioned if necessary, or the collar can be reversed to permit some flexion. This is a popular collar for whiplash injuries or postoperative support following a one- or two-level ACDF with instrumentation because cervical stability is provided by the cervical plate and interbody graft, as opposed to the orthosis. As well, this collar is inexpensive and generally very well tolerated. Biomechanically, it restricts only about 10% of cervical motion.[8] Most other cervical orthoses are made of more rigid composite materials.

Other common cervical orthoses include the Philadelphia (Fig. 10.2), C-Breeze (Fig. 10.3A,B) and Aspen (Fig. 10.4) collars. The Philadelphia collar is made of Plastazote with plastic reinforcing struts, and therefore, it can be worn in the shower. It is also fairly inexpensive, but may not be well tolerated. Additionally, it provides more restriction to motion than a soft collar. The Miami J is a two-piece orthosis. It has soft removable pads that line the plastic shell. Motion restriction is better than with the Philadelphia and soft collars. Similar to the Miami J, the Aspen collar has two pieces

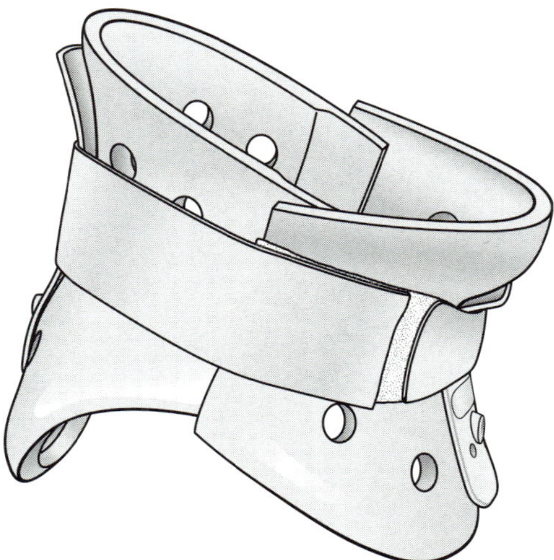

FIGURE 10.2. Philadelphia collar is made of a semirigid Plastazote that is reinforced by plastic struts.

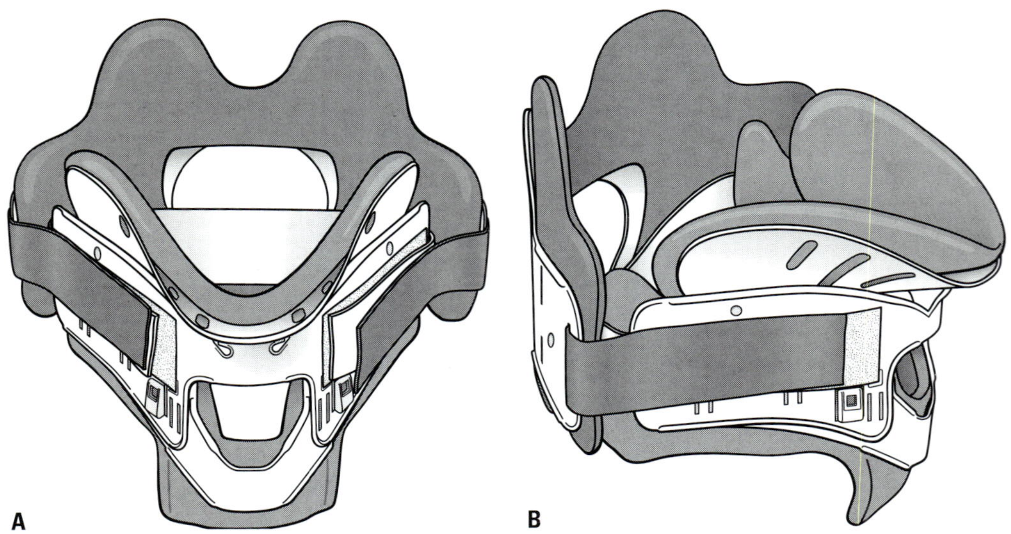

FIGURE 10.3. The C-Breeze orthosis is a two-piece design made of polyethylene and a soft liner.

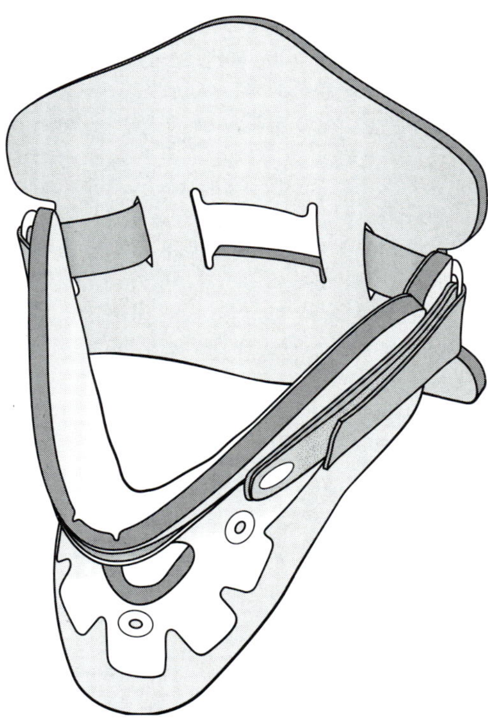

FIGURE 10.4. The Aspen orthosis is similar to the Miami J collar in that it is a two-piece design made of polyethylene.

and removable pads. It does not restrict motion as well as the Miami J, but it does offer a posterior cutout for posterior incisions and a thoracic extension if needed. The Miami J and Aspen collars are the primary collars used in our institution for prolonged cervical immobilization because their relative ease of wear.

Multiple studies have been completed using goniometry, roentgenography, and cineradiography to determine the residual cervical motion with various cervical orthoses.[3,7–9,17,29,30] Some authors consider roentgenography to be the most accurate methodology; however, conflicting studies have shown goniometry to be an adequate tool for general postimmobilzation range of motion.[7]

The first study to evaluate postimmobilization range of motion was conducted in 1960.[11] In this study, Jones examined both soft and rigid collars and found that none of the collars significantly restricted cervical motion, but, expectedly, hard collars were better than soft collars. Other studies have been performed since then using various methods to quantify motion.[4,5,7,11,25,28,30,32,33] The consensus from these studies is that flexion-extension is controlled better than lateral bending or axial rotation[5,7,9,17,28,33] (Fig. 10.5). For instance, in normal subjects, the Philadelphia collar has been

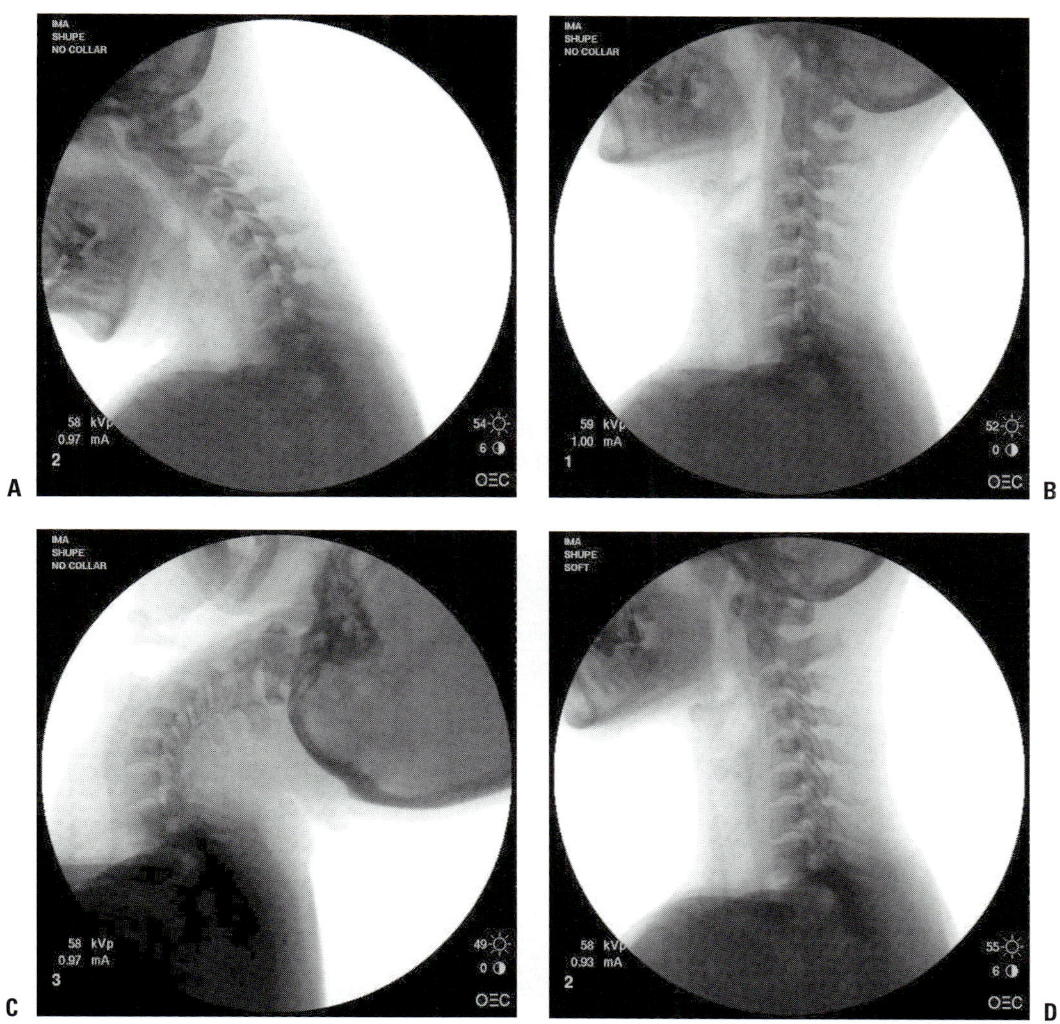

FIGURE 10.5. **A–C.** Lateral fluoroscopic radiograph (OEC, Salt Lake City, Utah) of flexion–lateral extension without a cervical orthosis, with a soft collar **(D–F)**, and with an Aspen collar **(G–I)**. Note that there is only a moderate decreased overall range of motion with the different orthoses. *(continued)*

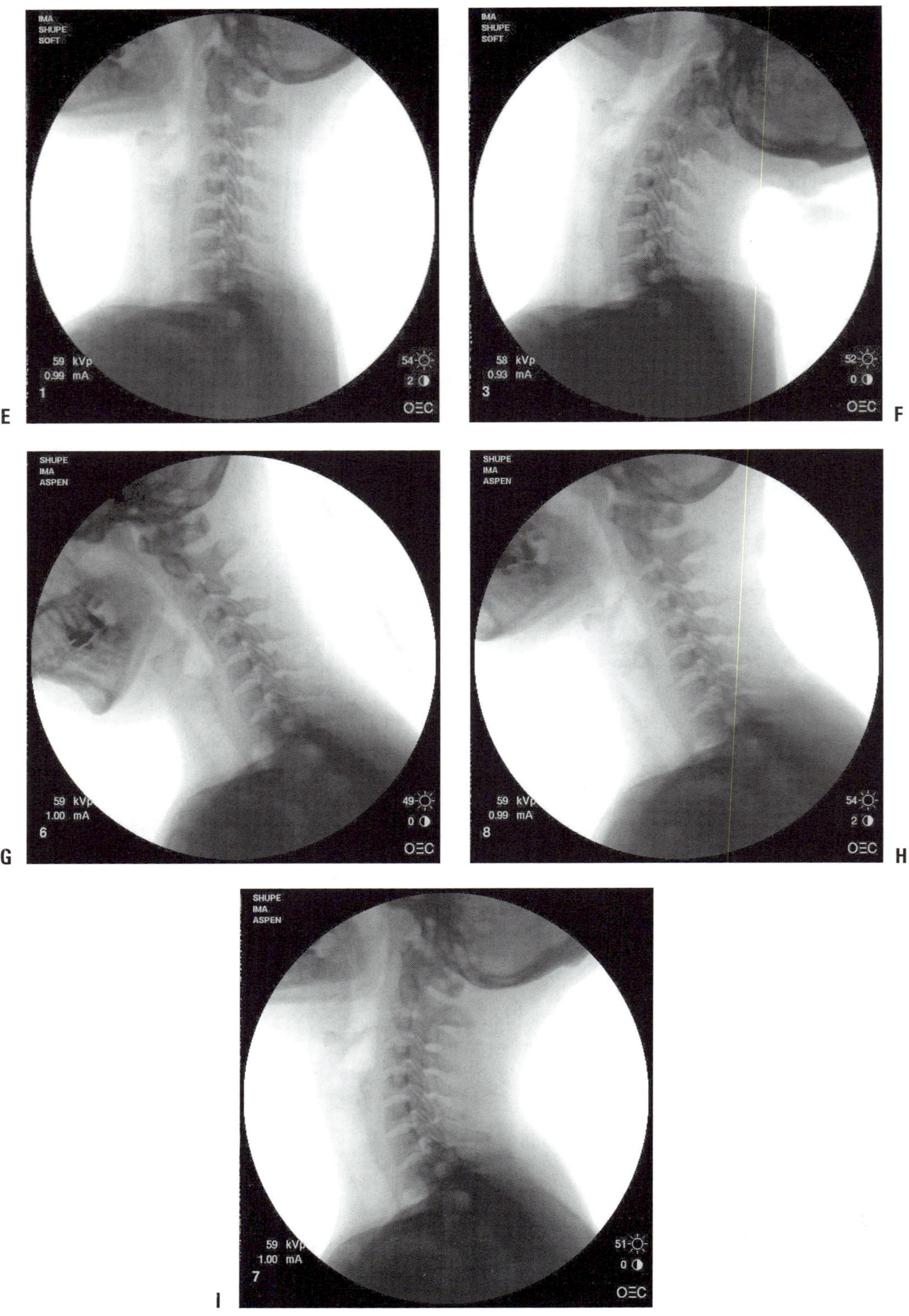

FIGURE 10.5. *(continued)*

shown to limit flexion-extension by 46%, lateral bending by 25%, and axial rotation by 29%.[28] In comparison, the NecLoc collar reduced flexion-extension by 62%, lateral bending by 43%, and axial rotation by 62%. The NecLoc collar, like the Stifneck collar, is a one-piece orthosis that is quite rigid and easy to store. The primary purpose of these collars is in prehospital transport of accident victims.[19] Similarly, in a separate study, four contemporary orthoses were studied: the Philadelphia collar, Miami J collar, Malibu collar, and Aspen collar.[31] In this study, the Malibu collar restricted cervical motion the best.

Additionally, occiput-C1 motion is increased with the use of cervical orthoses. Further, obese patients are more difficult to fit with a cervical orthosis, often requiring a more stout, short orthosis. None of these devices immobilize obese patients as well as thin patients.[17]

Complications

The most common problem from cervical orthoses is skin irritation or breakdown, especially with the rigid one-piece orthoses or in comatose or insensate individuals.[15] Therefore, these orthoses are primarily limited to prehospital transport of the injured. When necessary for long-term wear, skin irritation and breakdown can be reduced by trimming or shaving the hair beneath the brace on the posterior neck.[19] In a study using a sterno-occipito-mandibular immobilizer (SOMI) brace, skin contact pressures were noted to be in excess of the capillary closing pressure.[34] With adjustment, the pressures were reduced.

Other reported problems include local pain and rash and a continued sense of instability or inadequate immobilization. These problems are secondary to the inherent nature of the orthosis, as well as the varying anatomy of the soft tissues in individuals because customized fitting is not practical. Some patients are also "bothered" by the sense of a constricting device around the neck. Hair loss over the back of the occiput has also occurred following prolonged use as a result of the constant pressure, and muscle atrophy, soft tissue contracture, and decreased pulmonary function have been reported.[15]

Finally, perhaps the most common and least reported problem with cervical orthoses is noncompliance. It is extremely difficult to determine the incidence or effect of this "complication," but it is certainly significant. One means of reducing noncompliance is to ensure proper fit, which would minimize patient discomfort, minimize skin pressure, and limit skin breakdown problems.

CERVICOTHORACIC ORTHOSES

Cervicothoracic orthoses add an additional restriction of motion by providing supports that connect the mandible and occiput to the thorax. The primary effect is restriction of flexion-extension. Popular orthoses include the Yale brace, the SOMI brace, the Minerva brace, the halo vest and others. As well, the Aspen brace (see Fig. 10.4) can be converted to a cervicothoracic orthosis with an attachable thoracic extension. This has both anterior and posterior chest pads, as well as shoulder pads connected by straps. The SOMI has a solid anterior chest piece and shoulder supports that are attached by a strap, along with the mandible and occiput supports. It is best at restricting neck flexion, but not good at restricting extension. The Yale brace has both an anterior and posterior thorax piece, which is connected by a strap, but there are no shoulder supports.

Multiple studies have compared various cervical versus cervicothoracic orthoses. In a study comparing the Philadelphia collar, the Camp collar, a four-poster brace, and the SOMI, the four-poster brace was found to best immobilize the middle and lower cervical spine.[7] The SOMI best limited motion of the upper cervical spine. The Philadelphia collar performed the worst, especially from the occiput to C2. In a separate study, the best flexion-extension stability was found in the halo vest, followed by a cervicothoracic brace, a four-poster brace, a SOMI brace and Philadelphia collar, and a soft collar.[9] This was true at all cervical levels, and the halo vest was the only orthosis to control flexion-extension from the occiput to C2. However, not even halo vest immobilization is ideal. In a

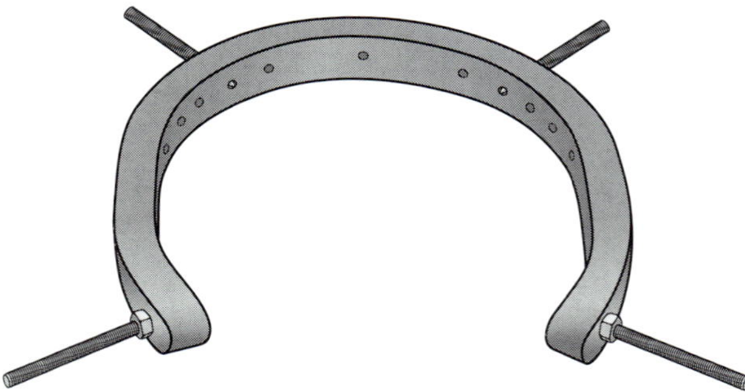

FIGURE 10.6. Halo "ring" or horseshoe.

study by Anderson et al.,[35] supine and upright lateral radiographs were obtained in 42 patients within 5 days after placement of a halo vest. The greatest motion occurred between the occiput and C1 (average 8 degrees), whereas other noninjured levels averaged 3 degrees, while injured levels averaged 7 degrees of motion and 1.7 mm of translation. The authors also found at least 3 degrees of motion and 1 mm of translation at 77% of the injured levels.[35] Similarly, in a halo cast study, C4-C5 was found to have an average of 7.2 degrees of motion.[36] Neck forces varied significantly from the supine to upright position.

The halo vest is the most rigid means of cervical immobilization, first being used in 1959 by attaching a halo ring to a cast by rods.[37] It was originally designed as a complete ring but is now generally used as an incomplete ring or horseshoe (Fig. 10.6). To date, it has been used for various traumas, infection, tumors, degenerative and inflammatory disorders, congenital malformation, and arthrodesis.[38–43] Various biomechanical studies have noted its excellent ability to immobilize the upper cervical spine, with residual motion in the middle and lower cervical spine.[32,36,44–49] As noted earlier, there is also a settling effect when moving from the supine to upright position, thus having little effect on axial loading.[36]

The halo vest is usually applied in the supine position, by placing the patient's head on a headboard that is suspended over the edge of the bed. This allows access to the posterior skull. If this is not possible, the pins can be placed in a more anterior position and later replaced. The ring should be sized just inferior to the equator of the skull and should permit at least 1 cm of clearance throughout. The pins should be placed alternately front and back to avoid asymmetric ring placement, and the patient's eyes should be closed. In adults, four pins are usually adequate and should be tightened to 8 in-lb with a torque wrench. For children, six to eight pins at 1 to 2 in-lb is recommended.[46,50,51] As well, the frontal pins should avoid the supraorbital and supratrochlear nerves and be placed in the safe zone or over the lateral two-thirds of the orbit (Fig. 10.7). If the patient is awake, the pin sites should be prepped and infiltrated with a local anesthetic. Hair should be removed from around the posterior pin sites. The vest is made of lightweight plastics and abundant padding, which is applied by log-rolling the patient with in-line cervical traction. Upright anteroposterior (AP) and lateral radiographs are obtained after placement. Current designs permit adjustments to the connecting rods if necessary. As a result of loosening, the pins should be retorqued within 24 to 48 hours after placement.

Complications

The most common complication is pin site infection, which is usually secondary to loosening.[50–52] Local wound care and oral antibiotics are usually adequate, but these should be aggressively managed to prevent an infection of the skull. The eyes should be closed during placement, but not too tightly. If not shut, then closure of the eyelids may not be possible, and if shut too tightly, it may be difficult to open the eyelids. Other reported complications include painful mas-

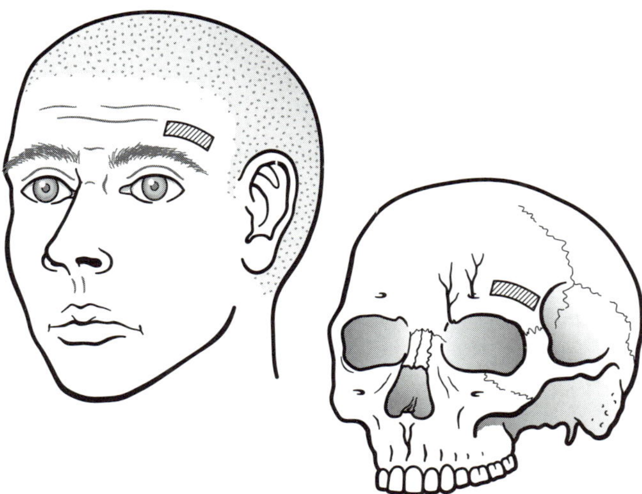

FIGURE 10.7. Schematic view of "safe zone" over the lateral two-thirds of the orbit. Note location of the supratrochlear and suprarobital nerves.

tication from placing the pins into the temporalis muscle, loss of fracture reduction, and graft displacement.[44,46,47,50–53]

CONCLUSION

Cervical orthoses have significantly advanced in the past 20 years secondary to the advances in materials engineering. However, at the same time, many cervical orthoses have not been well studied and, hence, their efficacy is not proven. Consequently, it is the duty of the prescribing spine specialist to fully understand the biomechanics of the cervical spine, injury mechanisms and forces, and biomechanical principles of various cervical orthoses to optimize their use.

REFERENCES

1. American Academy of Orthopaedic Surgeons: *Atlas of Orthotics.* St. Louis: CV Mosby, 1975.
2. Smith GE. The most ancient splints. *Br Med J* 1908;1:732.
3. Cline JR, Scheidel E, Bigsby EF. A comparison of methods of cervical immobilization used in patient extrication and transport. *J Trauma* 1985;25:649–653.
4. Colachis SC, Strohm BR. Radiographic studies of cervical spine motion in normal subjects. *Arch Phys Med Rehabil* 1965;46:753–760.
5. Colachis SC, Strohm BR, Ganter EL. Cervical spine motion in normal women: a radiographic study of effect of cervical collars. *Arch Phys Med Rehabil* 1973;54:161–169.
6. Fidler MW, Plasmans CMT. The effect of four types of support on the segmental mobility of the lumbosacral spine. *J Bone Joint Surg Am* 1983;65:943–947.
7. Fisher SV, Bower JF, Awad EA, et al. Cervical orthoses' effect on cervical spine motion: roentgenographic and goniometric method of study. *Arch Phys Med Rehabil* 1977;58:109–115.
8. Hartman JT, Palumbo F, Hill JB. Cineradiography of the braced normal cervical spine. *Clin Orthop* 1975;109:97–102.
9. Johnson RM, Hart DL, Simmons EF, et al. Cervical orthoses: a study comparing their effectiveness in restricting cervical motion in normal subjects. *J Bone Joint Surg Am* 1977;59:332–339.
10. Johnson RM, Owen JR, Hart DL, et al. Cervical orthoses. *Clin Orthop* 1981;154:34–45.
11. Jones MD. Cineradiographic studies of the collar-immobilized cervical spine. *J Neurosurg* 1960;17:633–637.
12. Lantz SA, Schultz AB. Lumbar spine orthosis wearing. *Spine* 1986;11:838–842.
13. Nachemson A, Schultz A, Anderson GB. Mechanical effectiveness of the lumbar spine orthoses. *Scand J Rehab Med Suppl* 1983;9:139–149.

14. Nakmura T, Oh-Hama M, Shingu H. A new orthosis for fixation of the cervical spine: fronto-occipito-zygomatic orthosis. *Orthot Prosthest* 1984;38:41.
15. Sypert GW. External spinal orthotics. *Neurosurgery* 1987;20:642–649.
16. Waters RL, Morris JM. Effect of spinal supports on the electrical activity of muscles of the trunk. *J Bone Joint Surg Am* 1970;52:51–60.
17. White AA, Panjabi MM. *Clinical Biomechanics of the Spine.* Toronto: JB Lippincott, 1978.
18. Zhang S, Wortley M, Clowers K, et al. Evaluation of efficacy and 3D kinematic characteristics of cervical orthoses. *Clin Biomech* 2005;20:264–269.
19. Anderson DG, Vaccaro AR, Gavin KF. *Cervical Orthoses and Cranioskeletal Traction.* New York: Lippincott Williams and Wilkins, 2005.
20. Richter D, Latta LL, Milne EL, et al. The stabilizing effects of different orthoses in the intact and unstable upper cervical spine: a cadaver study. *J Trauma* 50:848–854, 2001.
21. Barnes JW, Harwell AD. Technical note: the use of low heat thermoplastics in vacuum forming. *Orthot Prosthet* 1986;40:58.
22. Botte MJ, Garfin SR, Bergmann K, et al. *Spinal Orthoses for Traumatic and Degenerative Disease.* Philadelphia: WB Saunders, 1999.
23. Kottke FL, Mundle MO. Range of mobility of the cervical spine. *Arch Phys Med Rehabil* 1959;40:379–382.
24. Bhalla SK, Simmons EH. Normal ranges of intervertebral motion of the cervical spine. *Can J Surg* 1969;12: 181–187.
25. Fielding JW. Normal and selected abnormal motion of the cervical spine from the second cervical vertebra to the seventh cervical vertebra based on cineradiography. *J Bone Joint Surg Am* 1964;46:633–637.
26. Matsunaga S, Kabayama S, Yamamoto T, et al. Strain on intervertebral discs after anterior cervical decompression and fusion. *Spine* 1999;24:670–675.
27. Dmitriev A, Lehman RA, Kuklo TR. The effects of extending the length of a cervical arthrodesis on adjacent level range of motion: an in-vitro cadaveric study. Oral Poster Presentation. Fifty-Fifth Annual Meeting of the Congress of Neurological Surgeons Annual Meeting, Boston, Mass, October 8–13, 2005.
28. Kaufman WA, Lunsford TR, Lundsford BR, et al. Comparison of three prefabricated cervical collars. *Orthot Prosthet* 1986;39:21–28.
29. Morris JM, Lucas DB. Biomechanics of spinal bracing. *Ariz Med* 1964;2:170–176.
30. Podolsky S, Baraff LJ, Simon RR, et al. Efficacy of cervical spine immobilization methods. *J Trauma* 1983;23: 461–465.
31. Beavis A. Cervical orthoses. *Prosthet Orthot Int* 1989;13:6–13.
32. Lunsford TR, Davidson M, Lunsford BR. The effectiveness of four contemporary cervical orthoses in restricting cervical motion. *J Prosthet Orthot* 1994;6:93–99.
33. Plaisier B, Gabram SG, Schwartz RJ, et al. Prospective evaluation of craniofacial pressure in four different cervical orthoses. *J Trauma* 1994;37:714–720.
34. Fisher SV. Proper fitting of the cervical orthosis. *Arch Phys Med Rehabil* 1978;59:505–507.
35. Anderson PA, Budorick TE, Easton KB, et al. Failure of halo vest to prevent in vivo motion in patients with injured cervical spines. *Spine* 1991;16:S501–S505.
36. Koch RA, Nickel VL. The halo vest: an evaluation of motion and forces across the neck. *Spine* 1978;3: 103–107.
37. Perry J, Nickel VL. Total cervical-spine fusion for neck paralysis. *J Bone Joint Surg Am* 1959;41:37–59.
38. Abitbol JJ, Botte MJ, Garfin SR, et al. The treatment of multiple myeloma of the cervical spine with a halo vest. *J Spinal Disord* 1989;2:263–267.
39. Cooper PR, Maravilla KR, Sklar FH, et al. Halo immobilization of cervical spine fractures: indications and results. *J Neurosurg* 1979;50:603–610.
40. Ewald FC. Fracture of the odontoid process in a seventeen-month-old infant treated with a halo. *J Bone Joint Surg Am* 1971;53:1636–1640.
41. Garret A, Perry J, Nickel VL. Stabilization of the collapsing spine. *J Bone Joint Surg Am* 1961;43:474–484.
42. Kostuik JP. Indications for the use of the halo immobilization. *Clin Orthop* 1981;154:46–50.
43. Mubarek SJ, Camp JF, Vuletich W, et al. Halo application in the infant. *J Pediatr Orthop* 1989;9:612–614.
44. Botte MJ, Byrne TP, Garfin SR. Application of halo device for immobilization of the cervical spine utilizing an increased torque pressure. *J Bone Joint Surg Am* 1987;69:750–752.
45. Fukui Y, Krag M, Huston D, et al. 3D dynamic halo vest loads: full crossover comparison of three vest types. *Proc Cervical Spine Res Soc* 1994:131–133.
46. Garfin SR, Botte MJ, Centeno RS, et al. Osteology of the skull as it affects halo pin placement. *Spine* 1985;10: 696–698.
47. Johnson RM, Hart DL, Simmons EF, et al. Cervical orthoses: a study comparing the effectiveness in restricting cervical motion in normal subjects. *J Bone Joint Surg Am* 1977;59:332–339.
48. Walker PS, Lamser D, Hussey RW, et al. Forces in the halo-vest apparatus. *Spine* 1984;9:773–777.

49. Wang GJ, Moskal JT, Albert T, et al. The effect of halo vest length on stability of the cervical spine. *J Bone Joint Surg Am* 1988;70:357–360.
50. Whitesides TE, Mehserle WL, Hutton WC. The force exerted by the halo pin. *Spine* 1992;17:S413–S417.
51. Garfin SR, Botte MJ, Waters RL, et al. Complications in the use of halo fixation device. *J Bone Joint Surg Am* 1986;68:320–325.
52. Rizzolo SJ, Piazza MR, Cotler JM, et al. Effect of torque pressure on halo pin complication rates: a randomized, prospective study. *Spine* 1993;18:2163–2166.
53. Perry J. The halo in spinal abnormalities: practical factors and avoidance of complications. *Ortho Clinics North Am* 1972;3:69–80.

CHAPTER 11

Closed Skeleton Traction Techniques

Carson Campe and Alan Hilibrand

INTRODUCTION

First-line management of cervical spine trauma with malalignment is often accomplished through the use of closed skeleton axial traction. Despite advances in the techniques of surgical stabilization, closed traction can be used as definitive treatment or as an adjuvant to surgery. The goals of nonoperative management for cervical spine trauma include (1) reduction of spinal malalignment and restoration of the spinal canal architecture, (2) establishment of acceptable stability, (3) protection of neural and soft tissues from further injury, and (4) facilitation of both neurologic and functional recovery.

Closed reduction of cervical spine deformity with the use of axial skeletal traction has a long history dating to at least 3500 to 1800 BC, as recorded in the ancient Hindu epic *Srimad Bhagwat Mahapurana*.[1] Hippocrates recognized the value of closed reduction for both trauma and chronic deformity and in his treatise *On Joints* described several methods by which to treat these maladies.[2] In more modern times, Walton was the first to describe closed reduction of facet dislocation by manipulation in 1893.[3] Later, Taylor[4] used a sling to apply axial traction as an aid in his manipulation of facet dislocation.

Manipulation of the cervical spine to reduce malalignment has been met with mixed success and must be employed with extreme caution. In 1987, Cotler et al.[5] reported a series of 24 patients who underwent a combination of axial traction and awake manipulation. Of the 24 patients, 17 underwent successful reduction and 90% of patients with incomplete spinal cord injuries improved at least one Frankel grade following reduction. Ludwig et al.[6] later reported a case of awake manipulation to reduce facet dislocation, which resulted in the rapid development of complete motor quadriplegia secondary to spinal cord compression from an epidural hematoma that had formed at the level of injury. Manipulation under anesthesia (MUA) was introduced in the 1900s but is rarely employed; it is used only when necessary by experienced individuals as a secondary means of reducing spinal deformity.[7,8] Lee et al.,[9] in 1994, reported on the superiority of rapid axial traction in a case series comparing MUA to traction. His results demonstrated 73% successful reduction with MUA versus 88% success with traction. Furthermore, 16 of 91 patients (18%) in the MUA group died within 3 months of the initial injury compared to 9 of 119 patients (8%) in the traction group. More recently, Vital et al.[10] used a protocol in which patients were subjected first to closed reduction by traction, then reduction maneuvers under general anesthesia, and, finally, anterior surgical reduction. Neurologic deterioration was not reported for any of the patients, and reduction was achieved in 97% of the cases, with 30% of patients being reduced by MUA. Thus, in experienced hands, MUA appears to be an effective component of a closed reduction strategy, although complications are frequent and may be accompanied by severe morbidity.

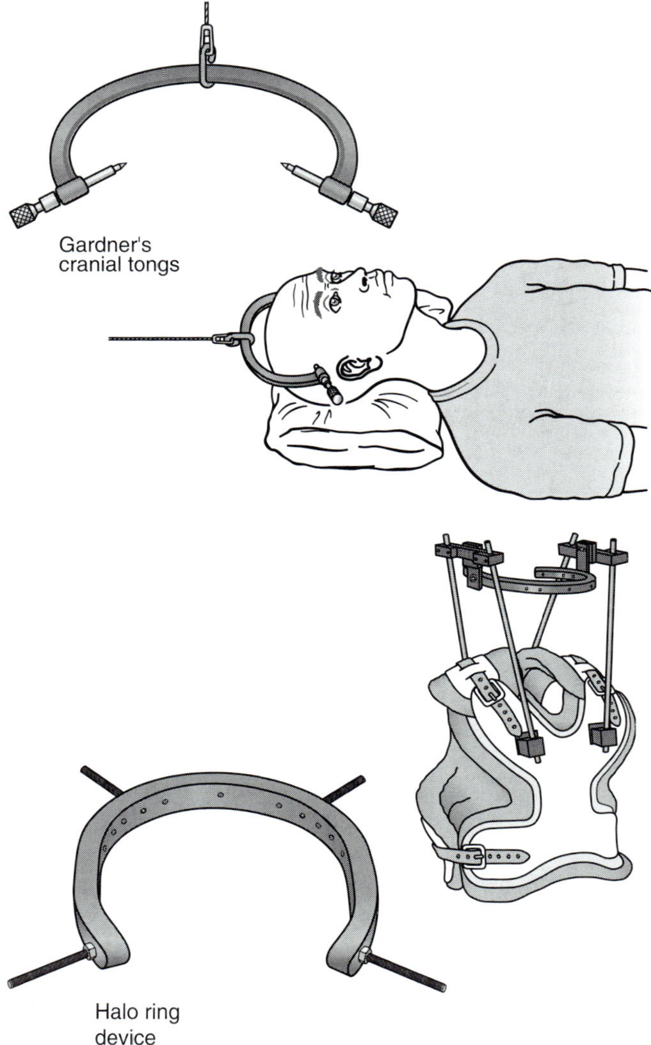

FIGURE 11.1. Gardner-Wells tongs placement and traction weight application.

The use of cranial tongs in the application of axial traction was first reported by Crutchfield[11] in 1933 when he modified Edmonton extension tongs for attachment to the skull. Multiple versions of the cranial tongs have been introduced since, although Gardner's 1973 design, which incorporated spring-loaded pins for fixation of the cranial tongs, is the most widely utilized today.[12] This design is favored because of its ease of application, low complication rate, and capacity to apply large traction forces (Fig. 11.1).

Halo-ring devices are also commonly used, especially since the incorporation of radiolucent materials into their construction and the design of open-ring devices that encircle only the anterior and lateral portions of the skull. The open posterior aspect obviates the need to lift the skull off of the bed during application and thus facilitates their use in a patient with an unstable cervical spine injury. Lerman et al.[13] reported on the pullout strength of halo rings compared to Gardner-Wells tongs, utilizing a copolymer skull model, and found halo pullout force to be 440 lb compared to 233 lb for the cranial tongs. Both of these pullout weights exceed the maximum traction force normally applied in reduction protocols, but the study suggests halo devices provide comparable, if not superior, strength for application of traction. Use of a halo device also facilitates transition from a traction setup to one of stabilization with the halo vest following successful reduction.

INDICATIONS

Cervical traction may be considered in any medically stable, awake, alert, and cooperative patient with an unstable cervical spine injury resulting from fracture or dislocation. However, absolute contraindications exist in some such patients, including those with an intracranial bleed, skull fracture, occipitocervical dissociation, or other complete ligamentous injuries of the cervical spine. Caution is advised in patients with ankylosing spondylitis or diffuse idiopathic skeletal hyperostosis because of an increased risk for displacement and overdistraction at the site of injury.[14]

METHOD

Before initiation of axial traction, a thorough baseline neurologic examination must be performed to establish the extent of the deficit, if any. This may include, but is not limited to, an American Spinal Injury Association (ASIA) impairment score and Frankel grade. Baseline plain films must be obtained to ascertain the nature and stability of the injury and to rule out the possibility of a significant ligamentous injury or occipitocervical dissociation. While adequate cervical spine stabilization is maintained, the patient can be transferred to a rotating bed with hardware appropriate for the application of traction. Use of a rotating bed decreases the incidence of complications that can arise secondary to prolonged immobility of the patient. Several authors suggest that rapid and early reduction of spinal column malalignment may facilitate neurologic recovery, as well as protect the patient from potential iatrogenic injury as the patient is transferred to various therapeutic and diagnostic procedures.[9,15–17] In light of this possibility, traction should be initiated as soon as possible after the patient's arrival in the emergency department. Following each application of additional traction weight, serial radiologic and neurologic evaluation of the patient must be performed to rule out the possibility of overdistraction or deterioration in neurologic status. Fluoroscopy can be used as a substitute for serial portable radiographs in an effort to ensure timely progression of the reduction protocol. Injuries to higher levels of the cervical spine, such as atlanto-occipital or atlantoaxial dislocations and axial fractures, appear to be more susceptible to overdistraction with the application of traction and must be monitored carefully during the procedure.[15,16] On the contrary, unilateral facet dislocations may require relatively larger traction forces to achieve reduction because of the resistance of supporting structures that remain intact surrounding the unaffected facet joint.[18]

There is some controversy surrounding the use of magnetic resonance imaging (MRI) before the initiation of closed traction, resulting from imaging data demonstrating the coincidence of disc herniation and/or rupture with traumatic cervical spine injury.[19,20] These data have led some surgeons to delay the initiation of closed traction until an MRI can be obtained for evaluation of the segments involved. Of interest, Vaccaro et al.[20] reported that although closed traction reduction appeared to increase the incidence of disc herniation, there was no associated neurologic deterioration of these patients. Grant et al.[21] also found that although a significant number of patients demonstrated disc herniation or disruption on postreduction MRI, these findings were not associated with decreased neurologic recovery. They were able to achieve realignment in study patients in an average of 2 hours from presentation and, as a result, advocated early closed reduction in place of waiting for MRI evaluation of the injury. Furthermore, Darsaut et al.[22] monitored closed reductions for cervical fracture dislocation with serial MRIs and found concomitant disc disruption in 88% of patient prereduction but demonstrated a return of disc material toward disc spaces in all patients as well as canal widening in 11 of 17 as reduction progressed. Thus, the acquisition of MRI studies before initiation of cervical traction remains controversial. In the neurologically intact, awake, alert, and cooperative patient, it is acceptable to proceed with closed traction reduction before obtaining an MRI as long as close attention to any changes in the patient's neurologic examination is undertaken.

HEAD HALTER

The head halter apparatus is the easiest traction device to apply and is noninvasive. Separate straps are placed under the chin and the occiput, and a small amount of weight is applied in traction. The technique is limited by the minimum amount of force that can be applied before the device fails or the patient becomes intolerant.

Complications include pressure ulcers, pullout with excessive weight, and temporomandibular joint pain with possible postprocedure dysfunction. Mandible fracture is an absolute contraindication to head halter application. Because of the limitations of this technique, it is seldom indicated in reduction of cervical spine injuries.

CRANIAL TONGS

Gardner-Wells tongs remain the most commonly used form of cranial tongs. They are usually fabricated from either stainless steel or MRI-compatible graphite and are shaped as a bow with threaded pins on opposite sides. The pins are angled rostrally to reduce pin migration and have a sharp taper that precludes the need for skin incision or predrilling of the cranial bone. Pin placement is crucial to avoid pullout and to ensure the spinal column is not subjected to asymmetric traction forces that could result in a rotational stress or unwanted flexion or extension moment. Care must also be taken to avoid irritation of the temporalis muscle, injury to the superficial temporal artery and vein, or piercing of the inner table in thinner areas of the calvarium below the temporal ridge. Pins are placed in line with the tragus or external auditory meatus and approximately 1 cm superior to the pinna or 3 cm superior to the external auditory meatus. This should locate the pins below the temporal ridge and the maximum biparietal diameter, reducing the incidence of pullout. Pin placement can be shifted anteriorly or posteriorly to place the cervical spine in slight extension or flexion, respectively, to aid in reduction of the deformity. For example, in the case of traumatically dislocated facet joints, Vital et al.[10] describe locating the pins in a line 1 cm posterior to the external auditory meatus to provide a flexion moment that theoretically aids in unlocking the facets as traction is applied. The scalp is prepared by cleansing the skin and hair with an antiseptic solution. There is no need to shave the pin insertion site if the area can be kept clean enough to prevent infection. The scalp is then injected with 1% lidocaine down to the level of the periosteum. The pins, which are kept sterile, are then tightened, piercing the skin, until 6 to 8 lb of torque or 30 to 35 lb of compressive force is applied. According to the manufacturer, the indicator stem will protrude 1 mm from the end of the spring-loaded pin when the desired force is attained, although the accuracy of this mechanism must be verified in heavily used tongs.[13] The pins are tightened progressively, simultaneously, or in alternating sequence, to maintain force and position symmetry. A sterile dressing is applied to the pin sites, and traction weights are added to the apparatus in line with the axial skeleton. The pins must be tightened again 24 hours after initial application and then left alone unless migration occurs. Pin insertion sites are cleaned daily with dilute hydrogen peroxide solution. The patient is bed-bound, required to lie supine, and cannot turn the head because of the lateral extension of both the tongs and pins.

To facilitate the MRI evaluation of a patient in Gardner-Wells tongs, a graphite tong with titanium pins was developed. Although MRI is successful with this device, Blumberg et al.[23] showed failure of the titanium pins at 60 to 100 lb of traction versus 160 to 250 lb of traction for stainless steel pins. Thus, the authors advised caution when using MRI-compatible tongs with weights greater than 50 lb.

Complications from cranial tong use include infection at the pin insertion sites, which is mostly avoided with sterile technique and proper cleansing; pin migration and pullout, which is most likely secondary to insufficient pin tightening, increased wear and dulling of the pin tips, or osteopenic bone,[24] and rarely, perforation of the inner table.[25]

HALO RING

Halo ring application for cervical traction is similar to that for cervical stabilization except for the attachment of a traction bow to enable the addition of weight for axial traction. Open-ring and crown-type designs permit the application of a halo ring without the need for raising the head or hanging it off the end of the bed. As with cranial tongs, the placement of the pins is crucial to prevent pullout. It is essential that the posterior portion of the ring be oriented slightly inferiorly to maintain pin placement below the equator of the calvarium and near the maximum biparietal diameter. Anterior pins are placed 1 cm superior to the orbital rim, above the lateral two thirds of the orbit, to avoid damage to the supratrochlear and supraorbital neurovascular bundles located medially and the zygomaticotemporal bundle located laterally.[26] Patients are instructed to close their eyes during application of the anterior pins to avoid tethering of the eyelid skin. Posterior pin placement does not directly endanger underlying structures and can be approximately diagonal to the opposite anterior pin. The posterior portion of the halo vest can be placed under the patient before the application of traction in anticipation of postreduction stabilization with the halo device. This decreases the amount a patient has to be moved after successful reduction. Further technique in the application of the halo ring for traction is identical to that used for stabilization.

In the event of a posteriorly displaced odontoid fracture, Rushton et al.[27] described the use of a halo device for the application of bivector traction in restoring the sagittal alignment of the dens. Traction is initially applied in two perpendicular vectors, anteriorly and superiorly, and adjusted to achieve reduction as evidenced by serial radiographs.

Complications from halo traction use are similar to those found with cranial tongs and include cranial pin loosening and pullout, infection at pin sites with potential for the development of a subdural abscess,[28] perforation of the inner table, and superficial nerve damage.

TRACTION WEIGHT

There is no consensus on the amount of weight necessary to provide adequate traction. Crutchfield[29] described the use of a graduated system of weight calculated based on the level of cervical spine injury. He applied 5 to 10 lb for an injury of the atlas and increased the weight in increments of 1 to 5 lb per vertebral level, with an injury of C7 receiving 18 to 35 lb of traction. Hadley et al.[30] proposed beginning at 3 lb per vertebral level superior to the injury and progressively increasing weight to a maximum of 12 lb per level. Vital et al.[10] applied baseline traction of 3 to 4 kg (6.5 to 9 lb) and added 2 kg (4.5 lb) per level. Similarly, Slucky et al.[31] suggested using a baseline of 10 lb for the occiput and adding 5 lb for each vertebral level. Jeanneret et al.[16] reported on five cases of overdistraction and recommended conservative application of traction weight, beginning with a baseline of 2 kg, regardless of the level of injury, and slowly increasing to a maximum total of 5 to 7 kg (11 to 15.5 lb). However, in Cotler's series of 24 patients with successful reduction,[32] he reported a final traction weight of greater than 50 lb in half of the subjects, with a maximum of 140 lb. Similarly, Lee et al.[9] reported using up to 150 lb without any evidence of morbidity in his cervical reduction series.

Most clinicians agree that weight must be added incrementally and time must be allowed between successive applications for relaxation of the muscle and soft tissue supporting structures of the bony spinal column. The author advocates the addition of 5 to 10 lb at intervals of 10 to 15 minutes as a reasonable strategy for the conservative attainment of reduction. As traction weights approach the weight of the patient, the bed may be placed in a reverse Trendelenburg position to counteract the force of traction and maintain the patient's position. Care must be taken to maintain traction in line with the axis of the spinal column as the bed is moved. Some clinicians also advocate the use of a nonsedating intravenous dose of muscle-relaxing agents, such as benzodiazepines, to accelerate the reduction process by reducing muscle spasm. Ideally, this procedure should be performed under close monitoring in the emergency room with frequent neurologic examinations and continuous availability of lateral radiographs. In the event of neurologic deterioration, intense pain, or evidence of overdistraction on radiographic analysis, traction weight is removed immediately and the patient examined thoroughly for the development of new neurologic deficits. Overdistraction may occur in an unstable injury with the addition of even 10 lb of weight.[18] Once traction has been removed, the patient must be stabilized conservatively in a halo apparatus or prepared for operative management of the injury.

Following successful reduction of the injury, traction weights are gradually decreased and either a stabilizing halo traction ring or a rigid cervical orthosis is applied to prevent displacement and further injury. A postreduction MRI study is indicated to assess the extent of canal restrictive cord compromise and determine if anterior decompressive surgery is necessary to relieve cord compression.[33] If closed traction fails to acceptably reduce the injury, traction weights are decreased and MRI studies are indicated for the continued evaluation of the patient's clinical status, as well as for planning of subsequent operative treatment.

REFERENCES

1. Sanan A, Rengachary SS. The history of spinal biomechanics. *Neurosurgery* 1996;39:657–668.
2. Marketos SG, Skinadas P. Hippocrates. *Spine* 1999;24:1381–1387.
3. Walton G. A new method of reducing dislocation of cervical vertebrae. *J Nerv Ment Dis* 1893;20:609–611.
4. Taylor AS. Fracture-dislocation of the neck: a method of treatment. *Arch Neurol Psychol* 1924;12:625.
5. Cotler HB, Miller LS, Delucia FA, et al. Closed reduction of cervical spine dislocations. *Clin Orthoped* 1987;214: 185–199.
6. Ludwig SC, Vaccaro AR, Balderston RA, et al. Immediate quadriparesis after manipulation for bilateral cervical facet subluxation: a case report. *J Bone Joint Surg Am* 1997;79:587–590.
7. Xiong XH, Bean A, Anthony A, et al. Manipulation for cervical spinal dislocation under general anesthesia: serial review for 4 years. *Spinal Cord* 1998;36:21–24.
8. Lu K, Lee TC, Chen HJ. Closed reduction of bilateral locked facets of the cervical spine under general anesthesia. *Acta Neurochir* 1998;140:1055–1061.
9. Lee AS, MacLean JC, Newton DA. Rapid traction for reduction of cervical spine dislocations. *J Bone Joint Surg Br* 1994;76:352–356.
10. Vital JM, Gille O, Senegas J, et al. Reduction technique for uni- and biarticular dislocations of the lower cervical spine. *Spine* 1998;23:949–955.
11. Crutchfield WG. Skeletal traction for dislocation of cervical spine: report of a case. *South Surg* 1933;2:156–159.
12. Gardner WJ. The principle of spring-loaded points for cervical traction: technical note. *J Neurosurg* 1973;39: 543–544.
13. Lerman JA, Haynes RJ, Koeneman EJ, et al. A biomechanical comparison of Gardner-Wells tongs and halo device used for cervical spine traction. *Spine* 1994;19:2403–2406.
14. Kwon BK, Hilibrand AS. Management of cervical fractures in patients with diffuse idiopathic skeletal hyperostosis. *Curr Opin Orthoped* 2003;14:187–192.
15. Gruenberg MF, Rechtine GR, Chrin AM, et al. Overdistraction of cervical spine injuries with the use of skull traction: a report of two cases. *J Trauma* 1997;42:1152–1156.
16. Jeanneret B, Magerl F, Ward JC. Overdistraction: a hazard of skull traction in the management of acute injuries of the cervical spine. *Arch Orthop Traum Surg* 1991;110:242–245.
17. Miller LS, Cotler HB, Delucia FA, et al. Biomechanical analysis of cervical distraction. *Spine* 1987;12:831–837.
18. Rizzolo SJ, Piazza MR, Cotler JM, et al. Intervertebral disc injury complicating cervical spine trauma. *Spine* 1991;16(suppl 6):S187–S189.
19. Doran SE, Papadopoulos SM, Ducker TB, et al. Magnetic resonance imaging documentation of coexistent traumatic locked facets of the cervical spine and disc herniation. *J Neurosurg* 1993;79:341–345.
20. Vaccaro AR, Falatyn SP, Flanders AE, et al. Magnetic resonance evaluation of the intervetebral disc, spinal ligaments, and spinal cord before and after closed traction reduction of cervical spine dislocations. *Spine* 1999;24: 1210–1217.
21. Grant GA, Mirza SK, Chapman JR, et al. Risk of early closed reduction in cervical spine subluxation injuries. *J Neurosurg* 1999;90(suppl 1):13–18.
22. Darsaut TE, Ashforth R, Bhargava R, et al. A pilot study of magnetic resonance imaging-guided closed reduction of cervical spine fractures. *Spine* 2006;31(18):2085–2090.
23. Blumberg KD, Catalano JB, Cotler JM, et al. The pullout strength of titanium alloy MRI-compatible and stainless steel MRI-incompatible Gardner-Wells tongs. *Spine* 1993;18:1895–1896.
24. Krag MH, Byrt W, Pope M. Pull-off strength of Gardner-Wells tongs from cadaveric crania. *Spine* 1989;14: 247–250.
25. Feldman RA, Khayyat GF. Perforation of the skull by a Gardner-Wells tong: case report. *J Neurosurg* 1976;44: 119–120.
26. Botte MJ, Byrne TP, Abrams RA, The halo skeletal fixator: current concepts of application and maintenance. *Orthopedics* 1995;18:463–471.
27. Rushton SA, Vaccaro AR, Levine MJ, et al. Bivector traction for unstable cervical spine fractures: a description of its application and preliminary results. *J Spin Disord* 1997;10:436–440.
28. Garfin SR, Botte MJ, Triggs KJ, et al. Subdural abscess associated with halo-pin traction. *J Bone Joint Surg Am* 1988;70:1338–1340.
29. Crutchfield WG. Skeletal traction in the treatment of injuries of the cervical spine. *JAMA* 1954;155:29–32.

30. Hadley MN, Fitzpatrick BC, Sonntag VK, et al. Facet fracture-dislocation injuries of the cervical spine. *Neurosurgery* 1992;30:661–666.
31. Slucky AV, Eismont FJ. Treatment of acute injury of the cervical spine. *Instr Course Lect* 1995;44:67–80.
32. Cotler JM, Herbison GJ, Nasuti JF, et al. Closed reduction of traumatic cervical spine dislocation using traction weights up to 140 lbs. *Spine* 1993;18:386–390.
33. Selden NR, Quint DJ, Patel N, et al. Emergency magnetic resonance imaging of cervical spinal cord injuries: clinical correlation and prognosis. *Neurosurgery* 1999;44:785–792.

CHAPTER 12

The Halo Vest

Hossein Elgafy and Charles Fisher

INTRODUCTION

Since its introduction by Perry and Nickel in 1959, the halo thoracic vest (HTV) has been well established as providing the most rigid immobilization of all the cervical orthotic devices. The HTV has been frequently used and extremely effective for a broad spectrum of cervical pathologic states, including trauma, tumor, and inflammatory conditions. The advancements in biomaterials, specifically cervical rod screw systems, and the emphasis on accelerated restoration of function have greatly diminished the indications for the HTV. Despite these advancements, the HTV remains an important component of the spine surgeon's armamentarium. This chapter will review the biomechanics, application, and clinical indications for the HTV in a trauma setting.

BIOMECHANICAL CONSIDERATIONS

Richter et al.[1] conducted a biomechanical study on fresh frozen cadavers to identify the stabilizing effects of different orthoses in the intact spine and unstable Anderson type II odontoid fracture. They compared the HTV, soft collar, prefabricated Minerva brace, and Miami J collar. All four orthoses reduced the range of motion at both C1-C2 and C2-C3 of the intact spine, with the HTV providing the most stability. The soft collar did not give any clinically relevant stability. The Miami J and Minerva brace provided better control of rotational forces than motion in the sagittal plane. The HTV did not allow any measurable motion in any plane. They concluded that the halo vest is the first choice for conservative treatment of unstable injuries of the upper or axial cervical spine.

Although the halo is the most stable orthosis for cervical spine immobilization, motion and variability in forces do occur with its use. These variations are dependent on patient position and activity, as well as the degree of spinal instability. Bending forward from a seated position or reaching sideways while lying down significantly alters forces across the cervical spine with the halo in place. The greatest absolute amount of motion is seen at the C4-C5 level (7.2 degrees); this has been referred to as the snaking phenomenon. Patients should therefore be cautioned against bending and twisting movements of the trunk. Medial lateral forces have been found to be small compared with vertical and anterior-posterior forces.[2,3] Because of the snaking phenomenon, HTV immobilization has few indications in subaxial injuries and should be used cautiously as an adjunct to surgical stabilization of unstable midcervical injuries.

COMPONENTS OF THE HALO THORACIC VEST

These include the ring, pins, vest, and connecting rods. Over the years modifications have been incorporated in the development of the current rings, which are composed of lightweight metals compatible with magnetic resonance imaging (MRI). The rings are now open posteriorly, so they encircle only part of the head and avoid the need to pass the head through a ring, thus facilitating application and improving safety. Lerman and Haynes[4] conducted a biomechanical study to compare the fixation strength between open versus closed halo rings. They reported that the closed halo ring provided distraction strength greater than that of the open rings, suggesting a more rigid system with the closed device. This biomechanical advantage, however, does not appear to be clinically relevant.

The halo pins are now titanium, which is lighter, stronger, and MRI compatible. Breakaway torque wrenches designed for one-time use are used to insert halo pins to the set torque amount of 8 in-lb. These wrenches have replaced the cumbersome standard wrenches and ease pin tightening. The halo vests are lightweight, easily applied, and adjustable. Cross-straps and supports stabilize the vest and decrease shear stress between the anterior and posterior components. The upright and horizontal connecting rods are low-profile, lightweight, radiolucent carbon fiber, and MRI compatible. Connecting bolts on the vest can be tightened with torque wrenches that ratchet and give way at a set amount of torque (28 ft-lb), thereby saving time and minimizing the chance of overtightening. Current plastic vests and connecting-rod systems allow cervical spine adjustment in multiple planes, thus assisting in maintaining optimal alignment of healing fractures.

HALO APPLICATION

The ring size selected should allow 2 cm of clearance around the head. The vest size is determined by measuring the chest circumference at the xiphoid process with a tape measure. With the newer "open" rings, the patient's head can remain on the bed. The closed ring necessitates that the head and shoulders be supported on folded towels or the head supported beyond the end of the bed, both of which potentially jeopardize spinal precautions. A three-person team is optimal for halo application, to ensure spinal precautions are maintained throughout the procedure. A crash cart with resuscitation equipment should be available.

The optimal position for placement of anterior halo pins is 1 cm cephalad to the lateral two thirds of eyebrow and below the greatest circumference of the skull. Placement of the pin above the supraorbital rim prevents displacement or penetration into the orbit. Placement of the pin below the level of the greatest skull diameter minimizes the tendency toward cephalad pin migration, which is especially important if traction is going to be applied. On the lateral aspect of the "safe zone" lies the temporalis muscle. Avoidance of the temporal area is desirable because the bone in this region is thin, which increases the risk for skull penetration or pin loosening. Penetration of the temporalis muscle by the halo pin is painful and impedes mandibular motion. On the medial aspect of the anterior safe zone lies the supraorbital and supratrochlear nerves and the underlying frontal sinus. During anterior pin advancement, the patient is asked to gently close the eyes and relax the forehead. This minimizes skin or eyebrow tenting or tethering, which hinders eyelid closing after pin insertion. The insertion sites of the posterior pins are less critical because neuromuscular structures are lacking and the skull is thicker and more uniform in this area. The posterior pins are optimally inserted about 1 cm cephalad to the ear. This site is inferior to the widest portion of the skull, yet superior enough to prevent ring impingement on the ear. Cyclic loading of pins inserted at different angles has demonstrated that perpendicular insertion is superior to placement at 15 or 30 degrees to the skull surface. A torque of 8 in-lb has been found safe and effective in lowering the incidence of pin loosening and infection compared with application at 6 in-lb. Pins are tightened in increments of 2 in-lb, alternating with the diagonal pin, until a torque of 8 in-lb is reached. After vest application, the head and neck are positioned and the bolts are secured. The halo screwdriver and wrench should be taped to the vest in case emergency removal of the vest is required.

Once the HTV is secure, a repeat clinical and radiographic evaluation should be completed. The pins should be retorqued 24 to 48 hours after the initial halo application. The pin sites are cleaned every 1 or 2 days with diluted hydrogen peroxide solution. Frequent radiographic assessment of the cervical spine is recommended to ensure appropriate alignment is maintained.[5]

INDICATIONS

The primary use of the HTV is in immobilization of unstable upper cervical spine injuries, specifically occiput to C3 injuries. There are, however, other injuries in which the HTV may be used as either a primary or supplementary form of treatment.

Acute Immobilization

Some surgeons suggest the HTV should be placed immediately in unstable atlanto-occipital dislocations. Some even suggest using the HTV as the initial mode of immobilization in high-risk trauma. Although this is probably not practical or necessary, it potentially facilitates transfer of the patient for imaging or surgery. Many of today's operating room tables allow for the attachment of skull clamps and halo rings, thus making turning the patient prone easier and probably safer.

Definitive Treatment

Atlanto-occipital Dislocation Early diagnosis and treatment are critical because patients are at high risk for neurologic injury or sudden death. Reduction of displacement can be performed cautiously with fluoroscopic guidance by carefully positioning the head with a bolster behind the thorax (for anterior displacement) or the occiput (for posterior displacement). Traction and collar immobilization can reproduce a distraction injury, precipitating neurologic injury, and accordingly should be avoided. For vertical displacement, reduction can be performed by providing gentle downward pressure or carefully elevating the head of the bed. The HTV can provide temporary immobilization, but surgical stabilization is usually necessary.[6]

Occipital Condyle Fractures Occipital condyle fractures are frequently diagnosed as a concurrent finding on head computed tomography (CT) scan done for trauma. They are commonly caused by an axial compression mechanism. The classification system described by Anderson and Montesano[7] is based on CT pattern and evaluates the potential for instability. A type I injury is a comminuted fracture of the condyle and is generally stable. A type II fracture is a condyle fracture with associated basilar skull fracture. This injury is stable except when the entire condyle is separated from the occiput. A type III injury is an avulsion fracture of the attachment of the alar ligament. This injury can be bilateral and occurs in 30% to 50% of patients with atlanto-occipital dislocations. Stable type I and II fractures should be treated in a cervical orthosis for 6 to 8 weeks. Displaced type II injuries should be treated in a halo vest for 8 to 12 weeks. Type III injuries are treated based on stability; stable nondisplaced injuries are treated in an orthosis, and minimally displaced injuries are treated in an HTV. Any evidence of anteroposterior (AP) displacement, joint incongruity, or abnormal diastasis makes the injury highly unstable, necessitating an occiput-C2 fusion.[6]

C1: Jefferson Fractures Nondisplaced or minimally displaced (<7 mm) burst fractures can be treated in either a cervical orthosis or HTV for 3 months and have a high union rate. A patient with a markedly displaced or unstable C1 burst fracture is treated by anatomic reduction using traction, followed by either prolonged traction and halo immobilization or surgery.[6,8] Some complex unstable fractures of C1 and C2 with significant bony comminution but reasonable alignment can be treated in an HTV to try to avoid C1-C2 fusion (Figs. 12.1 and 12.2). Long-term follow-up examination of patients with Jefferson fractures indicated that patients' status did not return to the level of their perceived preinjury health status or that of normative population controls. Those with other injuries and significant osseous displacement (≥7 mm total) may experience poorer long-term outcomes.[9]

C2 Fractures (Type II Hangman Fractures and Type III Odontoid Fractures) With the advent of the odontoid screw and the desire to avoid a C1-C2 fusion, most surgeons will manage type II odontoid fractures in patients with high risk for nonunion with odontoid screw fixation. There are, however, contraindications to direct odontoid fixation, such as comminuted and reverse

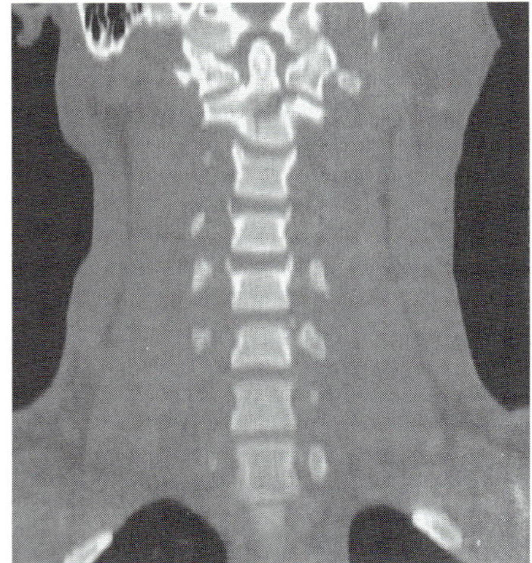
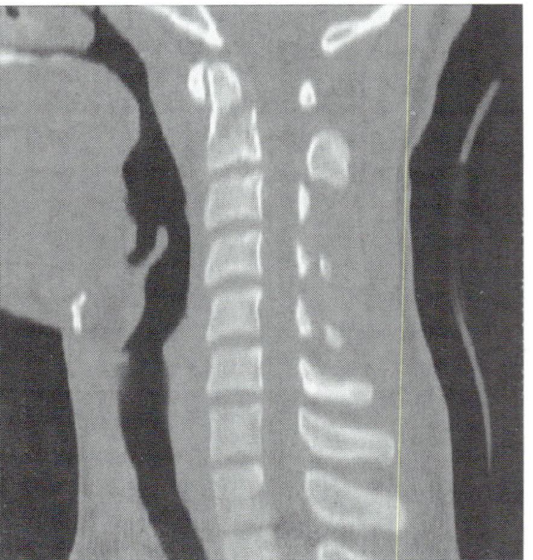

FIGURE 12.1. Coronal **(A)** and sagittal **(B)** computed tomography reformat of a college basketball player who suffered a complex C1-C2 fracture. The management options were halo thoracic vest (HTV) or occiput-C2 fusion. The patient was treated with HTV.

obliquity fractures. For these fractures the HTV becomes a viable alternative to try to avoid C1-C2 fusion, which causes significant impairment.[6,10,11]

Subaxial Fractures Halo immobilization has few indications in subaxial injuries because it does not provide enough stability to maintain reduction of unstable mid-cervical and low-cervical injuries. Fisher et al.[12] conducted a retrospective study comparing the outcome for two groups of patients with unstable cervical flexion teardrop fractures: those treated with HTVs and those treated with anterior corpectomy and plating. The study confirmed that the HTV was inferior to anterior corpectomy and plating in maintaining alignment. For other subaxial trauma, such as unilateral or bilateral facet injuries, surgical intervention is favored. Although not proven in a well-designed study, the relative efficacy and safety of both anterior and posterior procedures, in combination with the snaking phenomenon and the detrimental effects of prolonged immobilization, lend little support for the use of the HTV in these injuries.

Ankylosing Spondylitis Trauma Routine radiographs of the spine of patients with ankylosing spondylitis may fail to demonstrate a fracture or fracture-dislocation. Once the diagnosis is

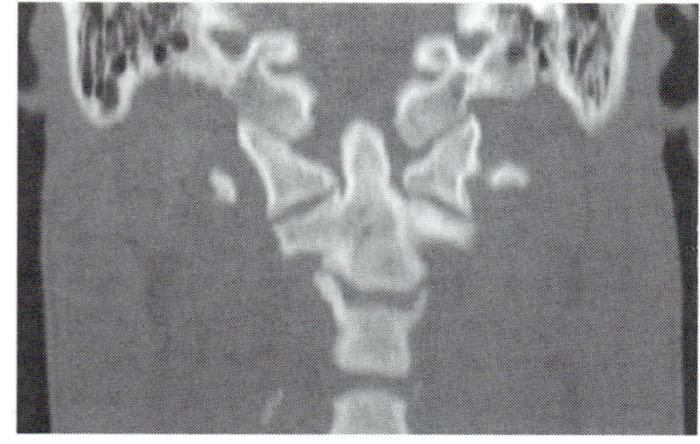
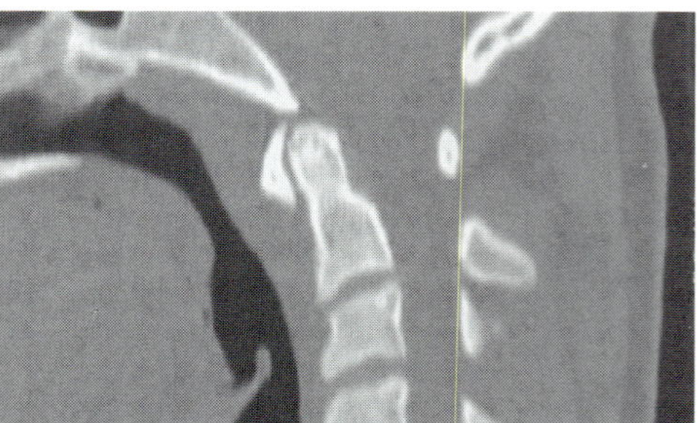

FIGURE 12.2 Coronal **(A)** and sagittal **(B)** CT reformat at 6 months of follow-up showed healed fracture in a good alignment. The patient returned to varsity basketball.

made, every effort should be made to prevent or minimize cord injury, especially in the presence of a complete transverse fracture, which converts the ankylosed spine into two rigid segments that move as independent units exerting large forces at the fracture site. If the displacement is slight and there is no neural involvement, immobilization by the HTV for approximately 12 weeks appears to be sufficient. In the presence of appreciable subluxation or instability, if surgical intervention is not possible, the HTV may be worn until the spine is stable for about 3 months. Traction must be adjusted with great care to ensure accurate restoration of the vertebral column alignment that was present before the injury.[13]

CONTRAINDICATIONS

The absolute contraindication for HTV is concomitant unstable skull fractures. There are relative contraindications, including traumatized skin overlying pin sites and obesity.[10]

COMPLICATIONS

The most common complications are pin site infection and loosening.[10,14] Pin loosening is reported in 36% to 60% of patients. The loose pin and remaining pins can be retightened once to 8 in-lb as long as resistance is met within the first few complete rotations of the pin. If no resistance is met, the pin should be removed after placement of a new pin in an adjacent location. Pin site infection is reported in 20% of patients. Management includes obtaining culture and sensitivity, starting oral antibiotics, and providing local pin care. If drainage does not respond to treatment, the pin should be removed after insertion of a new pin at a different site. If an abscess develops, incision and drainage should be performed, cultures taken, and parenteral antibiotic therapy instituted.[14]

Dural puncture is a rare but potentially serious problem that can occur after significant trauma to the halo, such as a blow or a fall onto the halo. Symptoms of dural puncture include leakage of clear cerebrospinal fluid around a loose or deeply seated pin, headache, malaise, and visual disturbances. Management includes hospitalization, head CT, neurosurgical consult, prophylactic antibiotics, and pin removal after placement of a new pin at a noninvolved site. Elevation of the head of the bed decreases intracranial pressure and helps improve leakage. The dural tear usually heals in few days. If the cerebrospinal fluid leak continues, a lumbar subarachnoid drain or surgical exploration and dural repair may be required. If a subdural abscess develops, surgical incision and drainage are indicated.[14]

Pin site bleeding is a rare complication, occurring in only 1% of patients, most of them receiving anticoagulation therapy. Pin site packing has been reported to be ineffective, and tapering or discontinuation of the anticoagulants may be necessary if bleeding persists.[10,14]

Loss of cervical reduction with the halo in place is reported in 10% of patients. Injuries to the posterior ligaments and facet fractures are likely to result in loss of reduction, especially in obese patients in whom the vest may not be long enough to exert sufficient control on the unstable cervical spine. Inability to maintain reduction with the halo is an indication for operative management.

Pressure sores under the vest are reported in 4% to 11% of patients as a result of insufficient padding or a poorly fitted vest. Pressure sores are best treated by prevention, with appropriate skin protection and vest padding. Patients with paralysis and poor protective sensibility require frequent turning, positioning, and skin inspection.

Dysphagia has been noted in 2% of patients as a result of exaggerated extension of the neck. Decreasing cervical extension may relieve the problem if this can be performed without compromising the cervical reduction.[10,14]

There is increasing recognition that the elderly may be more predisposed to complications from the HTV, with some studies noting that the elderly patient may have increased swallowing and airway problems, an increased rate of skin complications, and an increased acute mortality rate. Advanced age may be considered a relative contraindication to HTV use.[15,16]

CONCLUSION

The HTV provides the most rigid immobilization of all the cervical orthotic devices. Its effectiveness in the subaxial region is compromised by the snaking phenomenon and relative safety and efficacy of surgical treatment, thus limiting the majority of its indications to the upper cervical spine. As surgical techniques and spinal instrumentation continue to advance, the indications for the HTV will diminish. The HTV, however, will continue to have a role in unique clinical conditions in which the surgical impairment or risk is not justified when the safety, theoretical, and evidence-based advantages of the HTV are present.

REFERENCES

1. Richter D, Latta LL, Milne EL, et al. The stabilizing effects of different orthoses in the intact and unstable upper cervical spine: a cadaver study. *J Trauma* 2001;50:848–854.
2. Walker PS, Lamser D, Hussey RW, et al. Forces in the halo-vest apparatus. *Spine* 1984;9:773–777.
3. Lind B, Sihlbom H, Nordwall A. Forces and motions across the neck in patients treated with halo-vest. *Spine* 1988;13:162–167.
4. Lerman JA, Haynes RJ. Open versus closed halo rings: comparison of fixation strengths. *Spine* 2001;26:2102–2104.
5. Botte MJ, Garfin SR, Byrne TP, et al. The halo skeletal fixator: principles of application and maintenance. *Clin Orthop Relat Res* 1989;239:12–18.
6. Jackson RS, Banit DM, Rhyne AL III, et al. Upper cervical spine injuries. *J Am Acad Orthop Surg* 2002;10:271–280.
7. Anderson PA, Montesano PX. Morphology and treatment of occipital condyle fractures. *Spine* 1988;13:731–736.
8. Spence KF Jr, Decker S, Sell KW. Bursting atlantal fracture associated with rupture of the transverse ligament. *J Bone Joint Surg Am* 1970;52:543–549.
9. Dvorak MF, Johnson MG, Boyd M, et al. Long-term health-related quality of life outcomes following Jefferson-type burst fractures of the atlas. *J Neurosurg Spine* 2005;2:411–417.
10. Michael JB, Thomas P B, Reid AA, et al. Halo skeletal fixation: techniques of application and prevention of complications. *J Am Acad Orthop Surg* 1996;4:44–53.
11. Vaccaro AR, Madigan L, Bauerle WB, et al. Early halo immobilization of displaced traumatic spondylolisthesis of the axis. *Spine* 2002;27:2229–2233.
12. Fisher CG, Dvorak MF, Leith J, et al. Comparison of outcomes for unstable lower cervical flexion teardrop fractures managed with halo thoracic vest versus anterior corpectomy and plating. *Spine* 2002;27:160–166.
13. Grisolia A, Bell RL, Peltier LF. Fractures and dislocations of the spine complicating ankylosing spondylitis: a report of six cases. *Clin Orthop Relat Res* 2004;422:129–134.
14. Garfin SR, Botte MJ, Waters RL, et al. Complications in the use of the halo fixation device. *J Bone Joint Surg Am* 1986;68:320–325.
15. Majercik S, Tashjian RZ, Biffl WL, et al. Halo vest immobilization in the elderly: a death sentence? J Trauma 2005;59:350–356, discussion 6–8.
16. Tashjian RZ, Majercik S, Biffl WL, et al. Halo-vest immobilization increases early morbidity and mortality in elderly odontoid fractures. J Trauma 2006;60:199–203.

CHAPTER 13

Rehabilitation Following Orthosis Removal

Merrill Landers and Michael Daubs

INTRODUCTION

The overall goal of trauma care is to stabilize and restore function as quickly as possible. Modern internal fixation techniques allow rapid stabilization of most injuries, but there is still a need for immobilization in an orthosis for primary treatment and as a supplement to internal fixation. We know from the principles learned in the treatment of extremity fractures that prolonged immobilization causes capsular and ligamentous contractures and intrarticular adhesions that can result in severe limitations in range of motion. In addition, there is weakness secondary to disuse atrophy of the surrounding muscles.

Although the best method of prevention is to maximally stabilize the injury and allow early range-of-motion exercises, this is not always possible. The goal of physical therapy following orthosis removal is to safely restore strength and range of motion without causing further injury to the cervical spine. It is important that the physician and physical therapist work closely together to supervise a program that allows for the quickest and safest path back to function. It is with these goals in mind that the following recommendations for treatment are made.

TREATMENT PRINCIPLES

The specific rehabilitation program following cervical orthosis removal depends on the preinjury status of the patient, the mechanism and severity of the injury, the surgical stabilization, and the resultant impairment related to the immobilization. Overall, the emphasis of the rehabilitation should be placed on restoring function to preinjury levels, while at the same time avoiding adverse stress to healing tissue. As a general rule, it is recommended that rehabilitation should begin immediately after orthosis removal. However, aggressive rehabilitation (phase II discussed later) should begin only when the fracture or arthrodesis is healed or adequately stabilized. It is essential that the treating physician be involved in the decision for advancement into this phase of rehabilitation.

Although the efficacy of rehabilitation after orthosis removal has not been documented in the literature, the guidelines presented here are based on clinical experience and evidence from basic science and clinical trials related to the cervical spine.[1–19] Additionally, the following guidelines are for the uncomplicated patient after cervical orthosis removal. They are not intended to encompass the whole spectrum of individual variability commonly seen in this patient population.

This rehabilitation protocol is divided into 4 phases: (a) the protection phase, (b) the motion phase, (c) the strengthening phase, and (d) the return to activity phase. The estimated time frames for each of these phases are only guidelines. Progression from one phase to the next depends on meeting criteria, because individual patients will progress at different rates. Therefore, the physician and physical therapist should use sound clinical reasoning in determining when a patient's rehabilitation should be accelerated or decelerated.

REHABILITATION PHASES

PHASE I: PROTECTION (WEEKS 1 TO 3)

Following orthosis removal, there is a protective period of approximately 2 to 3 weeks. Patients are instructed to wear a soft collar and are encouraged to participate in a supervised rehabilitation program.

The initial trepidation experienced by the patient that follows orthosis removal is common. It is complicated by psychological dependence on the orthosis and the stress associated with the injury and surgical stabilization. Of the many psychological factors that complicate the progression of the patient in this early phase, the presence of anxiety and fear associated with movement needs particular attention. This phenomenon, known as fear-avoidance beliefs, suggests that there are two types of patients: confronters and avoiders.[20,21] In reality, most patients fall somewhere between these two extremes. However, either extreme poses its own unique concerns. *Confronters* are characterized by a strong desire to return to normal activities and work (a surgeon's dream patient). Additionally, they confront their own personal pain barriers. As a general rule, these patients typically progress normally and without complication. Occasionally, these patients need to be slowed down because their lack of fear may place adverse stress on the healing tissue. These patients need to be firmly educated to avoid deleterious movement or physical activity. *Avoiders* have an exaggerated fear of pain and will avoid any physical activity or movement that is anticipated to cause pain or aggravate their condition. It has been said that their fear of pain is more disabling than the condition itself.[22,23] This maladaptive coping strategy often stimulates self-imposed immobilization, which causes further fibrosis and atrophy. These patients should be identified early so appropriate coping treatment and education can be initiated.[22,24–26] The focus of treatment for patients with high fear-avoidance beliefs is to gain confidence with movement and physical activity through regular assurance and education from their physician and physical therapist.

Goals

The goals for phase I therapy are as follows:

- General:
  - Maintain the integrity of the healing tissue
  - Reestablish 75% of normal unloaded passive and active-assisted cervical range of motion with minimal discomfort
  - Decrease pain
  - Introduce upper extremity strengthening
- Range of motion:
  - Supine, passive cervical range of motion in all planes of motion with gentle axial traction (Fig. 13.1)
  - Supine, active-assisted cervical range of motion in all planes
  - Manual scapular mobilization in side-lying position
  - Upper extremity range of motion (rope and pulley)
- Strengthening:
  - Shoulder shrugs without resistance
  - Rows with minimal resistance

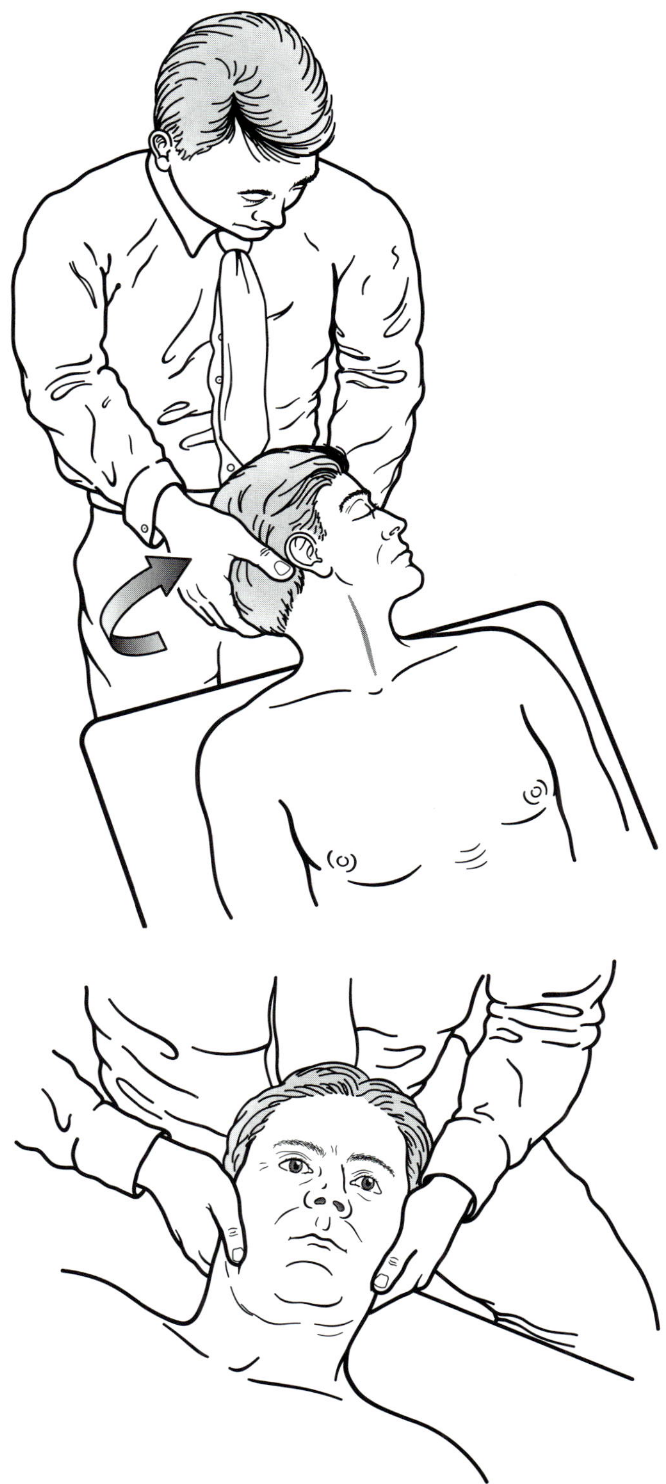

FIGURE 13.1. Supine, passive range of motion (rotation and side bending).

- Pain:
  - The decision to use physical agents must be based on the patient's presentation. They should be used only as an adjunct to therapy to promote better tolerance of exercise. These agents include moist heat, cryotherapy, and soft tissue mobilization. Electrical stimulation for pain control (transcutaneous electrical nerve stimulation [TENS]) or to reeducate or facilitate muscle contraction (high-voltage pulsed galvanic stimulation) may also be beneficial. TENS has been shown in one small randomized control trial to have a positive influence on pain-free range of motion in patients with neck pain.[27]
- Other:
  - Patients should be educated on good body biomechanics for safe and independent self-care (e.g., dressing, showering, sleeping, transfers).
- Home exercise program:
  - Gentle, pain-free, active, small-range movements performed 10 times every waking hour in each cardinal plane. These small-range movements should not go into tissue resistance.

PHASE II: MOTION (WEEKS 4 TO 6)

The criteria for progression to this phase are minimal discomfort with passive range of motion to 75% of normal and radiographic confirmation of cervical arthrodesis. Patients are gradually weaned from their soft collar and encouraged to participate in a more aggressive home exercise program. Essential to optimal recovery is early regaining of active range of motion. Therefore, the focus of this phase is to gradually progress the patient from passive and active-assisted motion to active motion. It is also important to be realistic with the patient's potential to regain range of motion by considering preinjury status, age, gender, and goals. As a general rule, it is unlikely that patients will regain full preinjury range of motion, particularly when there has been injury-related facet arthropathy.

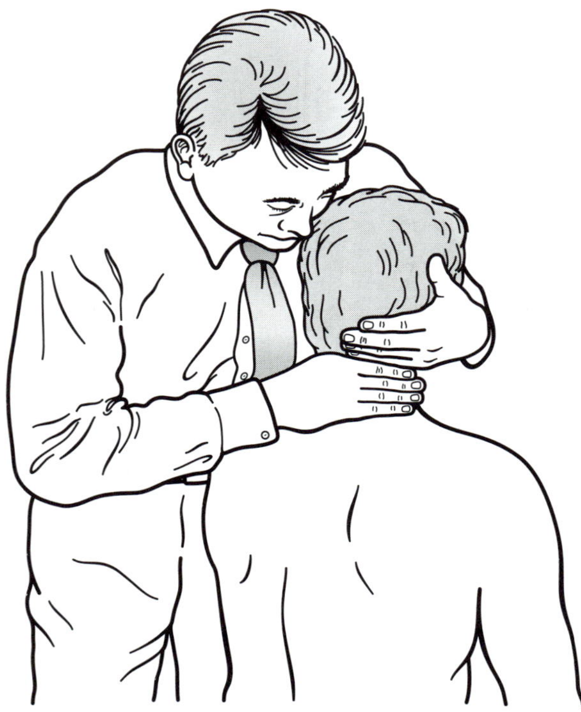

FIGURE 13.2. Loaded, active-assisted rotation range of motion.

Goals

The goals for phase II therapy are as follows:

- General
  - Reestablish full passive and active loaded cervical range of motion
  - Normalize arthrokinematics
  - Introduce cervical strengthening exercises
- Range of motion
  - Intersegmental mobilization, especially to hypomobile segments
  - Loaded, active-assisted, and active range of motion (Fig. 13.2)
  - Manual stretching of the upper trapezius, levator scapula, scalenes, and sternocleidomastoid (Fig. 13.3)

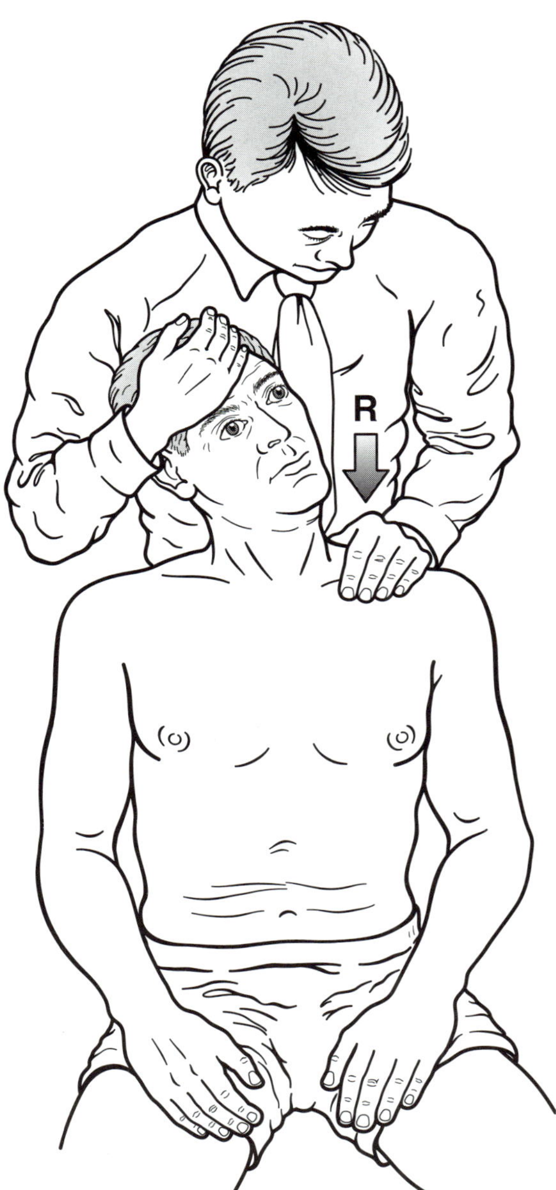

FIGURE 13.3. Manual stretching of the scalenes.

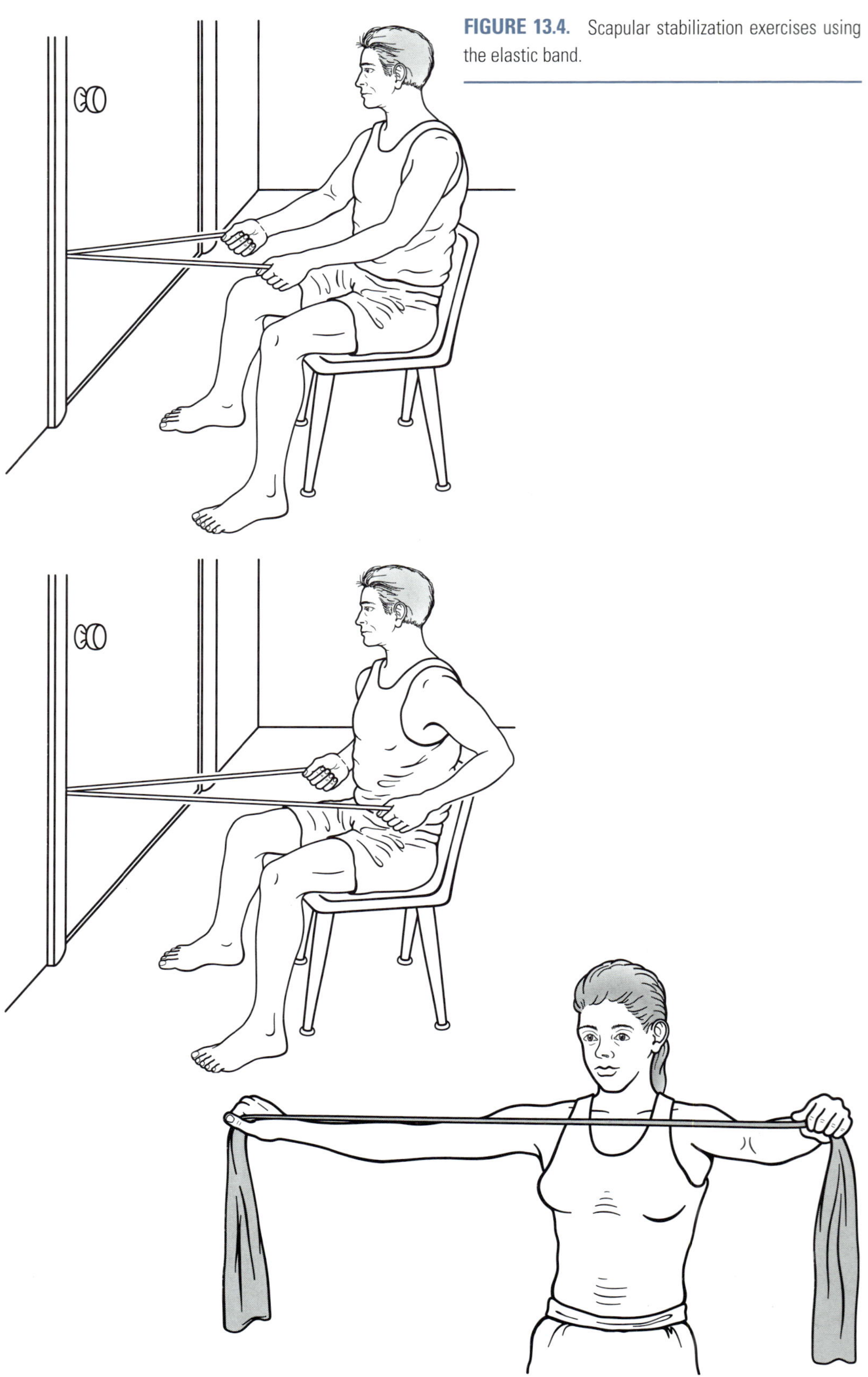

FIGURE 13.4. Scapular stabilization exercises using the elastic band.

- Stretching should not cause lingering discomfort.
- Be careful that gross stretching of the neck does not overstretch hypermobile segments.
- Strengthening
  - Gentle multidirectional cervical isometrics in supine
  - Retraining motor control and endurance of the deep cervical flexors
  - Trapezius, rhomboid, and levator scapula training with minimal resistance (shoulder shrugs, rows, scapular retraction with elastic band) (Fig. 13.4)
  - Cardiovascular conditioning (upper body ergometer) (Fig. 13.5)
- Pain
  - Passive modalities may continue into this phase. However, the patient should be weaned from these as soon as possible.
- Home exercise program
  - Towel rotation stretch (Fig. 13.6)
  - Towel traction
  - Side bending and flexion with light overpressure
  - Chin tucks

PHASE III: STRENGTHENING PHASE (WEEKS 7 TO 10)

The criteria for progression to this phase are near-normal pain-free active range of motion in all planes and good tolerance of gentle multidirectional isometrics. Now that near-normal active range of motion has been attained, in the next phase, we focus on progressive strengthening of the static neck stabilizers and the dynamic neck movers. The ideal program will consist of progressive strengthening exercises that target the major muscle groups of the neck, upper thoracic region, and scapula.

Goals

The goals for phase III are as follows:

- General
  - Reestablish dynamic stability and head control
  - Strengthen dynamic neck movers
  - Retard muscle disuse atrophy

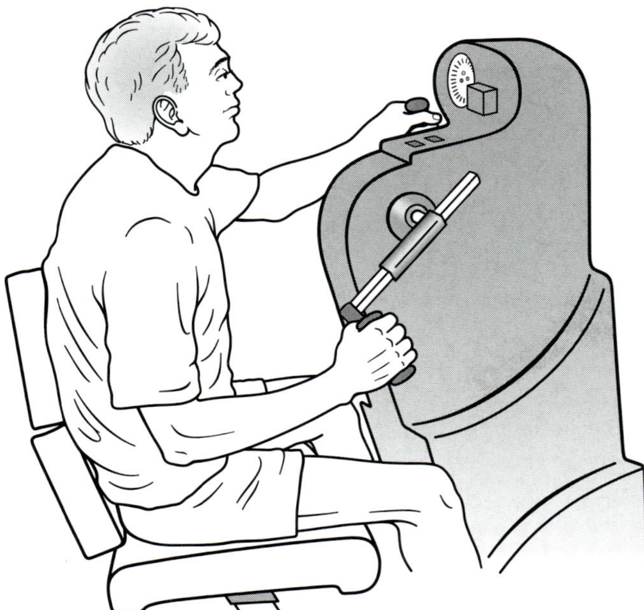

FIGURE 13.5. Upper body ergometer.

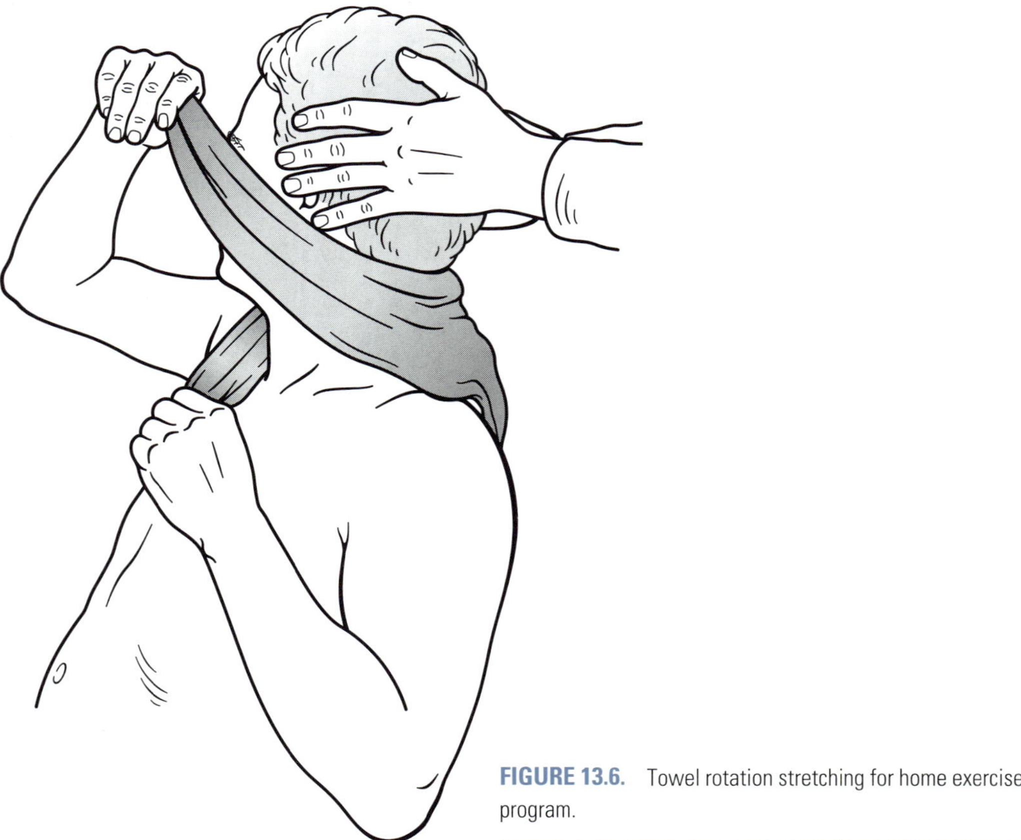

FIGURE 13.6. Towel rotation stretching for home exercise program.

- Range of motion
  - Manual stretching continues, to maintain the motion gained in the previous phase
- Strengthening
  - Cervical isometrics in sitting (Fig. 13.7)
  - Cocontraction of neck flexors and extensors
  - Concentric and eccentric cervical isotonics (Fig. 13.8)
  - Progressive resistive exercises of the scapular muscles (shrugs, rows, scapular retraction)
  - Wall push-ups
- Pain
  - Modalities should not be extended into this phase

PHASE IV: RETURN TO ACTIVITY PHASE (WEEKS 11 TO 16)

The criteria to progress to phase IV are minimal pain or discomfort with active range of motion in all planes and good motor control and strength (4 on a manual muscle test grading scale of 0 to 5) of the cervical musculature. In addition, the patient should consistently demonstrate good body mechanics without prompting and should tolerate almost all functional activities. The focus of this phase is to gradually introduce a functionally appropriate and suitably aggressive rehabilitation protocol that will prepare the patient for return to work, hobbies, and sports. The physician, physical therapist, and patient should work together to reach mutual agreement on realistic goals. Because these goals may vary dramatically from patient to patient, some may require more substantial training than others. However, a reasonable level of tolerance with functional activities (e.g., lifting, carrying, pulling, and reaching) should be expected for all patients. The resumption of more challenging physical activities (e.g., heavy lifting, repetitive lifting) should proceed with careful instruction.

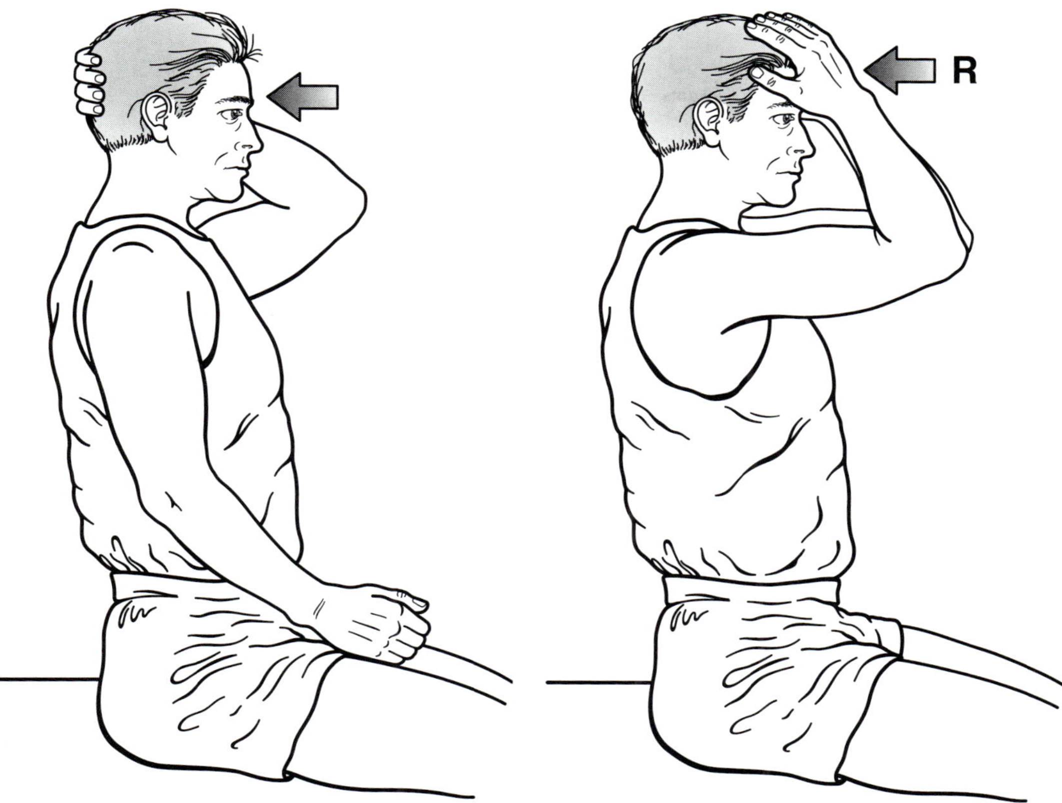

FIGURE 13.7. Cervical isometrics in sitting (extension and flexion).

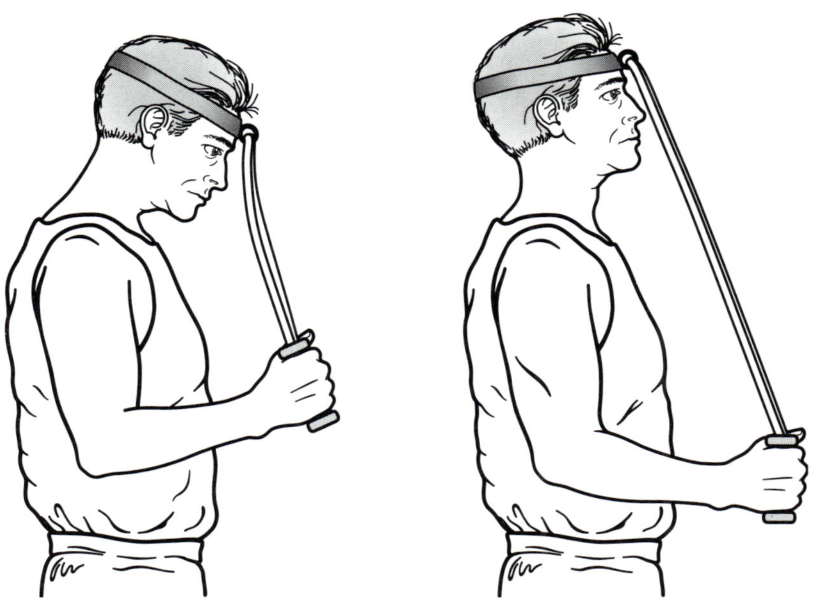

FIGURE 13.8. Cervical extension isotonic movements using the elastic band.

Goals

The goals for phase IV therapy include the following:

- General
  - Return to physical activities safely
- Range of motion
  - Stretching should continue into this phase, but should be done independently as part of a home exercise program.
- Strengthening
  - Weight ball toss with rebounder
  - Cardiovascular (upper body ergometer, jogging, cycling, swimming)
  - Progressive resistance exercises for lifting and carrying (e.g., ground to waist height, waist to overhead)
  - Progressive resistance exercises for pulling and reaching
  - Sport- or hobby-specific strengthening exercises
  - Work-hardening exercises

Criteria for Discharge to Full Activity

Criteria for discharge of the patient to full activity include the following:

- Consistent good body biomechanics
- Functional range of motion in all planes
- Full, pain-free functional strength of the cervical musculature
- Score of less than 5 on the Neck Disability Index
- Independence in a home exercise program

OUTCOME ASSESSMENT

An important component of rehabilitation is the assessment of the patient's progress. Impairment measures such as range of motion,[28] manual muscle testing, and visual analog scale for pain are recommended. Additionally, measures of neck function (e.g., Neck Disability Index,[29–31] Neck Pain and Disability Scale,[32,33] and Northwick Park Neck Pain Questionnaire[34])[35–37] play an important role in the assessment of patient outcome. Most important, these measures help when making clinical decisions about return to physical activity and work.

CONCLUSION

Rehabilitation following orthosis removal should be a team effort of the patient, physician, and therapist. It should be started by the treating physician as early as possible to prevent the permanent sequelae of prolonged immobilization. Communication among the physician and therapists is key to ensuring appropriate progress through the phases of rehabilitation. With a properly supervised program, a safe and rapid restoration of function to preinjury or near preinjury levels is possible.

REFERENCES

1. Levoska S, Keinanen-Kiukaanniemi S. Active or passive physiotherapy for occupational cervicobrachial disorders? A comparison of two treatment methods with a 1-year follow-up. *Arch Phys Med Rehabil* 1993;74:425–430.
2. Mealy K, Brennan H, Fenelon GC. Early mobilization of acute whiplash injuries. *Br Med J (Clin Res Ed)* 1986; 292:656–657.
3. Provinciali L, Baroni M, Illuminati L, et al. Multimodal treatment to prevent the late whiplash syndrome. *Scand J Rehabil Med* 1996;28:105–111.
4. McKinney LA. Early mobilisation and outcome in acute sprains of the neck. *BMJ* 1989;299:1006–1008.
5. McKinney LA, Dornan JO, Ryan M. The role of physiotherapy in the management of acute neck sprains following road-traffic accidents. *Arch Emerg Med* 1989;6:27–33.
6. O'Leary S, Falla D, Jull G. Recent advances in therapeutic exercise for the neck: implications for patients with head and neck pain. *Aust Endod J* 2003;29:138–142.

7. Falla D, Jull G, Rainoldi A, et al. Neck flexor muscle fatigue is side specific in patients with unilateral neck pain. *Eur J Pain* 2004;8:71–77.
8. Sterling M, Jull G, Vicenzino B, et al. Development of motor system dysfunction following whiplash injury. *Pain* 2003;103:65–73.
9. Falla D, Rainoldi A, Merletti R, et al. Myoelectric manifestations of sternocleidomastoid and anterior scalene muscle fatigue in chronic neck pain patients. *Clin Neurophysiol* 2003;114:488–495.
10. Sterling M, Jull G, Wright A. Cervical mobilisation: concurrent effects on pain, sympathetic nervous system activity and motor activity. *Man Ther* 2001;6:72–81.
11. Rosenfeld M, Gunnarsson R, Borenstein P. Early intervention in whiplash-associated disorders: a comparison of two treatment protocols. *Spine* 2000;25:1782–1787.
12. Borchgrevink GE, Kaasa A, McDonagh D, et al. Acute treatment of whiplash neck sprain injuries: a randomized trial of treatment during the first 14 days after a car accident. *Spine* 1998;23:25–31.
13. Salter RB. The physiologic basis of continuous passive motion for articular cartilage healing and regeneration. *Hand Clin* 1994;10:211–219.
14. Gross AR, Hoving JL, Haines TA, et al. A Cochrane review of manipulation and mobilization for mechanical neck disorders. *Spine* 2004;29:1541–1548.
15. Bronfort G, Haas M, Evans RL, et al. Efficacy of spinal manipulation and mobilization for low back pain and neck pain: a systematic review and best evidence synthesis. *Spine J* 2004;4:335–356.
16. Gross AR, Hoving JL, Haines TA, et al. Manipulation and mobilisation for mechanical neck disorders. *Cochrane Database Syst Rev* 2004:CD004249.
17. Wang WT, Olson SL, Campbell AH, et al. Effectiveness of physical therapy for patients with neck pain: an individualized approach using a clinical decision-making algorithm. *Am J Phys Med Rehabil* 2003;82:203–218, quiz 219–221.
18. Hoving JL, Koes BW, de Vet HC, et al. Manual therapy, physical therapy, or continued care by a general practitioner for patients with neck pain: a randomized, controlled trial. *Ann Intern Med* 2002;136:713–722.
19. Cervical Overview Group. Exercises for mechanical neck disorders. *Cochrane Database Syst Rev* 2005:CD004250.
20. Lethem J, Slade PD, Troup JD, et al. Outline of a fear-avoidance model of exaggerated pain perception. I. *Behav Res Ther* 1983;21:401–408.
21. Slade PD, Troup JD, Lethem J, etl. The fear-avoidance model of exaggerated pain perception. II. *Behav Res Ther* 1983;21:409–416.
22. Waddell G, Newton M, Henderson I, et al. A Fear-Avoidance Beliefs Questionnaire (FABQ) and the role of fear-avoidance beliefs in chronic low back pain and disability. *Pain* 1993;52:157–168.
23. Crombez G, Vlaeyen JW, Heuts PH, et al. Pain-related fear is more disabling than pain itself: evidence on the role of pain-related fear in chronic back pain disability. *Pain* 1999;80:329–339.
24. Nederhand MJ, Ijzerman MJ, Hermens HJ, et al. Predictive value of fear avoidance in developing chronic neck pain disability: consequences for clinical decision making. *Arch Phys Med Rehabil* 2004;85:496–501.
25. Swinkels-Meewisse IE, Roelofs J, Verbeek AL, et al. Fear of movement/(re)injury, disability and participation in acute low back pain. *Pain* 2003;105:371–379.
26. Symonds TL, Burton AK, Tillotson KM, et al. Absence resulting from low back trouble can be reduced by psychosocial intervention at the work place. *Spine* 1995;20:2738–2745.
27. Nordemar R, Thorner C. Treatment of acute cervical pain: a comparative group study. *Pain* 1981;10:93–101.
28. Sterling M, Jull G, Carlsson Y, et al. Are cervical physical outcome measures influenced by the presence of symptomatology? *Physiother Res Int* 2002;7:113–121.
29. Vernon H, Mior S. The Neck Disability Index: a study of reliability and validity. *J Manipulative Physiol Ther* 1991;14:409–415.
30. Riddle DL, Stratford PW. Use of generic versus region-specific functional status measures on patients with cervical spine disorders. *Phys Ther* 1998;78:951–963.
31. Kaale BR, Krakenes J, Albrektsen G, et al. Whiplash-associated disorders impairment rating: neck disability index score according to severity of MRI findings of ligaments and membranes in the upper cervical spine. *J Neurotrauma* 2005;22:466–475.
32. Goolkasian P, Wheeler AH, Gretz SS. The neck pain and disability scale: test-retest reliability and construct validity. *Clin J Pain* 2002;18:245–250.
33. Wheeler AH, Goolkasian P, Baird AC, et al. Development of the Neck Pain and Disability Scale. Item analysis, face, and criterion-related validity. *Spine* 1999;24:1290–1294.
34. Leak AM, Cooper J, Dyer S, et al. The Northwick Park Neck Pain Questionnaire, devised to measure neck pain and disability. *Br J Rheumatol* 1994;33:469–474.
35. Pietrobon R, Coeytaux RR, Carey TS, et al. Standard scales for measurement of functional outcome for cervical pain or dysfunction: a systematic review. *Spine* 2002;27:515–522.
36. Wlodyka-Demaille S, Poiraudeau S, Catanzariti JF, et al. The ability to change of three questionnaires for neck pain. *Joint Bone Spine* 2004;71:317–326.
37. Hoving JL, O'Leary EF, Niere KR, et al. Validity of the neck disability index, Northwick Park neck pain questionnaire, and problem elicitation technique for measuring disability associated with whiplash-associated disorders. *Pain* 2003;102:273–281.

SECTION VI

Surgical Treatment

CHAPTER 14

Neurophysiologic Monitoring

Nouzhan Sehati and Langston T. Holly

INTRODUCTION

The purpose of intraoperative spinal cord monitoring is to provide comprehensive information about the integrity of the neural structures that may be at risk during a surgical procedure. Since feasibility studies regarding electrophysiologic monitoring began surfacing in the literature nearly three decades ago, countless techniques and applications for monitoring the spinal cord and peripheral nervous system have been developed.[1–3] Furthermore, the evolving complexity of various instrumentation constructs has demanded the development of methods to reliably assess each neurologic element, with each successive monitoring method filling the information gap left by a previously established technique.[4–6]

Current intraoperative spinal cord monitoring techniques can be divided into three categories: somatosensory evoked potentials (SSEP), motor evoked potentials (MEP), and electromyography (EMG). SSEP monitoring remains the most widely used method in spinal surgery, mainly because of its comparative ease of application, relative familiarity with the method, and proven sensitivity to a wide range of variables.[2,7] With a 99.93% true-negative rate, this modality has become an important tool in providing reassurance, as well as a valuable means for the timely identification of a neurologic deficit during surgery.[8] There are, however, spinal cord pathologic conditions that are specific to motor tracts, without any disturbance of the sensory pathways.[9–11] Because SSEPs assess only the afferent pathways in the spinal cord, such lesions may go undetected during surgery, a limitation that led to the advent of MEP monitoring as an adjunct to the traditional techniques.[9,12,13] Another monitoring modality is intraoperative EMG testing. These data are myogenic responses that are recorded from skeletal muscles of the extremities where sufficient nerve root manipulation elicits an immediate response; therefore, EMG can be used in real time to monitor ongoing activity from muscle groups during a surgical procedure. This chapter provides an overview of these monitoring techniques.

MONITORING MODALITIES

SOMATOSENSORY EVOKED POTENTIALS

The SSEP is elicited by stimulating a peripheral nerve and recording the response at various points along the afferent pathway for that nerve and across the somatosensory cortex. Evoked potentials are small-amplitude responses that are not identifiable with a single stimulus. Therefore, instruments used to record these data typically amplify, filter, and average the signal from 300 to 500 trials to produce a measurable response (Figs. 14.1 and 14.2). This process takes about 60 seconds; evoked potentials are not real-time measurements and cannot be used as an indicator of what occurs moment to moment.

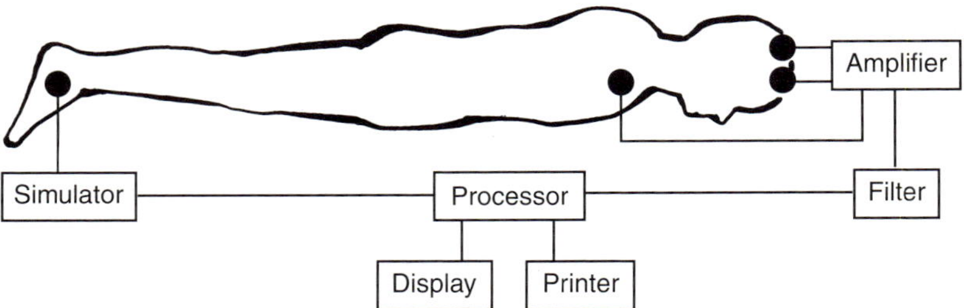

FIGURE 14.1. Diagram of the typical components of a somatosensory evoked potential monitor.

The electrical stimulation is delivered with a constant current at an intensity level that is twice that of the motor threshold.[14] For intraoperative monitoring, disposable subdermal needle electrodes are preferred over surface-type products because the former can be easily applied and provides excellent interelectrode impedance balance; the latter requires skin preparation to lower and balance impedance values, and the conductive gel used with surface electrodes must be checked frequently during surgery to maintain liquidity.[15]

Appropriate grounding, using ground patches, should be done in a location that is relatively free of muscle or surgically induced electrical noise. The need for single versus multiple ground sites is dictated by the specific equipment used for monitoring.[15]

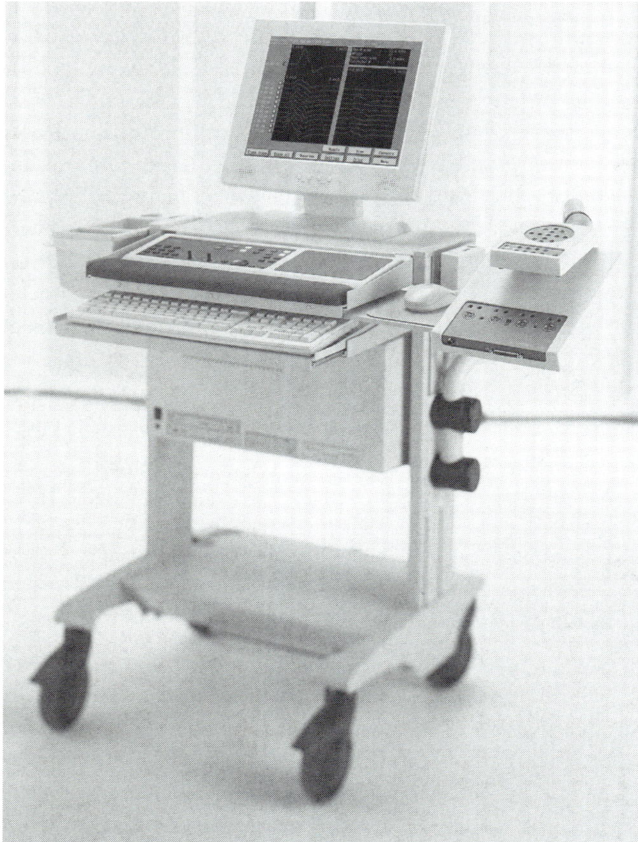

FIGURE 14.2. Various monitoring devices are commercially available that combine the necessary components of a somatosensory evoked potential monitor into a portable unit, such as this Keypoint SSEP Monitor™ by Dantec Instruments.

TABLE 14.1 Standard Somatosensory Evoked Potential Stimulation Locations

Nerve	Stimulation Site
Posterior tibial nerve	Medial malleolus
Peroneal nerve	Distal to the head of fibula
Femoral nerve	Midpoint between anterior iliac crest and pubis
Sciatic nerve	Popliteal fossa
Median nerve	Volar aspect of wrist
Ulnar nerve	Cubital tunnel

The choice of the specific nerve for stimulation is generally determined by the surgical approach and the spinal levels involved. The nerves usually used for stimulation and their corresponding stimulation sites are summarized in Table 14.1.

SSEP recordings typically appear as waveforms with predictable peaks and troughs, the amplitude and temporal spacing of which is used to interpret the results. Each peak corresponds to the arrival of the signal at a specific anatomic point that corresponds to a nearby recording site. The waveforms typically seen in an SSEP tracing are summarized in Table 14.2 and depicted in Figure 14.3.[16,17]

For procedures that involve the spinal levels T12-L4, the femoral nerve is typically used because it is more sensitive to the pathologic state of midlumbar roots, which may be overlooked by using tibial or peroneal SSEPs only. Furthermore, femoral nerve SSEPs can also detect excess retractor pressure on the iliopsoas muscle during anterior lumbar spine surgery, which, if undetected, can lead to femoral nerve palsy.[18]

Various authors have advocated the use of a secondary stimulating site that is not sensitive to pathologic conditions induced by the surgery, such as the use of an upper extremity stimulating site during thoracolumbar spine surgery.[19] This allows for an internal control that can help distinguish between iatrogenic neural injury and systemic variables such as anesthesia or blood pressure alterations as a source of SSEP change. In addition, upper extremity monitoring can permit early

TABLE 14.2 Standard Somatosensory Evoked Potential Peaks and the Corresponding Locations

Location	Waveform	Anatomic Site
Upper extremity	N10	Brachial plexus
	N12a/N12b	Segmental/ascending dorsal column
	N13a/N13b	Dorsal horn/cuneate nucleus
	N14	Medial lemniscus
	N20	Somatosensory cortex
Lower extremity	PV	Cauda equina/gracile tract
	N22/P22	Posterior horn (T10-L1)
	N29	Gracile tract nucleus
	P31	Medial lemniscus
	N34	Thalamus/brainstem
	P38/N38	Somatosensory cortex

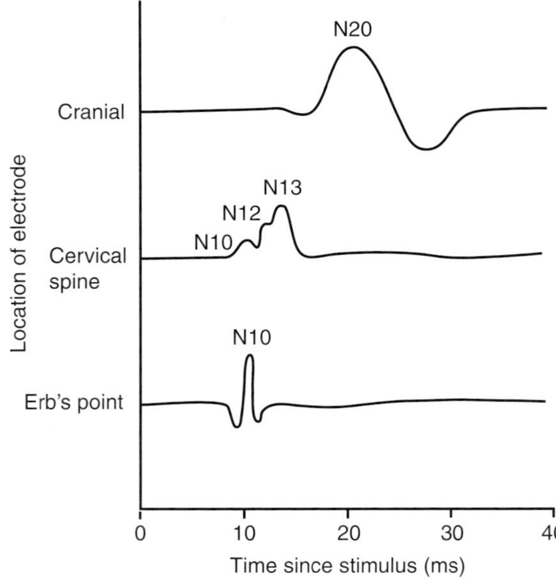

FIGURE 14.3. A typical somatosensory evoked potential recording from the ulnar nerve. Peak N10 corresponds to Erb's point, peak N12 corresponds to posterior column of the spinal cord, peak N13 corresponds to posterior column nuclei, and peak N20 corresponds to the thalamus or the primary sensory cortex.

detection of positioning-associated brachial plexus injury for cases in which the patient is placed prone on the operating table.[20]

SSEP recording sites typically consist of peripheral (popliteal fossa, sciatic notch, axilla, Erb's point), spinal (midspine and lower spine), subcortical (occiput), and cortical (C1,Cz, C2 for lower extremity, C3 for right upper extremity, and C4 for left upper extremity) locations, according to the International 10–20 System.[21] To assess encoding of the stimulus along the neural pathway, a peripheral recording site must be present for each nerve used for monitoring at a point between the primary stimulating spot and the surgical area. Such confirmation of the existence of adequate stimulation is critical in determining the presence of a neurologic problem during spinal surgery, as well as early detection of peripheral ischemia as a result of vascular compromise.

MOTOR EVOKED POTENTIALS

Since first described nearly two decades ago, transcranial magnetic stimulation (TCMS) has been used in various medical disciplines to produce peripheral myogenic responses. Magnetic stimulators are composed of a current source and a stimulating coil. The former produces sufficient current to generate a magnetic pulse within the stimulating coil that induces a current within cerebrospinal fluid and the cortex, thereby stimulating the cortical neurons and cranial nerves. The impulse that is subsequently created travels down the spinal cord and can be recorded from skeletal muscles in the extremities, typically from the tibialis anterior muscles.[15] In cases in which the spinal dura is exposed, responses can also be elicited from the spinal cord itself by using an epidural electrode.[22]

A safety concern with TCMS is its ability to cause seizures; however, studies have shown that such occurrences have been limited to patients with a prior history of seizures, making such a condition a contraindication for intraoperative MEP monitoring, as is the presence of a pacemakers, metal implants in the skull, or skull defects.[15]

Transcranial electrical stimulation (TCES) is another method currently in use for motor tract monitoring. TCES and TCMS are similar in that they both involve stimulation of the motor cortex, with both responses recorded myogenically. However, as the name implies, TCES uses direct electrical stimulation to elicit a response. Several protocols for electrical stimulation of the cortex exist. In one such protocol the active electrode is placed at Fz and the reference electrode over Cz.

Another method involves the use of one corkscrew electrode at Fz (active) and a circumferential surface electrode as reference.[23] The current required for TCES, generally in the order of 600 to 1200 volts, is typically supplied by an additional stimulator that interfaces with the existing monitoring equipment.[22]

TCMS and TCES are still in their early stages of development; thus, there are currently no standard characteristics and warning criteria. Change in amplitude and loss of response are generally considered to be sensitive indicators of subsequent neurologic deficit for both TCMS and TCES, although the choice of what constitutes significant decrease in data is, in most cases, arbitrary.[12,22,24] Despite the lack of consensus, TCES appears to be a more viable method of intraoperative MEP monitoring because of the lack of the many technical or anesthetic challenges that are seen with magnetic stimulation.

A third method of intraoperative MEP monitoring is through direct spinal cord stimulation with epidural or subarachnoid electrodes and recording of the responses from the distal spinal cord (spine to spine) or lower extremity muscles. The stimulating electrode is typically placed in the midline to allow for equal bilateral excitation of the spinal cord and avoidance of false identification of unilateral deficits.

One advantage of this method is that the obtained responses are typically robust and easily elicited, requiring minimal stimulation intensity because of the proximity of the stimulus source. Furthermore, if spine-to-spine recording is used, responses can be obtained under complete neuromuscular blockade. However, a disadvantage of this technique is that placement of stimulating and recording leads on the spinal cord can be fairly invasive, especially during spinal surgery, in which the laminotomy for electrode placement would be otherwise unnecessary.[15]

To overcome this limitation of the direct spinal cord stimulation, an alternative but similar method was introduced, called neurogenic motor evoked potential (NMEP). This involves the placement of a pair of 1-inch needle electrodes into adjacent spinous processes to stimulate the spinal cord with responses recorded neurogenically from the sciatic nerve at the ischial tuberosity or popliteal fossa.[25] Among the advantages of this method are results similar to those of direct spinal cord monitoring without the need for an unnecessary laminotomy for electrode placement and the ability to use intraoperative neuromuscular blockade during monitoring.

Variations of electrode placement for NMEP include percutaneous placement of 70- to 75-mm needle electrodes onto the base of two consecutive laminae, insertion of 1-inch needle electrodes into the disk space of consecutive spinal levels during anterior spinal surgery, and placement of an epidural catheter proximal to the surgical site.[15]

Regardless of the precise method of stimulation and recording, the NMEP response cannot be relied on as a very specific means of monitoring true motor activity because of the presence of antidromic sensory activity in the recorded response.[9,12] This has prompted some authors to refer to this method as neurogenic *mixed* evoked potential.[15]

NERVE ROOT MONITORING

The advent of spinal pedicle screw fixation has produced a new set of concerns for the intraoperative monitoring of neurologic integrity, namely that of the nerve root. Although SSEPs are of some benefit in this regard, the lower extremity somatosensory evoked response receives a contribution from multiple lumbar nerve roots, making this modality nonspecific for the individual nerve roots.

To address the concerns over nonspecificity of the traditional SSEPs, the use of dermatomal SSEPs (DSEPs) has been advocated as a method of intraoperative monitoring of the lumbar nerve roots.[26] This technique consists of stimulation of the specific dermatomal fields for the nerve roots of interest with subsequent recording of the responses across the somatosensory cortex.

One major disadvantage of this technique is the lack of a robust response compared to the SSEPs, making the identification and interpretation of the cortical DSEP data more difficult, with the subcortical and peripheral responses almost completely unidentifiable. Furthermore, this method suffers from the same limitations as the traditional SSEPs with regard to the restrictions on the use of volatile anesthetics. In addition, a growing body of evidence has suggested that the changes in intraoperative DSEP do not closely correlate with the observed postoperative neurologic status, suggesting that this method may not be a reliable means of intraoperative spinal cord monitoring.[27,28]

An alternative method for the intraoperative assessment of nerve root integrity is the spontaneous EMG. This method involves placement of an active electrode into the belly of the muscle innervated by the nerve root of interest, with a reference electrode inserted subcutaneously above the active electrode or in an adjacent tendon following adequate reversal of muscle relaxants. This allows for real-time continuous intraoperative monitoring because the stimulation of the nerve root evokes an immediate response from the corresponding myotome distribution.[29,30] Nerve roots that can be routinely monitored using this method and their corresponding muscle groups are listed in Table 14.3.

When a nerve root is activated for any reason, the consequent neurotonic discharge elicits changes on the tracing seen on the screen as well as auditory output that can be heard on the monitoring equipment. These responses are typically characterized as either *burst* or *sustained* activity. The former is the short-duration, large-amplitude response that is usually seen with sudden contact with a nerve root, as would occur when a nerve root is first retracted. Sustained or train activity is a more prolonged response that is typically an indicator of nerve root irritation or injury.[25,30–32]

Triggered electromyography, a modification of the spontaneous EMG, is a reliable means of nerve root monitoring during pedicle instrumentation. This method involves the electrical stimulation of metallic instruments (including the pedicle screw) that are placed inside of the pedicle opening for the screw, with subsequent recording of the response intensity in the muscle being monitored. A reading above a certain threshold would indicate intact pedicle borders. Although published articles have reported various threshold intensities consistent with intact versus perforated pedicle walls, a widely accepted standard guideline is currently lacking.[33,34] This is a static, stimulus-dependent technique, however, that is not capable of providing information over the course of an entire surgical procedure in the same manner as the spontaneous EMG. However, the value of the triggered EMG method for intraoperative nerve root monitoring has been extensively shown in various studies that have confirmed the results with postoperative computed tomography (CT), with a reported 98% accuracy for screw placement.[11]

TABLE 14.3 Electromyographic Recording Sites by Nerve Root

Nerve Root	Corresponding Myotome
C5	Deltoid and biceps
C6	Biceps and wrist extensors
C7	Triceps, wrist extensors, and wrist flexors
C8	Hand intrinsics and finger extensors
L2	Adductor longus and adductor magnus
L3	Adductors and vastus medialis
L4	Vastus medialis and vastus lateralis
L5	Anterior tibialis and extensor hallucis longus
S1	Medial gastrocnemius and peroneus longus
S2–S5	Perianal muscles

MONITORING PROTOCOLS

Regardless of the intraoperative monitoring technique, standard guidelines should be employed in the collection and storage of data during the procedure. Table 14.4 summarizes the recommended intraoperative monitoring modalities for some of the more common surgical procedures.[15] Typically, after induction of general anesthesia, baseline data are collected from all involved modalities before making an incision. This information is used as a baseline reference to which future data will be compared. Established warning criteria are then used to determine significant response degradation. These criteria should be sensitive to neural injury while minimizing the rate of false-positive findings.[15]

For the SSEP, the literature suggests that a change in amplitude of about 50% to 60% is a sensitive indicator of neurologic deficit, although latency of the response is also noted.[35]

Motor tract assessment using TCMS and TCES requires different criteria for significant change than those of SSEP; however, at present, further clinical studies are needed to establish reliable standards for these values.

The NMEP technique uses a degradation of 60% to 80% in amplitude as the reference point for significant neurologic injury, although, similar to the SSEP, changes in latency should also be monitored.[19,36]

Monitoring should be performed at appropriate intervals throughout the entire surgery, with more frequent data collection at critical periods, such as placement of instrumentation. Some have advocated the continuation of monitoring until postoperative neurologic status is assessed because of the possibility of a late-onset neurologic deficit.[15]

The individual performing the intraoperative monitoring must be responsible for meticulous recording and interpretation of the data. The surgical team should be made aware of true changes in data immediately, and appropriate steps should be taken to resolve the matter. Table 14.5 provides a troubleshooting guide for some of the routinely encountered intraoperative monitoring changes.[15] While interpreting the data, it should be considered that certain physiologic factors

TABLE 14.4 Recommended Intraoperative Monitoring Modalities for Various Surgical Procedures

Surgical Procedure	Monitoring Modality
Anterior cervical vertebrectomy	Median/ulnar/tibial SSEP Transcranial motor monitoring
C3-7 posterior fusion	Median/ulnar/tibial SSEP Triggered EMG Transcranial motor monitoring
T2-L3 posterior fusion	Tibial SSEP Motor tract monitoring Triggered EMG
L2-4 anterior fusion	Tibial/femoral SSEP
L3-S1 posterior decompression or fusion	Tibial SSEP Spontaneous/triggered EMG
L4-sacrum fusion	Tibial SSEP Spontaneous/triggered EMG

EMG, electromyelogram; SSEP, somatosensory evoked potential.

TABLE 14.5 Troubleshooting Guide for Selected Common Intraoperative Monitoring Changes

Monitoring Change	Possible Cause	Course of Action
Loss of SSEP from tibial nerve	Peripheral ischemia	Reposition limb or retractors
Loss of SSEP from ulnar nerve	Compression of brachial plexus	Reposition arm
Loss of cortical SSEP	Change in anesthesia	Inform anesthesiologist
	Cerebral ischemia	Finish surgery as soon as possible and initiate appropriate management
Loss of NMEP (Spinous process)	Pooling of fluid in wound	Remove excess fluid from wound
	Electrode contact with other metal	Reposition electrodes
	Neurologic deficit	Assess and reverse surgical cause
Loss of NMEP (Percutaneous)	Loss of electrode contact with lamina	Reposition electrodes
	Neurologic deficit	Place spinous process stimulating electrodes Assess and reverse surgical cause
Sustained EMG activity	Loss of recording electrodes	Reposition electrodes
	Nerve root irritation	Reposition retractors
No EMG response	Chemical muscle relaxation	Reverse muscle relaxation

EMG, electromyelogram; NMEP, neurogenic motor evoked potential; SSEP, somatosensory evoked potential.

lead to suboptimal responses, namely obesity, peripheral neuropathy, peripheral vascular disease, seizure disorders, cerebral palsy, and a history of head injury.[37,38]

In addition to systemic factors, the general anesthetic agents used can significantly affect cortically recorded or elicited data; therefore, continuous communication should exist between the monitoring technician and the anesthesiologist to ensure optimal monitoring conditions. Generally, narcotic agents are preferred over inhalation anesthetics, including nitrous oxide, for all types of intraoperative monitoring. For SSEP-monitored cases, however, the latter may be used at no more than 0.5% minimal alveolar concentrations. Conversely, when using TCMS monitoring, the use of any halogenated agents or propofol can create a marked decrease in the amplitude of the response. For this reason some authors have recommended the use of a combination of etomidate, fentanyl, and nitrous oxide for provision of anesthesia during the operation to create the optimal recording conditions with TCMS.[15]

With regard to the use of muscle relaxants, some degree of chemical paralysis may be necessary during certain critical stages of surgery because movement artifacts from TCMS or TCES can disrupt surgical maneuvers. For this reason, neuromuscular blockers can be carefully titrated to about one or two twitches in four, which minimizes patient movements while still allowing recording of a response. For EMG monitoring, however, three or four twitches are necessary because muscle fibers must be able to respond to smaller levels of neural excitement for this modality.[15]

MONITORING IN SPINAL TRAUMA

Spinal cord monitoring has been used extensively in experimental models of spinal cord injury. Several investigations have shown a time-dependent response to duration and severity of cord injury that is easily detectable with spinal cord monitoring techniques. Often the monitoring signals will recover before any clinical manifestations. The effects of decompression can be measured with somatosensory potentials again before clinical response. The use of this technique in humans with acute spinal cord injury is limited. To develop improved clinical and physiologic assessment after spinal cord injury, newer methods are being tested to measure responses distal to and at the zone of injury. These may demonstrate efficacy of new treatments or herald adverse events. For instance, loss of MEP over time has been shown to be diagnostic of posttraumatic syrinx. However, the clinical examination using American Spine Injury Association (ASIA) standards, as discussed in Chapter 7, has been shown to be as accurate as spinal cord monitoring to predict recovery.

CONCLUSION

Neurophysiologic monitoring in spinal trauma is currently used primarily for prevention of intraoperative neurologic deterioration and in experimental spinal cord injuries. The combined techniques of somatosensory and motor evoked potentials and EMG offer a more complete analysis of all modalities of spinal cord function. Standard monitoring techniques are widely available but require close communication among the surgeon, anesthesiologist, and neurophysiologist to understand the impact of any changes, as well as the strengths and limitations of the studies. Newer modalities may play a larger role in determining prognosis at an early stage following spinal trauma.

REFERENCES

1. Bradshaw K, Webb JK, Fraser AM. Clinical evaluation of spinal cord monitoring in scoliosis surgery. *Spine* 1984;9:636–643.
2. Dawson EG, Sherman JE, Kanim LE, et al. Spinal cord monitoring: results of the Scoliosis Research Society and the European Spinal Deformity Society survey. *Spine* 1991;16:S361–S364.
3. Mochida K, Shinomiya K, Komori H, et al. A new method of multisegment motor pathway monitoring using muscle potentials after train spinal stimulation. *Spine* 1995;20:2240–2246.
4. Ben-David B, Haller G, Taylor P. Anterior spinal fusion complicated by paraplegia: a case report of a false-negative somatosensory-evoked potential. *Spine* 1987;12:536–539.
5. Ben-David B, Taylor PD, Haller GS. Posterior spinal fusion complicated by posterior column injury: a case report of a false-negative wake-up test. *Spine* 1987;12:540–543.
6. Engler GL, Spielholz NJ, Bernhard WN, et al. Somatosensory evoked potentials during Harrington instrumentation for scoliosis. *J Bone Joint Surg Am* 1978;60:528-532, 1978.
7. Nuwer MR, Dawson EG, Carlson LG, et al. Somatosensory evoked potential spinal cord monitoring reduces neurologic deficits after scoliosis surgery: results of a large multicenter survey. *Electroencephalogr Clin Neurophysiol* 1995;96:6–11.
8. Potenza V, Weinstein SL, Neyt JG. Dysfunction of the spinal cord during spinal arthrodesis for scoliosis: recommendations for early detection and treatment: a case report. *J Bone Joint Surg Am* 1998;80:1679–1683.
9. Haghighi SS, York DH, Gaines RW, et al. Monitoring of motor tracts with spinal cord stimulation. *Spine* 1994;19:1518–1524.
10. Herron LD, Trippi AC, Gonyeau M. Intraoperative use of dermatomal somatosensory-evoked potentials in lumbar stenosis surgery. *Spine* 1987;12:379–383.
11. Lenke LG, Padberg AM, Russo MH, et al. Triggered electromyographic threshold for accuracy of pedicle screw placement: an animal model and clinical correlation. *Spine* 1995;20:1585–1591.
12. Edmonds HL Jr, Paloheimo MP, Backman MH, et al. Transcranial magnetic motor evoked potentials (tcMMEP) for functional monitoring of motor pathways during scoliosis surgery. *Spine* 1989;14:683–686.
13. Komanetsky RM, Padberg AM, Lenke LG, et al. Neurogenic motor evoked potentials: a prospective comparison of stimulation methods in spinal deformity surgery. *J Spinal Disord* 1998;11:21–28.
14. Prass R, Luders H. Constant-current versus constant-voltage stimulation. *J Neurosurg* 1985;62:622–623.
15. Padberg AM, Bridwell KH. Spinal cord monitoring: current state of the art. *Orthop Clin North Am* 1999;30: 407–433.

16. El Negamy E, Sedgwick EM. Delayed cervical somatosensory potentials in cervical spondylosis. *J Neurol Neurosurg Psychiatry* 1979;42:238–241.
17. Yu YL, Jones SJ. Somatosensory evoked potentials in cervical spondylosis: correlation of median, ulnar and posterior tibial nerve responses with clinical and radiological findings. *Brain* 1985;108(Part 2):273–300.
18. Robinson LR, Slimp JC, Anderson PA, et al. The efficacy of femoral nerve intraoperative somatosensory evoked potentials during surgical treatment of thoracolumbar fractures. *Spine* 1993;18:1793–1797.
19. Owen JH, Bridwell KH, Grubb R, et al. The clinical application of neurogenic motor evoked potentials to monitor spinal cord function during surgery. *Spine* 1991;16:S385–S390.
20. O'Brien MF, Lenke LG, Bridwell KH, et al. Evoked potential monitoring of the upper extremities during thoracic and lumbar spinal deformity surgery: a prospective study. *J Spinal Disord* 1994;7:277–284.
21. Klem GH, Luders HO, Jasper HH, et al. The ten-twenty electrode system of the International Federation: the International Federation of Clinical Neurophysiology. *Electroencephalogr Clin Neurophysiol Suppl* 1999;52:3–6.
22. Morota N, Deletis V, Constantini S, et al. The role of motor evoked potentials during surgery for intramedullary spinal cord tumors. *Neurosurgery* 1997;41:1327–1336.
23. Lang EW, Beutler AS, Chesnut RM, et al. Myogenic motor-evoked potential monitoring using partial neuromuscular blockade in surgery of the spine. *Spine* 1996;21:1676–1686.
24. Kalkman CJ, Ubags LH, Been HD, et al. Improved amplitude of myogenic motor evoked responses after paired transcranial electrical stimulation during sufentanil/nitrous oxide anesthesia. *Anesthesiology* 1995;83:270–276.
25. Owen JH, Naito M, Bridwell KH. Relationship among level of distraction, evoked potentials, spinal cord ischemia and integrity, and clinical status in animals. *Spine* 1990;15:852–857.
26. Machida M, Asai T, Sato K, et al. New approach for diagnosis in herniated lumbosacral disc: dermatomal somatosensory evoked potentials (DSSEPs). *Spine* 1986;11:380–384.
27. Toleikis JR, Carlvin AO, Shapiro DE, et al. The use of dermatomal evoked responses during surgical procedures that use intrapedicular fixation of the lumbosacral spine. *Spine* 1993;18:2401–2407.
28. Tsai RY, Yang RS, Nuwer MR, et al. Intraoperative dermatomal evoked potential monitoring fails to predict outcome from lumbar decompression surgery. *Spine* 1997;22:1970–1975.
29. Herdmann J, Deletis V, Edmonds HL Jr, et al. Spinal cord and nerve root monitoring in spine surgery and related procedures. *Spine* 1996;21:879–885.
30. Holland NR, Kostuik JP. Continuous electromyographic monitoring to detect nerve root injury during thoracolumbar scoliosis surgery. *Spine* 1997;22:2547–2550.
31. Hormes JT, Chappuis JL. Monitoring of lumbosacral nerve roots during spinal instrumentation. *Spine* 1993;18:2059–2062.
32. Owen JH, Kostuik JP, Gornet M, et al. The use of mechanically elicited electromyograms to protect nerve roots during surgery for spinal degeneration. *Spine* 1994;19:1704–1710.
33. Calancie B, Lebwohl N, Madsen P, et al. Intraoperative evoked EMG monitoring in an animal model: a new technique for evaluating pedicle screw placement. *Spine* 1992;17:1229–1235.
34. Calancie B, Madsen P, Lebwohl N. Stimulus-evoked EMG monitoring during transpedicular lumbosacral spine instrumentation: initial clinical results. *Spine* 1994;19:2780–2786.
35. Nagle KJ, Emerson RG, Adams DC, et al. Intraoperative monitoring of motor evoked potentials: a review of 116 cases. *Neurology* 1996;47:999–1004.
36. Padberg AM, Wilson-Holden TJ, Lenke LG, et al. Somatosensory- and motor-evoked potential monitoring without a wake-up test during idiopathic scoliosis surgery: an accepted standard of care. *Spine* 1998;23:1392–1400.
37. Ashkenaze D, Mudiyam R, Boachie-Adjei O, et al. Efficacy of spinal cord monitoring in neuromuscular scoliosis. *Spine* 1993;18:1627–1633.
38. Noordeen MH, Lee J, Gibbons CE, et al. Spinal cord monitoring in operations for neuromuscular scoliosis. *J Bone Joint Surg Br* 1997;79:53–57.

CHAPTER 15

Anterior Craniocervical Instrumentation

Daniel Fassett and Andrew T. Dailey

INTRODUCTION

The craniocervical junction (occiput, atlas, and axis) is a unique area of the spine with complex anatomy and biomechanics. Anterior approaches to the craniocervical junction are among the most technically challenging in spinal surgery, which accounts for a bias in treating unstable fractures in this area with posterior instrumentation. The mandible and multiple neurovascular structures significantly hinder the exposure to this area, and spinal surgeons often do not have significant experience with anterior exposures to the craniocervical junction. In addition, the biomechanics of the craniocervical junction favor posterior over anterior instrumentation to maximize stability in occipitocervical and atlantoaxial constructs.

With the exception of odontoid fractures, most traumatic injuries of the craniocervical junction are treated nonoperatively with halo immobilization or are surgically stabilized via posterior instrumentation. In rare situations with complex anatomy, such as a fracture in the setting of a congenital anomaly, anterior instrumentation may be used for atlantoaxial stabilization and, even more rarely, occipitocervical stabilization. Instrumentation designed for anterior approaches to the craniocervical junction is very limited and may require custom fabrication or surgeon ingenuity. This chapter will review odontoid screw fixation, anterior atlantoaxial transarticular screws, anterior atlantoaxial plating, and isolated anterior C1 fixation.

ODONTOID SCREW FIXATION

INDICATIONS

Odontoid fractures account for 10% to 20% of all cervical spine fractures and are the most common cervical spine fracture in patients over age 70.[1] Odontoid fractures may be treated conservatively with external orthosis, often with halo immobilization, but the risk for nonunion can be significant. Anderson and D'Alonzo[2] classified odontoid fractures into three clinically relevant types based on radiographic features. Type I fractures, which involve avulsion of the tip of the odontoid with the apical ligament, are extremely rare and typically do not need surgical intervention unless there is an associated atlanto-occipital dislocation. Type II fractures occur across the base of the dens and may have high nonunion rates (up to 60% to 90% in some studies) with halo immobilization. Factors predisposing a patient to nonunion include age greater than 40 years, fractures displaced more than 4 to 6 mm, or fractures angulated more than 10 degrees.[1,3–5] Type III fractures extend into the vertebral body of the axis and can be further subdivided into shallow type III fractures and more extensive fractures of the vertebral body. Type III fractures have a higher fusion rate with halo immobilization than type II fractures, and, thus, there is a bias toward conservative management with halo orthosis. However, shallow type III fractures may be more similar biomechanically and histologically to type II fractures, and, thus, some surgeons will consider odontoid screw fixation for shallow type III fractures.[6,7] Comminuted fractures of the body of C2 are generally a contraindication for screw fixation because the fractured body will not provide firm anchor for the screw head. While surgical indications for odontoid fractures remain controversial, many surgeons will consider odontoid screw fixation for type II and shallow type III fractures.

DESCRIPTION OF PROCEDURE

The key to odontoid screw fixation is the operative setup and optimization of the biplanar fluoroscopy, which is critical to any procedure performed without direct visualization of the surgical site. The patient is positioned supine in a slight reverse Trendelenburg position. Although the cervical spine should initially be kept in a neutral position, we recommend placing a folded blanket or towel beneath the patient's shoulders to maximize the potential for cervical extension, which could be required to obtain the trajectory needed for optimal odontoid screw placement. Two C-arms are preferred to provide simultaneous orthogonal images of the odontoid process without the need to move the C-arm many times through a 90-degree arc. The fluoroscopy units are brought in from opposite sides, and setup is easier if the C-arms are different sizes, with the smaller unit placed inside the larger (Fig. 15.1A). A radiolucent support (such as a bottle cork) is placed between the patient's upper and lower teeth to maintain an open-mouth anteroposterior (AP) fluoroscopic view.

Once true lateral and AP images are obtained, the cervical spine can be manipulated with lateral fluoroscopy to ensure that spinal canal compromise does not occur. An attempt should be made to maximize the extension of the cervical spine because this provides the best trajectory for screw placement. Without cervical extension, the chest tends to obstruct the trajectory for odontoid screw placement. A short neck, large "barrel chest," and loss of cervical lordosis are all relative contraindications to odontoid screw fixation because these factors can be associated with an obstructed screw trajectory. Careful attention should be paid to the lateral fluoroscopy as the cervical spine is extended, because this maneuver may displace the fractured dens into the spinal canal.

After careful positioning, the surgeon should confirm that a trajectory exists for odontoid screw placement by placing a Kirschner wire (K-wire) beside the patient's neck and confirming the trajectory on lateral fluoroscopy. A transverse incision is typically made on the right side of the patient's neck at the level of C5-C6, medial to the sternocleidomastoid for a standard Smith-Robinson approach to the prevertebral space. Blunt dissection is then performed in the prevertebral tissues up to the level of C2 with a side-to-side sweeping motion with a Kittner dissector to free the tissues over the screw entry point. One conventional retractor system, as described by Apfelbaum et al.[7] used Caspar-type blades placed under the longus colli muscle at C5 and an attachable up-angled blade to retract the pharyngeal tissues of the spine as far cephalad as the C1 level. New table-mounted tubular retractors have been used to eliminate the need for longus colli dissection and may provide better lateral protection of the surrounding soft tissues.[8,9]

Once the retractors are in place, the remainder of the procedure is performed with biplanar fluoroscopy guidance without direct visualization of the operative site. A K-wire is carefully guided to the anterior lip of the inferior endplate of C2 in the midline and gently tapped 3 to 4 mm into the body of C2 (Fig. 15.1B). Care is taken to make certain the starting point is in the inferior endplate of C2 and not along the anterior cortex of the C2 body, to prevent screw pull-out. A 7-mm-diameter drill is placed over the K-wire and advanced to the C2-C3 level to provide a trough in the C3 anterior cortex and allow better screw trajectory. A drill guide tube is inserted over the K-wire and gently advanced to the entry site on the inferior aspect of C2. A drill guide can be affixed to the C3 vertebral body, which then allows removal of the K-wire. A 3.0-mm drill bit is placed through the guide tube and a starter hole is drilled through the body of C2, across the fracture site, and into the dens including the distal cortex (Fig. 15.1C). The entire course of the screw should be drilled and tapped with

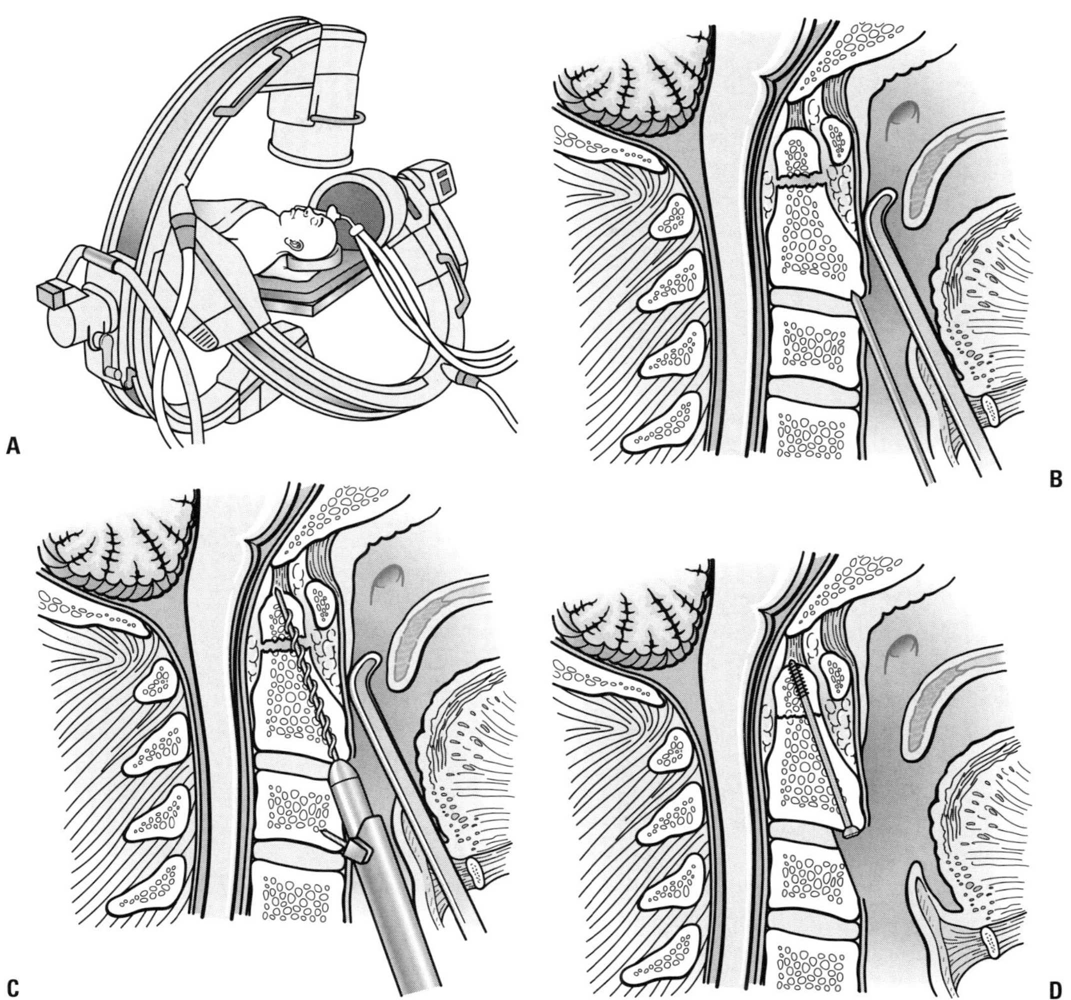

FIGURE 15.1. A. Odontoid screw placement is performed with fluoroscopic (preferably biplanar) guidance without direct visualization of the surgical site. **B.** A K-wire is guided to the midline of the inferior endplate of C2 and gently tapped into this endplate 1 to 2 mm behind the anterior wall of the vertebral body. **C.** After creating a trough in C3 with a hand drill, a drill-guide system is walked up the ventral cervical spine to the C3 level and a starter hole is drilled through the body of C2 across the fracture into the odontoid process. The drill is advanced under fluoroscopic guidance to the center of the odontoid tip in the anteroposterior and lateral planes. It is important to drill through the distal cortex of the odontoid to obtain bicortical purchase. **D.** The entire course of the screw is tapped, followed by placement of a lag screw (threaded only at the distal cortex to allow for reduction).

attention to include the distal cortex, which provides the majority of pull-out strength. Screw length is determined with the calibrated drill guide and tap. A lag screw is used to pull the fractured dens into approximation with the body of C2 to optimize bone healing (Fig. 15.1D). Some surgeons have advocated the use of two screws, but biomechanical and clinical studies have shown no benefit in two screws over one screw for odontoid fixation.[10,11] If two screws are to be placed, each screw should start approximately 3 to 4 mm off the midline at entry into the lower part of C2 and angle slightly medially to target the midline odontoid tip.

OUTCOMES AND COMPLICATIONS

Fusion rates for odontoid screw fixation are 81% to 92% for acute fractures (<6 months) in large reported series.[6,7,10] Horizontal and posterior oblique type II fractures have a better fusion rate than anterior oblique fractures, which are more likely to displace.[7] Many of these patients are older, with significant comorbidities, and, as a result, general complications such as myocardial infarction, pulmonary compromise, and general infections have been reported in up to 14% of these patients.[6] Surgery-specific complications include dysphagia, airway compromise from pharyngeal edema, esophageal injury, spinal cord injury, and hardware failure.[6,7]

ANTERIOR ATLANTOAXIAL TRANSARTICULAR SCREWS

INDICATIONS

Anterior atlantoaxial transarticular screws have been used in rare situations as a salvage technique after failed posterior C1-C2 arthrodesis, for complex fractures involving C1 and C2 that preclude posterior arthrodesis procedures, in patients who cannot tolerate prone positioning for posterior atlantoaxial arthrodesis, and as a salvage technique when an odontoid screw fails to gain purchase.[12,13]

DESCRIPTION OF PROCEDURE

This fixation technique was initially described via bilateral anterior prevascular retropharyngeal approaches,[13–17] but a standard Smith-Robinson approach with screw placement guided using biplanar fluoroscopy has also been reported.[18] Although the anterior retropharyngeal approach is more complex and requires bilateral approaches for screw placement, it provides better exposure of the C1-C2 articulation to allow for decortication of the facets and placement of bone graft.

In the anterior prevascular retropharyngeal approach, the patient is positioned supine with the neck extended as far as possible, and lateral fluoroscopy and neuromonitoring (somatosensory evoked potentials or motor evoked potentials) are used to ensure that spinal canal compromise does not occur. A submandibular incision is made from approximately 2 cm off the midline to the ipsilateral mastoid process (Fig. 15.2A). Subcutaneous tissues and the platysma are divided in this same dissection plane. Multiple superficial branches (greater auricular nerve and transverse cervical nerve) of the cervical plexus and the external jugular vein will be encountered and need to be divided. A careful dissection beneath the parotid gland is performed to protect the branches of the facial nerve contained within the gland. The digastric muscle and hypoglossal nerve are found deep to the parotid gland and, after careful dissection all of these structures, are gently retracted superiorly. The surgeon should exercise caution to protect the marginal mandibular nerve, a branch of the facial nerve that courses from the parotid gland along the inferior aspect of the mandible superficial to the vein. The facial vein is encountered coursing over the carotid bifurcation and is divided.

The lateral dissection is performed along the anterior margin of the sternocleidomastoid muscle and carotid sheath. Branches of the external carotid artery, usually the superior thyroid, lingual, and facial arteries, are found crossing the operative field at this level and can be ligated as necessary for exposure. The superior laryngeal nerve is identified posterior to the carotid artery running inferomedially and should be carefully mobilized and protected. The prevertebral tissues are visualized at this point, and the fascia can be incised to expose the longus colli muscles (Fig. 15.2B). A similar but smaller approach is performed on the contralateral side, and connection is made between the two sides. The longus colli muscles are elevated bilaterally to visualize the C1-C2 joints. Curettes and a high-speed drill are used to remove the articular cartilage and decorticate the surfaces of these joints. Morselized bone graft is placed within the decorticated C1-C2 articulation before placement of transarticular screws.

After the C1-C2 joints are prepared for arthrodesis, attention turns to placement of transarticular screws. Screws are best placed through the contralateral incisions (left screw placed through the right neck incision) to allow for the appropriate lateral screw angulation. The starting point for anterior transarticular screws is in the sulcus along the margin of the prominent C2 body where it joins the C2 lateral mass approximately midpoint on the sulcus (Fig. 15.2D). Cannulated and noncannulated systems have been used for this procedure. The screw trajectory is approximately 25 degrees laterally in the coronal plane and approximately 65 degrees superiorly in the sagittal plane (Fig. 15.2C,D). The optimum screw crosses perpendicular to the C1-C2 articulation to maximize the potential for lag screw compression across the joint and target the superior-posterolateral corner of the C1 lateral mass. Screw length is typically 15 to 25 mm, and care should be taken not to pass through the distal C1 cortex and into the occipital condyle–C1 lateral mass articulation.

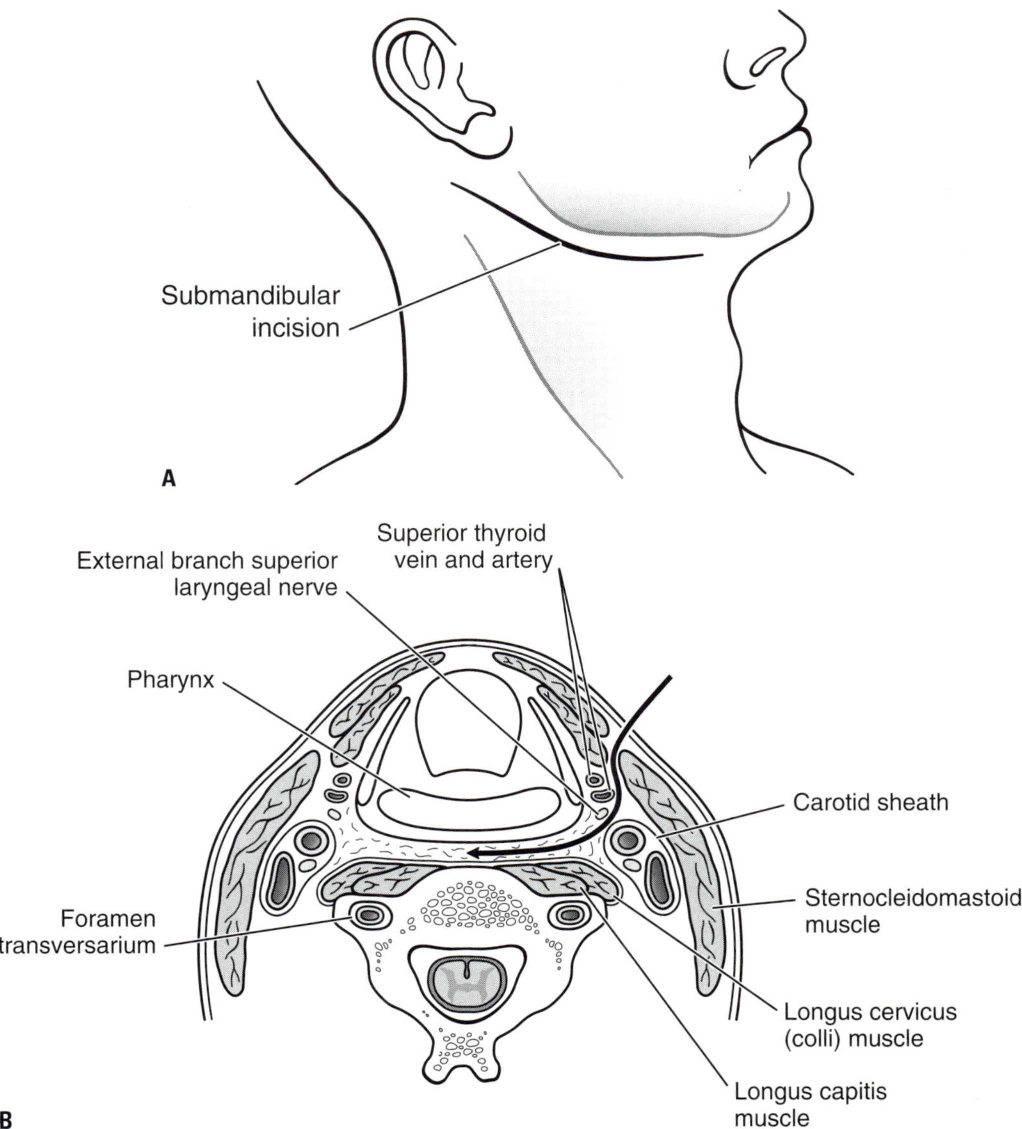

FIGURE 15.2. Anterior atlantoaxial transarticular screws. A bilateral prevascular retropharyngeal approach is often used to expose the spine for placement of anterior transarticular screws. **A.** Submandibular incision is used, and a dissection plane **(B)** is carried down to the prevertebral space ventral to the carotid sheath. *(continued)*

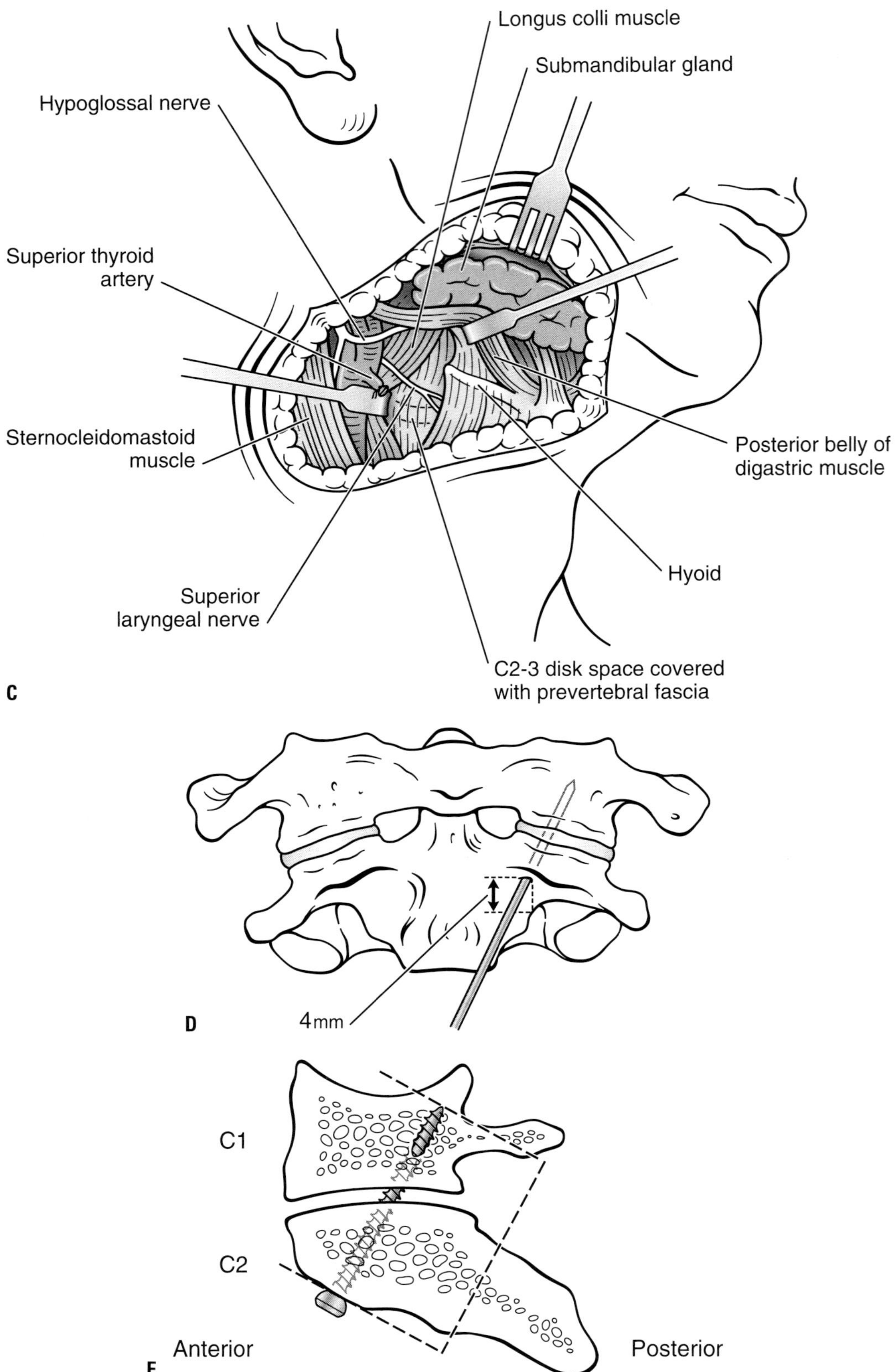

FIGURE 15.2. *(continued)* **(C)** After deep dissection with ligation of superior thyroid artery, the prevertebral space is exposed. Ventral **(D)** and lateral **(E)** views of anterior atlantoaxial transarticular screws placed through the C2 lateral masses across the atlantoaxial articulation into the C1 lateral masses.

OUTCOME AND COMPLICATIONS

Limited case reports have described success with this procedure, but sufficient numbers are lacking to report fusion rates to compare it with other C1-C2 arthrodesis procedures. Complications with this procedure have not been emphasized in the literature, but potential complications can include airway compromise; injury to hypoglossal, superior laryngeal, or marginal mandibular nerves; and vertebral artery injury.

C1-C2 ANTERIOR PLATE FIXATION

INDICATIONS

C1-C2 anterior plate fixation was originally developed by Harms et al.[19] for atlantoaxial stabilization after transoral odontoidectomy. Although it has mainly been used in degenerative or oncologic spinal conditions, it may have a role in cases of traumatic C1-C2 instability in which anterior decompression is needed, such as chronic odontoid nonunion with myelopathy.[20,21]

DESCRIPTION OF PROCEDURE

Transpharyngeal approaches, either standard transoral or mandibular splitting techniques, have been used most commonly with anterior atlantoaxial plating, but retropharyngeal approaches may also be used for this procedure. In transpharyngeal approaches, the posterior pharynx is exposed and the anterior tubercle of C1 is palpated as a reference landmark. The mucosa is opened in the midline from the clivus to the top of C3 (3.0 to 4.0 cm in length), and dissection is carried down to the anterior arch of C1 with Bovie cautery. Lateral dissection on top of the C1 arch and C2 body is carried laterally until the C1-C2 joints and screw entry points are exposed (usually 15 to 20 mm off the midline). The C1-C2 articular capsules are incised, and the articular cartilage is removed with curettes or a high-speed drill. If odontoidectomy is needed, the midline arch of C1 and odontoid are removed with a high-speed drill. The articular surfaces are packed with bone graft before plating.[12,22]

The Harms plate (Fig. 15.3A) has five screw fixation slots: one in each C1 lateral mass, one in each medial C2 lateral mass, and one in the midline C2 vertebral body. More recent plate designs such as the transoral atlantoaxial reduction plate (TARP) and subarticular atlantoaxial locking plate (SAALP) atlantoaxial plating systems (Fig. 15.3B,C) reported by Yin et al.[22] and Kandziora et al.[23] used a design similar to Harms plating, except for the screw-plate locking mechanisms and the fact that only two screws are placed into the vertebral body of C2 with the TARP system. The optimum entry point for C1 lateral mass screw placement is at the center of the C1 lateral mass, which is reported to be 16.8 ($\pm$1.5) mm off the midline and angled 10 to 15 degrees laterally.[22,24] The C1 articular mass screws are typically 20 to 24 mm in length and should not violate the posterior cortex of C1 to avoid potential vertebral artery injury.[24] Two of the C2 screws (usually 10 to 16 mm in length) are typically placed at the medial margin of the lateral masses and angled 5 to 10 degrees medially into the body of C2; in some systems a third screw is placed in the midline of the body of C2.[22,24,25]

OUTCOMES AND COMPLICATIONS

Few clinical data have been published on the efficacy of anterior atlantoaxial plating systems. Biomechanical studies have shown that the Harms anterior plate provides less stability than posterior atlantoaxial transarticular screws, but when supplemented by a Brooks posterior wiring construct, the Harms plate has stability similar to that provided by transarticular screws. In a limited clinical series, Kerschbaumer et al.[26] reported similar concerns with the Harms atlantoaxial plate when they noted screw pull-out in two of three patients treated with a Harms plate without a posterior wiring construct. In a subsequent study of 12 patients who had a Brooks wiring construct to supplement the Harms plate, the authors reported no hardware complications and a 100% fusion rate. Other biomechanical studies have shown that anterior atlantoaxial plating with locking screws provided more stability and was similar to posterior atlantoaxial transarticular screws in stiffness.[23] Yin et al.[22] reported no complications and a 100% fusion rate in five patients stabilized with the TARP system using a locking screw mechanism without posterior grafting.

A Harms plate

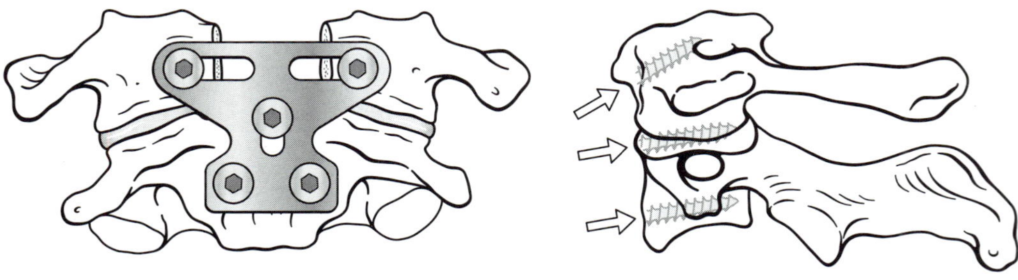

B SAALP plate (Subarticular atlantoaxial locking plate)

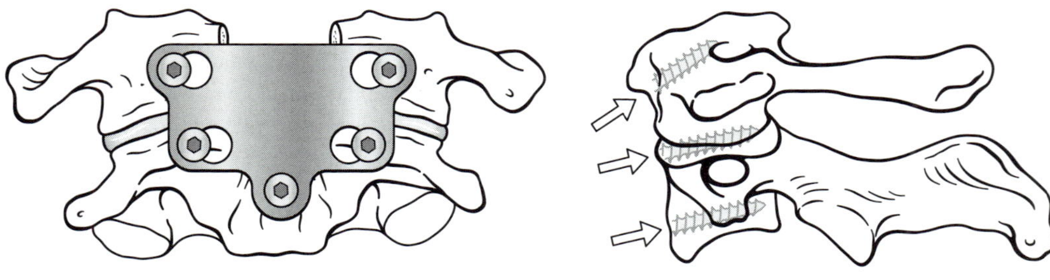

C TARP plate (Transoral atlantoaxial reduction plate)

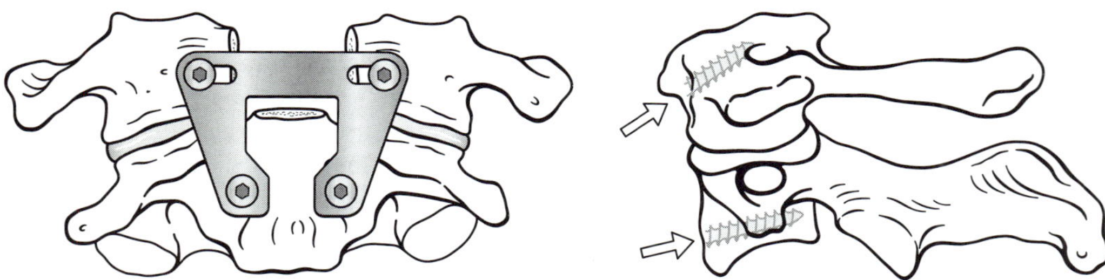

FIGURE 15.3. C1-C2 anterior plate fixation. Atlantoaxial plate fixation was originally described by Harms et al.[19] for anterior fixation after odontoidectomy. **A.** The Harms plate has two screws fixated into C1 lateral masses and three screws into C2. Subsequent modifications, by Kandziora et al.[23] and Yin et. al.,[22] have a screw-to-plate locking mechanism—SAALP plate **(B)** and TARP plate **(C)**—to improve stability and reduce complications resulting from screw pull-out.

Potential complications include the possibility of increased risk for infection with instrumentation placed through a transoral route, airway compromise, swallowing difficulty, and vertebral artery injury.

ISOLATED ANTERIOR ATLAS FIXATION

INDICATIONS

Stability of C1 burst fractures is determined by the integrity of the transverse ligament, and when unstable, management options vary. Some physicians will treat these fractures with reduction via traction followed by halo immobilization. On the other hand, because conservative treatment of

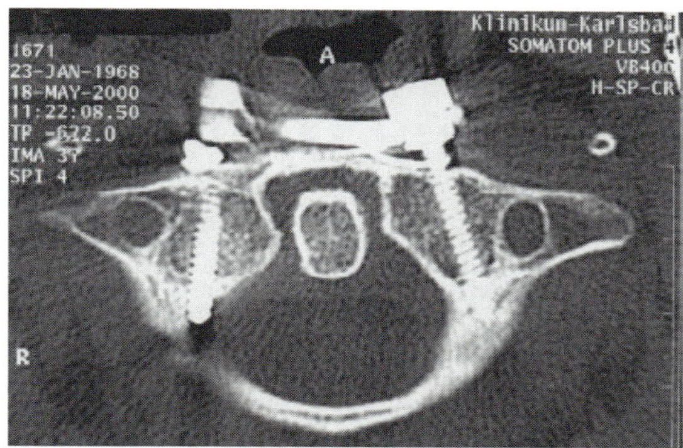

FIGURE 15.4. Anterior atlas fixation for treatment of C1 burst fractures. Although this procedure was originally performed by Harms with plate fixation of the atlas,[27] it was subsequently modified to bilateral anterior C1 lateral mass screws connected by a rod as shown. This procedure is typically placed through a transoral transpharyngeal approach.

unstable C1 burst fractures has a significant risk for persistent instability, some surgeons advocate primary C1-C2 fusion or occiput to C2 fusion to treat these fractures. With C1-C2 fusion, the loss of axial rotation range of motion is significant and degeneration in the cervical spine may be increased as a result. In addition, the occiput may need to be included in the construct unless the C1 lateral mass can accept direct fixation. As an alternative, Harms and colleagues proposed direct reduction and internal fixation of unstable C1 burst fractures to promote bone and ligament healing while maintaining mobility of the C1-C2 articulation.[27]

DESCRIPTION OF PROCEDURE

Patients are placed in traction to assist with reduction of the C1 lateral masses. The anterior arch and anterior aspect of the lateral masses of C1 are exposed by a transpharyngeal route as previously described. In their initial patients, Ruf et al.[27] used compression plates with screws placed into the bilateral lateral masses of C1. In subsequent patients, they used small polyaxial screws placed into the lateral masses of C1 and rods that allowed for improved reduction by compressing across the screws and locking the rod in place. The entry point for the screws is in the center of the lateral masses, which can be determined by palpating the margins of the lateral masses intraoperatively. Screw length is determined from preoperative computed tomography (CT) imaging and confirmed intraoperatively with lateral fluoroscopy.

OUTCOMES AND COMPLICATIONS

In 2004, Ruf et al.[27] reported that the average total lateral mass displacement in six patients treated with this technique was 13.5 mm before surgery and was reduced to 4.3 mm postoperatively. The average flexion-extension atlanto-dens interval difference in follow-up was 2.0 mm, and none of the patients needed subsequent fusion procedures for atlantoaxial instability. The authors noted one complication related to loosening of the screw-rod interface, which led to loss of reduction of one of the C1 lateral masses and may have resulted in a poor clinical outcome with chronic neck pain. All of the other patients showed a solid fusion of the C1 ring on follow-up CT imaging.

CONCLUSION

With the exception of odontoid screw fixation, anterior instrumentation of the craniocervical junction is technically challenging and limited to special circumstances in which posterior approaches are not feasible or ventral decompression is needed in addition to mechanical stabilization.

REFERENCES

1. Greene KA, Dickman CA, Marciano FF, et al. Acute axis fractures: analysis of management and outcome in 340 consecutive cases. *Spine* 1997;22:1843–1852.
2. Anderson LD, D'Alonzo RT. Fractures of the odontoid process of the axis. *J Bone Joint Surg Am* 1974;56: 1663–1674.
3. Apuzzo ML, Heiden JS, Weiss MH, et al. Acute fractures of the odontoid process: an analysis of 45 cases. *J Neurosurg* 1978;48:85–91.
4. Hadley MN, Browner C, Sonntag VK. Axis fractures: a comprehensive review of management and treatment in 107 cases. *Neurosurgery* 1985;17:281–290.
5. Dunn ME, Seljeskog EL. Experience in the management of odontoid process injuries: an analysis of 128 cases. *Neurosurgery* 1986;18:306–310.
6. Henry AD, Bohly J, Grosse A. Fixation of odontoid fractures by an anterior screw. *J Bone Joint Surg Br* 1999;81:472–477.
7. Apfelbaum RI, Lonser RR, Veres R, et al. Direct anterior screw fixation for recent and remote odontoid fractures. *J Neurosurg* 2000;93(suppl 2):227–236.
8. Hashizume H, Kawakame M, Kawai M, et al. A clinical case of endoscopically assisted anterior screw fixation for the type II odontoid fracture. *Spine* 2003;28:E102–E105.
9. Shalayev SG, Mun IK, Mallek GS, et al. Retrospective analysis and modifications of retractor systems for anterior odontoid screw fixation. *Neurosurg Focus*, 2004;16:E14.
10. Jenkins JD, Coric D, Branch CL Jr. A clinical comparison of one- and two-screw odontoid fixation. *J Neurosurg* 1998;89:366–370.
11. Doherty BJ, Heggeness MH, Esses SI. A biomechanical study of odontoid fractures and fracture fixation. *Spine* 1993;18:178–184.
12. Silber JS. C1-C2 transarticular screw fixation. In: Kim DH, Vaccaro AR, Fessler RG, eds. *Spinal Instrumentation.* New York: Thieme Medical Publishers, 2005:81–85.
13. Vaccaro AR, Lehman AP, Alhgren BD, et al. Anterior C1-C2 screw fixation and bony fusion through an anterior retropharyngeal approach. *Orthopedics* 1999;22:1165–1170.
14. de Andrade JR, Macnab I. Anterior occipito-cervical fusion using an extra-pharyngeal exposure. *J Bone Joint Surg Am* 1969;51:1621–1626.
15. Lu J, Ebraheim NA, Yang H. Anatomic considerations of anterior transarticular screw fixation for atlantoaxial instability. *Spine* 1998;23:1229–1235, discussion 1236.
16. Laus M, Pignatti G, Malaguti MC, et al. Anterior extraoral surgery to the upper cervical spine. *Spine* 1996;21:1687–1693.
17. McAfee PC, Bohlman HH, Riley LH Jr, et al. The anterior retropharyngeal approach to the upper part of the cervical spine. *J Bone Joint Surg Am* 1987;69:1371–1383.
18. Reindl R, Sen M, Aebi M. Anterior instrumentation for traumatic C1-C2 instability. *Spine* 2003;28:E329–E333.
19. Harms J, Schmelzle R, Stoltze D. Osteosynthsen im occipito-cervicalem Ubergang vom transoralen Zungang aus. In: XVII SICOT World Congress, Munich, 1987.
20. Subin B, Lui JF, Marshall GJ, et al. Transoral anterior decompression and fusion of chronic irreducible atlantoaxial dislocation with spinal cord compression. *Spine* 1995;20:1233–1240.
21. Silber JS. C1-C2 anterior plate fixation. In: Kim DH, Vaccaro AR, Fessler RG, eds. *Spinal Instrumentation.* New York: Thieme Medical Publishers, 2005:86–89.
22. Yin Q, Ai F, Zhang K, et al. Irreducible anterior atlantoaxial dislocation: one-stage treatment with a transoral atlantoaxial reduction plate fixation and fusion—report of 5 cases and review of the literature. *Spine* 2005;30: E375–E381.
23. Kandziora F, Phflugmacher R, Ludwig K, et al. Biomechanical comparison of four anterior atlantoaxial plate systems. *J Neurosurg* 2002;96(suppl 3):313–320.
24. Kandziora F, Kerschbaumer F, Starker M, et al. Biomechanical assessment of transoral plate fixation for atlantoaxial instability. *Spine* 2000;25:1555–1561.
25. Kandziora F, Schulze SN, Khodadadyan KC, et al. Screw placement in transoral atlantoaxial plate systems: an anatomical study. *J Neurosurg* 2001;95(suppl 1):80–87.
26. Kerschbaumer F, Kandziora F, Klein C, et al. Transoral decompression, anterior plate fixation, and posterior wire fusion for irreducible atlantoaxial kyphosis in rheumatoid arthritis. *Spine* 2000;25:2708–2715.
27. Ruf M, Melcher R, Harms J. Transoral reduction and osteosynthesis C1 as a function-preserving option in the treatment of unstable Jefferson fractures. *Spine* 2004;29:823–827.

CHAPTER 16

Posterior Craniocervical Instrumentation

K. Michael Webb, Mark G. Burnett, and Volker K. H. Sonntag

INTRODUCTION

Once traumatic occipitocervical instability has been established, the goals of surgical treatment are to restore normal alignment, to decompress neural elements, and to provide immediate stability to facilitate early rehabilitation and long-term bony fusion. The ideal construct should stabilize the craniocervical junction while minimizing fusion at normal levels and concomitant loss of cervical motion segments. This chapter describes occipitocervical screw-rod constructs, threaded Steinmann pin fixation, and two novel techniques that spare the atlantoaxial joint and preserve neck rotation.

POSITIONING

If not already wearing a halo brace, the patient is placed in the halo orthosis before positioning. Preoperative antibiotics are administered so that therapeutic levels are reached before the incision is made. Somatosensory evoked potential (SSEP) and motor evoked potential (MEP) leads are inserted, and baseline values are recorded to monitor spinal cord function during positioning and surgery.

The patient is log-rolled into the prone position on the operating table. The Mayfield head holder (Codman Inc., Raynham, MA) with a halo adapter is used to fix the head in a neutral position. This point is essential because significant disability can occur with fusion in lordosis or kyphosis. Fluoroscopy is used to evaluate the occipitocervical alignment. The iliac crest incision is then marked and prepared.

INCISION AND EXPOSURE

A midline incision is made from the inion to the midcervical spine. If C1-C2 transarticular screws will be used to fixate the upper cervical spine, the incision is extended to C7 or draping must accommodate percutaneous screw placement (Fig. 16.1).

Subperiosteal dissection with monopolar electrocauterization is used to expose the occipital squamosa from the foramen magnum to the inion, the spinous processes, and the laminae of the vertebrae to be fused. Laterally, we prefer gentle dissection with small periosteal elevators rather than electrocauterization because the former provides a better substrate for subsequent bony fusion. In most cases, the construct ends at C1 or C2. However, if a laminectomy is needed for decompression, we extend the fusion one level below the laminectomy.

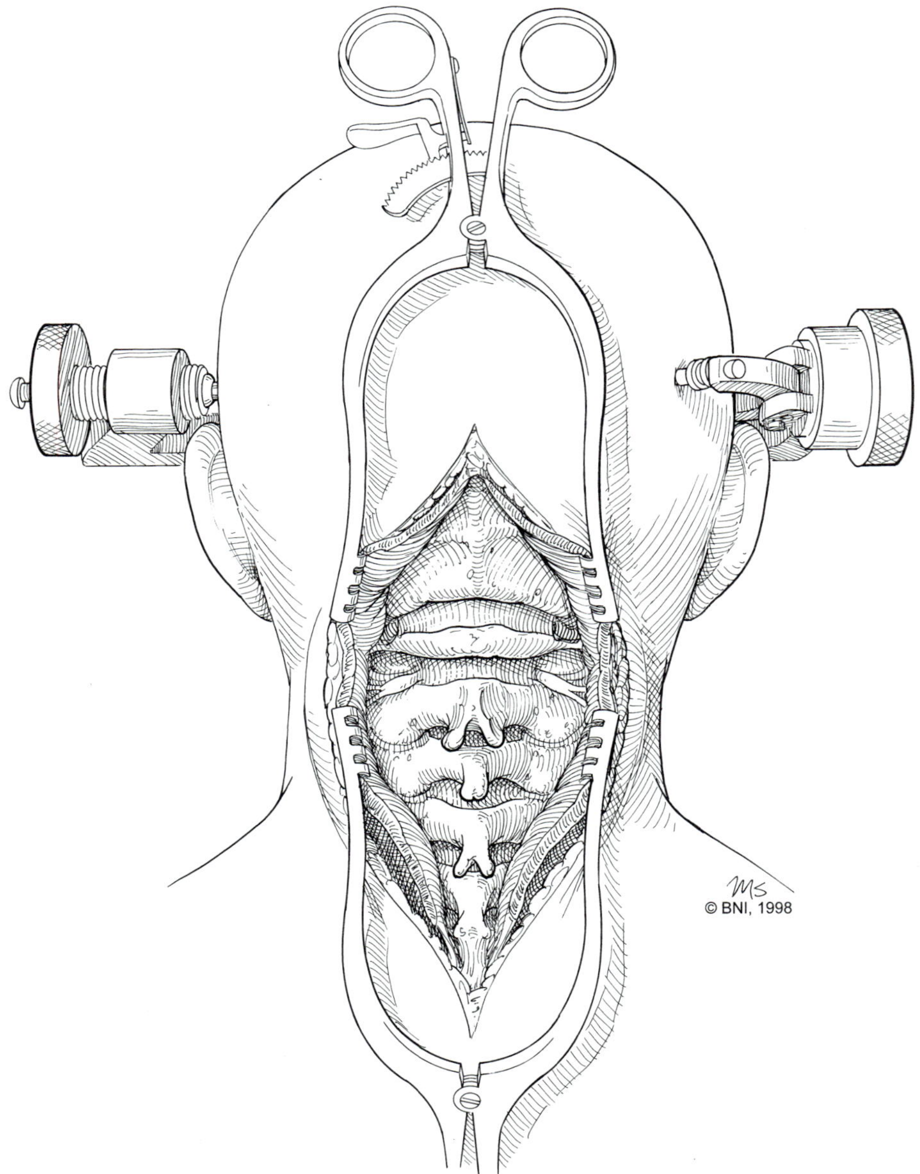

FIGURE 16.1. Surgical exposure required for most occipitocervical fusion procedures. (With permission from Barrow Neurological Institute.)

Two points of caution should be observed during the exposure. First, the ligaments attaching the occiput to the spine are damaged, making the area susceptible to abnormal movement during exposure. Gentle dissection must be used to avoid neurologic injury. Second, the vertebral artery courses on top of the arch of C1 before it enters the dura. This point is usually 1.5 cm lateral from the midline and far enough laterally to be of no practical significance during surgery for trauma. However, care must be taken during C1 exposure to avoid injury to the vertebral artery. The vertebral artery is surrounded by a venous plexus, bleeding from which heralds proximity to the vertebral artery. When the exposure is completed, the neural elements are decompressed if necessary.

OCCIPITOCERVICAL CONSTRUCTS

SCREW-ROD CONSTRUCTS

Screw-rod constructs have gained popularity as biomechanical studies have shown that they offer more stability than wiring or Steinmann pin techniques.[1–3] This increased stability allows the construct to span only the affected levels, thereby saving cervical motion segments. The most common constructs involve occipital screws joined to C1 lateral mass and C2 pars screws or to C1-C2 transarticular screws, the placement of which is described elsewhere (Fig. 16.2).[4–7]

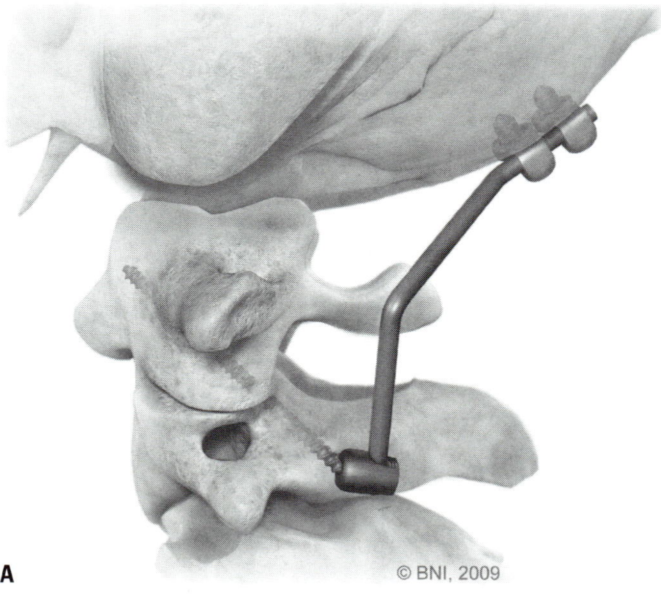

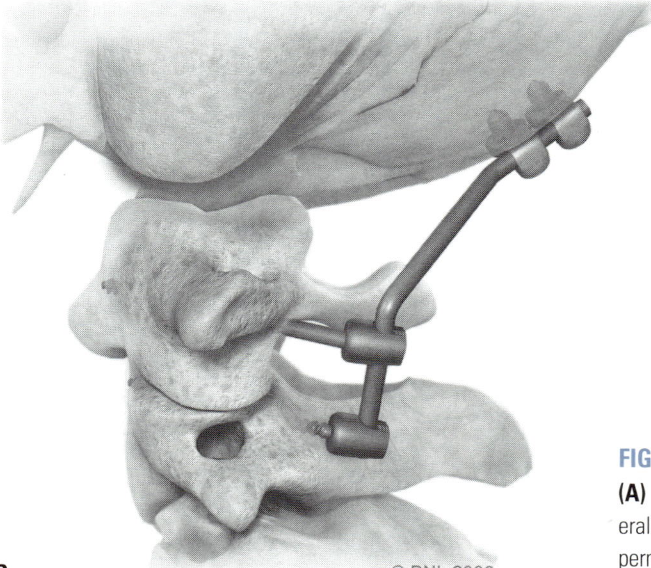

FIGURE 16.2. Occipitocervical fusion with **(A)** transarticular screws and with **(B)** C1 lateral mass and C2 pedicle/pars screws. (With permission from Barrow Neurological Institute.)

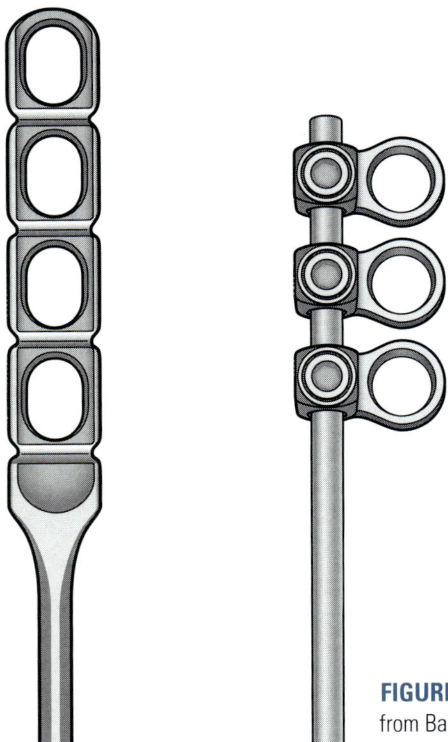

FIGURE 16.3. Rod implants for occipitocervical fusion. (With permission from Barrow Neurological Institute.)

Several implants are available to connect the occipital screws to the spine. One option is a combination rod-plate. Eyelet connectors also can be attached to a rod, through which occipital screws are placed (Fig. 16.3).

OCCIPITAL SCREW PLACEMENT

Because the suboccipital bone is thickest along its midline keel, occipital screws should be placed as medially as possible. It is often helpful first to bend and fit the rod to the occipitocervical junction to mark the location for the screw holes. A sterile endotracheal tube stylet can be used as a template.

A high-speed drill is used to create a hole in the suboccipital bone until the dura is exposed. This distance is measured and then tapped. The drill hole should be no larger than the minor diameter of the tap. If a dural tear occurs with cerebrospinal fluid leakage, a small piece of Gelfoam is inserted into the pilot hole, followed by screw placement.

VERTEBRAL ARTERY INJURY

If brisk arterial bleeding is encountered at any point during placement of the atlantoaxial screws, the vertebral artery has likely been damaged. Hemostasis is achieved by inserting the screw. However, it should be assumed that the involved vertebral artery no longer contributes to cerebral blood flow. Therefore, screw placement that could jeopardize the contralateral vertebral artery should be avoided. Postoperatively, a vascular study such as a computed tomography (CT) angiogram should be obtained to evaluate the vertebral artery for flow and for the presence of a pseudoaneurysm, fistula, or dissection. If one of these is present, endovascular repair using stents or balloon occlusion should be considered.

OCCIPUT-C1 FUSION TECHNIQUES

Although occipitocervical fixation using C1-C2 transarticular screws or C1 lateral mass/C2 pars screws offers excellent stability, both techniques involve fusion to C2. However, in some cases, the

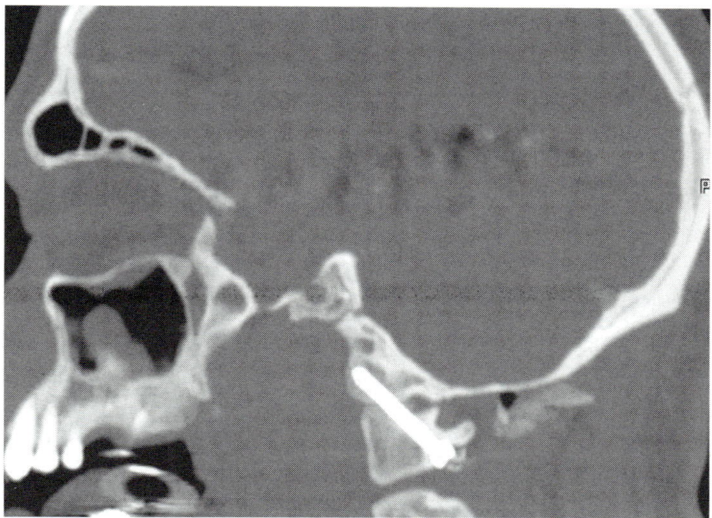

FIGURE 16.4. Lateral computed tomography scan after atlantocondylar screw placement. The hypoglossal canal is superior to the screw. (From Feiz-Erfan I, Gonzalez LF, Dickman CA. Atlantooccipital transarticular screw fixation for the treatment of traumatic occipitoatlantal dislocation. *J Neurosurg Spine* 2005;2:381–385. With permission from Journal of Neurosurgery.)

C1-C2 joint is stable. These cases would have intact alar ligaments and tectorial membranes. Two techniques have been described that provide occipitocervical stability and preserve neck rotation.

OCCIPUT-C1 TRANSARTICULAR SCREW FIXATION

First described by Grob in 2001, occipitoatlantal transarticular screws provide craniocervical stability while maintaining range of motion in the atlantoaxial joint.[8–10] After exposure, a pilot hole is drilled with a high-speed air drill midway along the mediolateral axis of the C1 lateral mass, just beneath where it joins the lamina. A Penfield No. 4 dissector is placed at the medial aspect of the atlantocondylar joint margin to mark the lateral border of the spinal canal and to serve as a landmark for the medial trajectory, which is approximately 10 degrees. Lateral fluoroscopy is used to determine the sagittal trajectory, which is toward the tip of the clivus.

A Kirschner wire (K-wire) is inserted along this trajectory under fluoroscopic guidance. A cannulated drill is used to prepare the screw pathway, which is then tapped, followed by placement of the appropriate length screw (Fig. 16.4).

Care must be taken to avoid damage to the hypoglossal nerve, which can occur if the screw is placed too laterally and superiorly. The position of the hypoglossal foramen should be assessed by preoperative CT before placement of this screw. Bleeding from the atlantoaxial joint veins can be controlled with careful subperiosteal dissection and topical hemostatic agents. Venous bleeding from the atlantocondylar joint veins can be controlled in the same fashion and is often aided by the use of the microscope.

OCCIPUT-C1 LATERAL MASS FIXATION

In another technique to fuse the occiput to C1 without involving C2, C1–lateral mass screws are placed and connected to occipital screws via a rod or plate (Fig. 16.5).[11]

WIRING TO A ROD

When a screw cannot be placed in the lateral mass or pedicle of a vertebral level to be fused (usually because of fracture), sublaminar wires can be passed and wired to the passing rod to provide extra stability (Horn et al., unpublished data; Fig. 16.6).

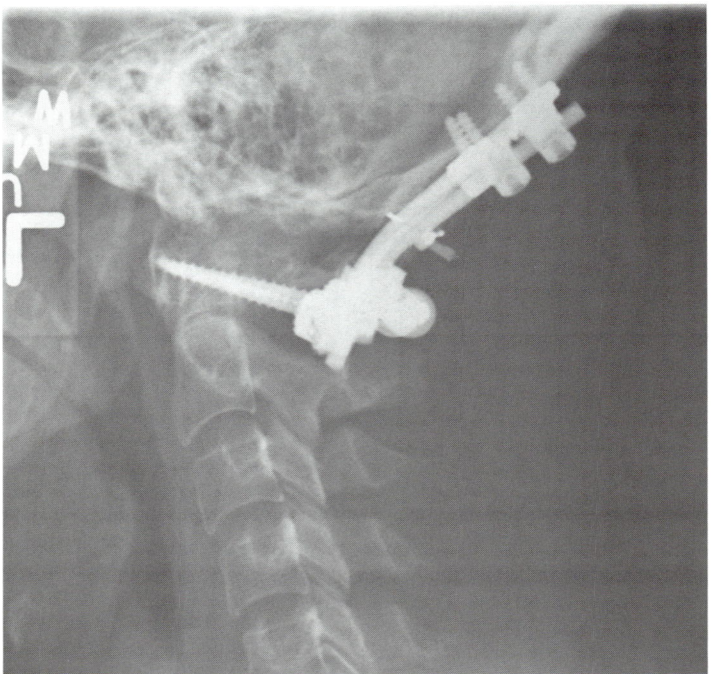

FIGURE 16.5. Lateral radiograph showing occipitocervical fusion with occipital keel screws and C1–lateral mass screws, sparing the atlantoaxial joint. (With permission from Barrow Neurological Institute.)

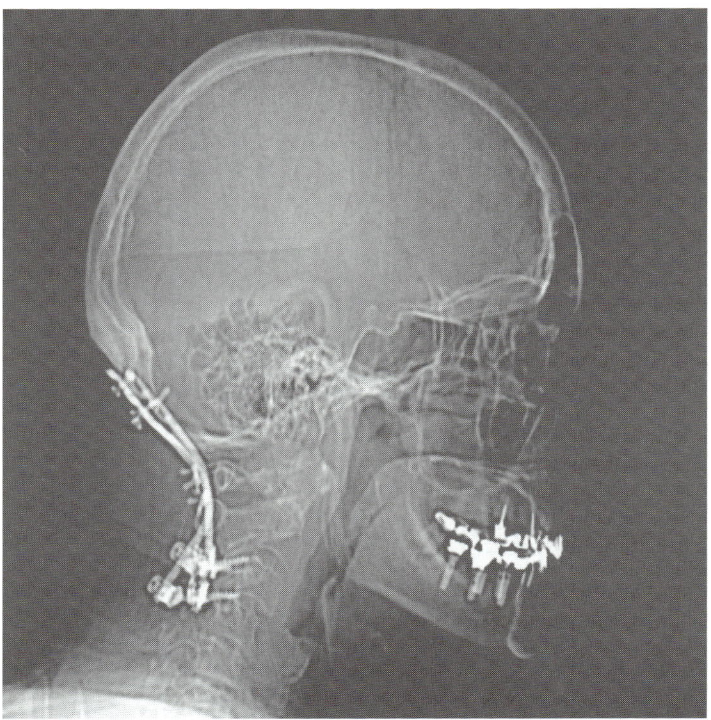

A

FIGURE 16.6. Lateral **(A)** and (*continued*)

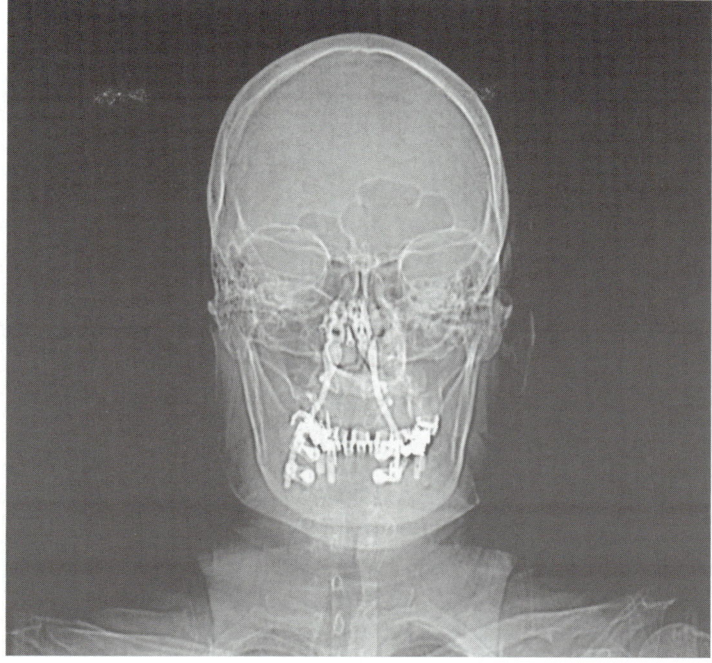

B

FIGURE 16.6. *(continued)* **(B)** anteroposterior radiographs after occiput-to-C4 fusion in a patient whose vertebral artery anatomy was unfavorable for C2 screw placement and sublaminar wiring of C1 and C2 to the rod for extra stability. (With permission from Barrow Neurological Institute.)

CONTOURED ROD FIXATION

A well-established technique is rod-wire fixation of the craniovertebral junction. This procedure is associated with an excellent rate of fusion and provides adequate stability.[12,13] The primary disadvantage is extension of the fusion to C2 or C3, which reduces the cervical range of motion.

A small suboccipital craniectomy is performed to widen the foramen magnum and to facilitate passage of the wires. A high-speed drill is used to create two or three burr holes on either side of the suboccipital midline keel. The blunt end of a 0-Vicryl needle is passed from each burr hole to the craniectomy. The suture can be threaded with a nerve hook, so that the sharp end of the needle does not traverse the dura. The suture is tied to a single-ended braided cable, which is passed using a two-handed feed-pull technique.

Next, the ligamentum flavum and atlanto-occipital membrane are detached from the lamina of C1, C2, and C3 with a curette. The safest place to pass the sublaminar cable is at the junction of the spinous process and lamina. A small laminotomy with a Kerrison punch can be made there to facilitate passage of the cable. Using the same 0-Vicryl needle technique as described above, a double-ended braided cable is passed under the lamina at each level. The cable is divided, and each end is moved laterally to the junction of the lamina and lateral mass.

A custom bending tool (BendMeister, Sofamor Danek, Memphis, TN) is used to shape a threaded Steinmann pin into a bent loop (Fig. 16.7C).[14] The loop must exactly fit the occipitocervical anatomy in neutral position to avoid occipitocervical lordosis or kyphosis when the cables are tightened to the Steinmann pin.

The cables are tightened to the loop to a tension of 20 to 40 Nm with the cable tightener and crimped. The cable is then trimmed at the level of the crimp (Fig. 16.7A–D).

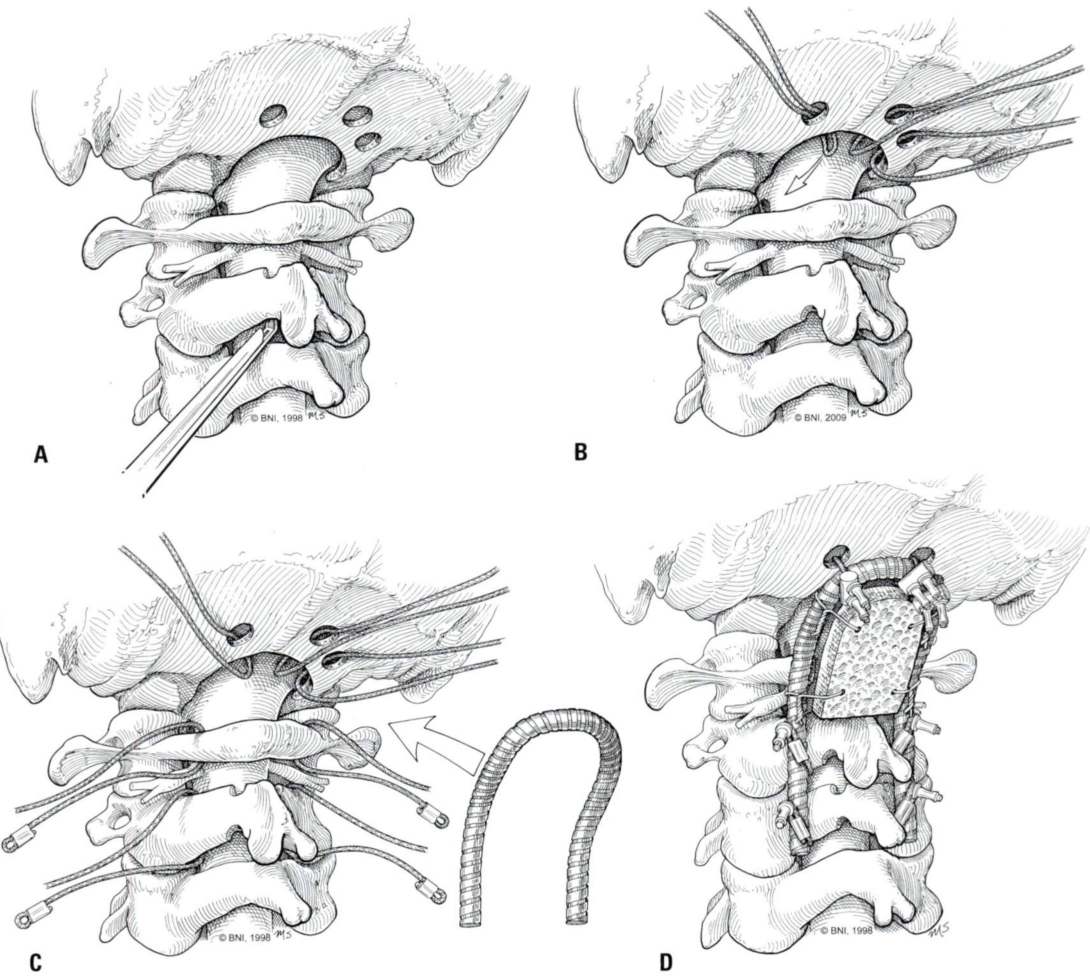

FIGURE 16.7. Threaded Steinmann pin fixation. **A.** Occipital bur holes and laminar notching to facilitate passage of sublaminar wires. **B.** Placement of suboccipital cables. **C.** Sublaminar cables and contoured Steinmann pin. **D.** Final construct and bone graft placement. (With permission from Barrow Neurological Institute.)

BONE GRAFT

The suboccipital bone, lamina, and spinous process are decorticated with a high-speed air drill. The C1-C2 facet joint is decorticated with curettage, drilling, or both. A bicortical or unicortical iliac crest graft is harvested from the iliac crest. Cancellous bone is packed in the facet joints and around the structural graft to facilitate fusion. In children it may be preferable to use autogenous rib grafts.

POSTOPERATIVE ORTHOSES

After surgery, the halo ring is removed unless the patient is thought to have poor bone quality or is at high risk for pseudarthrosis. Otherwise, the patient is placed in a Miami J cervical collar for 12 weeks after surgery. At 3 to 5 months after surgery, a thin-cut CT scan with reconstructions and flexion-extension radiographs are obtained to assess the status of the fusion, after which the orthosis is removed.

REFERENCES

1. Hurlbert RJ, Crawford NR, Choi WG, et al. A biomechanical evaluation of occipitocervical instrumentation: screw compared with wire fixation. *J Neurosurg* 1999;90:84–90.
2. Oda I, Abumi K, Sell LC, et al. Biomechanical evaluation of five different occipito-atlanto-axial fixation techniques. *Spine* 1999;24:2377–2382.
3. Shad A, Shariff SS, Teddy PJ, et al. Craniocervical fusion for rheumatoid arthritis: comparison of sublaminar wires and the lateral mass screw craniocervical fusion. *Br J Neurosurg* 2002;16:483–486.
4. Dickman CA, Foley KT, Sonntag VK, et al. Cannulated screws for odontoid screw fixation and atlantoaxial transarticular screw fixation: technical note. *J Neurosurg* 1995;83:1095–1100.
5. Goel A, Laheri V. Plate and screw fixation for atlanto-axial subluxation. *Acta Neurochir (Wien)* 1994;129:47–53.
6. Harms J, Melcher RP. Posterior C1-C2 fusion with polyaxial screw and rod fixation. *Spine* 2001;26:2467–2471.
7. Jeanneret B, Magerl F. Primary posterior fusion C1/2 in odontoid fractures: indications, technique, and results of transarticular screw fixation. *J Spinal Disord* 1992;5:464–475.
8. Feiz-Erfan I, Gonzalez LF, Dickman CA. Atlantooccipital transarticular screw fixation for the treatment of traumatic occipitoatlantal dislocation. Technical note. *J Neurosurg Spine* 2005;2:381–385.
9. Gonzalez LF, Crawford NR, Chamberlain RH, et al. Craniovertebral junction fixation with transarticular screws: biomechanical analysis of a novel technique. *J Neurosurg* 2003;98:202–209.
10. Grob D. Transarticular screw fixation for atlanto-occipital dislocation. *Spine* 2001;26:703–707.
11. Maughan PH, Horn EM, Theodore N, et al. Avulsion fracture of the foramen magnum treated with occiput-to-C1 fusion: case report. *Neurosurgery* 2005;57:E600.
12. Apostolides PJ, Dickman CA, Golfinos JG, et al. Threaded Steinmann pin fusion of the craniovertebral junction. *Spine* 1996;21:1630–1637.
13. Dickman CA, Douglas RA, Sonntag VKH. Occipitocervical fusion: posterior stabilization of the craniovertebral junction and upper cervical spine. *BNI Q* 1990;6:2–14.
14. Apostolides PJ, Karahalios DG, Yapp RA, et al. Use of the BendMeister rod bender for occipitocervical fusion: technical note. *Neurosurgery* 1998;43:389–390.

CHAPTER 17

Anterior Subaxial Instrumentation

Christian P. DiPaola and Robert W. Molinari

INTRODUCTION

The benefits of anterior cervical plating include increasing the stiffness of an arthrodesis, decreasing graft complications such as extrusion, and enhancing fusion rates. It also allows for decreased external immobilization. The ultimate goal is to enhance anatomic reconstruction with early mobilization.

Anterior cervical instrumentation is indicated in anterior and middle column injuries, as well as injuries that are rotationally unstable or have the tendency to develop late kyphosis or listhesis. Plating adds support to the anterior and middle column. The plate and screw construct acts as a tension band in extension and a buttress in flexion, especially with loss of vertebral body height and posterior ligamentous injury. Anterior cervical plating is also indicated after partial or complete corpectomy for spinal cord decompression. The technique of anterior bone grafting and plating in trauma has been shown to be reliable for both anterior and posterior injuries.[1]

Anterior plating is often contraindicated in the setting of infection and severe osteoporosis. Anterior cervical plating was first used in the setting of trauma and reported by Bohler[2] in 1967. It continues to be a mainstay among the treatment options for the surgical fixation of traumatic cervical spine instability. The instrumentation design and implementation have evolved over the years from simple long bone–type plates to anatomically designed load-bearing and load-sharing devices. Modifications have been made in each generation of implant to address specific complications or potential risks of the previous design. Both statically constrained, "locked" devices, which make a fixed-angle construct and "dynamic" plates are currently in widespread use.

It is important to understand that implant designs have evolved since their initial development. Modifications and progression in design have been driven by desire to increase safety and biomechanical stability. The use of instrumentation in anterior cervical discectomy and fusion (ACDF) for traumatic cervical spine instability has taken hold because of the poor outcomes and increased complications associated with fracture dislocations and attempted interbody dowel fusion. Bailey and Badgley[3] were the first to describe this technique. Cloward[4] and Smith and Robinson[5] improved on these techniques; however, they encountered high rates of pseudarthrosis in multilevel fusion and recurrent deformity. An important case report by Stauffer and Kelly[6] demonstrated a high rate of complications in all noninstrumented cervical fusions for traumatic instability. All patients in this study had postoperative instability and recurrence of deformity, and a majority required reoperation. Three patients had progressive neurologic deficit. The author recommended that noninstrumented fusions be contraindicated in cervical fractures with possible or confirmed posterior ligamentous disruption. This chapter will discuss the design rationales for plates in a progression from early designs to those currently in use.

ANTERIOR PLATING IN CERVICAL SPINE TRAUMA

The first report of anterior cervical plating was reported by Bohler.[2] He and others, such as Herrmann[7] and Orozco and Llovet,[8] described using an AO small fragment type plate and bone graft for fixation of unstable lower cervical spine fractures.[9,10] At that time others tried steel rods spanning bone graft and vertebral bodies, as well as a staple-shaped Kirschner wire (K-wire).[9,10] In 1970, Orozco and Llovet[8,11] described using the AO small fragment plate for ACDF in trauma and in 1971 designed and reported on the use of the first spine-specific "H" plate.[8,11] This later was developed as a standardized atlanto-occipital anterior cervical plate (Fig. 17.1). Bohler and Gaudernak[12] were the first to report on the benefits of the H plate in surgical fixation of the unstable cervical spine. In a 2-year period they noted that no patient needed postoperative external immobilization and there was no screw loosening or recurrence of deformity. All achieved solid fusion in this study.

In 1989, Caspar et al.[13,14] reported on a plating system that Caspar designed with a trapezoidal shape (Fig. 17.2). These plates were contoured to the anterior vertebral body. The H plate and the Caspar plate are considered "unrestricted backout" or "nonconstrained" implants. This means that the screw–plate interface is not fixed. Advantages to this design include high versatility for screw direction. Eccentric screw placement also allows for graft compression. Disadvantages include the need for bicortical screw penetration with possible risk of injury to dura or cord and screw loosening. There is also no fixed-angle or intrinsic construct stability, and intraoperative fluoroscopy is mandatory. Of note, biomechanical data on single-screw pull-out tests in cadaver models have not proven that bicortical purchase increases pull-out strength.[15] However, other studies have suggested that bicortical screw placement does enhance the overall rigidity of a construct, especially for long segment fusions.[15–17]

In the initial manuscript by Caspar et al.,[13] they described 60 trauma cases in which a 100% fusion rate was obtained. Other reports in the cervical spine trauma literature demonstrated favorable results

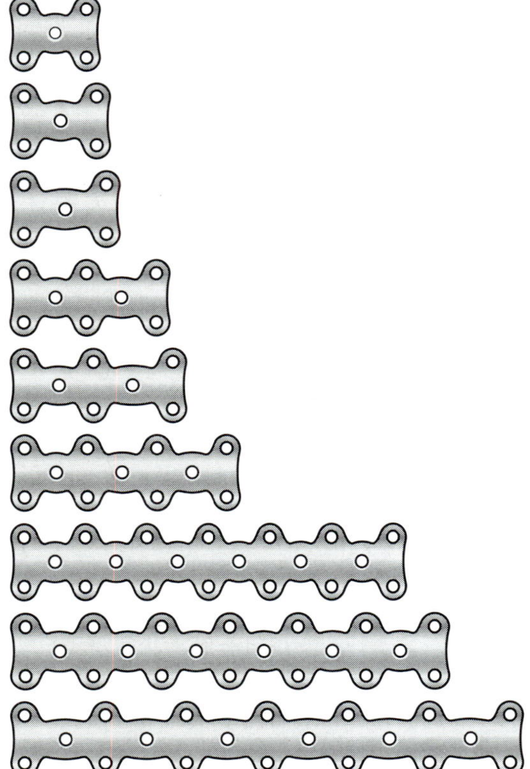

FIGURE 17.1. Initial Orozco cervical H plate used for anterior cervical stabilization. (From Bohler J, Gaudernak T. Anterior plate stabilization for fracture-dislocations of the lower cervical spine. *J Trauma* 1980;20:204, Figure 1.)

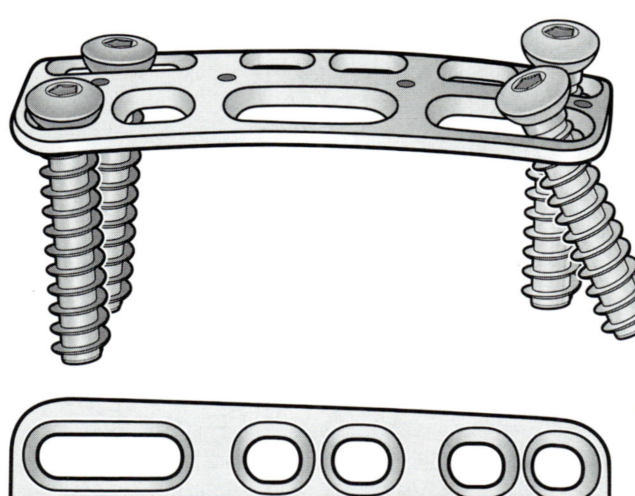

FIGURE 17.2. Caspar cervical plate with a trapezoidal shape, unrestricted screw back-out, and optional oval holes for screw–sliding and graft compression. (From Moftakhar R, Trost GR. Anterior cervical plates: a historical perspective. *Neurosurg Focus* 2004;16:E8, Figure 4).

with the Caspar plate, including a high rate of fusion and low rate of screw loosening or graft extrusion and excellent spinal realignment.[18–20] Bose[21] reported on a mixed population of patients using the Caspar plate and showed a high 97.91% fusion rate, but a 19% hardware complication rate. Most significant was the increased rate of screw fracture and pull-out. Seven patients underwent revision surgery. One screw had penetrated the posterior cortex but caused no neurologic injury.[21]

Despite the reported success of anterior plates in cervical trauma, controversy still exists over whether injuries with posterior ligamentous injury could be treated with anterior fusion surgery alone. Garvey et al.[22] recommended that when an anterior approach is necessary for decompression, Caspar plating can be used with bone graft and provides enough stability to eliminate posterior surgery in patients with posterior ligamentous injury. Aebi et al.[23] reported on use of the Orozco plate in 64 of 86 patients with posterior injury who were treated with anterior Orozco plating. They reported no nonunions, one loose screw, and one case of transient Horner syndrome. In the article they strongly advocate the use of anterior bone grafting and plating for posteriorly unstable cervical spine injuries. Ripa et al.,[24] in their series of 92 patients with traumatic cervical spine instability, also added to the evidence that these fractures can be treated with anterior plating and fusion. A recent report by Johnson et al.[25] cautions against being overly enthusiastic in certain circumstances for isolated anterior plating. They identified that patients with facet fracture dislocations have a high (13%) incidence of loss of postoperative radiographic alignment.

Hardware failures in nonconstrained plates continue to be a concern because of reports of screw loosening or back-out and subsequent possible pseudarthrosis or anterior soft tissue complications.[26] To address these shortcomings, some developers designed plating systems that created a constrained or restricted back-out construct. In 1986, Morscher[27] modified the Orozco plate to include an expansion bolt locking system that limited screw back-out. The hollow-headed screw is locked to the plate with a second, shorter locking screw.[26–28] This essentially creates a fixed-angle device and also obviates the need for bicortical screw purchase.[29,30] The other mechanical advantage offered is that the two rostral screw holes orient the screws rostrally and medially, which reduces the risk for screw plate back-out. The modifications on Morscher's design became known as the cervical spine locking plate (CSLP) (Synthes, West Chester, PA). The Orion plating system (Medronic Sofamor-Danek, Minneapolis, MN) was developed after the CSLP and incorporated modifications such as variable

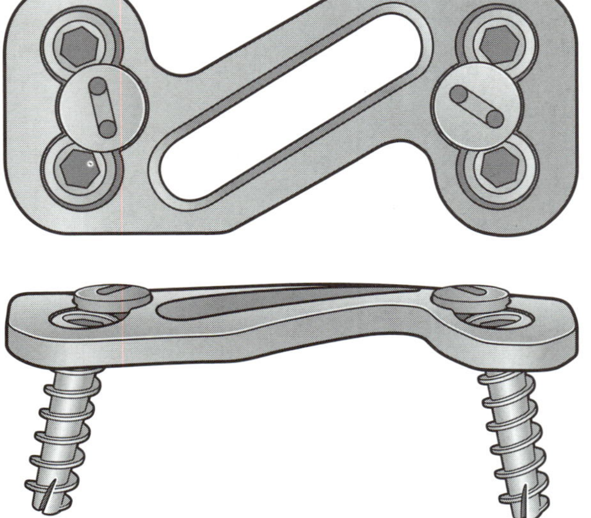

FIGURE 17.3. Orion cervical plate (Medronic Sofamor-Danek, Minneapolis, MN) that permits variable angle screw placement and also completely locks the screw to the plate. (From Lowery GL, McDonough RF. The significance of hardware failure in anterior cervical plate fixation: patients with 2- to 7-year follow-up. *Spine* 1998;23: 181–186, discussion 186–187, Figure 2.)

screw length, lordotic curvature, tapered screws, and a fixed-angled drill guide (Fig. 17.3). Other systems that completely lock the screw to the plate include the Reflex (Stryker, Kalamazoo, MI) and the fixed DOC plate (DePuy Acromed, Raynham, MA).

Razack et al.[31] reported on the management of single-level fracture dislocations with bone grafting and anterior plating using a locking plate with monocortical screw purchase. Only one patient in this study demonstrated instrumentation failure, and all eventually showed evidence of stability at the injured level. Lowery and McDonough[32] compared hardware failure in fusions with locking and nonlocking plates. This article also provides an excellent historical discussion of hardware complications in anterior cervical plating. They concluded that the nonconstrained plates had a much higher early and late hardware failure rate than locked plates. The early hardware failure is presumably due to the lack of initial construct stability, and late hardware failure is typically from pseudoarthrosis and screw pull-out (Fig. 17.4). In this study, longer constructs and allograft bone were also related to failure. When the CSLP and the Orion plate were directly compared, there were fewer plate failures in the Orion group. The authors attribute this finding to the increased thickness of the Orion plate. For the majority of cases, hardware failure did not result in clinical complications. Overall the authors felt that when patients are not symptomatic and when hardware is not prominent, hardware failure is relatively inconsequential. It should, however, increase the surgeon's suspicion of nonunion.[32]

Despite the apparent increased stability that a constrained plate offers, multiple studies have demonstrated the inadequacy of anterior fixation alone in long segment fusions.[33,34] These studies look at patients treated with two- or three-level corpectomies or discectomy with anterior bone grafting and plating. Both groups found an unacceptably high incidence of nonunion, graft, and hardware complications. The majority of patients in these series were being treated for degenerative conditions, but it stands to reason that trauma-induced instability would likely fare less well in the setting of isolated long segment anterior fusion and plating. The locking plate construct does not appear to confer additional stability to this clinical treatment dilemma.[33,34]

Rigid plate constructs offer the advantages of improved initial stability and decreased complications from graft dislodgement, endplate fracture, and kyphotic deformity.[9] However, it has been postulated that the rigidity of the constrained devices may inhibit bony healing by means of stress shielding mechanical load away from the graft.[35] There is evidence to suggest that less rigid fixation that allows some micromotion may enhance time to union.[36] The next generation in the design of anterior cervical plates incorporates this idea of dynamization. The goal is to transmit more load to the bone graft to permit union while also obtaining initial relative stability. Dynamic plates or semiconstrained plates can be subcategorized as rotational, translational, or mixed. They all incorporate

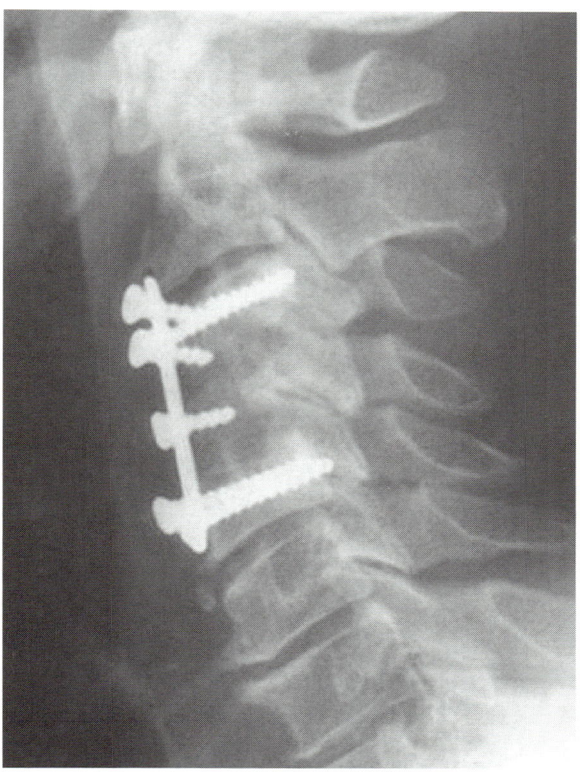

FIGURE 17.4. Screw backout from vertebral body and plate associated with unconstrained early cervical plating designs that did not permit screw–plate locking. (From Moftakhar R, Trost GR. Anterior cervical plates: a historical perspective. *Neurosurg Focus* 2004;16:E8, Figure 6, with permission.)

restricted screw back-out technology, but rotationally dynamic plates allow rotation at the plate–screw interface and translational plates allow axial translation. Mixed plates combine the two. Examples of rotational, semiconstrained plates include the Codman (Codman, Raynham, MA), Peak (DePuy), Acufix (Abbott Spine, Austin, TX), Zephir (Medtronic), and Atlantis (Medtronic) systems.[37]

As an example, the Codman plate uses a cam lock to prevent screw back-out but still allows screw rotation. Good short and intermediate segment fixation results have been reported; however, failures have occurred with long segment fusions and unstable cervical spines.[38] DePuy Acromed developed the first translational dynamic system, the DOC rod (Fig. 17.5). The cephalad screws were meant to slide along a rail, and the caudal screws remain rigid. Axial deformation can be controlled with a cross-fixator "stop" mechanism. The newest version of this implant, the DOC plate, uses a two-piece locking expansion screw system. The ABC plate, designed by Aesculap (South San Francisco, CA) combines axial translation and rotation (Fig. 17.6). The Atlantis system can be used with variable-angle or fixed-angle screws and allows rotation and axial translation.[37]

Although it has been shown that both dynamic and constrained plates are able to act as initial load-sharing devices, there is concern that as bone graft reabsorbs, more load will be transmitted to a rigid plate.[39] The dynamic plate designs attempt to account for this living, changing nature of bone and adapt to the graft collapse to a certain degree.

The role of dynamic plating in traumatic cervical spine instability remains to be determined. Biomechanics studies have recently been done to attempt to answer some of the concerns regarding dynamic anterior cervical plating and trauma. Dvorak et al.[40] studied human cadaver spinal units with experimentally induced posterior ligamentous destabilization and inferior facet excision. Anterior discectomy and iliac crest bone graft to match the disc space void was used and then plated. Strain was compared in the dynamic ABC and the CSLP in multiple bending and rotation modes to assess load sharing. Range of motion, bone mineral density, and endplate preparation techniques were also compared. Results were contrary to the original hypothesis, in that results between the two

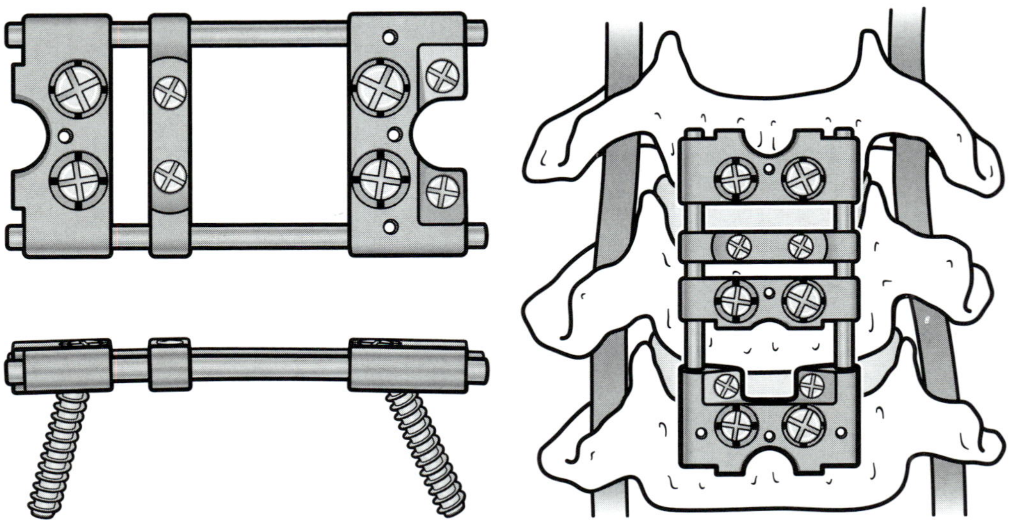

FIGURE 17.5. The first translational dynamic system, the DOC rod developed by DePuj Acromed. This system allows graft compression with screw–rod sliding. (From Moftakhar R, Trost GR. Anterior cervical plates: a historical perspective. *Neurosurg Focus* 2004;16:E8, Figure 7.)

plates were similar for construct range of motion and load sharing, except that the dynamic plate showed better stability in extension than the rigid plate. Endplate removal offered better stability with a dynamic plate and less stability for the rigid plate, and bone mineral density (BMD) correlated with stability of both constructs.[40] These findings are not fully understood, but it may be that dynamic plates offer better load sharing between the spinal segments and the graft. Brodke et al.[39] studied a corpectomy model in synthetic spinal segment models and cadavers without posterior instability. They looked at plating with a 10% undersized graft to simulate graft subsidence and reabsorption. Their conclusion was that all plates, constrained or nonconstrained, were able to load share effectively; however, dynamic plates load share better with undersized grafts than do locked plates. The ABC plate and CSLP were relatively similar in initial stiffness for flexion, extension, and lateral

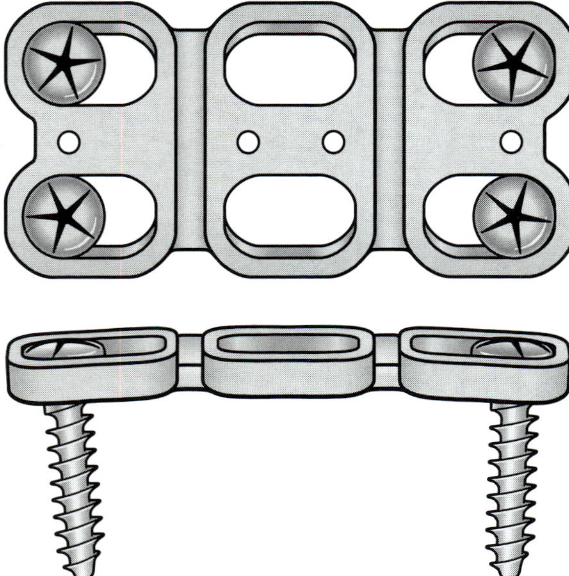

FIGURE 17.6. The ABC plate, a dynamic plating system designed by Aesculap (South San Francisco, CA), combines axial translation and rotation.

bending. The textured posterior aspect of the ABC plate appeared to offer more stiffness because of friction of the plate bone interface, whereas the DOC allows axial sliding and lateral bending with much less force.[39] Brodke et al.[39] state that this applies essentially all axial load to the graft and acts more as a "dynamic alignment guide." They conclude that the DOC and ABC plate may offer different healing microenvironments that have yet to be determined in the clinical arena. Reidy et al.[41] studied the Premier plate (Medtronic Sofamor-Danek) in both dynamic and static mode in a cadaver spinal segment corpectomy model. This study was performed with a height-adjustable graft and evaluated construct stability when posterior elements were both intact and removed. The authors concluded that the addition of a locked plate to an ACDF model stress shields the bone graft.[41] Dynamic plates increase load sharing with the graft. This is significant when the graft is undersized and when the posterior elements are removed. They caution that dynamic plates cannot fully compensate for undersized grafts, and thus the balance of load is transferred to the posterior elements. The undersized graft simulates poor grafting technique, graft reabsorption, and endplate subsidence. In the trauma setting, there is concern that use of dynamic plates with a reduced graft size will divert load from the graft to the plate and the injured posterior elements, which may decrease construct stability.

The majority of clinical literature in dynamic plating comes from case reports on reconstructions for degenerative disease, stenosis, myelopathy, and ossification of the posterior longitudinal ligament (OPLL).[42–44] Epstein[44] looked at 66 patients with myelopathy from OPLL who underwent multilevel anterior and posterior cervical corpectomy and fusion. Of these, 38 had a rigid plate and 28 had an ABC dynamic plate applied. Of fixed plates, 13% showed graft plate failures, compared to only 3.6% for the dynamic plates. Cephalad and caudad plate migration was measured on postoperative radiography for dynamic plates and was found to be 6.4 and 5.7 mm, respectively. Epstein[44] attributes the success of the dynamic plate to the ability to minimize graft shielding and facilitate compression. Epstein[42] reported a 9.5% failure rate for the ABC plate in patients who underwent a single-level corpectomy. This finding is high compared with other reports. However, it is lower than the author's initial experience with fixed plates.[42]

The authors identified morbid obesity as a risk factor for hardware failure and pseudarthrosis in single-level conditions treated anteriorly only and suggested the addition of posterior fusion or halo vest for supplemental fixation.[43,44] The indications for anterior dynamic plating in the unstable cervical spine have yet to be fully elucidated. It would appear that there is a role for dynamic plating for the benefits previously mentioned; however, it is possible that it may not be sufficient alone in the unstable cervical spine, with confirmed or questionable posterior ligamentous injury.

ANTERIOR CERVICAL SCREWS: BIOMECHANICS

Hitchon et al.[45] used a cadaver implant model and compared self-drilling and self-tapping screws for the Synthes expansion head locking screws. BMD and screw length were also compared. Pull-out strength strongly correlated to screw length. This suggested that, even though locking plates do not require bicortical purchase, the longest possible screws should be used to obtain the most stable construct. They also showed that there was no difference in self-drilling versus self-tapping screws. BMD and insertion torque and pull-out strength were also strongly correlated in the 14- and 16-mm screws. Pitzen et al.[46] showed that thicker core rescue screws did not increase pull-out strength compared to initial screws. Fenestrated screws are no longer used because of increased deformation and failure rate. Also, the bone ingrowth benefits have not been proven.[47]

SURGICAL TECHNIQUE

Before surgery it is important to thoroughly review all appropriate radiographic images for surgical planning. Special consideration should be given to need for reduction, amount of canal compromise, if applicable, and vertebral body dimensions. Preoperative planning should include patient positioning, need for traction, and method of transfer.

The anterior approach to the subaxial cervical spine has been well described in the literature and has gained the eponym Smith-Robinson approach.[4,5] For most operations a transverse skin incision can be made on the anterior neck corresponding to the proper level. In cases that may need additional exposure, an oblique incision is used along the medial border of the sternocleidomastoid. The platysma is then encountered and split in line with the direction of its fibers. At this point the surgeon palpates the carotid pulse and retracts the contents of the carotid sheath laterally. Blunt finger dissection is used to arrive at the prevertebral fascia. The longus colli muscles are elevated and retracted evenly. At this point, it is critical to define the midline and maintain the orientation throughout the case. The symmetric boarders of the longus colli muscles, as well as the uncinate processes, can provide landmarks to achieve this goal.

Interlocking dislocations of the facet joints can be reduced through the anterior approach. The disc spreader is inserted and distractive force applied until the facets disengage. The dislocated superior vertebra can then be pushed backward into its normal alignment.[12]

Once the appropriate procedure has been performed, that is, decompression and bone grafting, attention should turn to the plating construct. Measurements should be made from the midpoint of the cephalad vertebral body to the midpoint of the caudad vertebral body involved in the fusion. The correct plate should be selected and contoured as necessary with the aim of maintaining cervical lordosis. Newer plating systems come with a lordotic design built in. It is very important when fitting the plate that the disc spaces above and below are not violated or involved in the fusion construct, because this will lead to micromotion and eventual loosening.

CONCLUSION

A review of the literature supports an established role for anterior cervical plating in cervical spine trauma. Success has been reported with multiple generations of plating systems. Decreased complication rates have come from improved designs. The rates of complications with new plates are relatively low; however, the role of dynamic plates has yet to be defined in the setting of appropriate cervical spine trauma cases.

REFERENCES

1. Aebi M, Mohler J, Zach GA, et al. Indication, surgical technique, and results of 100 surgically-treated fractures and fracture-dislocations of the cervical spine. *Clin Orthop Relat Res* 1986;203:244–257.
2. Bohler J. Sofort-und Fruhnbehandlong traumatischer querschnitt lahmungen. *Zeitschr Orthapad Grenzgebiete* 1967;103:512–528.
3. Bailey RW, Badgley CE. Stabilization of the cervical spine by anterior fusion. *Am J Orthop* 1960;42A:565–594.
4. Cloward RB. Treatment of acute fractures and fracture-dislocations of the cervical spine by vertebral-body fusion: a report of eleven cases. *J Neurosurg* 1961;18:201–209.
5. Smith GW, Robinson RA. The treatment of certain cervical-spine disorders by anterior removal of the intervertebral disc and interbody fusion. *J Bone Joint Surg Am* 1958;40:607–624.
6. Stauffer ES, Kelly EG. Fracture-dislocations of the cervical spine: instability and recurrent deformity following treatment by anterior interbody fusion. *J Bone Joint Surg Am* 1977;59:45–48.
7. Herrmann HD. Metal plate fixation after anterior fusion of unstable fracture dislocations of the cervical spine. *Acta Neurochir (Wien)* 1975;32:101–111.
8. Orozco R, Llovet T. Osteosintesis en las fractures de raquis cervical. *Rev Ortop Traumatol* 1970;14:285–288.
9. Schurmann K, Busch G. [Treatment of cervical dislocation fractures using ventral fusion]. *Chirurg* 1970;41: 225–228.
10. Junghanns H. [Metal fixation of bone blocks of cervical spine]. *Chirurg* 1973;44:87–90.
11. Orozco R, Llovet T. Osteosintesis eb las lesiones traumaticas y degenerativas de la coluna cervical. *Cirurg Rehabil* 1971;1:45–52.
12. Bohler J, Gaudernak T. Anterior plate stabilization for fracture-dislocations of the lower cervical spine. *J Trauma* 1980;20:203–205.
13. Caspar W, Barbier DD, Klara PM. Anterior cervical fusion and Caspar plate stabilization for cervical trauma. *Neurosurgery* 1989;25:491–502.

14. Caspar W, Papavero L. The trapezial plate osteosynthesis: an advanced technology for anterior internal stabilization in cervical spine injuries and for the treatment of neck instability due to non traumatic causes. *Chir Organi Mov* 1992;77:87–99.
15. Maiman DJ, Pintar FA, Yoganandan N, et al. Pull-out strength of Caspar cervical screws. *Neurosurgery* 1992;31: 1097–101, discussion 101.
16. Tippets RH, Apfelbaum RI. Anterior cervical fusion with the Caspar instrumentation system. *Neurosurgery* 1988; 22:1008–1013.
17. Traynelis VC, Donaher PA, Roach RM, et al. Biomechanical comparison of anterior Caspar plate and three-level posterior fixation techniques in a human cadaveric model. *J Neurosurg* 1993;79:96–103.
18. Bremer AM, Nguyen TQ. Internal metal plate fixation combined with anterior interbody fusion in cases of cervical spine injury. *Neurosurgery* 1983;12:649–653.
19. Goffin J, Plets C, Van den Bergh R. Anterior cervical fusion and osteosynthetic stabilization according to Caspar: a prospective study of 41 patients with fractures and/or dislocations of the cervical spine. *Neurosurgery* 1989;25: 865–871.
20. Pasztor E, Lazar L, Benedek T, et al. Total body replacement with iliac bone graft and metal plate stabilization in lower cervical spine. *Acta Neurochir (Wien)* 1987;85:159–167.
21. Bose B. Anterior cervical fusion using Caspar plating: analysis of results and review of the literature. *Surg Neurol* 1998;49:25–31.
22. Garvey TA, Eismont FJ, Roberti LJ. Anterior decompression, structural bone grafting, and Caspar plate stabilization for unstable cervical spine fractures and/or dislocations. *Spine* 1992;17:S431–S435.
23. Aebi M, Zuber K, Marchesi D. Treatment of cervical spine injuries with anterior plating: indications, techniques, and results. *Spine* 1991;16:S38–S45.
24. Ripa DR, Kowall MG, Meyer PR Jr, et al. Series of ninety-two traumatic cervical spine injuries stabilized with anterior ASIF plate fusion technique. *Spine* 1991;16:S46–S55.
25. Johnson MG, Fisher CG, Boyd M, et al. The radiographic failure of single segment anterior cervical plate fixation in traumatic cervical flexion distraction injuries. *Spine* 2004;29:2815–2820.
26. Yee GK, Terry AF. Esophageal penetration by an anterior cervical fixation device: a case report. *Spine* 1993; 18:522–527.
27. Morscher E. [Indications and possibilities of patella wedge osteotomy]. *Orthopade* 1985;14:261–265.
28. Morscher E, Sutter F, Jenny H, et al. [Anterior plating of the cervical spine with the hollow screw-plate system of titanium]. *Chirurg* 1986;57:702–707.
29. Grubb MR, Currier BL, Shih JS, et al. Biomechanical evaluation of anterior cervical spine stabilization. *Spine* 1998;23:886–892.
30. Rechtine GR, Cahill DW, Gruenberg M, et al. The Synthes Cervical Spine Locking Plate in anterior fusion. *Tech Orthop* 1994;9:86–91.
31. Razack N, Green BA, Levi AD. The management of traumatic cervical bilateral facet fracture-dislocations with unicortical anterior plates. *J Spinal Disord* 2000;13:374–381.
32. Lowery GL, McDonough RF. The significance of hardware failure in anterior cervical plate fixation: patients with 2- to 7-year follow-up. *Spine* 1998;23:181–186, discussion 6–7.
33. Bolesta MJ, Rechtine GR 2nd, Chrin AM. Three- and four-level anterior cervical discectomy and fusion with plate fixation: a prospective study. *Spine* 2000;25:2040–2044, discussion 5–6.
34. Vaccaro AR, Falatyn SP, Scuderi GJ, et al. Early failure of long segment anterior cervical plate fixation. *J Spinal Disord* 1998;11:410–415.
35. Paramore CG, Dickman CA, Sonntag VK. Radiographic and clinical follow-up review of Caspar plates in 49 patients. *J Neurosurg* 1996;84:957–961.
36. Rubin CT, Lanyon LE. Regulation of bone formation by applied dynamic loads. *J Bone Joint Surg Am* 1984;66:397–402.
37. Moftakhar R, Trost GR. Anterior cervical plates: a historical perspective. *Neurosurg Focus* 2004;16:E8.
38. Haid RW Jr, McLaughlin MR. Neurosurgery of the spine in the year 2001: a four-year review. *Clin Neurosurg* 1999;45:153–159.
39. Brodke DS, Gollogly S, Alexander Mohr R, et al. Dynamic cervical plates: biomechanical evaluation of load sharing and stiffness. *Spine* 2001;26:1324–1329.
40. Dvorak MF, Pitzen T, Zhu Q, et al. Anterior cervical plate fixation: a biomechanical study to evaluate the effects of plate design, endplate preparation, and bone mineral density. *Spine* 2005;30:294–301.
41. Reidy D, Finkelstein J, Nagpurkar A, et al. Cervical spine loading characteristics in a cadaveric C5 corpectomy model using a static and dynamic plate. *J Spinal Disord Tech* 2004;17:117–122.
42. Epstein NE. Anterior cervical dynamic ABC plating with single level corpectomy and fusion in forty-two patients. *Spinal Cord* 2003;41:153–158.
43. Epstein NE. Anterior dynamic plates in complex cervical reconstructive surgeries. *J Spinal Disord Tech* 2002;15:221–227, discussion 227–228.

44. Epstein NE. Fixed vs dynamic plate complications following multilevel anterior cervical corpectomy and fusion with posterior stabilization. *Spinal Cord* 2003;41:379–384.
45. Hitchon PW, Brenton MD, Coppes JK, et al. Factors affecting the pullout strength of self-drilling and self-tapping anterior cervical screws. *Spine* 2003;28:9–13.
46. Pitzen T, Franta F, Barbier D, et al. Insertion torque and pullout force of rescue screws for anterior cervical plate fixation in a fatigued initial pilot hole. *J Neurosurg Spine* 2004;1:198–201.
47. Hollowell JP, Reinartz J, Pintar FA, et al. Failure of synthes anterior cervical fixation device by fracture of Morscher screws: a biomechanical study. *J Spinal Disord* 1994;7:120–125.

CHAPTER 18

Posterior Subaxial Instrumentation

Michael P. Steinmetz and Daniel K. Resnick

INTRODUCTION

Cervical trauma is the most common indication for posterior subaxial cervical spine instrumentation. In 1891, Hadra[1] described the process of spinous process wiring. This permitted the treatment of cervical trauma and other disorders without the need for long-term external immobilization. Following this description, many posterior subaxial fixation techniques were introduced. Many of these advanced on the prior techniques, permitting more effective and safe stabilization strategies.

Modern instrumentation systems permit multisegmental fixation. This allows for more rigid reconstruction of the spine that may allow for the involvement of fewer motion segments. The duration of immobilization with external orthoses has been considerably reduced, and in many cases, mobilization may begin immediately after fixation.

INDICATIONS

In general, posterior stabilization is indicated in pathology in which the spine is straight or ideally lordotic in alignment.[2] If the spine is kyphotic, an anterior procedure is often indicated as the primary reconstruction technique. Posterior stabilization alone is usually reserved for injuries in which there is reducible posterior ligamentous or bony injury. Facet dislocations are easily reduced from a posterior approach, and after successful closed reduction, posterior fixation may be used to maintain stability until fusion occurs.

SURGICAL OPTIONS AND TECHNIQUES

POSITIONING

The patient is positioned prone on the operating room table. The head is placed in a three-point head holder, a horseshoe, or a large foam cushion. If substantial instability is present, rigid fixation in a three-point head holder is ideal. Traction may also be applied for use during surgery. Utmost care must be used to avoid pressure on the eyes if the head is not placed into a three-point head holder.

EXPOSURE

The extent of exposure is determined based on the levels required for instrumentation. The spine is exposed through a posterior midline incision carried down to the cervical fascia. The fascia is opened in the midline raphe and not through the muscle. This permits a subperiostial exposure of the posterior elements without excessive blood loss. The muscles are reflected off the spinous processes, lamina, and facets. If the facets are to be used for fixation, the dissection is carried out over the joints to fully expose the lateral masses. A venous plexus is just lateral and deep to the lateral boundary of the facets. Bleeding may occur during dissection in this region. Such bleeding may be controlled with bipolar cautery or hemostatic sponges. Care must be taken around any fractured posterior elements. Neurologic injury or cerebrospinal fluid leak may occur if the thecal sac or spinal cord is injured during dissection.

SPINOUS PROCESS WIRING

The posterior subaxial spine is exposed as above. The spinous processes and laminae to be wired are completely cleared of muscle and soft tissue. The entire facet complex need not be exposed unless a facet fusion is planned. The rostral and caudal levels are identified. A hole is drilled in the cranial spinous process at its base or connection to the lamina (Fig. 18.1A). A towel clip may be used to widen the hole (Fig. 18.1B). A wire or cable is placed through the hole and wrapped around the caudal spinous process (Fig. 18.1B). Security may be increased by notching the caudal spinous process or double wrapping the cable around the process (Fig. 18.1C). Finally, the cable is tightened with care so as not to overtighten and potentially cut out of the bone. Alternatively a Steinman pin may be cut to the appropriate length and placed through a hole in the caudal spinous process; this will add security to the fixation. The wires are placed in a figure-of-8 configuration. If multiple levels are to be fused, cables should be wrapped around the intervening spinous processes. Failure to incorporate intervening levels may result in terminal bending moments applied to the spine that may result in loss of stability and persistent deformity. Alternative but biomechanically similar techniques to spinous process wiring include sublaminar wiring and facet wiring.

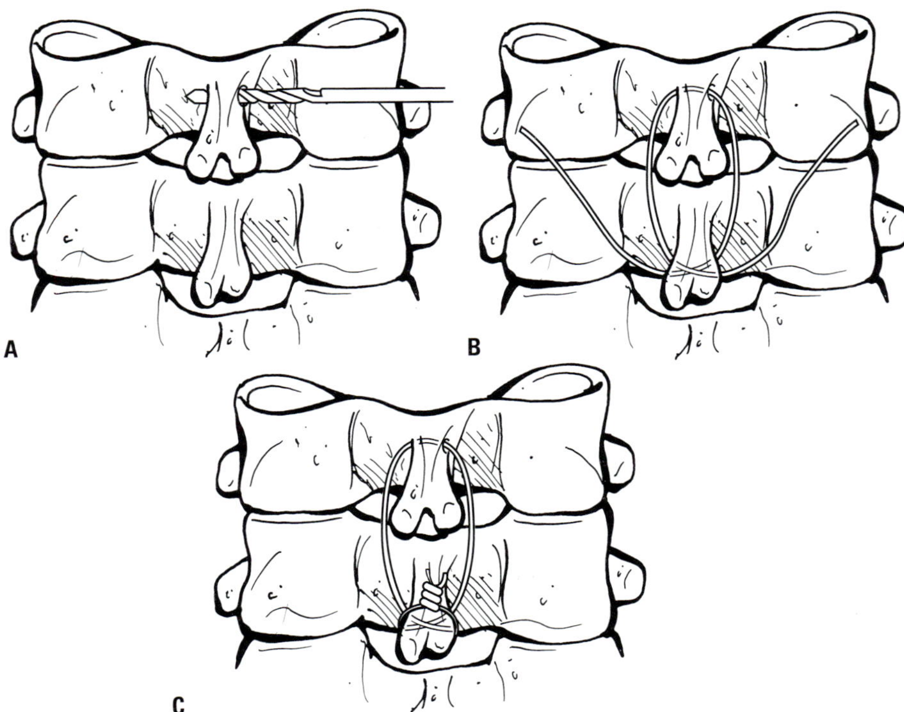

FIGURE 18.1. **A.** The spinous processes to be instrumented are exposed and cleaned of all soft tissue. A hole is drilled in the base of the cranial process. The hole is then expanded with a towel clip. **B.** The cable is placed through the cranial spinous process and then wrapped around the caudal process. **C.** To increase the stability of the purchase, the wire is double wrapped around the caudal spinous process.

HOOK FIXATION

Hook fixation may be used in the cervical spine, but with limited utility. Pedicle hooks may not be practically placed in the cervical spine. Moreover, sublaminar hooks placed in the midcervical spine may encroach on the spinal cord and lead to injury. Sublaminar hooks may be placed in the upper cervical spine in a claw configuration, while pedicle hooks and transverse process hooks may be placed in the upper thoracic spine. This creates a construct with good cranial and caudal fixation. Supplemental sublaminar wires may be placed in the midcervical spine; however, this technique is rarely used because of the potential for neurologic injury. This technique provides multiple points of fixation and substantially adds to the stability of the construct.

ROD AND CABLE FIXATION

Luque L rods or Luque rectangles (Zimmer, Warsaw, IN) may be placed in the posterior cervical spine. These devices are usually used for multilevel trauma and are useful when extended to the upper cervical spine or for spanning the cervicothoracic junction. Ideally, every level traversed is secured to the rod construct, but at a minimum, at least two levels above and below the level of injury should be included in the fixation.

The spine is exposed as above out to the lateral border of the facet joint. The appropriate-size rod construct is chosen and bent to the correct amount of lordosis. Sublaminar cables are passed (Fig. 18.2). The placement of sublaminar cables in the midcervical spine may be hazardous in the stenotic patient, and therefore, cables alternatively may be placed through the facet joints or spinous processes for fixation. In facet wiring, the facet joints are denuded of their articular cartilage at the levels selected for fixation. A hole is drilled in the midlateral mass into the facet joint. A Penfield dissector is placed into the joint so as not to drill too far through the joint. Once the wires or cables are placed, the rod construct is placed into the wound. The cables or wires are passed around the rods and sequentially tightened (Fig. 18.2). Tightening is done gradually, with opposite sides tightened concurrently. This will aid in the prevention of torsional forces.

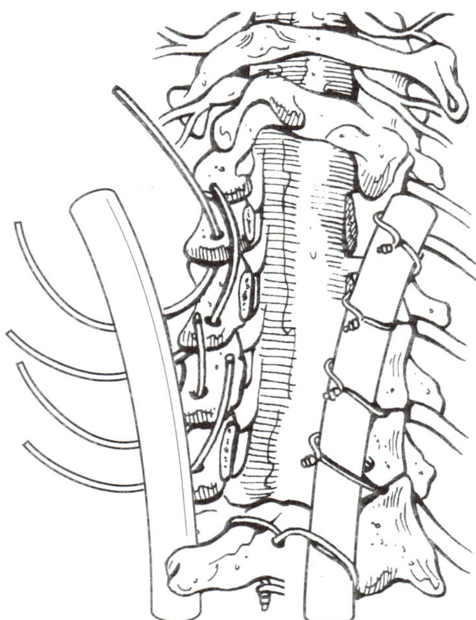

FIGURE 18.2. Sublaminar wire and rod construct may be used to stabilize traumatic pathology of the cervical spine. Sublaminar wires may be placed in the cervical spine, but with extreme caution, especially in the face of preexisting stenosis. In these circumstances, facet wiring may be used as depicted. The construct may be extended down to include the thoracic spine.

LATERAL MASS FIXATION

Plate Fixation

Wire and cable fixation of the cervical spine may be problematic. If bone is missing via decompression or fracture, such as laminar or facet fractures, cable fixation will not be possible. Furthermore, wire or cable may easily cut out of osteoporotic bone. The advent of screw fixation of the posterior cervical spine made fixation safer and faster, providing rigid multilevel fixation, such that complex forces may be applied to the spine if desired. These devices have proved superior to wire and cable constructs biomechanically.

The spine must be reduced before application of a lateral mass construct. This may be performed before surgery with traction or via an open reduction. Following reduction, the spine is exposed as above. The lateral edges of the instrumented lateral masses must be seen. The boundary of the lateral mass is identified for the appropriate levels. The lateral border is the lateral extent, the medial border is the valley created at the lateral mass/lamina junction. The superior and inferior borders are the facet joints. The facet joints should be denuded of their articular cartilage with a small curette or burr; this will aid in fusion and the determination of direction of the articular surfaces. The midportion of the lateral mass should be noted. Approximately 1 to 2 mm medial to this point marks the entry point for the lateral mass screw according to the Magerl technique (Fig. 18.3A). The plate should be sized, cut if necessary, and placed into the wound. The holes in the lateral masses should be placed in line with the holes in the plate so as to make application easier. The plate design is such that most holes will be accommodated equally. The same procedure should be performed on the opposite side.

The authors prefer to drill a pilot hole in the lateral mass with a high-speed drill before the formal drilling for screw placement. This aids in preventing the drill bit from slipping out of the appropriate trajectory during drilling. The trajectory for the pilot hole is 25 degrees divergent and 25 degrees cranial according to Magerl[3,4] (Fig. 18.3A,B). The hole is drilled with a 2.5-mm drill bit and may be done in several ways. A drill guide may be used and the hole drilled to a specific length. For example, all holes may be drilled to 14 mm and 14-mm screws placed. The guide has a stop to prevent plunging through the lateral mass. Alternatively, the hole may be drilled free-hand without a guide. The drill, in the proper trajectory, is simply "bounced" carefully while drilling proceeds. The drill is stopped once the distal cortex is breeched. A blunt tip probe is then inserted in the hole and the hole depth marked with a hemostat. This length is measured and the appropriate size screw chosen. The benefits of bicortical purchase should be weighed against the risks for potential neurologic injury; screw lengths should be selected based on the individual anatomy of the patient. After the hole is drilled, the outer cortex is tapped (usually a 3.5-mm tap) and the screw placed through the plate and into the lateral mass. The holes should always be drilled and tapped before placement of the plate, which will ensure accurate trajectory.

Roy-Camille et al.[5] described an alternative trajectory for lateral mass screws.[3] The trajectory is potentially more dangerous than in the Magerl technique, and shorter screws are used. Therefore, the Magerl technique is the preferred method. In the Roy-Camille trajectory, the lateral mass is divided into thirds. The hole is placed perpendicular to the dorsal cortex in the sagittal plane of the inferior articular facet. The starting point is at the junction of the upper and middle third of the lateral mass in the midline of the mass (Fig. 18.4A). The hole is drilled with a 10-degree lateral trajectory (Fig. 18.4B). As can be seen, there is an increased risk to damage to the exiting nerve root.

One disadvantage to plate fixation is that the screws are not rigidly affixed to the plate (nonfixed moment arm cantilever). Therefore, screw back-out and cut out are more common compared to the polyaxial screw rod constructs (see following discussion). A second disadvantage relates to the lack of coronal plane flexibility afforded by these plates. Transitioning to the upper thoracic or upper cervical spine may be difficult or impossible without the use of supplemental devices. This lack of coronal plane flexibility led to the development of screw and rod systems.

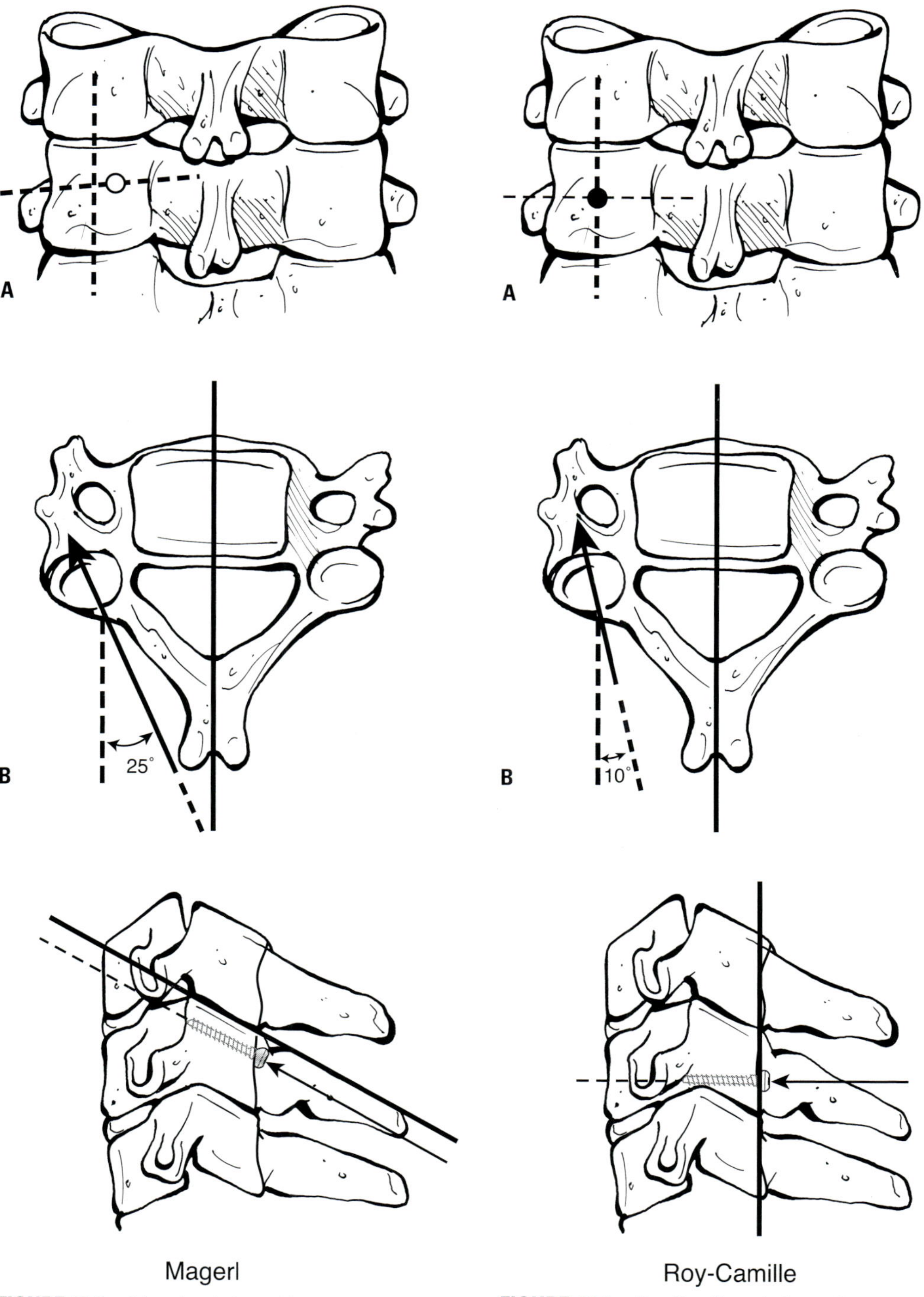

FIGURE 18.3. Magerl technique of lateral mass screw insertion. **A.** The starting point is 2 mm medial to the midpoint of the lateral mass. **B.** The trajectory is approximately 20 to 25 degrees divergent and 20 to 25 degrees cranial. This will be parallel to the articular surface of the facet joint.

FIGURE 18.4. Roy-Camille technique of lateral mass screw insertion. **A.** The starting point is at the junction of the upper and middle thirds of the lateral mass in the midline. **B.** The trajectory is perpendicular to the dorsal cortex in the sagittal plane and 10 degrees lateral.

Polyaxial Screw/Rod Fixation

The current posterior cervical spine instrumentation sets offer the placement of polyaxial screws that may be connected by rods, thus permitting segmental fixation. Screw placement technique is identical to that described previously; however, the polyaxial head allows more freedom to place screws in the anatomically ideal position without constraints placed by the plate. A further advantage of rod-based systems is the ability to place compressive and distractive forces within the construct. The screws are rigidly affixed to the longitudinal members (fixed-cantilever beam construct), which may be cross-linked, significantly adding to the stability of the construct.

POSTOPERATIVE MANAGEMENT

When rigid fixation systems are employed, patients may be mobilized as tolerated immediately. However, a hard cervical collar is often used for the first 6 to 12 weeks after surgery in the setting of cervical trauma.

COMPLICATIONS

After posterior cervical surgery, trauma patients frequently complain of significant cervical pain, often associated with muscle spasm. This resolves with the use of analgesics, muscle relaxants, and early mobilization. Wound hematoma or infection may occur, although this is not common. Meticulous hemostasis and attention to sterility will aid in the minimization of these events. Neurologic and vascular complications of lateral mass fixation are rare and are best avoided by a thorough understanding of the individual patient anatomy at the levels to be instrumented. Heller et al.[6] reported a 0.6% rate of nerve root injury during placement of lateral mass screws.

The spinal cord may be injured during sublaminar wire or hook placement. The best treatment is prevention. Careful attention should be given to the placement of cables and hooks, and they should be avoided in the stenotic spine. Other fixation techniques should then be employed. Spinal cord injury is rarely caused by lateral mass screw placement. This is due to the trajectory of the screw, which is away from the spinal cord. The spinal cord may be injured during screw placement as a result of inadvertent slippage of an instrument during drilling or screw tightening. For this reason, some surgeons do not perform any bony removal until all of the instrumentation has been placed. Other surgeons find that the presence of the instrumentation impedes their ability to accomplish a decompression.

There is a possibility of vertebral artery injury during screw placement. In the authors' experience, the incidence is extremely small. As with nerve root injury, proper screw trajectory will minimize this risk. If injury is suspected, the screw should be placed to limit bleeding. The instrumentation may be finished on the side with vessel injury, but contralateral instrumentation should not be performed. If the bleeding is not controlled with hemostatic agents and screw placement, the vertebral artery should be exposed for potential repair or sacrifice. If an injury is suspected and the patient hemodynamically stable, postoperative angiography for endovascular occlusion or stenting may be a possibility.

Hardware failure may occur. Wires or cables may break or cut out of bone, especially osteoporotic bone. Proper placement and multisegmental fixation will aid in the prevention of these complications. Screw breakage, cut, or pull-out or plate breakage may occur. Heller et al.[6] reported a 1.3% rate of plate breakage over a follow-up of 1.5 years. Modern rod and screw fixation systems have decreased the risk for these complications to some extent because of the rigidity of fixation.

CONCLUSION

Following trauma, posterior subaxial instrumentation is often employed. Many options exist, including the use of interspinous cables, sublaminar wire and cable fixation, and modern lateral mass fixation. The spine may be adequately stabilized with minimal morbidity. Furthermore, screw and rod systems may permit the application of complex forces to aid in traumatic deformity correction, if desired.

REFERENCES

1. Hadra BE. Wiring the vertebrae as a means of immobilization in fractures and Pott's disease. *Trans Am Orthop Assoc* 1981;4:206–211.
2. Benzel EC. *Biomechanics of Spine Stabilization.* 2nd ed. Rolling Meadows, Ill: American Association of Neurological Surgeons; 2001.
3. Heller JG, Carlson GD, Abitbol J-J, Garfin SR. Anatomic comparison of the Roy-Camille and Magerl techniques for screw placement in the lower cervical spine. *Spine* 1991;16:S552–S557.
4. Jeanneret B, Magerl F, Ward EH, et al. Posterior stabilization of the cervical spine with hook plates. *Spine* 1991;16:S56–S63.
5. Roy-Camille R, Saillant G, Mazel C. Internal fixation of the unstable cervical spine by a posterior osteosynthesis with plate and screws. In: Sherk H, Dunn E, Eismont F, et al., eds. *The Cervical Spine.* 2nd ed. Philadelphia: Lippincott-Raven, 1989:309.
6. Heller JG, Silcox H, Suterlin C III. Complications of posterior cervical plating. *Spine* 1995;20:2442–2448.

CHAPTER 19

Cervicothoracic Junction Instrumentation

Rick C. Sasso and Natalie M. Best

INTRODUCTION

The cervicothoracic junction is involved in 9% of all cervical trauma, and up to 80% of patients suffer a neurologic deficit.[1] This is a complex region characterized by a shift from the flexible lordotic cervical to the rigid kyphotic thoracic spine. Because of the anatomy and biomechanics at the cervicothoracic segment, successful stabilization is often a challenge and must address this change in configuration. In addition, imaging is complicated by the proximity of the shoulder girdle and rib cage. Plain lateral radiographs may insufficiently visualize the cervicothoracic junction (C6-T2). Missed and delayed diagnosis is often due to inadequate radiographs of the lower cervical spine. (Fig. 19.1). An adequate cervical spine series requires identification of the upper endplate of T1 and the C7-T1 facet joint. Shoulder pull-down views or swimmers view may increase visibility of this area. If these techniques prove inadequate, computed tomography (CT) (helical with sagittal and coronal reformation) is required. If spinal cord injury is apparent, magnetic resonance imaging (MRI) is essential.

Fracture treatment at the cervicothoracic junction includes several options. Standard resuscitation procedures are performed, and, if spinal cord injury is present, steroids may be administered. A steroid protocol, however, is controversial, and it is unclear whether they change the natural history of spinal cord recovery. The stability of the injury is determined by physical examination, radiography, CT, and MRI. The goals of treatment are to reduce and establish normal alignment of the spine and protect the spinal cord from further damage by stabilizing the injured segment. Closed reduction of subluxations and dislocations at the cervicothoracic junction usually require higher weights and are less successful than closed reduction techniques of the subaxial cervical spine. Nonoperative treatment of unstable fractures may include recumbent traction; however, the complications of bed rest are many including pulmonary embolus, skin problems, and respiratory difficulty, especially in patients with spinal cord injury. Also, halo vest immobilization may be considered, but this does not stabilize the cervicothoracic junction well. Because of the biomechanical disadvantage of the halo vest in this region of the spine, nonoperative treatment is recommended for only stable fractures in patients without neurologic deficits.

Surgical options depend on the characteristics of the injury. The surgical approach may be anterior or posterior. The anterior approach is particularly difficult due to both bone and soft tissue anatomic barriers. The manubrium, clavicle, and ribs are barriers to access, and careful attention must be made to the brachiocephalic vein, aortic arch, heart, recurrent laryngeal nerves, sympathetic ganglia, thoracic duct, trachea, lungs, and esophagus. Thus, anterior fixation is often avoided if possible. The posterior anatomy of the cervicothoracic junction is also difficult because of variable dimensions and angles of the lateral masses and pedicles. Inferiorly across the cervical spine to the

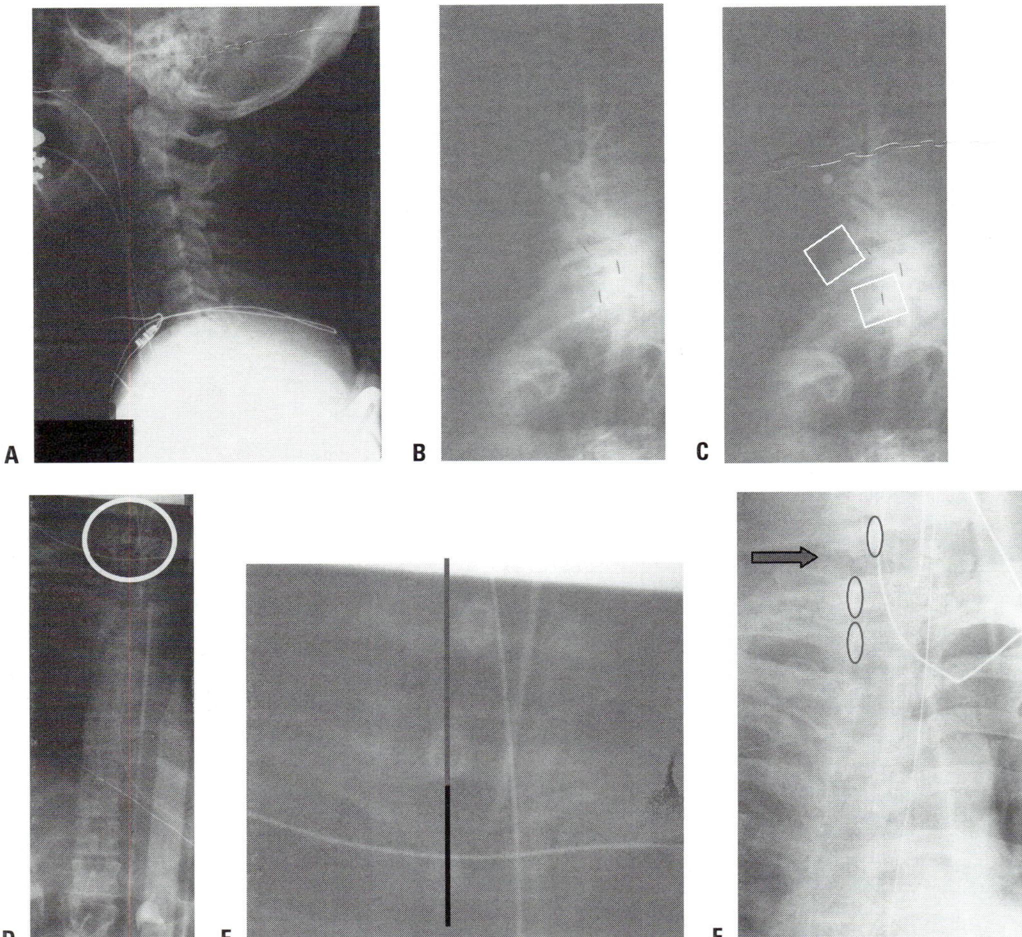

FIGURE 19.1. **A.** Lateral radiograph of cervical spine with inability to assess the 7th cervical vertebrae. Only C6 is seen. This is not adequate to clear the cervical spine. **B.** Lateral radiograph of cervicothoracic junction in same patient demonstrating a bilateral facet dislocation of C7-T1. **C.** The same lateral radiograph with the C7 and T1 vertebral bodies outlined in red. **D.** Anteroposterior (AP) radiograph of cervicothoracic junction and thoracic spine. The yellow circle surrounds the posterior spinous processes of the cervicothoracic region. **E.** AP radiograph in same patient demonstrating the lateral offset in the posterior spinous processes at the cervicothoracic junction. **F.** AP radiograph in the same patient with red arrow at C7-T1 dislocation and red ovals around the spinous processes at the cervicothoracic junction.

thoracic spine, the lateral masses narrow and the pedicles enlarge. The pedicle width increases from C6 to C7 to T1 and then decreases again caudal to T3; the vertebral axial length increases from C7 to T3 along with the laminae and pedicle axis thickness. This anatomy governs appropriate posterior instrumentation.

INDICATIONS

There are several indications for surgical treatment of the cervicothoracic spine. Instability and spinal cord compression causing a neurologic deficit are the most common reasons (Fig. 19.2). One of the most difficult issues is the determination of fracture stability. A detailed discussion of injury rendering the spine unstable and methods for evaluation of instability are beyond the scope of this manuscript, but careful evaluation of both anterior and posterior columns is mandatory. Surgery is

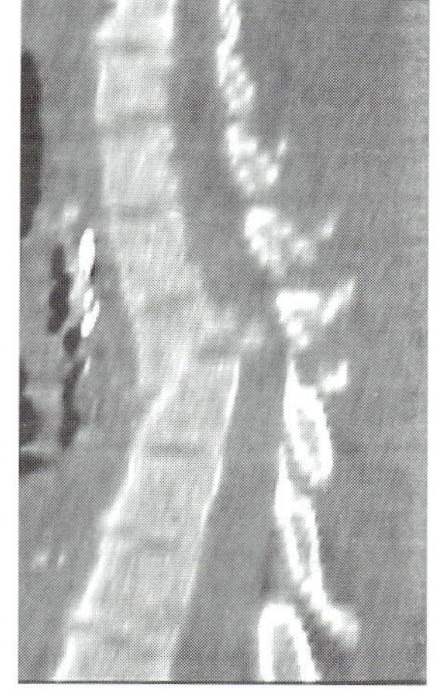

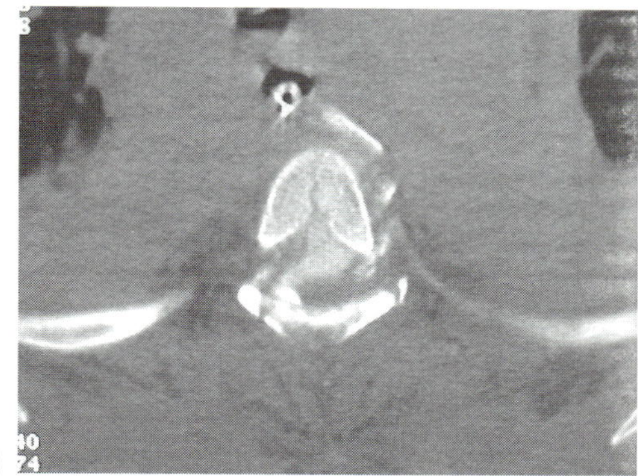

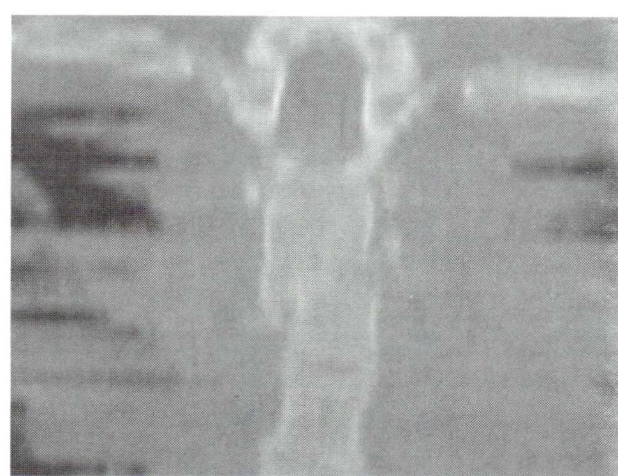

FIGURE 19.2. **A.** Sagittal reconstruction of helical computed tomography (CT) demonstration of a cervicothoracic fracture-dislocation. This is a very unstable injury with anterior and posterior column disruption, significant vertebral body fracture, and collapse. Bone is driven into the spinal canal, and a kyphotic deformity is present causing spinal cord compression. **B.** Axial CT image showing the profound spinal canal narrowing. **C.** Coronal reconstruction demonstrating the shear injury with lateral translation across this fracture. This signifies a very unstable spine.

often required for adequate nerve and spinal cord decompression, stabilization, restoration of alignment, and rapid rehabilitation. Decompression and stabilization may be performed from an anterior, posterior, or combined approach. If performed correctly, there is a high probability for a successful outcome.

ANTERIOR STABILIZATION

EXPOSURE AND APPROACH

The approach to the anterior cervicothoracic spine was first described in the late 1950s and was noted for being technically difficult. However, there may be indications necessitating this approach. These may include structural lesions of the ventral spine, such as burst fractures causing spinal cord compression and kyphotic deformities requiring reduction. The approach may be through an extension of the standard anterior approach to the cervical spine in the supine position or via a high thoracotomy with mobilization of the scapula in the lateral position.

To access this portion of the spine, extreme caution must be taken because of the complex anatomy at this junction. Several approaches have been described, including low cervical, transthoracic, transaxillary, combined cervical-thoracic, sternal splitting, and modified transsternal approaches. A transmanubrial approach creates a window in the manubrium and the medial clavicle. By resection of this bone at the caudal aspect of a traditional anterior approach to the cervical spine, additional caudal exposure is facilitated without the morbidity of splitting the sternum. A right-sided or left-sided approach can be performed. There is risk for injury to the right recurrent laryngeal nerve on the right side because of its variable course and risk for injury to the thoracic duct on the left side. This decision depends on surgeon preference. The esophagus and great vessels must be retracted for access to the upper thoracic spine. A standard approach to the cervical spine usually allows exposure down to T2, but placement of instrumentation may be difficult because of the clavicle or sternum. Extensile options include osteotomy of the clavicle or median sternotomy, which allows access as low as T4. The lung apex may be problematic, and the recurrent laryngeal nerve, thoracic duct, and great vessels are at risk.

Standard lateral thoracotomy with mobilization of the scapulae allows exposure up to T2, but the vertebral bodies are too small for application of noncustom anterior thoracic instrumentation. The transaxillary approach is an intrathoracic extrapleural approach via the third rib bed. It is a variant of the transthoracic approach with the advantages of a cosmetic axillary incision and avoidance of muscle division. It allows access to T1-T4; however, the disadvantages are that it is a very deep and very limited exposure, which does not allow easy insertion of instrumentation.

SURGICAL TECHNIQUE

Because of the anatomy at the cervicothoracic junction, inserting anterior instrumentation is difficult. A similar procedure to what is used in the cervical spine is often appropriate for the upper thoracic region through an extended anterior cervical approach. After adequate exposure has been obtained, lower cervical and upper thoracic corpectomies and discectomies can be performed as necessary. Once the lesion is removed, the endplates must be prepared parallel and the interbody space appropriately distracted. The interbody graft or cage must be sized for the resulting defect. It is placed into position and seated using a mallet. Common cages used in the cervicothoracic spine include Pyramesh (Medtronic Sofamor Danek, Memphis, TN) or Harms cage (J & J DePuy, Warsaw, IN).

A cervical plate can also provide stability to facilitate fusion and healing. A variety of plates can be used, including the Venture anterior cervical plate (Medtronic Sofamor Danek), Atlantis cervical plate (Medtronic Sofamor Danek), and many others. The most difficult issue regarding application of an anterior plate in the upper thoracic spine is the ability to drive the caudal screws into the vertebral body for correct placement. The clavicle, manubrium, and great vessels can prevent the surgeon's hand from dropping caudal enough to drill perpendicularly through the caudal plate holes. Cervical plates that allow significant angulation of the screws through the holes while ensuring proper functioning of the locking mechanism are optimal for the cervicothoracic junction. The screws can thus be driven with caudal angulation through the plate without hindrance because the surgeon's hand is positioned cranially.

If the exposure is performed via a high thoracotomy in the lateral position, internal fixation is hampered by the very small size of the upper thoracic vertebral bodies, which cannot accommodate standard anterior thoracic plates. Small posterior cervical screw-rod systems may be used in a single- or dual-rod fashion in the anterior vertebral bodies to provide stability at the cervicothoracic junction. Combining the small screw-rod construct with a strong interbody graft such as a well-sized and well-positioned titanium mesh cage (Fig. 19.3) can provide enough stability to afford an anterior stand-alone assembly. This obviates the need to perform a separate posterior cervicothoracic instrumentation and fusion to stabilize the anterior strut graft. Before stable anterior instrumentation was available, a circumferential approach was very common. This was required after completion of an anterior corpectomy to decompress the neural elements because the interbody strut graft by itself is not stable under shear and rotational loads. Anterior strut grafts are usually very stable under axial compressive loads, but tend to displace as a result of translational shear forces placed across the corpectomy segment. At the thoracolumbar junction, where most burst fractures occur, modern anterior thoracolumbar plate-screw devices provide excellent stability to allow a stand-alone anterior construct. The problem at the cervicothoracic junction, however, is that the size of the vertebral bodies is too small to allow proper positioning of these anterior plates. The advantage of the cervicothoracic junction is that the forces crossing this segment are less than at the thoracolumbar junction; thus, these smaller screw-rod constructs are quite adequate.[2]

A 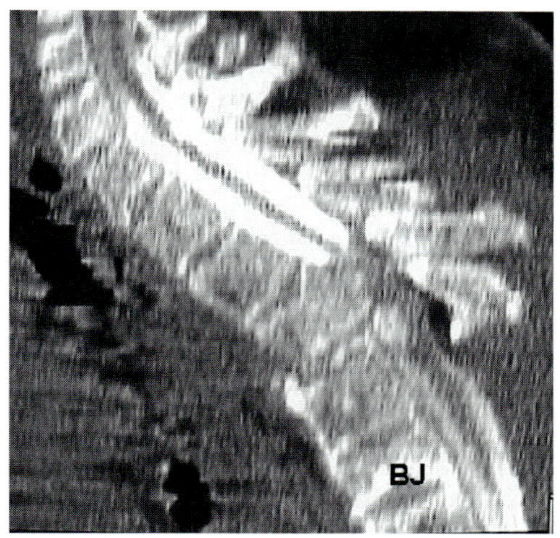

B 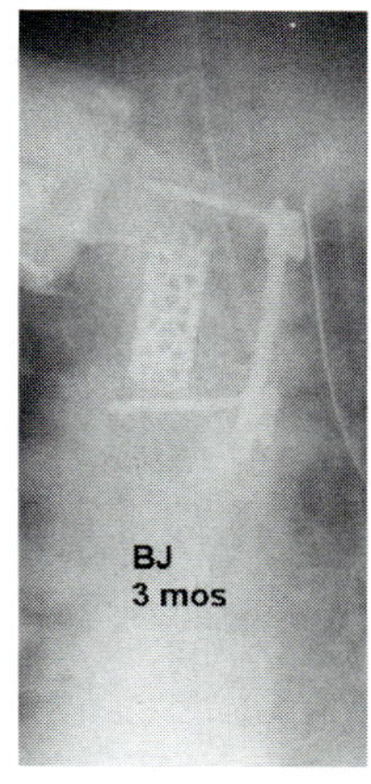

C 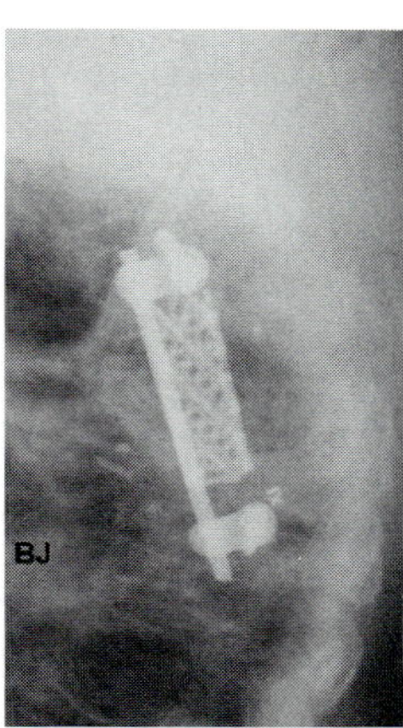

FIGURE 19.3. **A.** Sagittal reconstruction of computed tomography scan after myelography with complete block of contrast at cervicothoracic burst fracture. **B.** Anteroposterior radiograph after corpectomy and reconstruction with titanium mesh strut graft and screw-rod construct. **C.** Lateral radiograph of same construct.

POSTERIOR FIXATION

EXPOSURE AND APPROACH

A posterior approach is preferred because of the complex anatomy anterior to the spinal column at the cervicothoracic junction, both the bony and soft tissue structures. Posterior stabilization may be necessary in addition to anterior fixation to overcome the biomechanical challenge of connecting the highly mobile cervical spine to the anatomically different thoracic vertebrae.

Limited anterior decompression can also occur from various posterolateral approaches. The transpedicular approach has the advantages of a simple technique with less soft tissue and bony dissection than other posterolateral approaches, but suffers the disadvantages of a limited ventral exposure and it is not appropriate for multilevel pathology. Costotransversectomy is a technique in which the rib of interest is identified, isolated, divided at its angle, and disarticulated. The intercostal neurovascular bundle is isolated and followed to the foramen and thecal sac. One or two ribs are removed for adequate exposure, and the plane is developed between the endothoracic fascia and the parietal pleura. This plane is carried lateral to the vertebral body, and the parietal pleura is retracted ventrally. The main disadvantages are wound-related complications, neurovascular bundle sacrifice, potential pneumothorax, and cerebrovascular fluid leak. The ventral exposure is limited to the lateral two thirds of the vertebral body and is a difficult exposure for multilevel decompressions. The lateral extracavitary approach is carried out with a midline hockey-stick incision. A myocutaneous flap is developed superficial to the erector spinae muscle group and lateral to medial elevation of the erector spinae is performed, beginning at its lateral margin. The rib is resected and lateral thecal sac exposure ensured. The vertebral body resection, anterior reconstruction, and posterior instrumentation and fusion are performed simultaneously. The advantages are a simultaneous ventral and dorsal exposure, with the best access to ventral pathology of all posterolateral procedures. The disadvantages are extensive soft tissue exposure and the fact that visualization and decompression of the canal are less optimal than formal anterior thoracotomy. It is technically demanding, and the neurovascular bundle is sacrificed. Blood loss may be considerable after epidural decompression, and there is less ability to directly distract the anterior column and adequately seat the anterior construct. This can lead to difficulty placing anterior instrumentation.

Many different fixation constructs have been tried at the cervicothoracic junction. Hook and rod constructs were designed for the thoracolumbar spine, but hooks and sublaminar wires carry a significant risk for neurologic injury in the cervical canal. Standard fixation to the cervical spine is the lateral mass, but this is not an option in the thoracic spine. Screw fixation in the thoracic spine is through the pedicles or transverse processes. Screws placed lateral to the pedicle usually engage the base of the rib and are quite strong. The anatomy of C7 is different because it is a transitional vertebra. Important anatomic issues of C7 are (a) the lateral mass is smaller than the rest of the subaxial cervical spine, and, thus, lateral mass screws will be shorter and biomechanically weaker; (b) the pedicle is larger than the rest of the subaxial cervical spine and closer to the size of upper thoracic pedicles; and (c) the foramen transversarium does not usually contain the vertebral artery (be aware that 5% will harbor the vertebral artery). Thus pedicle screw placement is safer.[3]

SURGICAL TECHNIQUE

Several techniques can be performed posteriorly for fixation at this junction. Neural decompression is often performed in addition and can be through a laminectomy, laminoplasty, transpedicular decompression, costotransversectomy, or lateral extracavitary approach. The preference is to perform fixation before decompression, to limit passing instrumentation over the exposed dura and spinal cord. Lateral mass plating, lateral mass screws and rods, sublaminar wires, pedicle screws, lamina and pedicle hook placement, and combinations of these are all options for posterior fixation at the cervicothoracic junction. The purpose of this fixation must be stabilization, avoidance of future neurologic deficits, prevention of loss of reduction, and promotion of bone healing. Depending on the pathology and the resulting anatomy, different instrumentation may be indicated. The ultimate decision is based on surgeon preference and the bony elements available for fixation.

Wires have been the historical standard in posterior stabilization for the cervical spine. They function by creating a tension band posteriorly and limiting flexion loads; however, the anterior column must be intact for this construct to be stable. The wires provide limited shear, extension, and rotational stability. They are not rigid devices and should be used only in injuries with a stable anterior column. They are often inadequate at the cervicothoracic junction because a more rigid construct is required. The combination of sublaminar wires with a Luque rod improves the stability of wires alone, but this construct is weak under axial loads because the rod pistons through the wires. Also, passing wires in the sublaminar region is very dangerous below C1. Especially at the cervicothoracic junction, the spinal cord is relatively large compared to the canal and is at increased risk with intracanal instrumentation.

Lateral mass plating was first described by Roy-Camille with increased stability over wiring techniques. The screw was positioned perpendicularly through the plate hole and angled laterally 10 degrees. Magerl recommended a much steeper cranial angle to mimic the facet joint and angled laterally 30 degrees. This allowed for a much longer screw with increased biomechanical strength. This screw angle, however, is not normal to the plate hole and thus is not conducive to plating techniques. Because of the differing morphology across the cervical and thoracic spine, these plates are also very difficult to adequately place, particularly at the C6-T1 levels. The screws must be positioned to fit the predetermined holes and do not allow for variations in anatomy. The screws are not rigidly attached to the plate, so bicortical fixation is optimal to prevent screw toggle and back-out. C7 is a transitional vertebra with a relatively sparse lateral mass but a larger pedicle compared to the rest of the subaxial cervical spine. The upper thoracic vertebrae do not have a lateral mass, but rather the screws are placed into the larger and safer pedicles compared to the subaxial cervical spine. The trajectories of a lateral mass screw and a pedicle screw are much different, which becomes a very difficult problem when a plate is used for fixation across the cervicothoracic junction. The appropriate-length plate must be determined and then contoured to permit proper sagittal alignment. Several plates are available, including the Axis plate (Medtronic, Memphis, TN) and the atlanto-occipital reconstruction device (Synthes, Paoli, PA). Universal screw-rod systems have solved these problems with plates. The screws can be driven in exactly the perfect position without regard to plate-hole configuration, and because the screw is rigidly attached to the rod, unicortical fixation is as strong as bicortical purchase.[4]

The current preferred instrumentation for posterior fixation at the cervicothoracic junction is a screw and rod construct.[5] The screws may be placed independently of a plate and can adapt to variations in anatomy. Rods can be easily bent for proper cervicothoracic sagittal alignment. This is preferred over wiring techniques in that it provides rigid fixation and is resistant to rotation and extension. In addition, unlike wires, which create only a posterior tension band, screws and rods involve all three columns. Because of the anatomy across the cervicothoracic junction, lateral mass screws or pedicle screws may be indicated. The C7 vertebral body is a transitional segment from the lateral masses of the cervical spine to the transverse processes of the thoracic spine. C7 is therefore of particular interest. Some surgeons recommend the placement of pedicle screws at this level because of a narrow lateral mass and a wider pedicle. Additionally, the vertebral artery is normally outside of the vertebral foramen at C7 and is therefore less of a risk in pedicle screw placement. Cephalad to C7, lateral mass screws are often used because of the proximity of the spinal canal and vertebral artery to the pedicle and the ability to achieve strong fixation with the thicker lateral masses above C7. Caudal to C7, pedicle screws are indicated and allow for adequate purchase. Rod-screw systems are preferred because of their versatility in both the cervical and thoracic spines.[3]

Lateral mass screws should be placed before laminectomy at a point 1 mm medial to the center of the lateral mass, with a cephalad and lateral direction. This prevents injury to the vertebral artery and nerve roots. Pedicle screw insertion at C7 must be performed with caution because of the angle of the pedicle at this level. This is normally performed by angling the screw 25 to 30 degrees medially. In the thoracic spine, the angle is not as profound; the pedicle screw is normally inserted 10 to 15 degrees medially. Insertion is determined by the intersection of the middle of the facet joint and upper third of the transverse processes. Hooks may also be used but are not as strong as pedicle screws. Hooks can be placed around the cortical bone of the lamina, outer pedicle, or transverse process. Hooks can be easily combined with screw fixation through a universal rod construct.

After the anchors have been placed, a rod can be easily contoured to the anatomic lordotic and kyphotic sagittal configuration of the lower cervical and cervicothoracic junction. Lateral offset connectors may be necessary depending on the patient's anatomy and the resulting screw placement. The lateral offset connectors are helpful not only for attaching anchors translated medially or laterally from the rod but also to account for small differences in height of the screws. One of the most difficult screw combinations to capture on a rod is a lateral mass screw at C7 and a pedicle screw at T1 (Fig. 19.4). Because the lateral mass screw is angled up and out, the screw head is positioned down (close to T1) and medial. The T1 pedicle screw is angled medially; thus the head is lateral and almost at the same level horizontally. Lateral offset connectors allow achievement of this feat. The Vertex Reconstruction System (Medtronic Sofamor-Danek) improves on this by allowing the use of one rod with multiple multiaxial screws. The 3.2-mm rod often used in the cervical spine can be carried down into the midthoracic region, permitting the use of one rod across the cervicothoracic junction. The Vertex system includes several instrumentation options, including multiaxial screws, lateral offset connectors, hooks, lateral connectors, rod connectors, and attachment devices. This allows the surgeon to adapt the instrumentation to create sufficient fixation along the variable cervicothoracic junction.

CONCLUSION

Managing instability at the cervicothoracic junction can be quite challenging. Many injuries are often misdiagnosed or overlooked because of imaging difficulties in this region. The anatomy at the cervicothoracic junction is complex. In particular, the transition from the lordotic flexible cervical spine to the kyphotic rigid thoracic spine makes stabilization and fixation difficult. Anterior stabilization is complicated by the exposure of bony and soft tissue elements obstructing the cervicothoracic spine.

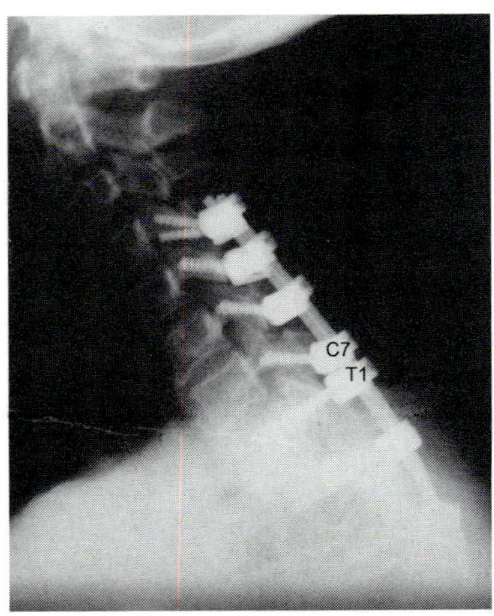

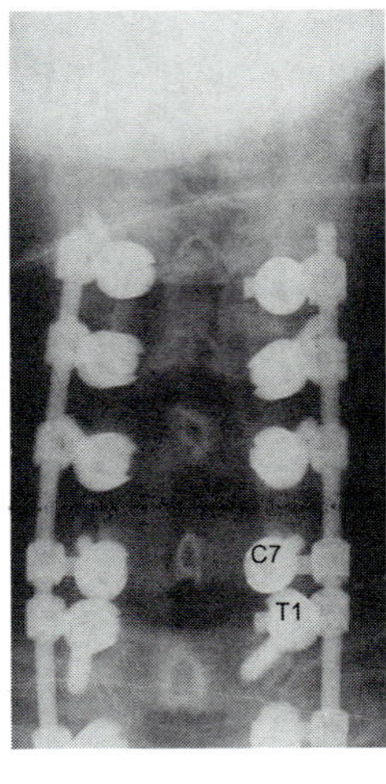

FIGURE 19.4. **A.** Lateral radiograph showing proximity of the screw heads at C7 (lateral mass) and T1 (pedicle) screws. **B.** Anteroposterior radiograph demonstrating the use of lateral offset connectors to allow capture of these screw heads onto the rod.

There are several indications for surgery at the cervicothoracic junction, including trauma. Posterior fixation is preferred if possible because of a less complicated exposure, and adequate fixation is often achieved with a posterior-only procedure.

Because of the number of interfering factors at these levels, instrumentation must be used that allows for both sufficient fixation and flexibility for the variable anatomic elements at these levels. Posterior screws and rods have become the best surgical treatment option for this junction. The first system was the Cervifix system (Synthes, Paoli, PA). However, this does not allow for rigid screw to rod attachment. An improvement was the Starlock system (Synthes, Paoli, PA), yet this does not permit variable medial-lateral screw variations. The Vertex Reconstruction System was the first universal polyaxial screw-rod system. Currently, many screw-rod systems are available that allow independent rigid placement of screws and also variable offset of the screw from the rod. These systems allow instrumentation options that can be used across both the cervical and thoracic spine, allowing for continuity and rigidity.

REFERENCES

1. An HS, Vaccaro A, Cotler JM, et al. Spinal disorders at the cervicothoracic junction. *Spine* 1994;19:2557–2564.
2. Boockvar JA, Philips MF, Telfeian AE, et al. Results and risk factors for anterior cervicothoracic junction surgery. *J Neurosurg (Spine 1)* 2001;94:12–17.
3. Stanescu S, Ebraheim NA, Yeasting R, et al. Morphometric evaluation of the cervico-thoracic junction: practical considerations for posterior fixation of the spine. *Spine* 1994;19:2082–2088.
4. Bueff HU, Lotz JC, Colliou OK, et al. Instrumentation of the cervicothoracic junction after destabilization. *Spine* 1995;20:1789–1792.
5. Kreshak JL, Kim DH, Lindsey DP, et al. Posterior stabilization at the cervicothoracic junction: a biomechanical study. *Spine* 2002;27:2763–2770.

SECTION VII

Cervical Spine Injuries

CHAPTER 20

Cervical Whiplash

Christopher M. Bono, Jared Toman, Kyle Cabbell, and Stephen M. Papadopoulos

INTRODUCTION

Although not a diagnosis itself, the term "whiplash" has become synonymous with the clinical sequelae of an acute hyperflexion or hyperextension injury of the cervical spine that may occur during a motor vehicle collision. As it is a collection of signs and symptoms, the term "whiplash associated disorder" (WAD) has been accepted as a description of the clinical condition. Of the roughly 13 million motor vehicle crashes every year, the estimated incidence of whiplash is 1,000,000 cases per year.[1,2] In Sweden, the incidence of WAD was approximately 0.1% between 1993 and 1995.[3]

Cervical whiplash injuries display minimal to no acute radiographic findings[4]; however, chronic pain is not uncommon. These and other factors make the management of whiplash sequelae challenging. Nonoperative measures are the mainstay of treatment. However, for recalcitrant pain, invasive modalities, such as radiofrequency neurotomy or, rarely, cervical fusion, might be helpful. This chapter will discuss these and other issues relevant to the management of whiplash injury.

MECHANISM OF INJURY

ANTERIOR STRUCTURES

The anterior longitudinal ligament (ALL) spans the ventral surface of the cervical vertebral bodies. It limits extension as a "check-rein" and can be injured with severe, abrupt hyperextension. Injury of the ALL occurs most commonly with acceleratory mechanisms, such as rear-end collisions. The anulus of the intervertebral disc supplements the ALL against these forces and can be similarly injured. Reports of intervertebral disc avulsion have been reported.[5,6] In addition, the outer anulus resists rotational forces and can be damaged with sudden torque, although this is not a common mechanism of whiplash. Muscular restraints to extension are also important. The sternocleidomastoid and longissimus muscles have demonstrated injuries in primate studies of acceleration and extension injuries.[1,7]

The nucleus pulposus is the gel-like core of the intervertebral disc. Contained by the fixed boundaries of the anulus, it becomes pressurized under compressive loads along the anterior spine. Abrupt hyperflexion can lead to pressures that exceed the capacity of the anulus to contain the nucleus. Microtears in this layered-wall structure can occur, but they are exceedingly difficult to detect acutely. Magnetic resonance imaging (MRI) results can be negative in the first few weeks.[8] In some cases, intradiscal degeneration can be detected as a so-called black disc on MRI, which may present weeks to months after the accident. It is commonly held that a posttraumatic degenerative disc can be a pain source. Anatomically, the disc receives nociceptive branches from the dorsal root ganglion.[9]

POSTERIOR STRUCTURES

With hyperflexion mechanisms, the facet capsule is stretched and may tear.[10] However, the facets are more frequently injured with hyperextension forces.[11] This briefly impacts the apposed articular surfaces. Articular cartilage damage can predispose to posttraumatic arthritis, which is often reported after whiplash injuries.[12–14] Sensory innervation from branches of the dorsal root ganglion can transmit arthritic pain. This is the proposed nociceptive pathway of posttraumatic facet arthritis after whiplash injury, evidenced by the effectiveness of anesthetic blocks injected into the zygapophyseal joints. Several randomized controlled studies have demonstrated significant pain relief with facet injections in some patients after whiplash.[12,15,16]

PREVENTION

Recent evidence has highlighted the importance of head restraint position and design in the prevention of hyperextension injuries to the cervical spine (Fig. 20.1). Welcher and Szabo[17] performed a human subject kinetic study of head and neck dynamics during simulated motor vehicle collisions. They found that the most influential factor was the distance between the head and restraint in both the horizontal and vertical planes. Notwithstanding vehicle speed change, Siegmund et al.[18] also found the relative head restraint position to be the most influential factor.

However, having occupants properly use the active safety systems has proven problematic. Fockler et al.[19] compared three methods of educating patients on correct adjustment of head restraints. These included a human interactive program, a passive video, and an interactive three-dimensional model. Although none of the three were extraordinarily effective, the human interactive program was best, prompting 28% of the participants to change their habits. These data highlight the futility of advancements in seat design if occupants do not use them correctly.

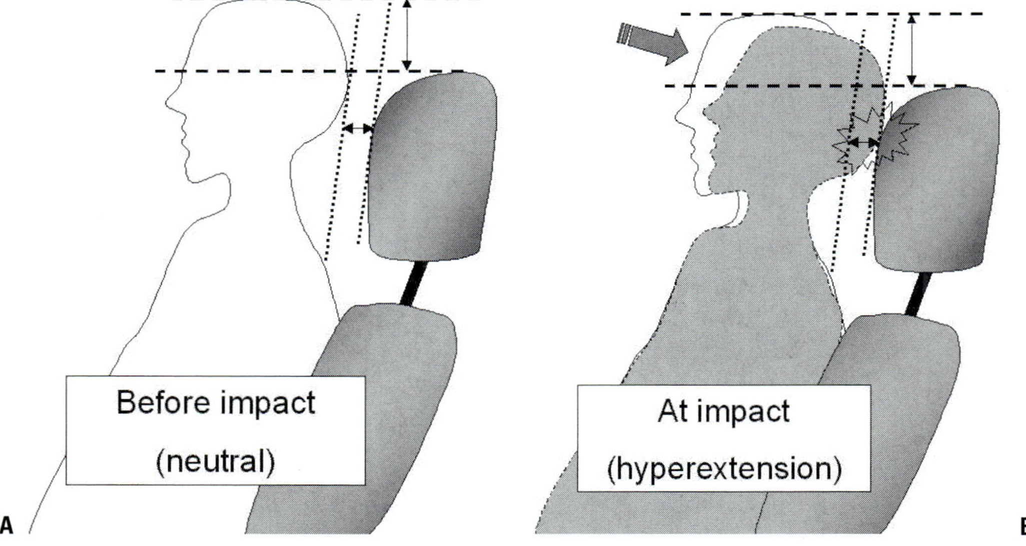

FIGURE 20.1. Diagram illustrating a motor vehicle occupant's head and neck in relation to the head restraint. The most important parameters are the horizontal and vertical distances *(double-sided arrows)* between the head and the restraint **(A)**. During a rear impact **(B)**, the head is thrust backward into the headrest. The greater the distance traveled, the greater is the speed at which the head hits the restraint and the greater is the degree of sudden deceleration imparted.

CLASSIFICATION

The most well-known and widely used classification system for WAD was developed by the Quebec Task Force.[20] Although grades III and IV are part of the classification, they represent injuries that most surgeons would not consider simple "whiplash" injuries, because they are associated with frank neurologic deficit or fracture and dislocation. Grades I and II are more characteristic of what one would consider a cervical whiplash injury. These are as follows:

- *Grade I:* Neck complaints of pain, stiffness, or tenderness
- *Grade II:* Neck complaints and musculoskeletal signs, including decreased range of motion and point tenderness

The utility of the Quebec Task Force classification has been examined. In a prospective 1-year follow-up study, Miettinen et al.[21] found that the WAD classification could predict the duration of work disability and long-term health damage. Sterling[22] performed a literature search and analysis of previous studies of whiplash injuries. Based on this analysis and his experience, he proposed a modification of the WAD classification, in which he subdivided grade II injuries into A, B, and C categories based on the presence and severity of psychological impairment parameters. Unfortunately, this modification has not been assessed prognostically, to the authors' knowledge.

CLINICAL PRESENTATION

Neck pain is the most common symptom reported after whiplash injury, with an incidence of 62% to 100%.[1,7,23–29] Pain may be localized more to the posterior or anterior neck. Pennie and Agambar[7] found that rear-end collisions led to more anterior neck pain. In contrast, Sturzenneger et al.[27] found that posterior neck pain was more common after this mechanism of injury.

Headaches are also a frequent complaint,[1] occurring in as many as 82% of cases. These complaints can be persistent; one study found that 80% of patients had continued headaches 6 months after the injury.[25,30] Vague neurologic symptoms are not infrequent. These can include upper extremity paresthesias, which may occur in up to 45% of patients.[31] True nerve root compression is rare, but may present with a cock-robin posture of the head.[27] Dizziness, vertigo, and cognitive and various visual and auditory complaints have been reported with varying frequency following whiplash injury.[1,7,23–29]

Other nonspecific complaints can also be present. Dysphagia, occurring in 7% to 18% of patients,[1,7,27,31] does not appear to persist as long as other symptoms. Most studies have found that it resolves within 0.5 to 8 years from the time of injury.[30–32]

PRETREATMENT ASSESSMENT

PHYSICAL EXAMINATION

In the acute setting, the patient must be carefully examined, including a systematic neurologic evaluation. Subtle signs, such as clonus or a Babinski response, can indicate spinal cord trauma without focal neurologic deficits. Radicular symptoms or signs can suggest foraminal encroachment. In most cases, cervical range of motion should not be tested at the time of injury. A hard cervical collar should remain in place until the initial pain and spasm subsides. Spasm can mask occult instability or subluxation of the vertebral column, which is more safely assessed 1 to 2 weeks after the injury. Palpation of the spine can reveal tenderness at the injured level.

PLAIN RADIOGRAPHY

In general, plain radiographs after whiplash are normal. In some cases, a loss of normal cervical kyphosis can be appreciated. It is thought that loss of kyphosis is secondary to muscular spasm after trauma. However, this may reflect normal variation in spinal posture. Matsumoto et al.[33] prospectively compared the radiographs of 488 whiplash-injured patients with those of 495 asymptomatic control subjects, finding no difference in the incidence of nonlordotic curves between the groups. Lateral flexion-extension views of the cervical spine can help detect dynamic instability not otherwise detectable on static films and should be considered before initiating an active, early range-of-motion program in a patient following a whiplash injury.

ADVANCED IMAGING

Although CT and MRI are of great benefit in cases of higher energy cervical trauma, their utility in the acute evaluation of whiplash injury has not been demonstrated. Without evidence of fracture on plain radiographs, there is little role for CT in evaluating whiplash injury.[34] Likewise, MRI is of low value in the early management of whiplash.[35,36] Because of its high sensitivity, a large number of false-positive MRI results are obtained immediately after the accident. Findings include muscle contusions, disc herniations, spondylosis, and disc changes.[35,36] Unfortunately, investigators have found that the MRI findings have little to no correlation with the clinical findings. Most authors would agree that MRI is best reserved for the chronic setting in patients with long-standing symptoms after whiplash injury.[36,37]

INITIAL (NONOPERATIVE) TREATMENT

Initial rest and immobilization in a soft collar seems a logical first step. Although this classic treatment is still used,[38,39] numerous studies have indicated that a program of early range-of-motion therapy is more beneficial. In a randomized controlled study, Rosenfeld et al.[40] found that an "active treatment protocol" (consisting of range-of-motion exercises) resulted in better pain control and cervical flexion when administered early rather than late. In a later study, Rosenfeld et al.[41] again found lower pain scores in addition to reduced sick leave with active versus standard treatment in a randomized controlled study of 97 patients after motor vehicle collisions. Likewise, McKinney et al.,[42] Mealy et al.,[43] and Schnabel et al.[44] found early mobilization to result in better range of motion and pain relief than standard treatment. Crawford et al.[45] found early mobilization led to earlier return to work, but no difference in functional outcomes.

Other nonoperative treatments have focused on the coordination of body movements and activities. Fitz-Ritson[46] reported lower pain and disability scores in whiplash patients who received so-called phasic exercises. These included exercises that reinforced the coordinated movements between the eyes and head and the neck and arms. Administration of nonsteroidal anti-inflammatory drugs (NSAIDs) can be of use for acute pain. This can follow a short prelude of narcotic analgesia. Although muscle relaxants are frequently prescribed for spasms, there is little evidence-based data to support their efficacy in this patient population.

DEFINITIVE TREATMENT

The indications for invasive treatments for whiplash injury are limited. They are usually reserved for the management of chronic pain and symptoms. Options can vary from trigger point injections to, rarely, fusion procedures. Although there are some limited data supporting these techniques for whiplash-associated pain, their definitive role remains unclear.

INJECTIONS

A variety of injections may be prescribed for a patient with chronic neck pain. These include epidural steroid injections, facet injections, and selective nerve root blocks. As the indications for these procedures are debated in the nonwhiplash population, there are no data, to the authors' knowledge, on injections as a treatment for whiplash-injured patients.

There are, however, some limited data on one specific type of trigger point injection. In a pilot study in patients with grade II WAD, Freund and Schwartz[47,48] found patients randomized to botulinum toxin-A intramuscular injection had statistically better pain improvement and range of motion compared to those with saline (control) injections. Although these results were encouraging, the number of patients was limited (n = 26), and a larger study, to the authors' knowledge, has not been performed.

RADIOFREQUENCY NEUROTOMY

The facet joint has been implicated as a major source of chronic pain after whiplash.[12] With radiographic and MRI evidence of posttraumatic articular degeneration, the diagnosis of facet arthritis can be strengthened with pain relief after selective injections of the joint.[15,16] Although injections can sometimes give long-lasting relief, minimally invasive neuroablative procedures have been developed for resistant cases. Radiofrequency neurotomy involves percutaneous insertion of an electrode that is directed toward the facet joint. The heat at the electrode can obliterate the sensory innervation from the medial branch of the primary dorsal rami and serve as a longer lasting facet injection.

Results with this technique for whiplash have been promising.[13,14] In a double-blind randomized study, Lord et al.[14] used this method in patients with chronic whiplash injury. Twelve patients who underwent the procedure had at least 50% pain relief for a median of 263 days, whereas the control group reported only 8 days. Of interest, some patients in the neurotomy group complained of numbness in the region of the procedure, which was most likely secondary to denervation of some of the dorsal rami branches to the posterior skin of the neck. A recent study also suggested that radiofrequency neurotomy has equivalent efficacy in litigant and nonlitigant patients with whiplash injuries.[49]

ANTERIOR DISCECTOMY AND FUSION

The rationale of anterior discectomy for whiplash injury sequelae relies on the hypothesis that the disc is the major pain generator. Although it is a rare indication, several authors have reported on the results of anterior cervical discectomy and fusion (ACDF) for whiplash injury.[30,50–54] Surgical outcomes have varied. Algers et al.[50] documented 4-year follow-up of 18 patients who underwent uninstrumented ACDF for painful sequelae after whiplash injury. Patients had a combination of isolated discogenic pain with or without radicular symptoms. Symptoms persisted between 1 and 25 years before surgery was contemplated. Preoperative discography was used in only two cases. The authors reported two good, eight fair, and eight poor results. Preinjury spondylosis can negatively influence the surgical results of anterior cervical fusion for postwhiplash disc degeneration.[55]

To determine the frequency that fusion is performed in whiplash-injured patients, Hamer et al.[51] retrospectively reviewed all cases of ACDF over a 3-year period. Of the 215 patients, 30 (14%) had a history of whiplash, which suggests that whiplash patients undergo surgery at a higher rate than the general population. In a long-term study of 146 patients, Hohl[30] found that three patients eventually underwent an anterior cervical fusion. Two had good pain relief, and one reported no improvement. Likewise, Squires et al.[54] reviewed the records of 40 cases of whiplash-injured patients. Two eventually underwent an anterior discectomy and fusion. One had complete alleviation of symptoms, and the other remained symptomatic.

It is the authors' belief that ACDF should be reserved for a select group of patients with pain secondary to whiplash injury. Better results are perhaps achieved in conjunction with discography that localizes the painful disc level.[55] With supportive discographic, MRI, and radiographic findings and failure of prolonged nonoperative and minimally invasive measures, including injections, ACDF may be contemplated. The authors usually wait at least 1 year before the first discussion of surgical options with the patient.

POSTERIOR FUSION

In the authors' review of the literature, there are no reports of isolated posterior fusion procedures in the treatment of whiplash injury. Some isolated reports of posterior laminectomy for decompression have been accompanied by ACDF.[30] There is a large body of evidence to support facet injury after whiplash. Facet injection and neurotomy studies have documented good pain relief. It is likely that some of the patients who have undergone ACDF have had concomitant facet pain. Fusion of the anterior spine probably diminishes motion in the posterior spine as well. Therefore, an ACDF could address facet arthritis in addition to discogenic pain. An important question is whether isolated facet pain without disc pathology, documented by MRI and discography, could be successfully treated with an isolated posterior fusion of the zygapophyseal joint. This option remains to be explored in a clinical study.

PROGNOSIS

The prognosis following a whiplash injury has been evaluated in many studies. A large number of studies have found that the number of signs and symptoms at presentation correlates with a poor prognosis, including paresthesias, thoracolumbar pain, prior history of neck pain, symptom onset within 12 hours, objective neurologic signs, neck stiffness, muscle spasms, and abnormal cervical curvature.[1,7,23,26–28,30–32,38,39] In a prospective study of 353 rear-end collision victims, Hartling et al.[58] found that increased age, number of initial physical symptoms, and early onset of upper back pain, upper extremity numbness or weakness, and vision complaints were risk factors for WAD. Likewise, Suissa et al.[56] found that women older than 60 years had a significantly longer recovery period than 20-year-old men. In addition, they also found that neck pain with palpation and numbness radiating from the neck to the arms were also poor prognostic factors.[57] Hendriks et al.[59] found that female gender, a lower level of education, high initial neck pain, and sleep difficulties were poor prognostic factors. However, the most predictive factors were neck pain intensity and work disability.

The nature of long-term morbidity with whiplash syndrome has also been examined. Foley-Nolan et al.[29] found that 59% of patients reported interference with activities of daily living. Balla[60] found that 26% of patients were not able to return to their preinjury activities after 6 months. In one study, 38% of patients were either unemployed or had taken some leave of absence after a whiplash-type injury.[61] Prognostically, a mean of 6 weeks off from work was found to be a poor predictive factor for recovery compared to a mean of 2 weeks missing work.[60] Norris and Watt[32] reported that 9.6% of affected individuals were permanently disabled secondary to their pain after whiplash injury.

Litigation is an unfortunate complicating factor in assessing whiplash patients. Counterintuitively, many studies have demonstrated that the presence of litigation may not significantly affect long-term outcomes.[26,30,32,39] Although litigation would seem to be a reason for symptom magnification and malingering, most litigant patients had continued symptoms following settlement of their cases.[26,30] Likewise, Sapir and Gorup[49] found the results of radiofrequency treatment of cervical facet pain to be unaffected by litigation.

Many have attempted to estimate prognosis using outcome instruments. Soderlund et al.[62] found patients who reported a low self-efficacy score (a measure of how confident a patient is in ability to complete activities of daily living despite pain) and a high disability index score were at highest risk for chronic symptoms. Olsson et al.[63] found that the West Haven-Yale Multidimensional Pain Inventory (MPI) could be used soon after injury to help predict those at risk for developing chronic neck pain after a traffic accident.

The age-old adage "time heals all wounds" may not apply to cervical whiplash injury. In one study from Finland, Miettinen et al.[64] found the frequency of symptoms and care-seeking for those symptoms was similar 1 and 3 years after the injury. In contrast to these findings, Olivegren et al.[65] found that patients could continue to improve up to 2 years after injury.

COMPLICATIONS

In general, the complications of whiplash injury are related to the development of a chronic pain syndrome. Other complications may be related to the type of treatment. The complications of injections are local infections, discitis, or neurologic deficit, although they occur rarely. Radiofrequency neurotomy most often can lead to numbness over the posterior skin of the neck or upper back. The potential complications of anterior and posterior cervical fusion are numerous and lie beyond the scope of this chapter. They include swallowing difficulty, recurrent laryngeal nerve injury (anterior surgery), wound infection (posterior surgery), and pseudarthrosis.

CONCLUSION

WAD is a set of symptoms that occur following neck injury, usually from vehicular trauma. Grades I and II reflect absence of observable bone or neurologic injury. The prognosis is variable, with risk factors for chronic pain and disability being severity of initial symptoms, multiple physical findings at initial presentation, older age, and female gender. Approximately 30% of patients will progress to chronic pain and disability. Initial treatment should be reassurance and emphasis on early range of motion and activities. Chronic symptoms can be investigated for facet-mediated pain using anesthetic facet and medial branch blocks. Radiofrequency rhizotomy may be efficacious in patients who have two positive anesthetic blocks.

In patients with isolated disc disease and chronic pain, anterior cervical discectomy and fusion may be beneficial. However, identification or confirmation of the level is difficult even using discography. Psychological impairments are frequent, occurring within 3 months of injury, but do not appear to be preexisting as originally thought. Similarly, compensation does not appear to play as negative role as once thought.

REFERENCES

1. Evans R. Some observations on whiplash injuries. *Neurol Clin* 1992;10:975–997.
2. O'Neill B, Haddon W, Kelly A, et al. Automobile head restraints-frequency of neck injury claims in relation to the presence of head restraints. *Am J Public Health* 1972;62:403.
3. Herrstrom P, Lannerbro-Geijer G, Hogstedt B. Whiplash injuries from car accidents in a Swedish middle-sized town during 1993–95. *Scand J Primary Care* 2000;18:154–158.
4. McDowell G, Cammisa F, Eismont F. Hyperextension injuries of the cervical spine. In: Levine A, Eismont F, Garfin S, et al., eds. *Spine Trauma.* Philadelphia: WB Saunders, 1998:380–384.
5. Davis S, Teresi L, Bradley W, et al. Cervical spine hyperextension injuries: MR findings. *Radiology* 1991;180: 245–251.
6. LaRocca H, Butler J, Whitecloud T. Cervical acceleration injuries: diagnosis, treatment, and long-term outcome. In: Frymoyer J, ed. *The Adult Spine.* 2nd ed. Philadelphia: Lippincott-Raven, 1997:1235–1243.
7. Pennie B, Agambar L. Whiplash injuries: a trial of early management. *J Bone Joint Surg Br* 1990;72:277–279.
8. Ronnen H, deKorte P, Brink P, et al. Acute whiplash injury: is there a role for MR imaging? A prospective study of 100 patients. *Radiology* 1996;201:93–96.
9. Bogduk N, Windsor M, Omgos A. The innervation of the cervical intervertebral discs. *Spine* 1988;13:2–8.
10. Winkelstein B, Nightingale R, Richardson W, et al. The cervical facet capsule and its role in whiplash injury: a biomechanical investigation. *Spine* 2000;25:1238–1246.
11. Yoganandan N, Pintar F, Klienberger M. Cervical spine vertebral and facet joint kinematics under whiplash. *J Biomech Eng* 1998;120:305–307.
12. Lord S, Barnsley L, Wallis B, et al. Chronic cervical zygapophysial joint pain after whiplash. *Spine* 1996;21: 1737–1745.
13. Lord SM, Barnsley L, Bogduk N. Percutaneous radiofrequency neurotomy in the treatment of cervical zygapophysial joint pain: a caution. *Neurosurgery* 1995;36:732–739.
14. Lord SM, Barnsley L, Wallis BJ, et al. Percutaneous radio-frequency neurotomy for chronic cervical zygapophyseal-joint pain [see comments]. *N Engl J Med* 1996;335:1721–1726.
15. Barnsley L, Lord S, Bogduk N. Comparative local anaesthetic blocks in the diagnosis of cervical zygapophyseal joint pain. *Pain* 1993;55:99–106.
16. Barnsley L, Lord S, Wallis B, et al. The prevalence of chronic cervical zygapophysial joint pain after whiplash. *Spine* 1995;20:20–25.
17. Welcher JB, Szabo TJ. Relationships between seat properties and human subject kinematics in rear impact tests. *Accid Anal Prev* 2001;33:289–304.
18. Siegmund GP, Heinrichs BE, Wheeler JB. The influence of head restraint and occupant factors on peak head/neck kinematics in low-speed rear-end collisions. *Accid Anal Prev* 1999;31:393–407.

19. Fockler SK, Vavrik J, Kristiansen L. Motivating drivers to correctly adjust head restraints: assessing effectiveness of three different interventions. *Accid Anal Prev* 1998;30:773–780.
20. Spitzer WO, Skovron ML, Salmi LR, et al. Scientific monograph of the Quebec Task Force on Whiplash-Associated Disorders: redefining "whiplash" and its management. *Spine* 1995;20:1S–73S.
21. Miettinen T, Lindgren KA, Airaksinen O, et al. Whiplash injuries in Finland: a prospective 1-year follow-up study. *Clin Exp Rheumatol* 2002;20:399–402.
22. Sterling M. A proposed new classification system for whiplash associated disorders: implications for assessment and management. *Manual Therapeutics* 2004;9:60–70.
23. Deans G, Magalliard J, Kerr M, et al. Neck sprain: a major cause of disability following car accidents. *Injury* 1987;18:10–12.
24. Galasco C, Murray P, Pitcher M, et al. Neck sprains after road traffic accidents: a modern epidemic. *Injury* 1993;24:155–157.
25. Maimaris C, Barnes M, Allen M. "Whiplash injuries" of the neck. *Injury* 1988;19:393–396.
26. Parmar H, Raymakers R. Neck injuries from rear impact road traffic accidents: prognosis in person seeking compensation. *Injury* 1993;24:75–78.
27. Sturzenneger M, Distenafo G, Radanov B, et al. Presenting symptoms and signs after whiplash injury: the influence of accident mechanisms. *Neurology* 1994;44:688–693.
28. Watkinson A, Gargan M, Bannister G. Prognostic factors in soft tissue injuries of the cervical spine. *Injury* 1991;22:307–309.
29. Foley-Nolan D, Moore K, Codd M, et al. Low energy high frequency pulsed electromagnetic therapy for acute whiplash injuries: a double blind randomized controlled study. *Scand J Rehab Med* 1992;24:51–59.
30. Hohl M. Soft tissue injuries of the neck in automobile accidents: factors influencing prognosis. *J Bone Joint Surg Am* 1974;56:1675–1682.
31. Gargan M, Bannister G. Long-term prognosis of soft-tissue injuries of the neck. *J Bone Joint Surg Br* 1990;72: 901–903.
32. Norris S, Watt I. The prognosis of neck injuries resulting from rear-end vehicle collisions. *J Bone Joint Surg Br* 1983;65:608–611.
33. Matsumoto M, Fujimura Y, Suzuki N, et al. Cervical curvature in acute whiplash injuries: prospective comparative study with asymptomatic subjects. *Injury* 1998;29:775–778.
34. van Goethem J, Biltjes I, Hauwe LVD, et al. Whiplash injuries: is there a role for imaging? *Eur J Radiol* 1996;22:30–37.
35. Borchgrevink G, Smevik O, Nordby A, et al. MR imaging and radiography of patients with cervical hyperextension-flexion injuries after car accidents. *Acta Radiol* 1995;36:425–428.
36. Pettersson K, Hildingsson C, Toolanene G, et al. MRI and neurology in acute whiplash trauma: no correlation in prospective examination of 39 cases. *Acta Orthop Scand* 1994;65:525–528.
37. Pettersson K, Hildingsson C, Toolanen G, et al. Disc pathology after whiplash injury: a prospective magnetic resonance imaging and clinical investigation. *Spine* 1997;22:283–287.
38. Hirsch S, Hirsch P, Hiramoto H, et al. Whiplash syndrome: fact or fiction? *Orthop Clin North Am* 1988;19: 791–795.
39. McNab J. Acceleration extension injuries of the cervical spine. In: Rothman R, Simeone F, eds. *The Spine.* Philadelphia: WB Saunders, 1982:647–660.
40. Rosenfeld M, Gunnarsson R, Borenstein P. Early intervention in whiplash-associated disorders: a comparison of two treatment protocols. *Spine* 2000;15:1782–787.
41. Rosenfeld M SA, Carlsson J, Gunnarsson R. Active intervention in patients with whiplash-associated disorders improves long-term prognosis: a randomized controlled clinical trial. *Spine* 2003;15:2491–2498.
42. McKinney LA, Dornan JO, Ryan M. The role of physiotherapy in the management of acute neck sprains following road-traffic accidents. *Arch Emerg Med* 1989;6:27–33.
43. Mealy K, Brennan H, Fenelon GC. Early mobilization of acute whiplash injuries. *Br Med J (Clin Res Ed)* 1986;292:656–657.
44. Schnabel M, Ferrari R, Vassiliou T, et al. Randomised, controlled outcome study of active mobilisation compared with collar therapy for whiplash injury. *Emerg Med J* 2004;21:306–310.
45. Crawford JR, Khan RJ, Varley GW. Early management and outcome following soft tissue injuries of the neck: a randomised controlled trial. *Injury* 2004;35:891–895.
46. Fitz-Ritson D. Phasic exercises for cervical rehabilitation after "whiplash" trauma. *J Manipulative Physiol Ther* 1995;18:21–24.
47. Freund BJ, Schwartz M. Treatment of chronic cervical-associated headache with botulinum toxin A: a pilot study. *Headache* 2000;40:231–236.
48. Freund BJ, Schwartz M. Treatment of whiplash associated neck pain [corrected] with botulinum toxin-A: a pilot study. *J Rheumatol* 2000;27:481–484.
49. Sapir DA, Gorup JM. Radiofrequency medial branch neurotomy in litigant and nonlitigant patients with cervical whiplash: a prospective study. *Spine* 2001;26:E268–E273.

50. Algers G, Pettersson K, Hildingsson C, et al. Surgery for chronic symptoms after whiplash injury: follow-up of 20 cases. *Acta Orthop Scand* 1993;64:654–656.
51. Hamer AJ, Gargan MF, Bannister GC, et al. Whiplash injury and surgically treated cervical disc disease [see comments]. *Injury* 1993;24:549–550.
52. Muzumdar DP, Deopujari CE, Bhojraj SY. Bilateral vocal cord paralysis after anterior cervical discoidectomy and fusion in a case of whiplash cervical spine injury: a case report. *Surg Neurol* 2000;53:586–588.
53. Senter BS. Cervical discogenic syndrome: a cause of chronic head and neck pain. *J Miss State Med Assoc* 1995;36:231–234.
54. Squires B, Gargan M, Bannister G. Soft-tissue injuries of the cervical spine. *J Bone Joint Surg Br* 1996;78:955–957.
55. Siebenrock K, Aebi M. Cervical discography in discogenic pain syndrome and its predictive value for cervical fusion. *Arch Orthop Trauma Surg* 1994;113:199–203.
56. Suissa S, Harder S, Veilleux M. The relation between initial symptoms and signs and the prognosis of whiplash. *Eur Spine J* 2001;10:44–49.
57. Suissa S. Risk factors of poor prognosis after whiplash injury. *Pain Res Manage* 2003;8:69–75.
58. Hartling L, Pickett W, Brison RJ. Derivation of a clinical decision rule for whiplash associated disorders among individuals involved in rear-end collisions. *Accid Anal Prev* 2002;34:531–539.
59. Hendriks EJ, Scholten-Peeters GG, van der Windt DA, et al. Prognostic factors for poor recovery in acute whiplash patients. *Pain* 2005;114:408–416.
60. Balla J. The late whiplash syndrome. *Aust N Z J Surg* 1980;50:610–614.
61. Deans G, Magaillard J, Kerr M, et al. Neck sprain: a major cause of disability following car accidents. *Injury* 1987;18:10–12.
62. Soderlund A, Olerud C, Lindberg P. Acute whiplash-associated disorders (WAD): the effects of early mobilization and prognostic factors in long-term symptomatology. *Clin Rehabil* 2000;14:457–467.
63. Olsson I, Bunketorp O, Carlsson SG, et al. Prediction of outcome in whiplash-associated disorders using West Haven-Yale Multidimensional Pain Inventory. *Clin J Pain* 2002;18:238–244.
64. Miettinen T, Leino E, Airaksinen O, et al. Whiplash injuries in Finland: the situation 3 years later. *Eur Spine J* 2004;13:415–418.
65. Olivegren HJ, Jerkvall N, Hagstrom Y, et al. The long-term prognosis of whiplash-associated disorders (WAD). *Eur Spine J* 1999;8:366–370.

CHAPTER 21A

Spinal Cord Injury and Pathophysiology

Darryl C. Baptiste and Michael G. Fehlings

INTRODUCTION

Spinal cord injury (SCI) occurs with a varied regional estimated incidence of 11.5 to 57.8 spinal cord–injured persons per million population each year, with the most common causes including motor vehicle crashes, sports- and recreational-related injuries, and workplace accidents. Although relatively uncommon, SCI can leave the individual with significant deficits in motor, sensory, and autonomic functions. Moreover, SCI represents a major cause of morbidity and mortality, with considerably burdening societal expenses associated with the medical management and lost earnings.

Pathophysiologically, the mechanical forces imparted to the spinal cord cause primary damage to the neural tissue and elicit a complex cascade of events, including ischemia, ionic derangements, lipid peroxidation, glutamatergic excitotoxicity, inflammation, and apoptosis, that jeopardize adjacent, initially spared tissue to secondary damage. Scientific researchers today have focused their attention on these secondary processes of SCI in hope to not only define more clearly the mechanism(s) involved in neurologic destruction, but also to discover novel approaches that can be applied to attenuate this secondary damage. The focus of this review will be to highlight some of the events associated with SCI secondary pathologic change, including the role of such processes as vascular insult, ischemia-reperfusion and ionic disturbances, and inflammation.

EPIDEMIOLOGY AND PATHOGENESIS OF SPINAL CORD INJURY

SCI is a relatively rare disorder, afflicting 11.5 to 57.8 cases per million people worldwide each year. The highest incidence of SCI in all countries occurs in persons 20 to 40 years of age.[1,2] Thus, considering the debilitating nature of SCI coupled with the relatively high frequency of SCI in society's highest earning potential substrata, SCI places a significant monetary burden on our health care system.

The major causes of SCI include motor vehicle collisions, work-related injuries, sports or aquatics-related injuries, falls, and violence-related injuries (gunshot, stabbing; Table 21A.1).[1,3] People who have had the misfortune of sustaining an SCI rarely have the force of the mechanical insult result in complete physical transection of the cord.[4] This is true even when the injury leaves the victim with complete loss of neurologic, sensory, and/or autonomic function. Rather, the majority of SCIs leave behind some nervous tissue and a pial rim, which surrounds the injury epicenter. The resulting neurologic deficits associated with SCI occur as a result of physical disruption of spinal cord axons through the injury epicenter.

TABLE 21A.1 Major Etiologies of Acute Spinal Cord Injury

Cause of Injury	Incidence (%)
Motor vehicle collisions (also including bicycle and pedestrian)	40–50
Work	10–25
Sports/aquatics recreation	10–25
Falls	20
Violence (gunshot/stab)	10–25

Modified with permission from Sekhon LH, Fehlings MG. Epidemiology, demographics, and pathophysiology of acute spinal cord injury. *Spine* 2001;26:S2–12.

Animal modeling has permitted further understanding of the pathologic sequelae following SCI. At present it is widely accepted that two major pathophysiologic events account for the neurologic deficits associated with SCI: primary and secondary injury.[4,5] Recently we reviewed the status of prospective randomized clinical trials for pharmacologic compounds designed to intervene at a specific pathologic event within the secondary injurious cascade of acute SCI.[6] At present, no acute treatment or rehabilitative therapy exists, although modest improvements in neurologic function have been reported from the National Acute Spinal Cord Injury Studies (NASCIS) II and III[7–9] and the Maryland and Sygen GM-1 ganglioside trials.[10,11] Continued research involving clinically relevant animal models of SCI will likely lead to improved understanding of the pathobiology of SCI together with further identification of novel pharmacologic compounds with better ability to prevent the spread of neurodegeneration within the injured spinal cord.

PRIMARY AND SECONDARY SPINAL CORD INJURY

The most common underlying primary injury mechanism of trauma-induced paralysis results from the acute compression and contusion of the spinal cord resulting from bone or disc displacement within the spinal column following fracture-dislocation or burst fracture of the spine (Table 21A.2).[3] Primary mechanical trauma to the spinal cord, along with subsequent persistent compression, triggers a secondary pathologic cascade of biochemical and neurologic events that may continue to progress on the order of minutes to months. Secondary damage occurs as a consequence of numerous interwoven autodestructive events, fueled by the actions of each other generating a positive feedback loop to amplify spinal cord pathology and neurologic deficit.[12] The spatial extent of secondary injury events spreads both radially and longitudinally along the spinal cord in a rostral-caudal manner (Fig. 21A.1). Consequently, the final outcome of SCI is directly correlated to the degree of the initial traumatic insult and the secondary events that follow resulting in nerve cell death and cavitation of central gray matter.

Physical trauma to the central nervous system culminates in neurologic deficit as a result of damage to nerve fibers or axons, with blockade of nerve impulse transduction along the nerve fiber. Ultimately, this axonal dysfunction may be attributable to a physical discontinuity in the axon in which loss of ionic homeostasis occurs as a result of membrane disruption.[13]

CELL DEATH MECHANISMS

Cell death following SCI occurs by necrosis and apoptosis. Although necrosis predominates immediately after the primary traumatic episode, delayed stages of subacute spinal cord pathology induce apoptosis predominantly of oligodendrocytes and to a lesser extent neurons.[14] Apoptotic oligodendrocyte death is associated with axonal degeneration at and adjacent to the injury site, as well as with the ensuing wallerian degeneration of ascending and descending spinal tracts in white matter. The

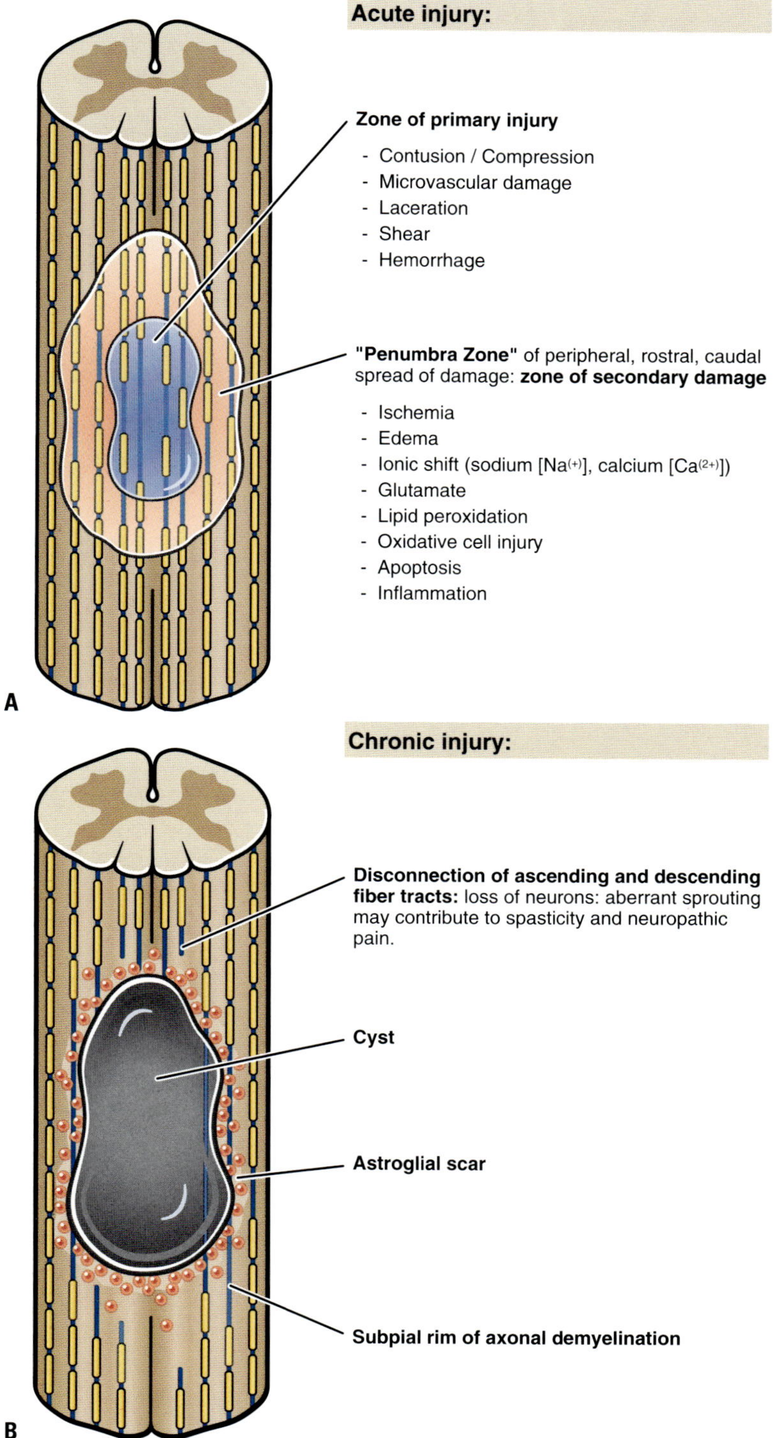

FIGURE 21A.1. A. Rostral-caudal spread of acute spinal cord injury. Mechanical trauma to the spinal cord at the time of injury causes immediate tissue disruption known as primary injury. Primary injury rarely results in a complete transection of the spinal cord; rather, the act of primary injury leaves behind a compromised but viable and intact rim of neural tissue that is vulnerable to **(B)** secondary acute pathophysiologic processes (i.e., vascular disruption and ischemia, glutamate-mediated excitotoxicity, and inflammation). These secondary injury events are capable of initiating processes that contribute to the necrotic and apoptotic death of cells within the spinal cord.

TABLE 21A.2 Pathobiology of Acute Spinal Cord Injury

Primary Mechanisms		
Compression	Iatrogenic vertebral distraction	
Contusion	Acceleration-deceleration	
Shear	Bone or disc displacement	
Laceration	Fracture-dislocation	
Acute stretching	Burst fracture	
Secondary Mechanisms		
Systemic events:	systemic shock	hypoxia
	spinal shock	hyperthermia
Extracellular factors:	microcirculatory vascular damage	tissue swelling
	ischemia	cytokine-mediated inflammation
	hemorrhage	
Intracellular factors:	ischemic cascade	lipid peroxidation
	electrolyte shifts	free radical injury
	edema	neurotrophic factor deprivation
	neutrotransmitter excess	
	glutamate excitotoxicity	apoptosis

Modified with permission from Sekhon LH, Fehlings MG. Epidemiology, demographics, and pathophysiology of acute spinal cord injury. *Spine* 2001;26:S2–S12.

mechanisms of apoptosis likely involve microglial activation with activation of the Fas death receptor and the p75 low-affinity neurotrophin receptor (Fig. 21A.2).[14] Using terminal deoxynucleotidyl transferase–mediated dUTP in situ nick end labeling (TUNEL) and immunohistochemistry, Emery et al.[15] provided morphologic evidence for apoptosis and caspase-3 activation along the pia rim surrounding the lesion epicenter in 14 of 15 traumatized human postmortem spinal cords and in oligodendrocytes in white matter tracts to support wallerian degeneration.

Potential triggers of apoptosis within the injured spinal cord may include, but are certainly not limited to, vascular abnormalities, ischemia-reperfusion, glutamate-mediated excitotoxicity and ionic imbalance, generation of free radicals and reactive oxygen species (ROS), and inflammation. These events may operate on their own or in concert and provide a window of opportunity for applied pharmacologic intervention to prevent the neuropathologic consequences of SCI. The remainder of this review will focus on the potentially important apoptotic initiating events following SCI.

VASCULAR ABNORMALITIES

SCI compromises the spinal cord vasculature directly and initiates a cascade of events that alter the integrity of the blood–spinal cord barrier (BSCB), the tight junctions formed between endothelial cells lining the vessels surrounding the spinal cord to physiologically impede transcellular transport.[16] Following mechanical trauma to the cord, the traumatic event disrupts the BSCB to effectively loosen the endothelial junctions to allow a pathologic increase in BSCB permeability, transendothelial vesicular transport, and immune cell extravasation.

In addition to weakening of the BSCB, traumatic injury to the spinal cord induces progressive pathologic change. Recent investigations into the exact mechanism(s) involved in BSCB dissolution following SCI have implicated matrix metalloproteinases (MMPs) as the chief enzymes involved. In

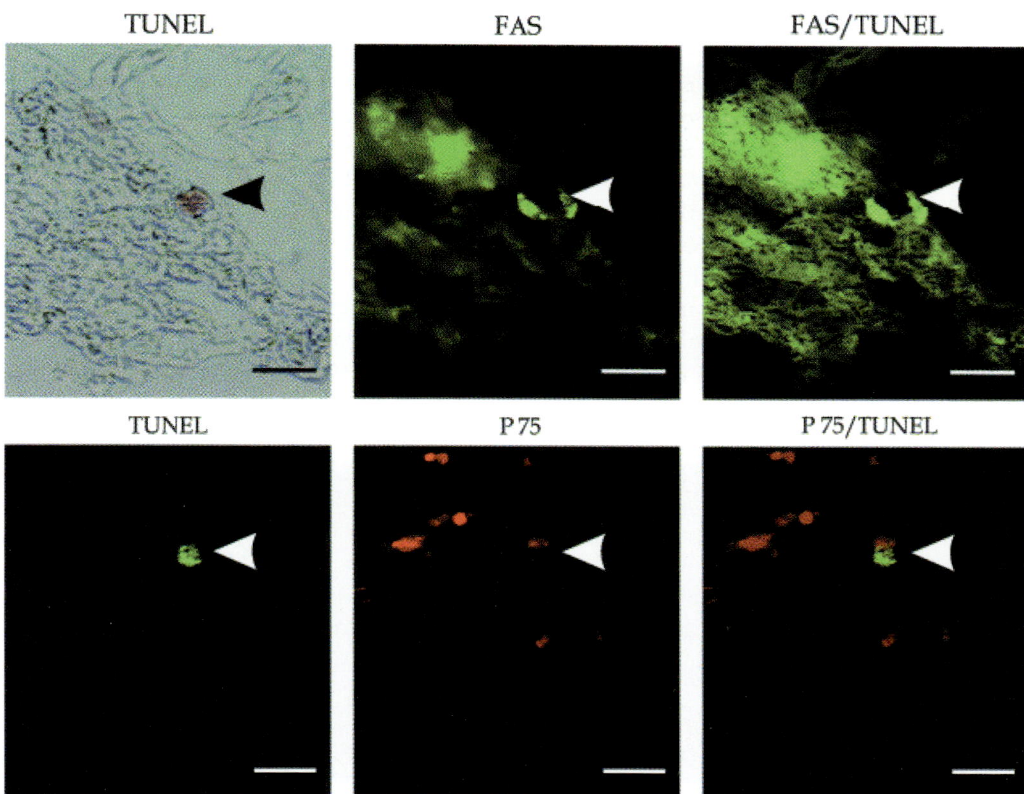

FIGURE 21A.2. Death receptor expression on apoptotic glia following spinal cord injury. Double-labeling immunohistochemistry with TUNEL was used to examine the expression of Fas and p75 on apoptotic cells. **Top panels:** Fas labeling *(center: FITC)* and TUNEL *(left: HRP)* colocalized *(right)* in many instances during the first week following injury; however, unlabeled TUNEL-positive cells were also seen. **Lower panel:** Similarly, p75 *(center–Texas Red)* and TUNEL *(left–FITC)* were seen to colocalize *(right)* in some cells at times 1 and 2 weeks postinjury. *Arrows* indicate double-labeled cells. Scale Bars = 20 μm. (Figure republished with permission from Casha S, Yu WR, Fehlings MG. Oligodendroglial apoptosis occurs along degenerating axons and is associated with FAS and p75 expression following spinal cord injury in the rat. *Neuroscience* 2001;103:203–218.)

one study, researchers compared the neurologic recovery following weight drop injury in wild-type and MMP knockout mice.[17] The results of this study demonstrated that there was decreased permeability of the BSCB and reduced microglial and macrophage density in MMP-12 null mice compared with wild-type controls. Moreover, the Basso-Beattie-Bresnahan (BBB) locomotor rating scale and the inclined plane test demonstrated that MMP-12 null mice exhibited significantly improved functional recovery compared with wild-type controls.[17] Furthermore, in a rat contusion model of SCI, a preincubation with either MMP-2 or MMP-9 antibodies significantly decreased the MMP-mediated gelatinase activity pattern, suggesting the involvement of at least both MMPs in SCI, while concomitantly supporting MMPs as a potential therapeutic target.[18]

ISCHEMIA-REPERFUSION AND IONIC DISTURBANCES

Mechanical trauma to the spinal cord causes immediate vasospasm of the superficial vessels and intraparenchymal hemorrhage, which is initially localized in the highly vascularized central gray matter. Immediate mechanical damage to the gray matter microvasculature impairs microcirculation and impedes perfusion, especially within the venules and capillaries, leading to a profound reduction of spinal cord blood flow accompanied by a loss of autoregulation to maintain constant blood flow over a wide range of pressures. Moreover, this may worsen the magnitude of ischemic injury through neurogenic shock or may exacerbate hemorrhage with spikes in systemic blood pressure.[19] Still, the impaired spinal cord blood flow may be further compromised by systemic responses, including bradycardia and reduced cardiac output, all of which work to exacerbate ischemic damage. Therefore, ischemia occurs as a direct result of vascular injury and is likely secondary to pathologic reductions in spinal cord blood flow from thrombosis, vasospasm, and a loss of microcirculation or systemic hypoperfusion, along with loss of autoregulatory homeostasis.[19]

Following traumatic SCI, reoxygenation-reperfusion injury to ischemic spinal cord regions threatens to impose further nervous cell damage. ROS, including superoxide, hydroxyl radical, and nitric oxide, are produced during ischemia.[20,21] Moreover, there is a notable increase in the levels of ROS during early reperfusion periods.[22] The presence of these oxygen species contributes to oxidative stress and the secondary pathologic sequela that occurs in SCI. Once the endogenous antioxidant capacity is surpassed by the increasing efforts of ROS, proteins, lipids, and nucleic acids are oxidized. Furthermore, mitochondrial adenosine triphosphate (ATP) synthesis is disrupted, leading to energy failure and increased levels of extracellular glutamate, which arise as a result of disruption of normal energy-dependant glutamate reuptake mechanisms.[23–26] Elevated extracellular concentrations of glutamate can be toxic to neurons. In 1969, Olney et al.[27] described this form of neuronal death as a process of overexcitation and coined the term excitotoxicity.

GLUTAMATERGIC EXCITOTOXICITY

Glutamate-mediated neuropathology has been noted in SCI as well as a variety of other CNS disorders, including stroke, amyotrophic lateral sclerosis, Alzheimer disease, Parkinson disease, and Huntington disease.[24,27–29] Elevations in extracellular glutamate concentrations lead to excessive activation of glutamate receptors (GluRs), including the three ionotropic GluRs: (1) N-methyl-D-aspartate (NMDA); (2) 2-amino-3-(3-hydroxy-5-methylisoxazol-4-yl) propionate (AMPA); and (3) kainate (KA) receptor subtypes. Activation of the ionotropic GluR subtypes leads to increased intracellular concentrations of Ca^{2+}, sodium (Na^+), and chloride (Cl^-) ions.[30,31] Moreover, using an in vitro model of traumatic SCI, Mills et al.[32] were able to demonstrate that shortly after localized mechanical spinal cord trauma, astroglial and oligodendrocyte calcium signals transiently rise rapidly to very high levels and spread along white matter tracts (Fig. 21A.3). Increases in these ions contribute to neuronal death through the activation of proteases,[33] the uncoupling of mitochondrial oxidative phosphorylation, and the release of ROS (Fig. 21A.4).[31,34] Inhibition of the NMDA receptors has been demonstrated to provide neuroprotection following ischemic insults in vitro[35]; however, pharmacologic blockade of NMDA receptors with preintravenous and postintravenous infusion of MK801 in spinally injured rats inhibited evoked potentials but failed to improve spinal cord blood flow or cord edema.[36]

Although the term glutamate excitotoxicity is usually applied to neurons, where glutamate has excitatory effects, it is also widely used in glial cell research,[37] despite the fact that these cells normally do not exhibit a true excitability because of the absence of action potentials.[31] Extracellular excitatory amino acid concentrations increase to neurotoxic levels within minutes after SCI.[38,39] The observed rise in glutamate is responsible for excessive activation of glutamate receptors in the central nervous system, resulting in neuronal cell death.[29] Furthermore, prior histologic examination of healthy spinal cord tissues that had received an exogenously applied amount of glutamate comparable to extracellular concentrations achieved following traumatic SCI clearly demonstrated the extensive glutamatergic neuronal death within the gray matter.[40]

Although this demonstrates a role for gray matter pathophysiology, an increasing number of studies have revealed glutamate-mediated excitotoxicity as a significant contributor to secondary injury

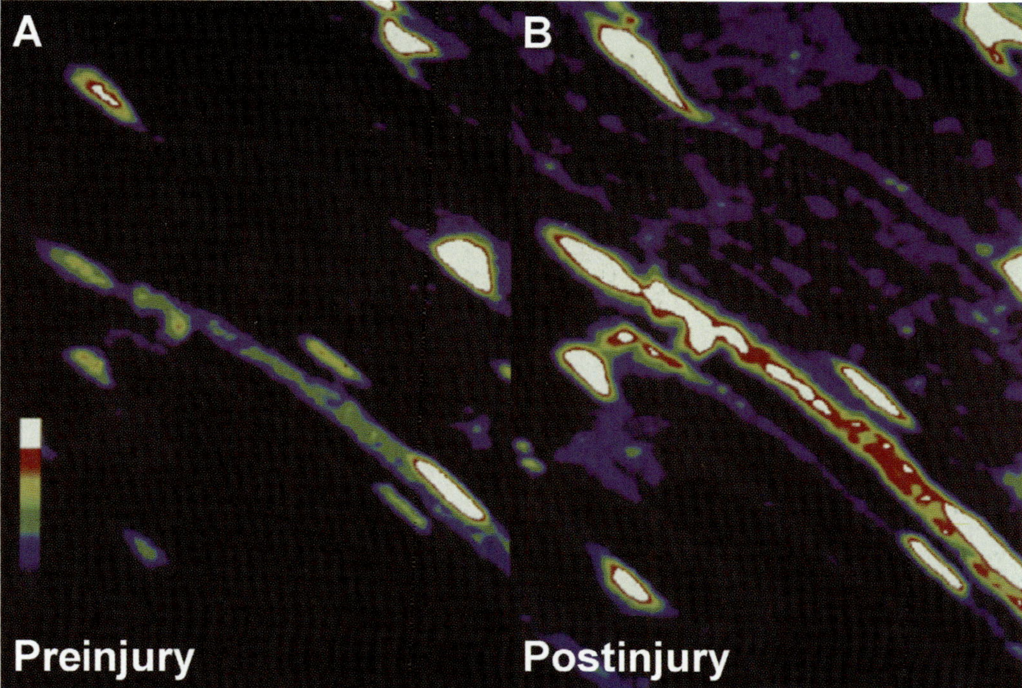

FIGURE 21A.3. Confocal imaging of intracellular calcium rise following acute spinal cord injury. **A.** Preinjury confocal settings were adjusted to keep subsequent images below saturation *(white areas)* where possible, so spinal cord intracellular calcium (Ca_i^{2+}) levels were only barely detectable before clip compression spinal cord injury in adult female Wistar rats. **B.** At 0.5 min after injury, Ca_i^{2+} levels have risen markedly within the cord. (Modified with permission from: Mills LR, Velumian AA, Agrawal SK, et al. Confocal imaging of changes in glial calcium dynamics and homeostasis after mechanical injury in rat spinal cord white matter. *Neuroimage* 2004;21:1069–1082.)

mechanisms in white matter tissue as well.[41,42] Evidence indicates that the group I metabotropic glutamate receptors (mGluRs) play a role in glutamate release after SCI,[43–45] presumably via modulation of presynaptic glutamate release.[46] However, given the lack of synaptic connections in white matter, glutamate release via Ca^{2+}-dependent presynaptic release after trauma[47] does not provide an adequate explanation for its role in white matter injury. Alternatively, heightened extracellular glutamate levels may lead to the activation of resident microglial cells, which may be responsible for inflicting Fas/p75 receptor–mediated injury to oligodendroglial cell populations.[48,49] Thus, ischemia-mediated increases in extracellular glutamate concentrations and resulting glutamatergic excitotoxicity are likely coupled to inflammatory responses following SCI.

INFLAMMATION

Secondary pathologic aberrations following SCI also involve actions of inflammatory cells. Despite the fact that the host inflammatory response is required for repair of injured tissues as well, as host defense versus infection, an unregulated inflammatory response may exacerbate the neuropathology after SCI.[50] Microglia, leukocytes (lymphocytes, neutrophils, and monocytes), and astrocytes contribute to the cellular inflammatory response after experimental SCI. Inflammation following SCI has been shown to promote secondary cell death within the lesion penumbra. By 24 hours postinjury, both resident microglia and infiltrating macrophages become activated and can be seen within the lesion and penumbra, increasing in number by 48 hours postinjury.[51] Although microglia and

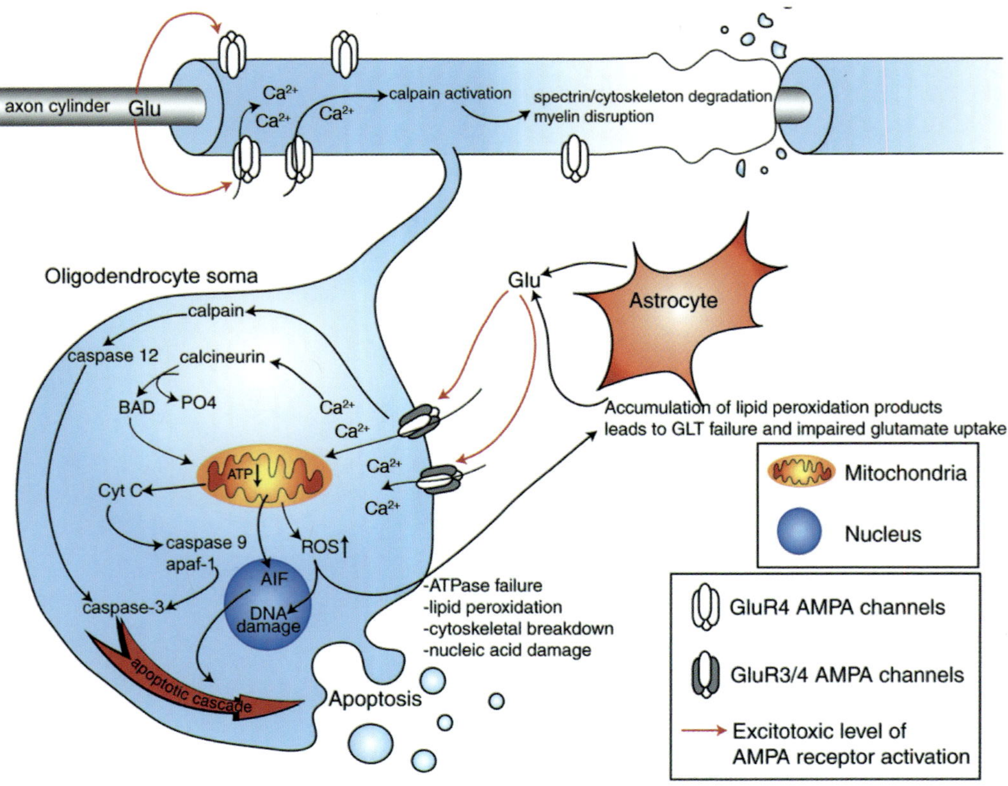

FIGURE 21A.4. Excitotoxicity and apoptosis in oligodendrocytes. Glutamate released from axonal cylinders and astrocytes can raise extracellular glutamate concentration to excitotoxic levels. Calcium (Ca^{2+}) permeable glutamate receptor (GluR) 4 expressing 2-amino-3-(3-hydroxy-5-methylisoxazol-4-yl) propionate (AMPA) receptors on myelin sheaths could activate Ca^{2+}-sensitive proteases such as calpain, resulting in cytoskeletal degradation and subsequent myelin disruption. Ca^{2+} permeable GluR3/4 expressing AMPA receptors on oligodendrocyte somata are potential entry routes for Ca^{2+} that initiate a host of molecular cascades, including activation of calpain and subsequent procaspase-12 activation, dephosphorylation of Bcl-2 associated death protein (BAD) by calcineurin contributing to mitochondrial dysfunction, and generation of reactive oxygen species (ROS), which can affect both intracellular mechanisms or potentially neighbouring astrocytes by inhibiting glutamate uptake. Ca^{2+} may also be responsible for saturating the Ca^{2+} buffering capability of mitochondria at the expense of ATP generation. Mitochondrial dysfunction results in release of proapoptotic factors including cytochrome (Cyt) C, which is required for the binding of apoptosis protease activating factor-1 (Apaf-1) to procaspases-9, as well as apoptosis-inducing factor (AIF), which exerts proapoptotic events in the nucleus. (Figure republished with permission from Park E, Velumian AA, Fehlings MG. The role of excitotoxicity in secondary mechanisms of spinal cord injury: a review with an emphasis on the implications for white matter degeneration. *J Neurotrauma* 2004;21:754–774.)

macrophages are thought to engage in mainly phagocytic activity within the lesion, they are often found adjacent to apoptotic oligodendroglia in the penumbra and may play a role in the death of these cells even weeks after injury.[14,48,52] Cytokines such as tumor necrosis factor-alpha (TNF-α) and Fas are thought to promote and enhance microglial-mediated cell death.[14,48]

Although the latter paragraph describes a pathologic role for inflammatory responses following SCI, it is still unclear whether inflammation possesses any protective qualities following traumatic CNS injury; lymphocyte populations previously thought to be injurious and encephalitogenic, as determined within the demylinating autoimmune animal model known as experimetal autoimmune encephalomyelitis (EAE), have demonstrated ability to provide protection and promote improved neurologic recovery in the injured spinal cord. Through exploring mechanisms of central nervous system regeneration, researchers have identified the myelin-associated protein neurite outgrowth (Nogo)-A as an inhibitor to neurite outgrowth.[53] Additional studies have demonstrated that macrophage and T lymphocyte activation following traumatic central nervous system injury is a physiologic response generated to facilitate protection, repair, and regeneration.[54] On noting neuroprotection of the spinal cord with systemic intraperitoneal administration of autoimmune T lymphocytes specific to myelin basic protein (MBP), it soon became clear that myelin-associated antigens were responsible for triggering a protective "self-reaction" by T lymphocytes after traumatic insult to the spinal cord.[54] Most impressive, Hauben et al.[54] found that passive immunization was effective in promoting functional recovery even when treatment was delayed 1 week after SCI. Moreover, active immunization with MBP emulsified within incomplete Freud's adjuvant 1 week before induction of SCI resulted in enhanced functional recovery in comparison to nonimmunized controls.[54]

Recently, this same group demonstrated that vaccination with dendritic cells pulsed with MBP-derived peptides mediates neuroprotection when administered up to 12 days after SCI.[54] However, despite the success of therapeutic vaccination in animal models of SCI, it is evident that further testing is required before this approach can be translated to humans, because a recent report by Jones et al.[55] could not validate the putative neuroprotective effects mediated by myelin-reactive T-lymphocyte vaccination; rather their data supports a role for myelin-reactive T-cells as effectors of central nervous system pathology to induce EAE.

CONCLUSION

SCI leads to devastating disability. The global estimates of the number of annual new cases range from 8 to 58 per million. The current pharmacologic treatment for SCI is limited to administration of high-dose methylprednisolone, but this therapy has limited effectiveness[7–9] and thus remains controversial.[56] The prospect for improved therapies must come from improved understanding of the secondary injury mechanisms causing neuronal death after SCI, for which we are almost entirely dependant on clinically relevant animal models.

To date, such preclinical research has helped aid the discovery of potentially promising therapeutic strategies that may be translated into useful clinical treatment options. Two examples of novel approaches currently under clinical investigation to treat acute SCI include the Rho pathway antagonist Cethrin (Aseres Pharmaceuticals, Inc., Hopkinton, MA) and the neurite outgrowth inhibitor antagonist ATI355 (Novartis Pharma AG, Basel, Switzerland) in patients with thoracic and cervical SCI. Additionally, enthusiasm exists within the SCI community over the potential application of tissue engineering and stem-cell strategies, which may potentially improve neurologic recovery and plasticity following traumatic central nervous system injury through enhanced regeneration of neurons and support cells. However, considering the heterogeneous and multifactorial nature of acute SCI, effective therapeutic strategies in the future will need to involve combinations of surgical approaches (early decompression, stabilization), pharmacologic strategies, and possibly tissue engineering and cell-based techniques.

REFERENCES

1. Ackery A, Tator C, Krassioukov A. A global perspective on spinal cord injury epidemiology. *J Neurotrauma* 2004;21:1355–1370.
2. Albert T, Ravaud JF. Rehabilitation of spinal cord injury in France: a nationwide multicentre study of incidence and regional disparities. *Spinal Cord* 2005;43:357–365.
3. Sekhon LH, Fehlings MG. Epidemiology, demographics, and pathophysiology of acute spinal cord injury. *Spine* 2001;26:S2–S12.
4. Tator CH, Fehlings MG. Review of the secondary injury theory of acute spinal cord trauma with emphasis on vascular mechanisms. *J Neurosurg* 1991;75:15–26.

5. Tator CH. Update on the pathophysiology and pathology of acute spinal cord injury. *Brain Pathol* 1995;5:407–413.
6. Fehlings MG, Baptiste DC. Current status of clinical trials for acute spinal cord injury. *Injury* 2006;36(suppl 2):B113–B122.
7. Bracken MB, Shepard MJ, Collins WF Jr, et al. Methylprednisolone or naloxone treatment after acute spinal cord injury: 1-year follow-up data: results of the second National Acute Spinal Cord Injury Study. *J Neurosurg* 1992;76:23–31.
8. Bracken MB, Holford TR. Effects of timing of methylprednisolone or naloxone administration on recovery of segmental and long-tract neurological function in NASCIS 2. *J Neurosurg* 1003;79:500–507.
9. Bracken MB, Shepard MJ, Holford TR, et al. Administration of methylprednisolone for 24 or 48 hours or tirilazad mesylate for 48 hours in the treatment of acute spinal cord injury: results of the Third National Acute Spinal Cord Injury Randomized Controlled Trial. National Acute Spinal Cord Injury Study. *JAMA* 1997;277:1597–1604.
10. Geisler FH, Dorsey FC, Coleman WP. Recovery of motor function after spinal cord injury: a randomized, placebo-controlled trial with GM-1 ganglioside. *N Engl J Med* 1991;324:1829–1838.
11. Geisler FH, Coleman WP, Grieco G, et al. The Sygen multicenter acute spinal cord injury study. *Spine* 2001;26:S87–S98.
12. Schwartz G, Fehlings MG. Evaluation of the neuroprotective effects of sodium channel blockers after spinal cord injury: improved behavioral and neuroanatomical recovery with riluzole. *J Neurosurg Spine* 2005;94:245–256.
13. Stys PK. White matter injury mechanisms. *Curr Mol Med* 2004;4:113–130.
14. Casha S, Yu WR, Fehlings MG. Oligodendroglial apoptosis occurs along degenerating axons and is associated with FAS and p75 expression following spinal cord injury in the rat. *Neuroscience* 2001;103:203–218.
15. Emery E, Aldana P, Bunge MB, et al. Apoptosis after traumatic human spinal cord injury. *J Neurosurg* 1998; 89:911–912.
16. Whetstone WD, Hsu JY, Eisenberg M, et al. Blood-spinal cord barrier after spinal cord injury: relation to revascularization and wound healing. *J Neurosci Res* 2003;74:227–239.
17. Wells JE, Rice TK, Nuttall RK, et al. An adverse role for matrix metalloproteinase 12 after spinal cord injury in mice. *J Neurosci* 2003;23:10107–10115.
18. Duchossoy Y, Arnaud S, Feldblum S. Matrix metalloproteinases: potential therapeutic target in spinal cord injury. *Clin Chem Lab Med* 2001;39:362–367.
19. Dumont RJ, Okonkwo DO, Verma S, et al. Acute spinal cord injury. Part I: pathophysiologic mechanisms. *Clin Neuropharmacol* 2001;24:254–264.
20. Takahashi G, Sakurai M, Abe K, et al. MCI-186 prevents spinal cord damage and affects enzyme levels of nitric oxide synthase and Cu/Zn superoxide dismutase after transient ischemia in rabbits. *J Thorac Cardiovasc Surg* 2003;126:1461–1466.
21. Ilhan A, Yilmaz HR, Armutcu F, et al. The protective effect of nebivolol on ischemia/reperfusion injury in rabbit spinal cord. *Prog Neuropsychopharmacol Biol Psychiatry* 2004;28:1153–1160.
22. Chan PH. Mitochondria and neuronal death/survival signaling pathways in cerebral ischemia. *Neurochem Res* 2004;29:1943–1949.
23. Rothstein JD, Martin LJ, Kuncl RW. Decreased glutamate transport by the brain and spinal cord in amyotrophic lateral sclerosis. *N Engl J Med* 1992;326:1464–1468.
24. Rothstein JD, Van Kammen M, Levey AI, et al. Selective loss of glial glutamate transporter GLT-1 in amyotrophic lateral sclerosis. *Ann Neurol* 1995;38:73–84.
25. Milton ID, Banner SJ, Ince PG, et al. Expression of the glial glutamate transporter EAAT2 in the human CNS: an immunohistochemical study. *Brain Res Mol Brain Res* 1997;52:17–31.
26. Massieu L, Garcia O. The role of excitotoxicity and metabolic failure in the pathogenesis of neurological disorders. *Neurobiology (Bp)* 1998;6:99–108.
27. Olney JW, Zorumski CF, Stewart GR, et al. Excitotoxicity of L-dopa and 6-OH-dopa: implications for Parkinson's and Huntington's diseases. *Exp Neurol* 1990;108:269–272.
28. Mattson MP. Calcium and neuronal injury in Alzheimer's disease: contributions of beta-amyloid precursor protein mismetabolism, free radicals, and metabolic compromise. *Ann N Y Acad Sci* 1994;747:50–76.
29. Lipton SA, Rosenberg PA. Excitatory amino acids as a final common pathway for neurologic disorders. *N Engl J Med* 1994;330:613–622.
30. Choi DW. Ionic dependence of glutamate neurotoxicity. *J Neurosci* 1987;7:369–379.
31. Park E, Velumian AA, Fehlings MG. The role of excitotoxicity in secondary mechanisms of spinal cord injury: a review with an emphasis on the implications for white matter degeneration. *J Neurotrauma* 2004;21:754–774.
32. Mills LR, Velumian AA, Agrawal SK, et al. Confocal imaging of changes in glial calcium dynamics and homeostasis after mechanical injury in rat spinal cord white matter. *Neuroimage* 2004;21:1069–1082.
33. Leist M, Volbracht C, Kuhnle S, et al. Caspase-mediated apoptosis in neuronal excitotoxicity triggered by nitric oxide. *Mol Med* 1997;3:750–764.

34. Rego AC, Oliveira CR. Mitochondrial dysfunction and reactive oxygen species in excitotoxicity and apoptosis: implications for the pathogenesis of neurodegenerative diseases. *Neurochem Res* 2003;28:1563–1574.
35. Pringle AK, Iannotti F, Wilde GJ. Neuroprotection by both NMDA and non-NMDA receptor antagonists in in vitro ischemia. *Brain Res* 1997;755:36–46.
36. Li S, Tator CH. Effects of MK801 on evoked potentials, spinal cord blood flow and cord edema in acute spinal cord injury in rats. *Spinal Cord* 1999;37:820–832.
37. Li Z, Hogan EL, Banik NL. Role of calpain in spinal cord injury: increased calpain immunoreactivity in spinal cord after compression injury in the rat. *Neurochem Int* 1995;27:425–432.
38. Liu D, Thangnipon W, McAdoo DJ. Excitatory amino acids rise to toxic levels upon impact injury to the rat spinal cord. *Brain Res* 1991;547:344–348.
39. Farooque M, Hillered L, Holtz A, et al. Changes of extracellular levels of amino acids after graded compression trauma to the spinal cord: an experimental study in the rat using microdialysis. *J Neurotrauma* 1996;13:537–548.
40. Liu D, Xu GY, Pan E, et al. Neurotoxicity of glutamate at the concentration released upon spinal cord injury. *Neuroscience* 1999;93:1383–1389.
41. Wrathall JR, Choiniere D, Teng YD. Dose-dependent reduction of tissue loss and functional impairment after spinal cord trauma with the AMPA/kainate antagonist NBQX. *J Neurosci* 1994;14:6598–6607.
42. Agrawal SK, Fehlings MG. Role of NMDA and non-NMDA ionotropic glutamate receptors in traumatic spinal cord axonal injury. *J Neurosci* 1997;17:1055–1063.
43. Agrawal SK, Theriault E, Fehlings MG. Role of group I metabotropic glutamate receptors in traumatic spinal cord white matter injury. *J Neurotrauma* 1998;15:929–941.
44. Mills CD, Xu GY, Johnson KM, et al. AIDA reduces glutamate release and attenuates mechanical allodynia after spinal cord injury. *Neuroreport* 2000;11:3067–3070.
45. Mills CD, Xu GY, McAdoo DJ, et al. Involvement of metabotropic glutamate receptors in excitatory amino acid and GABA release following spinal cord injury in rat. *J Neurochem* 2001;79:835–848.
46. Herrero I, Miras-Portugal MT, Sanchez-Prieto J. Positive feedback of glutamate exocytosis by metabotropic presynaptic receptor stimulation. *Nature* 1992;360:163–166.
47. Katayama Y, Kawamata T, Tamura T, et al. Calcium-dependent glutamate release concomitant with massive potassium flux during cerebral ischemia in vivo. *Brain Res* 1991;558:136–140.
48. Beattie MS, Hermann GE, Rogers RC, et al. Cell death in models of spinal cord injury. *Prog Brain Res* 2002;137:37–47.
49. Stirling DP, Khodarahmi K, Liu J, et al. Minocycline treatment reduces delayed oligodendrocyte death, attenuates axonal dieback, and improves functional outcome after spinal cord injury. *J Neurosci* 2005;24:2182–2190.
50. Popovich PG, Stuckman S, Gienapp IE, et al. Alterations in immune cell phenotype and function after experimental spinal cord injury. *J Neurotrauma* 2001;18:957–966.
51. Popovich PG, Hickey WF. Bone marrow chimeric rats reveal the unique distribution of resident and recruited macrophages in the contused rat spinal cord. *J Neuropathol Exp Neurol* 2001;60:676–685.
52. Shuman SL, Bresnahan JC, Beattie MS. Apoptosis of microglia and oligodendrocytes after spinal cord contusion in rats. *J Neurosci Res* 1997;50:798–808.
53. Jacobs WB, Fehlings MG. The molecular basis of neural regeneration. *Neurosurgery* 2003;53:943–948, discussion 948–950.
54. Hauben E, Butovsky O, Nevo U, et al. Passive or active immunization with myelin basic protein promotes recovery from spinal cord contusion. *J Neurosci* 2000;20:6421–6430.
55. Jones TB, Ankeny DP, Guan Z, et al. Passive or active immunization with myelin basic protein impairs neurological function and exacerbates neuropathology after spinal cord injury in rats. *J Neurosci* 2004;24:3752–3761.
56. Hurlbert RJ. The role of steroids in acute spinal cord injury: an evidence-based analysis. *Spine* 2001;26:S39–S46.

CHAPTER 21B

Spinal Cord Injury and Pathophysiology: Cord Syndromes

Vivek Joseph and Y. Raja Rampersaud

INTRODUCTION

The initial clinical evaluation of a patient with acute spinal cord injury (SCI) is one of the most important steps in their management. In addition to following Advanced Trauma Life Support (ATLS) guidelines, ensuring a detailed neurologic examination in the patient with SCI is essential to accurately classifying the neurologic injury. Classification of the SCI is crucial to acute management decisions and strongly reflects the neurologic prognosis of the patient. Numerous studies have shown that the degree and type of neurologic injury is one of the most important predictors of neurologic recovery.[1–5]

Accurate serial neurologic assessment and classification is required to enable assessment of the effect of medical and surgical management on the natural history of SCI. The 1996 American Spinal Injury Association (ASIA) recommendations for international standards of neurologic and functional classification of SCI include ASIA scales (consisting of the ASIA scores, including the motor index scores, sensory scores, and the ASIA impairment scale) and is currently the most commonly used system for neurologic assessment.[6]

COMPLETE VERSUS INCOMPLETE ACUTE SPINAL CORD INJURY

The distinction between complete and incomplete injury is paramount in acute management decisions and prediction of outcome. The ASIA grading scale improves the ability to distinguish between complete and incomplete injuries (Table 21B.1). To make this distinction, it is necessary to test touch and pin-prick sensation in the sacral dermatomes at the perianal mucocutaneous junction, as well as deep anal sensation. Voluntary contraction of the external anal sphincter must also be tested by digital examination. As originally described by Waters et al.,[7] a complete injury (ASIA grade A) is defined as the absence of sensory and motor function in the lowest sacral segment.

INCIDENCE AND PROGNOSIS

Complete injuries are reported to occur in 44.7% to 67% of acute SCI.[5,8–11] A review of over 1600 spinal cord–injured patients shows that, unfortunately, more than half of patients at the time of initial assessment have complete injuries (58%).[12] This group of patients has the worst prognosis for recovery and the highest mortality rate. A small (12%) group of these patients may regain some ability to perceive pressure, and an even smaller number (4.5%) may regain the ability to ambulate. Although a small number of patients show significant recovery, total recovery from a complete injury is an extremely rare event.[13] Misinterpretation of recovery from a "complete SCI" may occur as a result of the relatively common inability to accurately assess the degree of SCI because of confounders such as an altered level of consciousness (e.g., inebriation, drugs, or concomitant head injury), spinal shock, or significant distracting injuries.

The prognosis for neurologic recovery is significantly better for incomplete SCI compared to complete injuries at all levels of the spinal cord.[12,14] Nearly 50% of patients with some preserved sensation only (ASIA B) may eventually walk. Patients with some preserved motor power (ASIA C) have up to an 80% chance of ambulating, and patients with retained useful motor function have the best prognosis with more than a 95% chance of ambulating.[12]

INCOMPLETE ACUTE SPINAL CORD INJURY SYNDROMES

Several different types of incomplete acute neurologic syndromes occur in SCI (Table 21B.1). The various traumatic cord syndromes can be differentiated according to the neurologic examination and knowledge of the major ascending and descending tracts in the spinal cord. Further, these findings indicate the dominant area of injury in the transverse plane of the spinal cord (Fig. 21B.1).[15] However, it must be noted that a significant number (25% to 30%) of incomplete SCI may not be definable to a specific syndrome.[9]

In addition to grading patients according to the ASIA scale, it is also useful to categorize the patients with incomplete SCI according to the location (i.e., specific syndrome) of the injury in the spinal cord. This is of prognostic importance because the various categories of incomplete SCI injury have differing prognoses for recovery. This distinction may also provide some information about the mechanism of injury.

At the level of the cervical spinal cord, the traumatic incomplete SCI syndromes of importance are central cord and the related cervicomedullary cord syndromes, anterior cord syndrome, Brown-Séquard syndrome, and posterior cord syndrome.

ACUTE TRAUMATIC CENTRAL CORD SYNDROME

History and Clinical Features

Schneider et al.[16,17] first described acute central cervical cord syndrome as being characterized by a disproportionally greater loss of motor power in the upper extremities than the lower extremities with varying degrees of sensory loss. In addition, there is predominant distal upper extremity weakness and variable degrees of bladder, bowel, and sexual dysfunction.

Various theories have been postulated as to why there is more injury to the central regions of the cervical spinal cord with relative sparing of the peripheral region. The majority of theories have been

TABLE 21B.1 Acute Cervical Spinal Cord Injury Syndromes in Trauma Patients

General Category of Neurologic Injury	Specific Type of Neurologic Injury
Complete spinal cord injury	Unilevel: No zone of partial preservation
ASIA grade A	Multiple level: Zone of partial preservation
Incomplete spinal cord injury	Anterior cord syndrome
ASIA grades B, C, and D	Central cord syndrome
	Cervicomedullary syndrome
	Brown-Séquard syndrome
	Posterior cord syndrome
Transient syndromes	Cord concussion

based on Foerster's presumption that there was somatotopic organization in the lateral corticospinal tract similar to the fasciculi cuneatus or gracilis and the lateral spinothalamic tract.[18] Accordingly, the medially (i.e., centrally located) placed corticospinal fibers that were thought to subserve arm and hand function would thus have to be differentially injured to produce the clinical findings of the "central cord syndrome." Consequently, acute traumatic central cord syndrome (ATCCS) has been classically felt to be the result of compression of the cervical cord between the posterior infolding of ligamentum flavum and the anterior bony spurs because of hyperextension in a patient with cervical spondylosis. This mechanism could lead to greater injury to the central region of the cord and the medial corticospinal tract as a result of combination of both mechanical and vascular factors (Fig. 21B.2).[16,17,19–22] Reduced flow from the anterior spinal artery may result in selective ischemia of the central region of the spinal cord. This is secondary to the watershed zone of cord blood supply from the terminal branches of the anterior spinal, posterior spinal, and radicular arteries.[16,20] In addition, Turnbull[20] also noted that because of their transverse orientation, the small vessels supplying the lateral column and gray matter are more affected by the presence of preexisting spinal cord anterior-posterior compression (e.g., secondary to cervical spondylosis) and cannot respond to additional anterior-to-posterior compression. Schneider et al.[16] also postulated that this area is more prone to microvascular damage because of thin-walled veins at the interface of firmer and denser

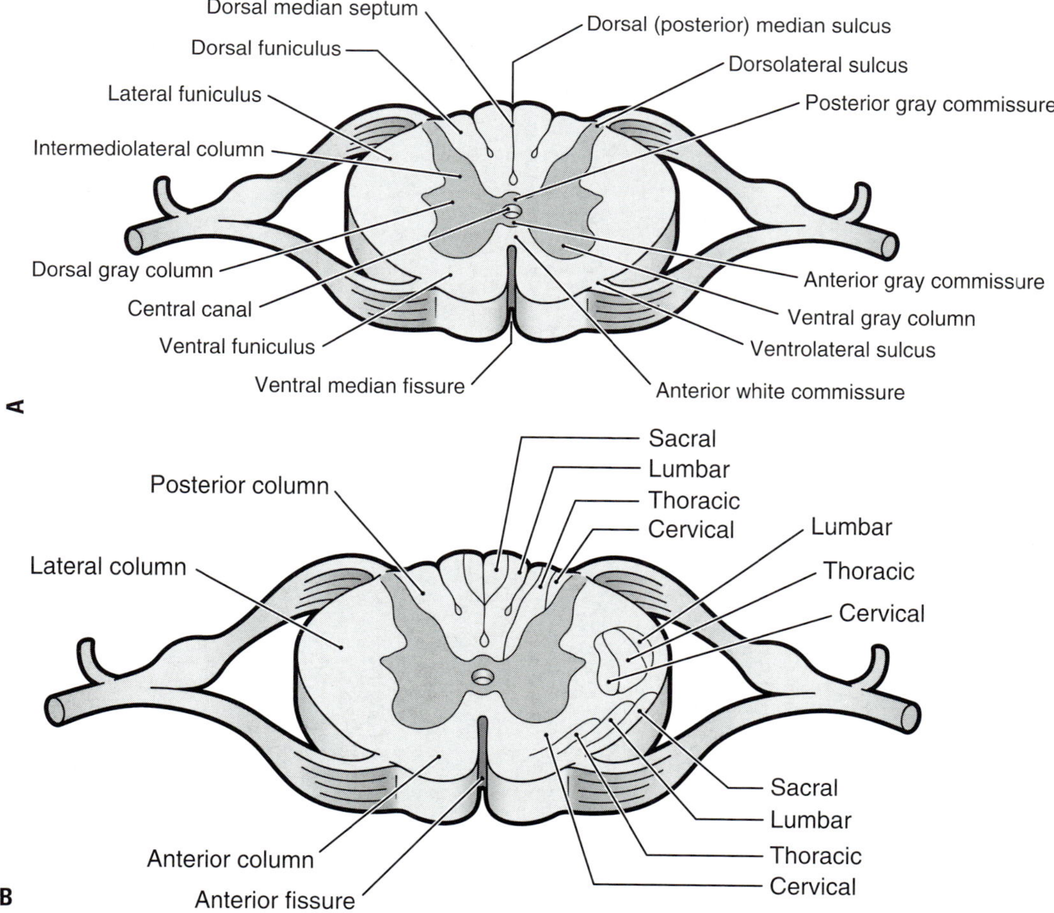

FIGURE 21B.1. Cross section of the normal cervical spinal cord. **A.** The normal white matter funiculi and gray matter columns. **B.** The somatotopic arrangement in the white matter tracts of the posterior, lateral, and anterior columns are shown. *(continued)*

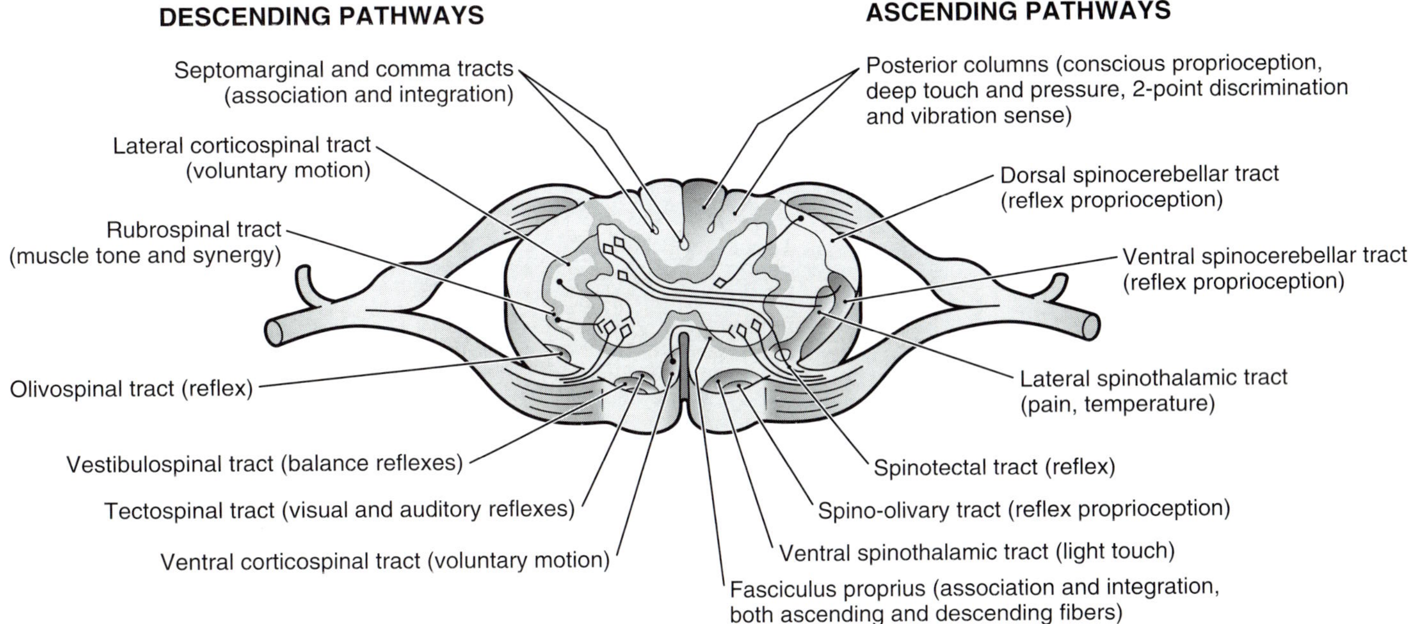

FIGURE 21B.1. *(continued)* **C.** The normal location and function of the various ascending and descending tracts in the spinal cord are shown. (From O'Brien MF. Nervous system. In DeWald RL, ed. *Spinal Deformities: The Comprehensive Text.* New York: Thieme Medical Publishers, 2003:97, with permission.)

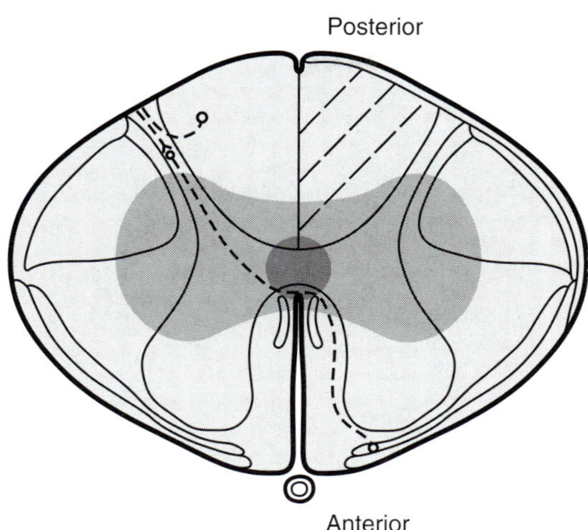

FIGURE 21B.2. Area of injury in acute traumatic central cord syndrome. The central portion of the cord with maximal injury and hematomyelia is shown with a surrounding area of microvascular damage and edema. The damaged area includes the medial segments of the corticospinal tracts previously thought to be the somatotopic organization of upper limb fibers; however, recent evidence suggests that the majority of the corticospinal tract subserves hand and upper limb function. (From Engler GL, Cole J, Merton LW, eds. *Spinal Cord Diseases: Diagnosis and Treatment.* New York: Marcel Dekker, 1998:130–131, with permission.)

white matter and the more friable and flexible gray matter. McVeigh's experimental work[17,23] supports the hypothesis that the relatively looser texture and less supporting strength of the central gray matter may enable the development and longitudinal progression of central hematomyelia causing compression of the adjacent white matter (Figs. 21B.1 and 21B.2).

It is now thought that the greater weakness in the arms compared to the legs occurs because the lateral corticospinal tract subserves mainly hand and upper limb function. Therefore, when this area is the primary site of damage, the functional deficits would be more pronounced in the hands.[24,25] In a recent histopathologic analysis of the spinal cords of five patients with documented evidence of ATCCS, the authors concluded that hand dysfunction in ATCCS resulted from a primary injury involving the large fibers of the lateral corticospinal tract and could occur in the absence of motor neuron loss supplying the hand musculature. Reduction in the hand motor neuron pool occurred in the chronic low cervical injury where the epicenter of injury was adjacent to this area.[25]

The most common clinical scenario that results in a central cord syndrome is a hyperextension injury in an older patient (>50 years) with preexisting spinal canal stenosis. In these patients, cervical hyperextension results in clinically significant compression of the cord between anterior osteochondral bars and posteriorly infolded ligamentum flavum. This can occur without evidence of bony or ligamentous injury. In the younger patients (<50 years), this syndrome typically is caused by spinal cord compression from fractures of the anterior column.[3]

Incidence and Prognosis

ATCCS is the most common incomplete traumatic cervical cord syndrome. ATCCS accounts for 16% to 20% of all cervical spinal cord injuries.[3,11,26] Fortunately, most patients with central cord syndrome improve. Motor recovery typically follows a pattern of lower extremities recovering first, followed by bladder function, and finally the upper extremities with finger movements recovering last. Improvement in hand function, bowel and bladder function, and independence is reported to occur in 50% to 86% of patients.[1,3,4,11,16,17,26] However, even though the motor function may improve significantly, many patients may have significant residual disability and are less functional than the general population.[1] A lower initial ASIA score, lower level of formal education, increased medical comorbidities, older age, and the development of spasticity have been shown to be negative predictors of outcome.[1,3,26,27]

Historically, Schneider et al.[16,17] were against operating on individuals with central cord syndrome, because some of their patients showed very rapid spontaneous clinical recovery and a few deteriorated following laminectomy. Other reports of increased morbidity and neurologic deterioration after early

TABLE 21B.2 Central Cord Versus Cervicomedullary Syndrome

Clinical Parameters	Central Cord Syndrome	Cervicomedullary Syndrome
Site of lesions	Mid to lower cervical cord Anterior horn cells Lateral corticospinal tract	Anterior aspect of lower medulla and upper cervical cord Corticospinal decussation caudal to the pyramids
Clinical manifestations	Arms weaker than legs Flaccid arms acutely Legs normal or variably weak Lower motor neuron deficits in upper limbs persist	Arms weaker than legs Flaccid arms acutely Legs normal or variably weak Upper motor neuron deficits in upper limbs develop ± Trigeminal sensory deficit (onion skin, spinal tract of cranial nerve V) ± Cranial nerve dysfunction (cranial nerve IX, X, or XI)
Magnetic resonance imaging	Lesion in mid-lower cervical spine	Lesion in cervicomedullary junction
Prognosis for neurologic recovery	Variable, but usually favorable	Usually good

surgery have long maintained this approach to the acute management of SCI.[28–32] However, the majority of these historically reported concerns were more likely due to difficulties in critical care, neuroanaesthesia (e.g., blood pressure control), and surgical techniques at the time. Certainly in the scenario in which a patient has a stable spine with no static ongoing compression and/or progressive neurologic improvement, nonsurgical management is still advocated. However, in the presence of persistent compression, instability, or lack of neurologic improvement or neurologic deterioration, acute surgery is a valuable safe option.[10,34–36]

Injuries occurring in the upper cervical spine can also present with a similar neurologic picture; however, there are distinct clinical and prognostic differences between SCI in the upper (cervicomedullary syndrome) and lower spinal cord (Table 21B.2).

CERVICOMEDULLARY SYNDROME

History and Clinical Features

Cervicomedullary syndrome is a term used to describe the syndromes involving injury to the upper cervical cord and brainstem. Nielsen[37] first described cervicomedullary syndrome in 1941. Historically, the localization of the syndrome was placed at the corticospinal tract to the upper limbs at the pyramid. The decussating fibers for the upper limbs were thought to be cephalad to and more ventral, medial, and superficial to those of the lower limbs. The odontoid process lies near the level of the medially decussating upper limb fibers; thus, fractures and other lesions of the odontoid could explain this syndrome. As already described, an alternative hypotheses has been suggested based on evidence that the corticospinal tract in primates is critical for hand function, but not for locomotion.[24,25] Therefore, injury to the corticospinal tract at the cervicomedullary junction and cervical levels of the spinal cord tends to cause greater hand and upper limb weakness compared to lower limb weakness.

This syndrome can occur in acute SCI as a result of traction injury secondary to subluxation or dislocation at the occipital-cervical junction or C1-C2 or direct compression from fracture. As a result of improved management at the trauma scene, a larger number of patients are surviving these historically fatal injuries and are subsequently requiring intensive medical and surgical management.

Because of the relative infrequency of cervicomedullary syndrome, many clinicians are not as familiar with the clinical features of this SCI syndrome. Clinically, the essential features include respiratory insufficiency or arrest, hypotension, and varying degrees of quadriparesis, with the upper limbs more severely affected. Sensory features include hyperesthesia from C1-C4 and onion skin or Déjerine pattern of sensory loss over the face.[17,38] The more severe manifestations tend to occur with higher lesions. As recommended by Schneider et al., testing facial sensation in all patients with cervical SCI is important.[17,38] In this scenario, a loss of facial sensation denotes damage to the fibers of the descending spinal tract or cell bodies within the nucleus of the trigeminal nerve, which begins in the pons and medulla and extends downward to at least the C4 cervical segment. Because of the onion skin or Déjerine pattern of topographic representation, a perioral distribution of sensory loss denotes a lesion in the lower medulla and upper cervical cord, whereas a more peripheral facial distribution of sensory loss involving the forehead, ear, and chin denotes a lesion in the cord at C3-C4. Cervicomedullary injuries often mimic the central cord syndrome because of a greater weakness in the arm than the leg; however, careful assessment of the cranial nerves can make the clinical diagnosis (Table 21B.2). Furthermore, the level of injury as determined by imaging will anatomically differentiate between a central cord syndrome (lesion to either the mid or lower cervical spine) and cervicomedullary syndrome.[39]

Incidence and Prognosis

Dickman et al.[39] identified a cohort of 14 patients with isolated upper cervical spinal cord injury, resulting in cruciate paralysis over a 5-year period. This represented approximately 2% of all cervical spine injuries and 4% of all cervical spine–injured patients over the same period of time. Upper limb weakness was bilateral and symmetric in 57%, bilateral and asymmetric in 21.5%, and unilateral in 21.5%. All patients had severe upper limb weakness with less severe or no lower limb weakness. At mean follow-up of 21.6 months for the 14 patients (range 4 to 58 months), all had progressive neurologic improvement and 8 recovered completely. The 5 patients with incomplete recovery had mild residual spastic weakness involving one or both upper limbs. Only one patient had residual gait spasticity. There was one death in a postoperative patient (out of 5 surgical patients) at 6 months postinjury from pneumonia. From this limited series, the prognosis in patients with cervicomedullary syndrome is seemingly good. Most patients demonstrate complete recovery, and residual deficits are usually mild.

ANTERIOR CORD SYNDROME

History and Clinical Features

Schneider[40] originally described this syndrome in two patients with acute cervical trauma. In his article, Schneider states, "This is characterized by immediate complete paralysis, with hypesthesia and hypalgesia to the level of the lesion, and with the preservation of motion, position, and vibration sense." Both patients had ruptured disks, and both had good recovery following surgical decompression of the cord. Schneider felt that this was "a syndrome for which early operative intervention is indicated."

In this syndrome, the anterior aspect of the spinal cord is injured with sparing of the posterior columns (Fig. 21B.3). Therefore, there is loss of motor function and the sensations of pain and temperature (subserved by the spinothalamic tract) below the level of injury. Sensations of touch, vibration, and joint position, subserved by the posterior columns, are relatively preserved. The anterior cord syndrome is usually associated with cervical flexion-distraction injuries producing a fracture dislocation or axial loading injuries producing a burst fracture.

Anterior Cord Syndrome

Posterior

Anterior

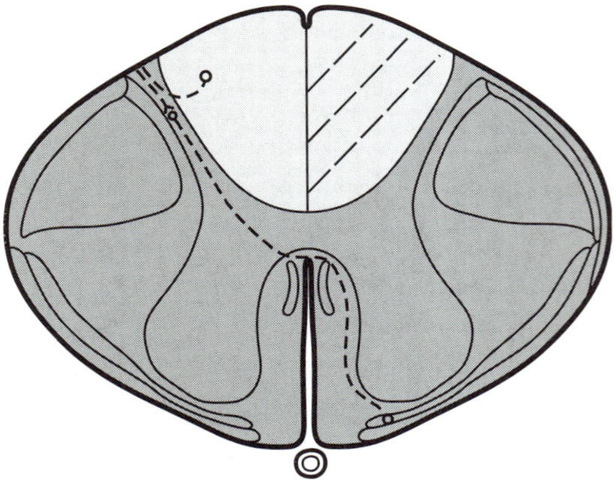

FIGURE 21B.3. Area of injury that would result in anterior cord syndrome. (From Engler GL, Cole J, Merton LW, eds. *Spinal Cord Diseases: Diagnosis and Treatment.* New York: Marcel Dekker, 1998:130–131, with permission.)

There are typically two components to this syndrome. First, there is direct damage to the anterior part of the cervical spinal cord by the compressive bone fragment or herniated disk. Second, there also may be varying degrees of vascular insufficiency produced by the occlusion of the anterior spinal artery. The anterior spinal artery is responsible for the perfusion of the anterolateral two thirds of the spinal cord.[41]

Incidence and Prognosis

The anterior cord syndrome occurs in approximately 20% of incomplete spinal cord injuries and is the second most common traumatic incomplete spinal cord syndrome.[8,11] These patients classically have a severe motor deficit with posterior column sparing; thus, they typically fall into the ASIA B group. The prognosis, despite the historically good recovery reported by Schneider,[40] is typically poor. Bosch et al.,[11] reported on a group of 12 patients with anterior cervical cord syndrome in which all were nonambulatory at admission and remained nonambulatory at an average of 5 years and 4 months of follow-up. Hand function was present in only two cases of low cervical lesions, but no functional return occurred in any case. Bladder and bowel control was also absent on admission and at the last follow-up in all cases.

BROWN-SÉQUARD SYNDROME

History and Clinical Features

The syndrome was first described by Charles Edouard Brown-Séquard (1817–1894) in 1849. His description was based on numerous animal experiments and collected human cases with autopsy confirmation. When he returned to the subject in *The Lancet* in 1869, he stated that, "a lesion in one of the lateral halves of the spinal cord produces: 1st, paralysis of voluntary movements in the same side; 2nd, anaesthesia to touch, tickling, painful impressions, and changes of temperature in the opposite side; 3rd, paralysis of the muscular sense in the same side."[42]

Brown-Séquard syndrome is defined as an incomplete lesion of the spinal cord characterized by ipsilateral upper motor neuron paralysis and loss of proprioception with contralateral loss of pain and temperature sensation. A zone of partial preservation or segmental ipsilateral lower motor neuron weakness and analgesia may also be noted. Loss of ipsilateral autonomic function can result in Horner syndrome.

The Brown-Séquard, or hemicord, syndrome results from a lesion affecting the lateral half of the spinal cord (Fig. 21B.4). This type of injury results in damage to the corticospinal, spinothalamic, and posterior column in half of the spinal cord. A variety of injury mechanisms, including

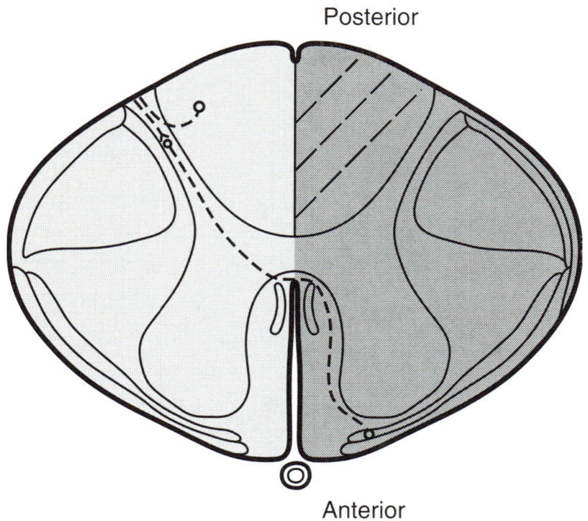

FIGURE 21B.4. Area of the cord injured in Brown-Séquard syndrome, also known as the hemicord syndrome. (From Engler GL, Cole J, Merton LW, eds. *Spinal Cord Diseases: Diagnosis and Treatment.* New York: Marcel Dekker, 1998:130–131, with permission.)

penetrating trauma, can cause the Brown-Séquard syndrome or the Brown-Séquard–plus syndrome (more than half of the cord involved).[43–45] In the series by Roth et al.,[44] of 38 patients with Brown-Séquard syndrome or the Brown-Séquard–plus syndrome, 22 injuries were caused by road traffic accidents, 8 by penetrating injuries, 5 by diving injuries, and 3 by other causes. In the series by Braakman and Penning,[45] this syndrome was most commonly seen with hyperextension injuries; however, flexion injuries, locked facets, and compression fractures were also noted. Brown-Séquard syndrome may be present at the onset of injury or become apparent in a delayed manner following the gradual evolution of a bilateral incomplete injury. Combinations of Brown-Séquard and other incomplete spinal cord syndromes can also occur. As an incomplete spinal cord syndrome, the clinical presentation of Brown-Séquard syndrome may range from mild to severe neurologic deficits.

The pathoanatomy of Brown-Séquard syndrome is damage or loss of ascending and descending spinal cord tracts on one side of the spinal cord. The descending motor fibers of the corticospinal tracts cross at the junction of the medulla and spinal cord (i.e., above the injury). The ascending dorsal column carrying sensation of vibration and position runs ipsilateral to the roots of entry and crosses above the spinal cord in the medulla. The ascending spinothalamic tracts cross at or within several levels above their entry into the spinal cord. Therefore the spinothalamic tracts convey sensations of pain, temperature, and crude touch from the contralateral side of the body below the level of the spinal cord injury. At the site of spinal cord injury (SCI), nerve roots or anterior horn cells also may be affected (i.e., concomitant lower motor neuron injury).

Incidence and Prognosis

Brown-Séquard syndrome occurs in about 8% to 10% of incomplete traumatic spinal cord injuries.[11] Because it is an incomplete injury affecting half of the cord, the prognosis is usually good. In the series by Roth et al.,[44] all 38 patients showed early functional improvement, with 29 walking independently. In the incomplete cervical SCI series from Bosch et al.,[11] 5 patients presented with Brown-Séquard syndrome. At admission, 3 of 5 were ambulating, all had bladder control, and 1 had nonfunctional use of the hand. At 5.33 years follow-up, all were ambulating (except 1 for medical reasons), with functional hand and bladder control.

POSTERIOR CORD SYNDROME

Posterior cord syndrome is a rare type of incomplete SCI syndrome. In fact, many researchers have actually doubted its existence in traumatic SCI. It anecdotally occurs after injury to the posterior aspect of the cord but with residual functioning spinal cord tissue anteriorly (Fig. 21B.5). The

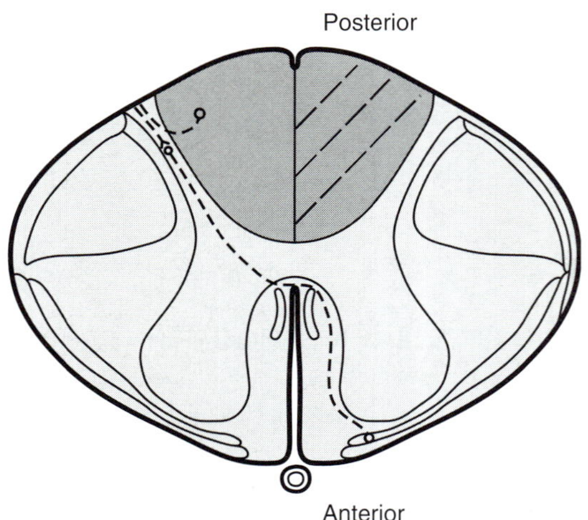

FIGURE 21B.5 Area of the spinal cord (posterior columns) primarily injured in posterior cord syndrome. Some authors feel that the adjacent corticospinal tracts in the posterior aspect of the lateral columns are also injured in this syndrome. (From Engler GL, Cole J, Merton LW, eds. *Spinal Cord Diseases: Diagnosis and Treatment.* New York: Marcel Dekker, 1998:130–131, with permission.)

reported clinical presentation is variable and may be isolated to loss of vibration and position sense as a result of injury of the posterior columns as described by Bosch et al.[11] or may also include loss of motor function with concomitant injury to the lateral columns, as noted by Tator.[14] Posterior cord syndrome was reported in only 1% of incomplete injuries in the NASCIS II study.[8] Bosch et al.[11] found only 1 case among 60 with incomplete cervical cord injury. This patient was ambulatory at admission and continued to ambulate, despite the loss of posterior column sensation. Hand function was not significantly involved, and bladder and bowel control were present at admission.

CONCLUSION

The difference in prognosis between complete and incomplete spinal cord injury is dramatically different. Complete spinal cord injuries are associated with a very poor overall prognosis. For incomplete spinal cord injuries, the degree of spinal cord impairment and the associated type of spinal cord syndrome are very important clinical prognostic indicators. Incomplete cervical spinal cord syndromes include central cord, cervicomedullary, anterior cord, Brown-Séquard, and posterior cord syndromes. With the exception of the anterior cord syndrome, most incomplete SCIs are associated with a good to excellent prognosis for ambulation and overall functional recovery. In-depth knowledge of these various incomplete spinal cord syndromes gives additional information regarding the anatomic location of maximal injury and the possible mechanism of injury. Consequently, it is mandatory to perform a detailed neurologic examination that includes cranial nerve assessment in all patients with spinal cord injury. Also, the importance of examining sensation at the perianal mucocutaneous junction and performing a digital rectal examination in a patient with an apparent "complete" SCI cannot be overemphasized. The use of a valid neurologic grading system for SCI, such as the ASIA grading system, is strongly recommended. This system provides an objective assessment tool and serves as a common language among the numerous disciplines caring for patients with SCI.

CLASSIC REFERENCES

American Spinal Injury Association, International Medical Society of Paraplegia. *International Standards for Neurological and Functional Classification of Spinal Cord Injury.* Revised 1996. Chicago: American Spinal Injury Association, 1996.

Bosch A, Stauffer S, Nickel VL. Incomplete traumatic quadriplegia: a ten year review. *JAMA* 1971:216;473–478.

Jimenez O, Marcillo A, Levi ADO. A histopathological analysis of the human cervical spinal cord in patients with acute traumatic central cord syndrome. *Spinal Cord* 2000:38;532–537.

Schneider RC, Crosby EC, Russo EH, et al. Traumatic spinal cord syndromes and their management. *Clin Neurosurg* 1973:20;424–492.

Waters RL, Adkins RH, Yakura JS. Definition of complete spinal cord injury. *Paraplegia* 1991:29;573–581.

REFERENCES

1. Dvorak MF, Fisher CG, Hoekema J, et al. Factors predicting motor recovery and functional outcome after traumatic central cord syndrome: a long-term follow-up. *Spine* 2005;30:2303–2311.
2. Pollard ME, Apple DF. Factors associated with improved neurologic outcomes in patients with incomplete tetraplegia [clinical case series]. *Spine* 2003;28:33–38.
3. Newey ML, Sen PK, Fraser RD. The long-term outcome after central cord syndrome: a study of the natural history. *J Bone Joint Surg Br* 2000;82:851–855.
4. Merriam WF, Taylor TKF, Ruff SJ, et al. A reappraisal of acute traumatic central cord syndrome. *J Bone Joint Surg Br* 1986;68:708–713.
5. Maynard FM, Reynolds GG, Fountain S, et al. Neurological prognosis after traumatic quadriplegia: three year experience of California Regional Spinal Cord Injury Care System. *J Neurosurg* 1979;50:611–616.
6. American Spinal Injury Association, International Medical Society of Paraplegia. *International Standards for Neurological and Functional Classification of Spinal Cord Injury.* Revised 1996. Chicago: American Spinal Injury Association, 1996.
7. Waters RL, Adkins RH, Yakura JS: Definition of complete spinal cord injury. *Paraplegia* 1991;29:573–581.
8. Bracken MB, Shepard MJ, Collins WF, et al. A randomized, controlled trial of methylprednisolone or naloxone in the treatment of acute spinal cord injury: results of the second National Acute Spinal Cord Injury Study. *N Engl J Med* 1990;322:1405–1411.
9. Bracken MB, Shepard MJ, Holford TR. Administration of methylprednisolone for 24 or 48 hours or tirilazad mesylate for 48 hours in the treatment of acute spinal cord injury: results of the Third National Acute Spinal Cord Injury Randomized Controlled Trial. *JAMA* 1997;277:1597–1604.
10. Tator CH, Duncan EG, Edmonds VE, et al. Comparison of surgical and conservative management in 208 patients with acute spinal cord injury. *Can J Neurol Sci* 1987;14:60–69.
11. Bosch A, Stauffer S, Nickel VL. Incomplete traumatic quadriplegia: a ten year review. *JAMA* 1971;216:473–478.
12. Piepmie JM, Collins WF. Recovery of function following spinal cord injury. In: Vinken PJ, Bruyn GW, Klawans HL, et al. *Handbook of Clinical Neurology.* Vol 61. Amsterdam: Elsevier Science, 1992:421–433.
13. Hansebout RR. A comprehensive review of methods of improving cord recovery after acute spinal cord injury. In: Tator CH, ed. *Early Management of Acute Spinal Cord Injury.* New York: Raven Press, 1982:181–196.
14. Tator CH. Classification of spinal cord injury based on neurological presentation. In: Narayan RK, Wilberger JE Jr, Povlishock JT, eds. *Neurotrauma.* New York: McGraw-Hill, 1996:1053–1073.
15. Tator CH. Spine-spinal cord relationships in spinal cord trauma. *Clin Neurosurg* 1983;30:479–494.
16. Schneider RC, Crosby EC, Russo EH, et al. Traumatic spinal cord syndromes and their management. *Clin Neurosurg* 1973;20:424–492.
17. Schneider RC, Cherry G, Pantek H. The syndrome of acute central cervical spinal cord injury. *J Neurosurg* 1954;11:546–577.
18. Foerster O. Symptomatologie der erkrankungen des rückenmarks und seiner wurzeln. In Bumke O, Foerster O, eds. *Handbook of Neurology.* Vol. 5. Berlin: Springer, 1936:83.
19. Taylor AR. The mechanism of injury to the spinal cord in the neck without damage to the vertebral column. *J Bone Joint Surg Br* 1951;30:543–547.
20. Turnbull IM. Blood supply of the spinal cord: normal and pathological considerations. *Clin Neurosurg* 1973; 20:56–84.
21. Ducker TB, Kindt GW, Kempe LG. Pathologic findings in acute experimental cord trauma. *J Neurosurg* 1971; 35:700–708.
22. Goodkin R, Campbell JB. Sequential pathological changes in spinal cord injury: a prelimnary report. *Surg Forum* 1969;20:430–432.
23. McVeigh JF. Experimental cord crushes with special reference to the mechanical factors involved and subsequent changes in the areas of the cord affected. *Arch Surg Chicago* 1923;7:573–600.
24. Levi ADO, Tator CH, Bunge RP. Clinical syndromes associated with disproportionate weakness of the upper versus the lower extremities after cervical spinal cord injury. *Neurosurgery* 1996:38;179–185.
25. Jimenez O, Marcillo A, Levi ADO. A histopathological analysis of the human cervical spinal cord in patients with acute traumatic central cord syndrome. *Spinal Cord* 2000;38:532–537.
26. Roth EJ, Lawler MH, Yarkony GM. Traumatic central cord syndrome: clinical features and functional outcomes. *Arch Phys Med Rehabil* 1990;71:18–23.

27. Penrod LE, Hegde SK, Ditunno JF. Age effect on prognosis for functional recovery in acute, traumatic central cord syndrome. *Arch Phys Med Rehabil* 1990;71:963–968.
28. Marshall LF, Knowlton S, Garfin SR, et al. Deterioration following spinal cord injury: a multicenter study. *J Neurosurg* 1987;66:400–404.
29. Collins WF. A review and update of experiment and clinical studies of spinal cord injury. *Paraplegia* 1983;21: 204–219.
30. Bedbrook GM, Sakae T. A review of cervical spine injuries with neurological dysfunction. *Paraplegia* 1982;20: 321–333.
31. Bedbrook GM, Sedgley GI. The management of spinal injuries: past and present. *Int Rehabil Med* 1980;2:45–61.
32. Bedbrook GM. Spinal injuries with tetraplegia and paraplegia. *J Bone Joint Surg Br* 1979;61:267–284.
33. Vale FL, Burns J, Jackson AB, et al. Combined medical and surgical treatment after acute spinal cord injury: results of a prospective pilot study to assess the merits of aggressive medical resuscitation and blood pressure management. *J Neurosurg* 1997;87:239–246.
34. Levi L, Wolf A, Belzberg H. Hemodynamic parameters in patients with acute cervical cord trauma: description, intervention, and prediction of outcome. *Neurosurgery* 1993;33:1007–1017.
35. Benzel EC, Larson SJ. Functional recovery after decompressive operation for thoracic and lumbar spine fractures. *Neurosurgery* 1986;19:772–778.
36. Rosner MJ, Elias Z, Coley I. New principles of resuscitation for brain and spinal injury. *N C Med J* 1984;45: 701–708.
37. Nielsen JM. *A Text Book of Clinical Neurology*. New York: Paul B Hoeber, 1941:149–168.
38. Schneider RC. Concomitant craniocerebral and spinal trauma, with special reference to the cervicomedullary region. *Clin Neurosurg* 1970;17:266–309.
39. Dickman CA, Hadley MN, Pappas CTE, et al. Cruciate paralysis: a clinical and radiographic analysis of injuries to the cervicomedullary junction. *J Neurosurg* 1990;73:850–858.
40. Schneider RC. A syndrome in acute cervical injuries for which early operation is indicated. *J Neurosurg* 1951; 8:360–367.
41. Engler GL, Cole J, Merton LW, eds. *Spinal Cord Diseases: Diagnosis and Treatment.* New York: Marcel Dekker, 1998:1–14.
42. Brown-Séquard CE. Lectures on the physiology and pathology of the nervous system and on the treatment of organic nervous affections: Lecture II, part 1. *Lancet* 1869;i:1–3.
43. McCarron MO, Flynn PA, Pang KA, et al. Traumatic Brown-Séquard-plus syndrome. *Arch Neurol* 2001; 58:1470–1472.
44. Roth EJ, Park T, Pang T, et al. Traumatic cervical Brown-Séquard and Brown-Séquard-plus syndromes: the spectrum of presentations and outcomes. *Paraplegia* 1991;29:582–589.

CHAPTER 21C

Spinal Cord Injury and Pathophysiology: Timing of Intervention in the Treatment of Spinal Cord Injuries

Gordon K. T. Chu and Michael G. Fehlings

INTRODUCTION

There are approximately 10,000 to 12,000 new spinal cord injuries (SCIs) in the United States each year, with approximately 280,000 people currently living with SCI.[1–3] In 1995, the direct costs associated with SCI were $7.7 billion. With newer surgical, anesthetic, critical care, and rehabilitation techniques, these costs will surely rise because there will be more SCI survivors who live longer.[4] Furthermore, a large proportion of these victims are young people who will spend the rest of their lives tetraplegic or paraplegic. Therefore, the effort to improve the neurologic outcome for these patients is of utmost importance.

SCI has been recognized as a disease entity since the time of the ancient Egyptians, but many aspects of its treatment remain controversial. The pathophysiology of SCI has been reviewed elsewhere, so this chapter will provide only a brief summary.[1,5,6] SCI can be divided into primary and secondary injury mechanisms. The primary injury involves the initial mechanical deformation and destruction of spinal cord tissue at the time of injury. This is generally thought to be irreversible and not amenable to treatment. Secondary injury mechanisms are initiated by the primary injury and continue the destruction of spinal cord tissue. Secondary injury mechanisms can be further subdivided into the following groups, which include but are not limited to: (a) vascular changes, (b) biochemical and electrolyte derangements, and (c) cellular and molecular changes. Vascular changes include ischemia, loss of autoregulation, and hemorrhage. Biochemical and electrolyte changes include calcium and sodium influx, increased extracellular concentration of potassium, and excitatory neurotransmitters such as glutamate, serotonin, and catecholamines. Cellular and molecular changes include infiltration of inflammatory cells, loss of mitochondrial potential, and activation of caspase proteins leading to forms of programmed cell death including apoptosis. This understanding of the secondary injury mechanisms led to developments of possible therapeutic agents. The two National Acute Spinal Cord Injury Studies (NASCIS II and III) demonstrated that methylprednisolone may confer a modest benefit with regard to neurologic improvement if given within 8 hours of the SCI.[7,8] The course of treatment is shortened if the drug is administered within 3 hours of injury. Treatment with methylprednisolone remains controversial, but it is still the only neuroprotective agent that is in widespread use after SCI.

The NASCIS trials were the first randomized double-blinded controlled trials in humans that demonstrated that there is a time window after SCI in which interventions targeting secondary injury mechanisms may be instituted that could improve the outcome of SCI. It has been suggested that persistent compression of the spinal cord is a potential secondary injury mechanism that may exacerbate the effects of the other secondary injury mechanisms. Given that there is a time window for pharmacologic intervention, it is only logical to hypothesize that there may be one for surgical intervention, in particular decompression. This chapter summarizes data culled from several systematic reviews performed by the senior author, which are referenced.[9–13]

ANIMAL STUDIES OF EARLY DECOMPRESSION

The initial studies demonstrating efficacy of methylprednisolone were conducted with animal models of SCI. Similarly, there is strong evidence in animal models that suggest that early decompression of the spinal cord can lead to neurologic improvement. Experiments conducted on primates, cats, dogs, and rodents using various methods of SCI have demonstrated improved neurologic recovery with early decompression within minutes to hours of the spinal cord.[14–17] Dimar et al.[16] used a weight drop injury followed by placement of epidural spacers to simulate persistent cord compression in the rat thoracic spinal cord. The cord compression was relieved at 0, 2, 6, 24, and 72 hours after the primary injury. The rodents demonstrated improved neurologic recovery that was inversely proportional to the time of compression. Similarly, Carlson et al.[15] reported that dogs that had early decompression showed greater neurologic improvement.

THE ROLE OF NONSURGICAL INTERVENTION IN SPINAL CORD INJURY

The role of surgery in SCI has been only recently accepted as common practice. Traditionally, the treatment of SCI has been nonsurgical because of the poor results after laminectomies and the long-held view that there is no recovery after SCI.[18–21] Furthermore, there was a higher incidence of neurologic complications after surgery. This argument may still have some merit with regard to patients with central cord syndrome; however, with the modern advances in neuroanesthesia, critical care, and surgical techniques, nonoperative treatment of SCI is no longer the preferred treatment option. However, it is still important to note the outcomes in nonoperative patients to carefully gauge the positive or negative impact of surgical intervention. In 1969, Frankel et al.[23] reported on the results of conservative management on 612 patients with SCI. In his series, 29% of the patients with a Frankel A grading improved at least one grade neurologically. Only four patients developed delayed instability. Others have also reported neurologic improvement with nonoperative treatment. All of the studies involving only conservative management would be considered class III evidence (Table 21C.1), consisting mainly of retrospective studies or case series. Although some reports have noted spontaneous improvement from nonoperative treatment, one report has also shown up to 10% of patients with incomplete cervical cord injury may deteriorate with conservative treatment.[24]

TABLE 21C.1 Classification of Medical Evidence

Class of Evidence	Type of Study
Randomized controlled clinical trial	I
Prospective, nonrandomized studies	II
Retrospective studies, case series, expert opinion	III

CLINICAL STUDIES OF EARLY DECOMPRESSION IN SPINAL CORD INJURY

Currently, there are no published reports at the level of class I evidence that demonstrate that early decompression improves neurologic outcome after SCI. Class II evidence from prospective nonrandomized studies with respect to surgical treatment of SCI have demonstrated that it is possible to do early decompression safely.[25–27] Tator el al.[28] demonstrated that surgery resulted in a lower mortality rate in spite of a higher thromboembolic rate in a prospective nonrandomized case-control study of 208 patients with SCI or cauda equina injury. No difference in neurologic recovery was noted between the two groups. However, the question of timing of the decompression was not addressed. Similarly, Waters et al.[25] showed that delayed surgery (>14 days) did not improve neurologic outcome. One prospective, randomized clinical trial examined the question of timing of surgical decompression.[29] Vaccaro et al.[29] demonstrated no difference in neurologic recovery between early (<72 hours) and delayed (>5 days) surgery. However, it can be argued that 72 hours is too long a delay to be considered "early" surgery. Furthermore, nearly one third of the patients in the study were lost to follow-up. Therefore, this study could be treated as class II evidence as opposed to class I. Using NASCIS II data, Duh et al.[30] concluded that early surgery (<25 hours) had better outcomes compared to nonsurgical management, although the results were not statistically significant. Of interest, this same study noted that delayed surgery (>200 hours) may also show benefit. More recently, Papadopoulos et al.[26] reported a study of 91 patients with cervical SCI. They demonstrated that the group of patients who underwent early (<10 hours) surgery through a protocol had a greater percentage of patients with improved neurologic recovery compared to the control group. They also demonstrated the feasibility of early decompressive surgery because all but one patient was admitted within 9 hours of surgery. This study was a prospective nonrandomized trial. In contrast, Pointillart et al.[31] in another prospective nonrandomized study could not detect any difference in neurologic recovery between the group with surgery less than 8 hours and the group with surgery greater than 8 hours in 106 patients, 49 of whom had early decompression. However, the intent of the study was to look at differences between methylprednisolone, nimodipine, and no medical treatment, not early decompression. In a retrospective review, Aebi et al.[32] demonstrated that 75% of the patients who recovered were reduced by closed or open reduction in the first 6 hours. In the study by Papadopolos et al.,[26] patients who had closed reduction (mean time for decompression 6 hours) had even better outcomes than those who had open reduction (mean time 12.6 hours). However, Tator et al.,[13] in a multicenter retrospective study, noted an 8.1% rate of neurologic deterioration in 585 cases of closed reduction.

For the special case of fracture dislocations of the cervical spine, there may be sufficient evidence to support a recommendation for urgent reduction for bilateral locked facets in patients with incomplete injury. Burke and Berryman[33] presented a study of 76 patients with unilateral or bilateral facet dislocations. Half of the patients were admitted under 8 hours, and the authors concluded that early reduction improved the neurologic outcome in patients with incomplete SCI. Several other class II studies reached the same general conclusion.

La Rosa et al.[34] attempted to perform a meta-analysis of studies from 1966 to 2000 that dealt with early versus late decompression. Their goal was "to determine whether neurological outcome is improved in traumatic spinal cord injured patients who had surgery within 24 hours as compared with those who had late surgery or conservative treatment." Additionally, they wished to quantify the effect of early decompression after SCI. They analyzed data from 1687 patients, dividing them into three groups: (a) early decompression (<24 hours), (b) late decompression (>24 hours), and (c) conservative management. They concluded that statistically patients who underwent decompression early had better outcomes compared to late treatment. However, they also concluded that, because of the heterogeneity of their data, only results from patients with incomplete neurologic deficits who had early surgery were reliable.

Late decompression has also been suggested for treatment of SCI.[35] This practice continues because of concerns regarding increased medical complications secondary to early surgery.[36] Moreover, there has been class III evidence mainly from retrospective studies and case series that decompression in a delayed fashion may also lead to some neurologic improvement.[30,37–40]

The question of the potential benefit of early decompression remains unanswered. It is with this question in mind that our institution in collaboration with colleagues at Thomas Jefferson University and the Spine Trauma Study Group (STSG) has helped create a multicenter, prospective trial to evaluate early (<24 hours) versus late (24 hours) decompressive surgery for cervical SCI (Surgical Timing in Acute Spinal Cord Injury Study [STASCIS]). A total of 450 patients are required for this study, which is currently open for enrollment.

CONCLUSION

The concept of the secondary injury in the pathophysiology of SCI has led to the idea of a possible time window for the preservation and protection of spinal cord tissue. The NASCIS trials have shown that this time window may exist in humans. Animal studies have also shown that early decompression can lead to improved neurologic function. However, it is unclear whether surgical decompression in humans would provide a similar time window, if indeed one exists. Studies of class II level evidence have demonstrated that early surgery can be done effectively and safely. To date, there have been no definitive clinical studies that have shown the benefit of early decompression.

Therefore, early decompression for SCI remains only as a surgical option but no stronger recommendations can be made at this time (Table 21C.2). It is hoped that future studies such as STASCIS can help clarify the answer to this important question.

TABLE 21C.2 Evidence-based Recommendations Regarding the Role and Timing of Decompression in Acute Spinal Cord Injury

Level of Recommendation	Class of Evidence	Details
Standards		No standards exist regarding the role and timing of decompression in acute SCI.
Guidelines	II	Early surgery (<72 hours) can be done safely in patients with SCI if they are hemodynamically optimized. Data exist to support a recommendation for urgent reduction of bilateral locked facets in a patient with incomplete tetraplegia. Data exist to support a recommendation for urgent decompression in a patient with SCI experiencing neurologic deterioration.
Options	III	Decompression is a reasonable practice option in acute cervical SCI; when possible (excluding patients with life-threatening multisystem trauma), it is recommended that urgent decompression be performed within 24 hours of SCI. Class III evidence exists that early (<24 hours) surgery reduces length of stay in patients with acute SCI and may reduce postinjury medical complications.

Reproduced with modifications from Fehlings M, Perrin RG. The timing of surgical intervention in the management of spinal cord injury: a systematic review of recent clinical evidence. *Spine* 2006;31:S28–S35, with permission.

REFERENCES

1. DeVivo MJ. Causes and costs of spinal cord injury in the United States. *Spinal Cord* 1997;35:809–813.
2. Kraus JF, Franti CF, Riggins RS, et al. Incidence of traumatic spinal cord lesions. *J Chronic Dis* 1975;28:471–492.
3. Sekhon LH, Fehlings MG. Epidemiology, demographics, and pathophysiology of acute spinal cord injury. *Spine* 2001;26:S2–S12.
4. Tator CH, Duncan EG, Edmonds VE, et al. Neurological recovery, mortality and length of stay after acute spinal cord injury associated with changes in management. *Paraplegia* 1995;33:254–262.
5. Povlishock JT, Christman CW. The pathobiology of traumatically induced axonal injury in animals and humans: a review of current thoughts. *J Neurotrauma* 1995;12:555–564.
6. Tator CH, Fehlings MG. Review of the secondary injury theory of acute spinal cord trauma with emphasis on vascular mechanisms. *J Neurosurg* 1991;75:15–26.
7. Bracken MB, Shephard MJ, Collins WF, et al. A randomized, controlled trial of methylprednisolone or naloxone in the treatment of acute spinal-cord injury: results of the Second National Acute Spinal Cord Injury Study. *N Engl J Med* 1990;322:1405–1411.
8. Bracken MB, Shephard MH, Holford TR, et al. Administration of methylprednisolone for 24 or 48 hours or tirilazad mesylate for 48 hours in the treatment of acute spinal cord injury: results of the Third National Acute Spinal Cord Injury Randomized Controlled Trial. National Acute Spinal Cord Injury Study. *JAMA* 1997; 277:1597–1604.
9. Fehlings MG, Perrin RG. The role and timing of early decompression for cervical spinal cord injury: update with a review of recent clinical evidence. *Injury* 2005;36(suppl 2):B13–B26.
10. Fehlings M, Perrin RG. The timing of surgical intervention in the management of spinal cord injury: a systematic review of recent clinical evidence. *Spine* 2006;31:S28–S35.
11. Fehlings MG, Tator CH. An evidence-based review of decompressive surgery in acute spinal cord injury: rationale, indications, and timing based on experimental and clinical studies. *J Neurosurg* 1999;91:1–11.
12. Fehlings MG, Sekhon LHS, Tator C, et al. The role and timing of decompression in acute spinal cord injury: what do we know? What should we do? *Spine* 2001;26:S101–S110.
13. Tator CH, Fehlings M, Thorpe K, et al. Current use and timing of spinal surgery for management of acute spinal surgery for management of acute spinal cord injury in North America: results of a retrospective multicenter study. *J Neurosurg* 1999;91:12–18.
14. Brodkey JS, Richards DE, Blasingame JP, et al. Reversible spinal cord trauma in cats: additive effects of direct pressure and ischemia. *J Neurosurg* 1972;37:591–593.
15. Carlson GD, Gorden CD, Oliff HS, et al. Sustained spinal cord compression. I: Time-dependent effect on long-term pathophysiology. *J Bone Joint Surg Am* 2003;85:86–94.
16. Dimar JR 2nd, Glassman SD, Raque GH, et al. The influence of spinal canal narrowing and timing of decompression on neurologic recovery after spinal cord contusion in a rat model. *Spine* 1999;24:1623–1633.
17. Kobrine AI, Evans DE, Rizzoli HV, et al. Experimental acute balloon compression of the spinal cord: factors affecting disappearance and return of the spinal evoked response. *J Neurosurg* 1979;51:841–845.
19. Bedbrook GM. Spinal injuries with tetraplegia and paraplegia. *J Bone Joint Surg Br* 1979;61:267–284.
20. Bedbrook GM, Sedgley GI. The management of spinal injuries: past and present. *Int Rehabil Med* 1980;2:45–61.
21. Bedbrook GM, Sakae T. A review of cervical spine injuries with neurological dysfunction. *Paraplegia* 1982;20: 321–333.
22. Collins WF. A review and update of experiment and clinical studies of spinal cord injury. *Paraplegia* 2003;21: 204–219.
23. Frankel HL, Hancock DO, Hyslop G, et al. The value of postural reduction in the initial management of closed injuries of the spine with paraplegia and tetraplegia. I. *Paraplegia* 1969;7:179–192.
24. Katoh S, El-Masry WS, Jaffray D, et al. Neurologic outcome in conservatively treated patients with incomplete closed traumatic cervical spinal cord injuries. *Spine* 1996;21:2345–2351.
25. Ng WP, Fehlings MG, Cuddy B, et al. Surgical treatment for acute spinal cord injury study pilot study #2: evaluation of protocol for decompressive surgery within 8 hours of injury. *Neurosurg Focus* 1999;6:3.
26. Papadopoulos SM, Selden NR, Quint DJ, et al. Immediate spinal cord decompression for cervical spinal cord injury: feasibility and outcome. *J Trauma* 2002;52:323–332.
27. Waters RL, Meyers PR, Adkins RH, et al. Emergency, acute, and surgical management of spine trauma. *Arch Phys Med Rehabil* 1999;80:1383–1390.
28. Tator CH, Duncan EG, Edmonds VE, et al. Comparison of surgical and conservative management in 208 patients with acute spinal cord injury. *Can J Neurol Sci* 1987;14:60–69.
29. Vaccaro AR, Daugherty RJ, Sheehan TP, et al. Neurologic outcome of early versus late surgery for cervical spinal cord injury. *Spine* 1997;22:2609–2613.
30. Duh MS, Shephard MJ, Wilberger JE, et al. The effectiveness of surgery on the treatment of acute spinal cord injury and its relation to pharmacological treatment. *Neurosurgery* 1994;35:240–248, discussion 248–249.

31. Pointillart V, Dixmerias F, Wiart L, et al. Pharmacological therapy of spinal cord injury during the acute phase. *Spinal Cord* 2000;38:71–76.
32. Aebi M, Zuber K, Marchesi D, et al. Indication, surgical technique, and results of 100 surgically-treated fractures and fracture-dislocations of the cervical spine. *Clin Orthop Relat Res* 1986;203:244–257.
33. Burke DC, Berryman D. The place of closed manipulation in the management of flexion-rotation dislocations of the cervical spine. *J Bone Joint Surg Br* 1971;53:165–182.
34. La Rosa G, Conti A, Cardali S, et al. Does early decompression improve neurological outcome of spinal cord injured patients? Appraisal of the literature using a meta-analytical approach. *Spinal Cord* 2004;42:503–512.
35. Larson SJ, Holst RA, Hemmy DC, et al. Lateral extracavitary approach to traumatic lesions of the thoracic and lumbar spine. *J Neurosurg* 1976;45:628–637.
36. Marshall LF, Knowlton S, Garfin SR, et al. Deterioration following spinal cord injury: a multicenter study. *J Neurosurg* 1987;66:400–404.
37. Anderson PA, Bohlman HH. Anterior decompression and arthrodesis of the cervical spine: long-term motor improvement. II: Improvement in complete traumatic quadriplegia. *J Bone Joint Surg Am* 1992;74:683–692.
38. Bohlman HH, Anderson PA. Anterior decompression and arthrodesis of the cervical spine: long-term motor improvement. II: Improvement in incomplete traumatic quadriparesis. *J Bone Joint Surg Am* 1992;74:671–682.
39. Brodkey JS, Miller CF Jr, Harmody RM, et al. The syndrome of acute central cervical spinal cord injury revisited. *Surg Neurol* 1980;14:251–257.
40. Transfeldt EE, White D, Bradford DS, et al. Delayed anterior decompression in patients with spinal cord and cauda equina injuries of the thoracolumbar spine. *Spine* 1990;15:953–957.

CHAPTER 21D

Spinal Cord Injury and Pathophysiology: Pharmacotherapy for Spinal Cord Injury

Steven Casha, Joseph Silvaggio, and R. John Hurlbert

INTRODUCTION

The pharmacologic management of acute spinal cord injury (ASCI) remains the source of significant controversy. Optimism that a greater understanding of the pathogenesis of ASCI would lead to effective pharmacologic treatment strategies, aimed at mitigating secondary injury, has been met with disappointment in the clinical arena. In March 2002, the American Association of Neurological Surgeons/Congress of Neurological Surgeons Joint Section on Disorders of the Spine and Peripheral Nerves, with the collaboration of the Joint Section on Trauma, published the *Guidelines for the Management of Acute Cervical Spine and Spinal Cord Injury*. The document, representing enormous effort and collaboration, was generally well accepted and praised. Clearly, however, the most controversial chapter dealt with pharmacologic therapy after acute cervical SCI. The prechapter editor's comment, advising readers to "carefully review the available data and comments . . . to establish their own perspective on this evolving matter," demonstrates the controversial and politically sensitive nature of this topic. In this chapter the various pharmacologic agents that have been investigated in the treatment of human ASCI are reviewed, focusing on evidence for their use. The wealth of animal studies that have not reached clinical investigation, as well as treatment strategies aimed at neuroaugmentation and neuroregeneration (recently reviewed[1]), are beyond the scope of this discussion.

METHYLPREDNISOLONE

Steroids have been anecdotally administered to patients with ASCI for many years and in various forms and dosages. However, following publication of the NASCIS II results, a degree of scientific credibility became associated with methylprednisolone administration that very quickly led many centers to adopt it as a standard of care. However, independent reevaluation of the published NASCIS results consistently suggests that this reputation was not deserved.[2–5] Indeed, a recent survey of Canadian Spinal Surgeons confirms that only 17% prescribe methylprednisolone because they believe it has a therapeutic benefit and 83% prescribe it because of peer pressure or for fear of litigation.[6]

TABLE 21D.1 Level of Evidence for Clinical Studies Using Steroids for Spinal Cord Injury

Author	Year	Design	Level	Agent	Result*
Bracken et al.[86] (NASCIS I)	1984	Prospective, randomized, double-blind	I	Methylprednisolone	Negative
Bracken et al.[8,9] (NASCIS II)	1990 1992	Prospective, randomized, double-blind	I	Methylprednisolone	Positive
Bracken et al.[10,11] (NASCIS III)	1997 1998	Prospective, randomized, double-blind	I	Methylprednisolone/ tirilazad	Positive
Otani et al.[12]	1994	Prospective, randomized, no blinding	I	Methylprednisolone	Positive
Pointillart et al.[64]	2000	Prospective, randomized, blinded	I	Methylprednisolone/ nimodipine	Negative
Kiwerski[13]	1993	Retrospective, concurrent case control	II-2	Dexamethasone	Positive
Poynton et al.[84]	1997	Retrospective, concurrent case control	II-2	Methylprednisolone	Negative
George et al.[83]	1995	Retrospective, historical case control	II-3	Methylprednisolone	Negative
Gerhart et al.[82]	1995	Retrospective, historical case control	II-3	Methylprednisolone	Negative
Prendergast et al.[85]	1994	Retrospective, historical case control	II-3	Methylprednisolone	Negative

*As reported by the authors.

Several published studies besides the NASICS trials have attempted to establish the usefulness of steroids in ASCI. They are summarized in tabular form and ranked by level of evidence in Table 21D.1. Briefly, level I evidence is gained through prospective randomized trials. Level II evidence arises from prospective nonrandomized trials or retrospective studies that make use of concurrent or historical case controls. Level III evidence is gained from descriptive uncontrolled studies or through expert opinion.[7] Level I evidence is generally required to establish a treatment as a "standard of care," level II evidence defines a treatment as "recommended," and level III evidence generally supports the treatment as a therapeutic "option." However, despite the rigorous structure of this classification, proper weighting can become problematic because of flaws in data harvesting, reporting, or analyses that are independent of trial design.[4]

NASCIS II AND III

Results of NASCIS II and III form the highest level of evidence arguing for the use of methylprednisolone in ASCI.[8–11] The 6-month data were released initially for each study, followed by publication of the 12-month data under separate cover. Both trials were well designed and executed. Patient follow-up was meticulous. Without dispute, the primary analyses looking for a steroid treatment effect was negative in both studies. Only post-hoc analyses revealed potential and admittedly minor treatment effects on motor scores at 1 year and when therapy was initiated within 8 and 3 to 8 hours for NASCIS II and III, respectively (Fig. 21D.1). Statistical testing probability was slightly greater than 0.05 for 1-year motor scores in the NASCIS III 48-hour steroid group (mean change in motor score 19, $p = 0.053$). If we are to accept this as a significant finding however, we must also accept

TABLE 21D.2 Level of Evidence for Clinical Studies Using Nonsteroid Medications for Spinal Cord Injury

Author	Year	Design	Level	Agent	Result*
Geisler et al.[20]	1991	Prospective, randomized, double-blind	I	GM-1 ganglioside	Positive
Geisler et al.[21]	2001	Prospective, randomized, double-blind	I	GM-1 ganglioside	Negative
Bracken et al.[8] (NASCIS II)	1990 1992	Prospective, randomized, double-blind	I	Naloxone	Negative
Flamm et al.[44]	1985	Prospective feasibility/ safety study	III	Naloxone	N/A
Pitts et al.[45]	1995	Prospective, randomized, double-blind	I	Thyrotropin-releasing hormone	Positive
Tadié et al.[55] (abstract only)	1999	Prospective, randomized, double-blind	†	Gacyclidine	Negative
Pointillart et al.[64]	2000	Prospective, randomized, blinded	I	Nimodipine	Negative

*As reported by the authors

†To our knowledge, this study has not been published in the peer-reviewed literature and has only been presented in abstract form. Therefore, level of evidence is not assigned.

that this treatment increased mortality resulting from respiratory failure with a comparable $p = 0.056$ (0.6% and 3.6% incidence for 24- and 48-hour methylprednisolone treatment, respectively). None of the sensory scores were different between treatment groups in either study.

Several questions remain unanswered about the post-hoc analyses of NASCIS II and III, casting serious doubt that even a small benefit might be provided to SCI patients by methylprednisolone

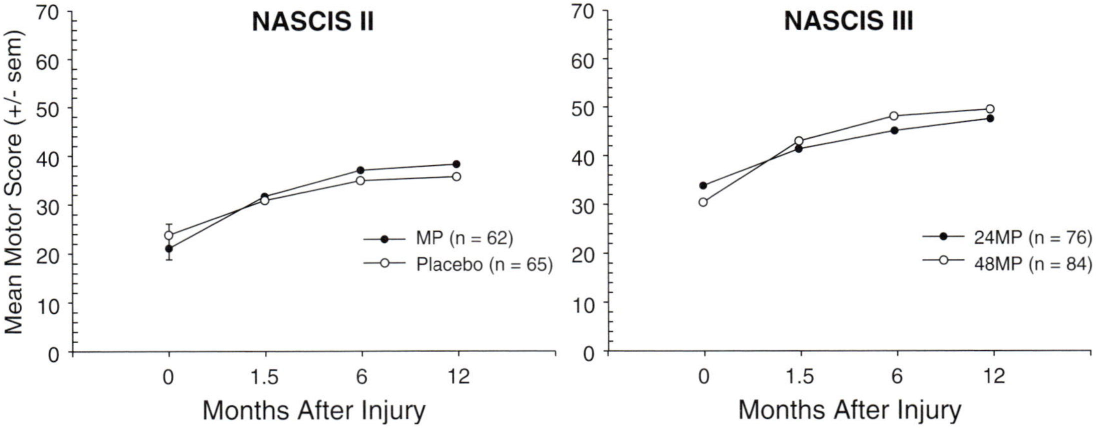

FIGURE 21D.1. Summary of positive post-hoc results reported in the NASCIS II and NASCIS III trials. No differences were observed in any primary outcome measures. Post-hoc sensory scores were no different among treatment groups. Only relative improvement in motor score was reported as significantly improved in 24-hour MP patients (NASCIS II) and 48-hour MP patients (NASCIS III) at 12 months. Although reported as statistically significant, the actual differences observed between treatment and control groups are not compelling.

administration. The left-sided motor scores were never published but reported as "similar." Right-sided scores were reported representing only half the available data. No attempt was made to correct for multiple statistical comparisons. More than 65 *t*-tests were performed in NASCIS II and more than 100 *t*-tests in NASCIS III (ignoring naloxone and tirilazad comparisons). Hence, the likelihood of encountering statistical significance through random chance alone is high (type 1 error). Furthermore, the rationale behind an 8-hour subanalysis in NASCIS II is uncertain. It has been claimed that the post-hoc 8-hour therapeutic window for steroid administration was based on median time to treatment. Analysis of a true median time to treatment (8.5 hours) should assign 50% of patients (244 of 487) before cutoff and 50% after. However within the 8-hour window, only 38% of patients (183 of 487) were included in the post-hoc analysis, thereby excluding well over half the randomized patients. Similarly, the justification of a 3- to 8-hour window in NASCIS III is obscure. Finally, improvement in function meaningful to the patient was not documented in either study.

OTHER EVIDENCE

In 1994, Otani et al.[12] published a prospective trial investigating methylprednisolone administration using the NASCIS II dosing regimen. Although the trial was randomized, the investigators were not blinded to treatment. In addition, the control group was allowed to receive alternative steroids at the physicians' discretion. Of 158 patients entered, 117 were analyzed. Primary outcome measures (American Spinal Injury Association [ASIA] motor and sensory scores) were not different between treatment groups. Post-hoc analyses suggested that more patients improved on the NASCIS II steroid regimen than did controls. However, these analyses ignored the fact that for a greater number of steroid-treated patients to improve, the fewer control patients who also improved must have demonstrated a larger magnitude of recovery (because overall change in ASIA motor and sensory score were no different between groups). Thus on closer inspection, such post-hoc analyses become conflicting and therefore meaningless.

The only other study claiming to demonstrate a benefit to steroid administration was a retrospective study with concurrent case controls from Poland, published in 1993.[13] The dose of dexamethasone was left up to the discretion of the attending physician. Treatment was instituted within 24 hours of injury. Length of follow-up was not specified. A novel but unvalidated neurologic grading system was used for assessment. The author reported that the percentage of patients improved was significantly higher in the steroid-treated group compared to controls. However, closer examination of the data demonstrated higher mortality rates within the control group, suggesting this group may have been more severely injured and perhaps subject to selection bias (Fig. 21D.2). The magnitude of the mortality rates themselves is cause for concern.

In summary, there exists no level I evidence to suggest that methylprednisolone or any other steroid is beneficial in the treatment of ASCI. Weak post-hoc analyses are proposed to show a small effect on motor function in the three level I trials. However, all of these analyses contain significant flaws, rendering conclusions of efficacy dubious. Furthermore, there is no compelling level II or level III evidence further supporting the role of methylprednisolone in ASCI. These observations have led two national organizations to classify methylprednisolone administration as a treatment option rather than as a standard of care or recommended treatment.[14,15]

GANGLIOSIDES

Gangliosides are sialic acid–containing glycophosphosphingolipids found in high concentration in the outer cell membranes of central nervous system cells, especially in the vicinity of synapses. Although their exact function is unknown, they appear to play a role in neural development and plasticity. The proposed mechanisms of action of exogenously administered gangliosides include antiexcitotoxic activities, prevention of apoptosis, augmentation of neurite outgrowth, and induction of neuronal sprouting and regeneration.[16–19]

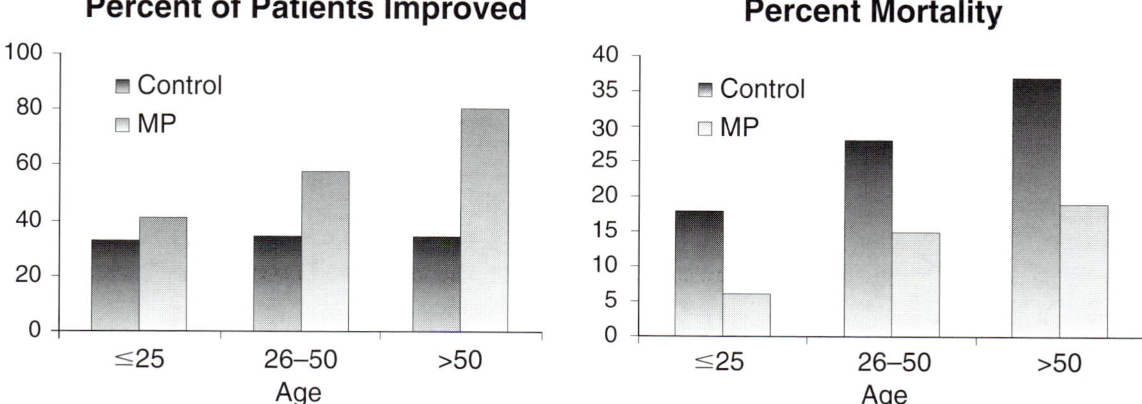

FIGURE 21D.2. Graphical representation of Kiwerski data demonstrating that more patients in the steroid-treated group improved neurologically compared to controls. However, when one examines mortality data, approximately twice as many patients in the control group died. The results suggest that the control group was more seriously injured than the steroid-treated group. In addition, the high mortality rates observed overall suggest that the study population may not be representative and the results not generalizable.

GM-1 ganglioside has been evaluated in both animal and human studies of ASCI. In 1991, the first of two prospective randomized placebo-controlled trials studying the efficacy of GM-1 ganglioside in the treatment of ASCI was published.[20] Thirty-seven patients were enrolled, and 1-year follow-up was available for 34 patients. All patients received a 250-mg bolus of methylprednisolone, followed by 125 mg every 6 hours for 72 hours. Patients were administered 100 mg intravenous GM-1 ganglioside or placebo daily for 18 to 32 days, with the first dose given within 72 hours of injury. Neurologic recovery was assessed using the Frankel scale and the ASIA motor score. The authors reported a significant difference between groups with improvement of Frankel grades from baseline at 1 year ($p = 0.034$). The GM-1–treated patients also had a significantly greater mean improvement in ASIA motor score from baseline to 1-year follow-up than the placebo-treated patients ($p = 0.047$). When recovery of individual muscles was analyzed, the increased recovery in the GM-1–treated group was attributed to recovery of useful strength in initially paralyzed muscle groups, rather than to strengthening of paretic muscles. There were no reported adverse effects attributed to the administration of the study drug. The authors concluded that their small study provided evidence that GM-1 enhances recovery of neurologic function 1 year after ASCI in humans. They recommended a larger study examining the safety and efficacy of GM-1 in ASCI.

In 1992, a larger GM-1 ganglioside ASCI study was initiated.[21] The study was designed as a prospective, multicenter, double-blind, randomized trial. When the study was closed in 1997, 797 patients had been enrolled. All patients received methylprednisolone according to NASCIS II protocol. Patients were randomized into three groups: (a) placebo, (b) low-dose GM-1 (300-mg loading dose then 100 mg/day for 56 days), (c) and high-dose GM-1 (600-mg loading dose then 200 mg/day for 56 days). Study medication (placebo or GM-1) was initiated at the completion of the 23-hour methylprednisolone infusion. Clinical outcomes were assessed using the modified Benzel Classification and the ASIA motor and sensory examinations at 4, 8, 16, 26, and 52 weeks after injury. The primary efficacy assessment was the proportion of patients who demonstrated marked improvement (at least two grades of the modified Benzel score) from baseline, at week 26 of the study. Secondary outcomes included timing of recovery, the ASIA motor score and the ASIA sensory evaluations, relative and absolute sensory levels of impairment, and assessments of bladder and bowel function. A planned interim evaluation after the first 180 patients resulted in discontinuation of the high-dose treatment strategy because of an early trend toward higher mortality. At the conclusion of the study, 760 patients remained for primary efficacy analysis. The results of the trial were published in 2001.[21] The authors found no significant difference in mortality between the groups. The GM-1–treated group did not have a significantly higher proportion of patients with marked recovery at 26 weeks compared to placebo-treated patients. The time course of recovery suggested earlier attainment of marked recovery in GM-1–treated patients, regardless of baseline severity. The authors also reported that there was a large, consistent, and, at some points, significant effect in the primary outcome in the subgroup of nonoperated patients through week 26. The ASIA motor, light touch, and pin-prick scores showed a consistent trend in favor of GM-1, as did bladder function, bowel function sacral sensation, and anal contraction. The authors concluded that despite the lack of statistical significance in the primary analysis, numerous positive secondary analyses indicate that GM-1 ganglioside may be a useful drug in the management of severe ASCI.

In summary, the available evidence does not support a significant, lasting, clinical benefit from the administration of GM-1 ganglioside in the treatment of patients after ASCI. Two North American randomized controlled trials have been completed.[20,21] Improvement in neurologic recovery with the administration of GM-1 ganglioside following ASCI has been suggested but not convincingly proven.

OPIATE ANTAGONISTS

Shock and microcirculatory collapse are thought to negatively influence SCI by adding an ischemic insult to the spinal cord. Hypovolemic and spinal shock syndromes in the polytrauma patient as well as microcirculatory collapse contribute to this phenomenon. Opiate receptor antagonists and physiologic opiate antagonists improve blood pressure and survival following traumatic shock.[22] Furthermore, animal studies have demonstrated release of endogenous opioid peptides after ASCI.[23,24] Dynorphin, through the kappa opioid receptor, decreases microcirculatory blood flow in the spinal cord and may contribute directly to neurotoxicity, possibly through the N-methyl-D-aspartate (NMDA) receptor.[25–27] These observations have led to exploration of the role of opioid antagonists in neuroprotection after ASCI. Three agents have shown neuroprotective effects in animal models: naloxone, nalmefene, and thyrotropin-releasing hormone (TRH).[23,28–28] Conversely, however, some studies of naloxone have failed to show neuroprotection.[39–42]

In human studies, naloxone was included as one of the treatment arms in NASCIS II.[8] The 154-patient naloxone group was given a 5.4-mg/kg bolus followed by a 23-hour, 4-mg/kg per hour infusion and compared to the 171-patient placebo group. Motor and sensory functions were assessed by systematic neurologic examination on admission and 6 weeks and 6 months after injury. This study failed to demonstrate a therapeutic benefit.[8,9] Subsequent post-hoc reanalysis indicated that although there was no effect on neurologic recovery at the level of the lesion, there was an effect on long tract recovery when naloxone was administered within 8 hours of injury, suggesting that this effect may warrant further study.[43]

Flamm et al.[44] conducted a phase I study of naloxone in ASCI before the NASCIS II investigation. Two groups were included in the study. A group of 20 patients received a low dose of naloxone (0.14 to 1.43 mg/kg loading followed by 20% of loading 47-hour infusion), whereas the other group of 9 patients received a high dose (2.7 to 5.4 mg/kg loading dose followed by 75% of loading 23-hour infusion). The study was designed with an escalating dose because patients were enrolled so as to explore safety and feasibility of the medication over a dose range. The high- and low-dose groups also differed in that more patients in the low-dose group had complete injuries (85% versus 44%) and initiated their treatment later (average 12.9 hours versus 6.6 hours). The low-dose group showed no improvement in neurologic examination or somatosensory evoked potentials (SSEPs). In the high-dose group a small number of patients demonstrated neurologic improvement and improvement in SSEPs, which was sustained and progressive months later. This study was designed as a phase I study and as such did not have the appropriate placebo group or statistical power to examine drug efficacy. The observed improvements were encouraging but not statistically validated. The authors were able to show that the high doses of naloxone indicated by animal studies of ASCI would be tolerated clinically with minimal side effects.

TRH has been the subject of one human study.[45] Twenty patients with ASCI subclassified as complete and incomplete injury were administered TRH (0.2-mg/kg bolus followed by 0.2 mg/kg per hour 6-hour infusion) or placebo within 12 hours of injury. No discernible treatment effect was found in patients with complete injuries (6 patients), whereas at 4 months, in the incomplete injury subgroup (11 patients), TRH treatment was associated with significantly higher motor and sensory recovery and Sunnybrook Cord Injury Scale scores. The small sample size in this study led the authors to recommend caution in interpreting their statistical evaluation, and they were unwilling to confidently dismiss the null hypothesis.

In summary, to date, opioid receptor antagonism has shown experimental promise but the limited human trials do not support the role in the current management of ASCI. Three human studies have been conducted that have produced preliminary evidence supporting further study. Some animal studies have suggested a bell-shaped efficacy curve for naloxone, necessitating further determination of optimal dosing before definitive human randomized placebo control studies.[32]

EXCITATORY AMINO ACID RECEPTOR ANTAGONISTS

Excitotoxicity has been a key biochemical process implicated in secondary injury following ASCI. Animal evidence points to an increase in extracellular glutamate and aspartate after injury,[46,47] leading to toxicity of both neurons and glia through ligand gated ionotropic receptors, as well as G-protein coupled metabotropic receptors.[48–52] Inhibition of these mechanisms in rodents has resulted in improved behavioral and histologic outcomes.[48,53,54] However, the application of these observations to clinical studies has been difficult. Glutamate is a ubiquitous excitatory neurotransmitter in the central nervous system, and as such its inhibition is fraught with adverse reactions. Furthermore, the rise in excitatory amino acids seen after injury occurs early and is transient (likely complete within 2 hours), suggesting that the therapeutic window is small.[46]

To date, one clinical study of the compound gacyclidine, an inhibitor of NMDA-type ionotropic glutamate receptors, failed to show efficacy.[55,56] This study succeeded in enrolling 280 patients with ASCI within 2 hours of injury. Patients received 0.005 mg/kg, 0.01 mg/kg, or 0.02 mg/kg gacyclidine or placebo at randomization and 4 hours later. Although the 1-month data showed a nonsignificant trend to better outcome in the high-dose group, this effect was not sustained at 1 year.[55] Of the patient group, 72% suffered complete injuries. There was a suggestion in the data of a more promising effect in the incomplete-injury group.

Thus, amino acid excitotoxicity has long been established as a key secondary injury mechanism following neural trauma. Animal data suggest that inhibitors are likely to be efficacious in the treatment of ASCI; however, the therapeutic window after injury may be very short. A single human study has been completed, which did not show efficacy.

CALCIUM CHANNEL BLOCKERS

Dysregulation of calcium homeostasis and in particular rise in cytoplasmic calcium is thought to be an event common to many pathways leading to cell death.[57] Calcium is frequently employed by the cell for intracellular signaling and enzyme regulation. A host of calcium-dependant proteases, nucleases, and lipases have been identified, which together with other less directly calcium-regulated cellular events (e.g., increased free radical production) contribute to cellular demise after injury.[57] In the setting of neural trauma, calcium channel blockers may have a direct effect in ameliorating these calcium fluxes and thus decreasing cell death. In addition, they may also be effective through vascular smooth muscle by decreasing injury-induced vasospasm. This potentially advantageous effect on spinal cord perfusion must be balanced with the potential hypotensive effect caused by peripheral vascular dilatation seen with these drugs. In animal models, calcium channel blockade has been neuroprotective[58–61] and has been shown to increase posttraumatic spinal blood flow.[62,63]

In human SCI a single randomized placebo controlled trail of the calcium channel blocker nimodepine has been published.[64,65] A total of 106 patients with ASCI were administered methylprednisolone (NASCIS II protocol), nimodipine (0.015 mg/kg per hour for 2 hours, followed by 0.03 mg/kg per hour for 7 days), both agents, or placebo. No difference in blinded neurologic recovery (ASIA score) was found among these groups at 1 year.

Thus, to date, cellular calcium fluxes are thought to be a key event in secondary injury after neural trauma and remain a popular topic in the scientific literature. However, the application of calcium channel antagonists to human SCI has been limited to a single study, which did not show efficacy.

ANTIOXIDANTS AND FREE RADICAL SCAVENGERS

Following neural trauma, several conditions promote formation of free radicals. Increased cytosolic calcium induces several free radical–producing pathways, including xanthane oxidase, nitrous oxide synthetase, and the phospholipase A2–cyclooxygenase pathway.[66] Free radicals (superoxide) are also produced through the Fe^{2+}-dependent Fenton and Haber-Weiss reactions.[66] Alterations in the inner mitochondrial membrane proteins (removal, release, or inactivation) may reduce the efficiency of the electron transport chain, leading to increased production of superoxide radical.[66,67] Activated inflammatory cells yield reactive oxygen species.[66] The resultant increased production of free radicals overwhelms the cell's free radical scavenging systems (e.g., superoxide dismutases—catalases, glutathione, ascorbic acid) leading to oxidation of lipids, proteins, and nucleic acids. This in turn may lead to cell death.[68]

Several animal studies provide good evidence for the involvement of free radicals and peroxidation reactions in the pathophysiology of ASCI. Studies have demonstrated increases in specific free radicals,[69–72] evidence of increased macromolecular oxidation after,[70,73–75] and evidence that free radical scavenging compounds, decreased free radical production, and increased free radical scavenging are neuroprotective.[70,76–80]

In human studies, the mechanism of action of methylprednisolone, which was the subject of the NASCIS studies, likely includes inhibition of peroxidation reactions. As discussed earlier, these studies have not shown conclusively that this agent is useful in the treatment of ASCI. Tirilazad mesylate is believed to inhibit iron-dependent lipid peroxidation in central nervous system tissue and was also included in the NASCIS III investigation.[81] In the tirilazad group, 166 patients received a 2.5-mg/kg bolus infusion every 6 hours for 48 hours after their 30-mg/kg methylprednisolone bolus (administered before randomization). When compared with the control group in this study, which received methylprednisolone 5.4 mg/kg per hour for 24 hours, no difference in motor recovery was found.[10,11] This study indicates that tirilazad mesylate is equally effective as methylprednisolone in the treatment of ASCI. Given the lack of conclusion regarding the role of methylprednisolone (as discussed previously), the role of both of these agents in the treatment of ASCI will require further scrutiny.

In summary, although macromolecular peroxidation likely contributes to cell death and neurologic dysfunction, as supported by animal studies in ASCI, the human data to date on methylprednisolone and tirilazad mesylate, which are believed to decrease peroxidation, do not support conclusively their use in the treatment of ASCI.

CONCLUSION

From the generally accepted injury model of SCI stems the hypothesis that amelioration of either primary or secondary injury mechanisms will decrease tissue damage in the spinal cord and lead to improved neurologic outcome. Animal studies addressing the large array of secondary injury mechanisms have significantly improved our understanding of these phenomena and have yielded encouraging behavioral and histologic results. Some of this basic research has been successfully translated into human clinical trials through admirably complex protocols in multiple centers. Unfortunately, the results of these studies to date, although encouraging, have not yielded any clearly effective therapies for the treatment of ASCI.

It is reasonable to expect that manipulation of a single pathway in the large milieu of secondary injury mechanisms will have only a small overall effect in a system as complex as the central nervous system. Ultimately, a treatment strategy of multiple agents with broad specificity will likely evolve from our present efforts. The task of proving efficacy in human ASCI is made more difficult by the reality that the injury is heterogeneous, unlike the uniform injury of animal models used in the laboratory. Interventions shown to be efficacious in animals may produce similar effects in human tissue, but perhaps on a scale too small to measure with the crude clinical tools presently available. Nonetheless, the encouraging results and broad scope of activities in animal models combined with a now well-established track record in the execution of complex clinical trials secures an exciting arena in which the goal of effective pharmacologic strategies in ASCI will ultimately be achieved.

REFERENCES

1. Deumens R, Koopmans GC, Joosten EA. Regeneration of descending axon tracts after spinal cord injury. *Prog Neurobiol* 2005;77:57–89.
2. Nesathurai S. Steroids and spinal cord injury: revisiting the NASCIS 2 and NASCIS 3 trials. *J Trauma* 1998;45:1088–1093.
3. Coleman WP, Benzel D, Cahill DW, et al. A critical appraisal of the reporting of the National Acute Spinal Cord Injury Studies (II and III) of methylprednisolone in acute spinal cord injury. *J Spinal Disord* 2000;13:185–199.
4. Hurlbert RJ. Methylprednisolone for acute spinal cord injury: an inappropriate standard of care. *J Neurosurg* 2000;93:1–7.
5. Short DJ, El Masry WS, Jones PW. High dose methylprednisolone in the management of acute spinal cord injury: a systematic review from a clinical perspective. *Spinal Cord* 2000;38:273–286.
6. Hurlbert RJ, Moulton R. Why do you prescribe methylprednisolone for acute spinal cord injury? A Canadian perspective and a position statement. *Can J Neurol Sci* 2002;29:236–239.
7. Woolf SH, Battista RN, Anderson GM, et al. Assessing the clinical effectiveness of preventive maneuvers: analytic principles and systematic methods in reviewing evidence and developing clinical practice recommendations: a report by the Canadian Task Force on the Periodic Health Examination. *J Clin Epidemiol* 1990;43:891–905.
8. Bracken MB, Shephard MJ, Collins WF, et al. A randomized, controlled trial of methylprednisolone or naloxone in the treatment of acute spinal-cord injury: results of the Second National Acute Spinal Cord Injury Study. *N Engl J Med* 1990;322:1405–1411.
9. Bracken MB, Shephard MJ, Collins WF, et al. Methylprednisolone or naloxone treatment after acute spinal cord injury: 1-year follow-up data—results of the second National Acute Spinal Cord Injury Study. *J Neurosurg* 1992;76:23–31.
10. Bracken MB, Shephard MJ, Holford TR, et al. Administration of methylprednisolone for 24 or 48 hours or tirilazad mesylate for 48 hours in the treatment of acute spinal cord injury: results of the Third National Acute Spinal Cord Injury Randomized Controlled Trial. National Acute Spinal Cord Injury Study. *JAMA* 1997;277:1597–1604.
11. Bracken MB, Shephard MJ, Hellenbrand KG, et al. Methylprednisolone or tirilazad mesylate administration after acute spinal cord injury: 1-year follow up: results of the third National Acute Spinal Cord Injury randomized controlled trial. *J Neurosurg* 1998;89:699–706.
12. Otani K, Abe H, Kadoya S. Beneficial effect of methylprednisolone sodium succinate in the treatment of acute spinal cord injury. *Sekitsui Sekizui J* 1994;7:633–647.
13. Kiwerski JE. Application of dexamethasone in the treatment of acute spinal cord injury. *Injury* 1993;24:457–460.
14. Hugenholtz H, Cass DE, Dvorack MF, et al. High-dose methylprednisolone for acute closed spinal cord injury: only a treatment option. *Can J Neurol Sci* 2002;29:227–235.
15. Hadley MN, Walters BC. Guidelines for the management of acute cervical spine and spinal cord injuries: pharmacological therapy after acute cervical spinal cord injury. *Neurosurgery* 2002;50:S63–S72.
16. Zeller CB, Marchase RB. Gangliosides as modulators of cell function. *Am J Physiol* 1992;262:C1341–C1355.
17. Rahmann H. Brain gangliosides and memory formation. *Behav Brain Res* 1995;66:105–116.
18. Sabel BA, Stein DG. Pharmacological treatment of central nervous system injury. *Nature* 1986;323:493.
19. Gorio A. Gangliosides as a possible treatment affecting neuronal repair processes. *Adv Neurol* 1988;47:523–530.
20. Geisler FH, Dorsey FC, Coleman WP. Recovery of motor function after spinal-cord injury: a randomized, placebo-controlled trial with GM-1 ganglioside. *N Engl J Med* 1991;324:1829–1838.
21. Geisler FH, Coleman WP, Grieco G, et al. The Sygen multicenter acute spinal cord injury study. *Spine* 2001; 26:S87–S98.
22. McIntosh TK, Faden AI. Opiate antagonist in traumatic shock. *Ann Emerg Med* 1986;15:1462–1465.
23. Faden AI, Jacobs TP, Mougey E, et al. Endorphins in experimental spinal injury: therapeutic effect of naloxone. *Ann Neurol* 1981;10:326–332.
24. Faden AI, Holaday JW. A role for endorphins in the pathophysiology of spinal cord injury. *Adv Biochem Psychopharmacol* 1981;28:435–446.

25. Winkler T, Sharma T, Gordh RD, et al. Topical application of dynorphin A (1-17) antiserum attenuates trauma induced alterations in spinal cord evoked potentials, microvascular permeability disturbances, edema formation and cell injury: an experimental study in the rat using electrophysiological and morphological approaches. *Amino Acids* 2002;23:273–281.
26. Hauser KF, Knapp PE, Turbek CS. Structure-activity analysis of dynorphin A toxicity in spinal cord neurons: intrinsic neurotoxicity of dynorphin A and its carboxyl-terminal, nonopioid metabolites. *Exp Neurol* 2001;168:78–87.
27. Hu WH, Lee FC, Wan XS, et al. Dynorphin neurotoxicity induced nitric oxide synthase expression in ventral horn cells of rat spinal cord. *Neurosci Lett* 1996;203:13–16.
28. Behrmann DL, Bresnahan JC, Beattie MS. A comparison of YM-14673, U-50488H, and nalmefene after spinal cord injury in the rat. *Exp Neurol* 1993;119:258–267.
29. Benzel EC, Khare V, Fowler MR. Effects of naloxone and nalmefene in rat spinal cord injury induced by the ventral compression technique. *J Spinal Disord* 1992;5:75–77.
30. Akdemir H, Pasaoglu A, Ozturk F, et al. Histopathology of experimental spinal cord trauma: comparison of treatment with TRH, naloxone, and dexamethasone. *Res Exp Med (Berl)* 1992;192:177–183.
31. Hashimoto T, Fukuda N. Effect of thyrotropin-releasing hormone on the neurologic impairment in rats with spinal cord injury: treatment starting 24 h and 7 days after injury. *Eur J Pharmacol* 1991;203:25–32.
32. Benzel EC, Hoffpauir GM, Thomas MM, et al. Dose-dependent effects of naloxone and methylprednisolone in the ventral compression model of spinal cord injury. *J Spinal Disord* 1990;3:339–344.
33. Faden AI, Sacksen I, Noble LJ. Opiate-receptor antagonist nalmefene improves neurological recovery after traumatic spinal cord injury in rats through a central mechanism. *J Pharmacol Exp Ther* 1988;45:742–748.
34. Arias MJ. Treatment of experimental spinal cord injury with TRH, naloxone, and dexamethasone. *Surg Neurol* 1987;28:335–338.
35. Arias MJ. Effect of naloxone on functional recovery after experimental spinal cord injury in the rat. *Surg Neurol* 1985;23:440–442.
36. Flamm ES, Young W, Demopoulos HB, et al. Experimental spinal cord injury: treatment with naloxone. *Neurosurgery* 1982;10:227–231.
37. Faden AI, Jacobs TP, Holaday JW. Opiate antagonist improves neurologic recovery after spinal injury. *Science* 1981;211:493–494.
38. Faden AI, Jacobs TP, Holaday JW. Thyrotropin-releasing hormone improves neurologic recovery after spinal trauma in cats. *N Engl J Med* 1981;305:1063–1067.
39. Black P, Markowitz RS, Gillespie JA, et al. Naloxone and experimental spinal cord injury: effect of varying dose and intensity of injury. *J Neurotrauma* 1991;8:157–171.
40. Black P, Markowitz RS, Keller S, et al. Naloxone and experimental spinal cord injury. II: Megadose treatment in a dynamic load injury model. *Neurosurgery* 1986;19:909–913.
41. Black P, et al. Naloxone and experimental spinal cord injury. I: High dose administration in a static load compression model. *Neurosurgery* 1986;19:905–908.
42. Wallace MC, Tator CH. Failure of blood transfusion or naloxone to improve clinical recovery after experimental spinal cord injury. *Neurosurgery* 1986;19:489–494.
43. Bracken MB, Holford TR. Effects of timing of methylprednisolone or naloxone administration on recovery of segmental and long-tract neurological function in NASCIS 2. *J Neurosurg* 1993;79:500–507.
44. Flamm ES, et al. A phase I trial of naloxone treatment in acute spinal cord injury. *J Neurosurg* 1985;63:390–397.
45. Pitts LH, Ross A, Chase GA, et al. Treatment with thyrotropin-releasing hormone (TRH) in patients with traumatic spinal cord injuries. *J Neurotrauma* 1995;12:235–243.
46. Farooque M, Hillered L, Holtz A, et al. Changes of extracellular levels of amino acids after graded compression trauma to the spinal cord: an experimental study in the rat using microdialysis. *J Neurotrauma* 1996;13:537–548.
47. Panter SS, Yum SW, Faden AI. Alteration in extracellular amino acids after traumatic spinal cord injury. *Ann Neurol* 1990;27:96–99.
48. Mills CD, Johnson KM, Hulsebosch CE. Group I metabotropic glutamate receptors in spinal cord injury: roles in neuroprotection and the development of chronic central pain. *J Neurotrauma* 2002;19:23–42.
49. Liu D, Xu GY, Pan E, et al. Neurotoxicity of glutamate at the concentration released upon spinal cord injury. *Neuroscience* 1999;93:1383–1389.
50. Liu D. An experimental model combining microdialysis with electrophysiology, histology, and neurochemistry for studying excitotoxicity in spinal cord injury: effect of NMDA and kainate. *Mol Chem Neuropathol* 1994;23:77–92.
51. Agrawal SK, Fehlings MG. Role of NMDA and non-NMDA ionotropic glutamate receptors in traumatic spinal cord axonal injury. *J Neurosci* 1997;17:1055–1063.
52. Agrawal SK, Theriault E, Fehlings MG. Role of group I metabotropic glutamate receptors in traumatic spinal cord white matter injury. *J Neurotrauma* 1998;15:929–941.
53. Lang-Lazdunski L, Heurteaux C, Vaillant N, et al. Riluzole prevents ischemic spinal cord injury caused by aortic crossclamping. *J Thorac Cardiovasc Surg* 1999;117:881–889.
54. Wrathall JR, Choiniere D, Teng YD. Dose-dependent reduction of tissue loss and functional impairment after spinal cord trauma with the AMPA/kainate antagonist NBQX. *J Neurosci* 1994;14:6598–6607.

55. Tadié M, d'Arbigny P, Mathé JF, et al. Acute spinal cord injury: early care and treatment in a multicenter study with gacyclidine. *Soc Neurosci Abstr.* Abstr. 444.2. Part 1, 1090. Miami: Society for Neuroscience, 1999.
56. Mitha AP, Maynard KI. Gacyclidine (Beaufour-Ipsen). *Curr Opin Investig Drugs* 2001;2:814–819.
57. Tymianski M, Tator CH. Normal and abnormal calcium homeostasis in neurons: a basis for the pathophysiology of traumatic and ischemic central nervous system injury. *Neurosurgery* 1996;38:1176–1195.
58. Ross IB, Tator CH, Theriault E. Effect of nimodipine or methylprednisolone on recovery from acute experimental spinal cord injury in rats. *Surg Neurol* 1993;40:461–470.
59. Agrawal SK, Nashmi R, Fehlings MG. Role of L- and N-type calcium channels in the pathophysiology of traumatic spinal cord white matter injury. *Neuroscience* 2000;99:179–188.
60. Pointillart V, Gense D, Gross C, et al. Effects of nimodipine on posttraumatic spinal cord ischemia in baboons. *J Neurotrauma* 1993;10:201–213.
61. De Ley G, Leybaert L. Effect of flunarizine and methylprednisolone on functional recovery after experimental spinal injury. *J Neurotrauma* 1993;10:25–35.
62. Ross IB, Tator CH. Spinal cord blood flow and evoked potential responses after treatment with nimodipine or methylprednisolone in spinal cord-injured rats. *Neurosurgery* 1993;33:470–476.
63. Guha A, Tator CH, Piper I. Effect of a calcium channel blocker on posttraumatic spinal cord blood flow. *J Neurosurg* 1987;66:423–430.
64. Pointillart V, et al. Pharmacological therapy of spinal cord injury during the acute phase. *Spinal Cord* 2000;38:71–76.
65. Petitjean ME, Pointillart V, Dixmerias F, et al. Medical treatment of spinal cord injury in the acute stage. *Ann Fr Anesth Reanim* 1998;17:114–122.
66. Lewen A, Matz P, Chan PH. Free radical pathways in CNS injury. *J Neurotrauma* 2000;17:871–890.
67. Kowaltowski AJ, Castilho RF, Vercesi AE. Ca(2+)-induced mitochondrial membrane permeabilization: role of coenzyme Q redox state. *Am J Physiol* 1995;269:C141–147.
68. Gardner AM, Xu FH, Fady C, et al. Apoptotic vs. nonapoptotic cytotoxicity induced by hydrogen peroxide. *Free Radic Biol Med* 1997;22:73–83.
69. Liu D, Ling X, Wen J, et al. The role of reactive nitrogen species in secondary spinal cord injury: formation of nitric oxide, peroxynitrite, and nitrated protein. *J Neurochem* 2000;75:2144–2154.
70. Liu D, Li L, Augustus L. Prostaglandin release by spinal cord injury mediates production of hydroxyl radical, malondialdehyde and cell death: a site of the neuroprotective action of methylprednisolone. *J Neurochem* 2001; 77:1036–1047.
71. Liu D, Liu J, Wen J. Elevation of hydrogen peroxide after spinal cord injury detected by using the Fenton reaction. *Free Radic Biol Med* 1999;27:478–482.
72. Liu D, Sybert TE, Qian H, et al. Superoxide production after spinal injury detected by microperfusion of cytochrome c. *Free Radic Biol Med* 1998;25:298–304.
73. Leski ML, et al. Protein and DNA oxidation in spinal injury: neurofilaments: an oxidation target. *Free Radic Biol Med* 2001;30:613–624.
74. Springer JE, et al. 4-hydroxynonenal, a lipid peroxidation product, rapidly accumulates following traumatic spinal cord injury and inhibits glutamate uptake. *J Neurochem* 1997;68:2469–2476.
75. Barut S, Canbolat A, Bilge T, et al. Lipid peroxidation in experimental spinal cord injury: time-level relationship. *Neurosurg Rev* 1993;16:539. (1993).
76. Kaptanoglu E, Sen S, Beskonackli E, et al. Antioxidant actions and early ultrastructural findings of thiopental and propofol in experimental spinal cord injury. *J Neurosurg Anesthesiol* 2002;14:114–122.
77. Farooque M, Isaksson J, Olsson Y. Improved recovery after spinal cord injury in neuronal nitric oxide synthase-deficient mice but not in TNF-alpha-deficient mice. *J Neurotrauma* 2001;18:105–114.
78. Fujimoto T, Nakamura T, Ikeda T, et al. Effects of EPC-K1 on lipid peroxidation in experimental spinal cord injury. *Spine* 2000;25:24–29.
79. Katoh D, Ikata T, Katoh S, Effect of dietary vitamin C on compression injury of the spinal cord in a rat mutant unable to synthesize ascorbic acid and its correlation with that of vitamin E. *Spinal Cord* 1996;34:234–238.
80. Naftchi NE. Treatment of mammalian spinal cord injury with antioxidants. *Int J Dev Neurosci* 1991;9:113–126.
81. Kavanagh RJ, Kam PC. Lazaroids: efficacy and mechanism of action of the 21-aminosteroids in neuroprotection. *Br J Anaesth* 2001;86:110–119.
82. Gerhart KA, Johnson RL, Menconi J, et al. Utilization and effectiveness of methylprednisolone in a population-based sample of spinal cord injured persons. *Paraplegia* 1995;33:316–321.
83. George ER, et al. Failure of methylprednisolone to improve the outcome of spinal cord injuries. *Am Surg* 1995;61:659–663, discussion 663–664.
84. Poynton AR, O'Farrell DA, Shannon F, et al. An evaluation of the factors affecting neurological recovery following spinal cord injury. *Injury* 1997;28:545–548.
85. Prendergast MR, Saxe JM, Ledgerwood AM, et al. Massive steroids do not reduce the zone of injury after penetrating spinal cord injury. *J Trauma* 1994;37:576–579.
86. Bracken MB, Collins WF, Freeman DF, et al. Efficacy of methylprednisolone in acute spinal cord injury. *JAMA* 1984;251:45–52.

CHAPTER 21E

Spinal Cord Injury and Pathophysiology: Spinal Cord Injury Regeneration Strategies

Brian K. Kwon, Scott Paquette, and Michael C. Boyd

INTRODUCTION

Scientific progress over the past two decades in our understanding of the neurobiology of spinal cord injury has prompted hope that therapies might soon be developed to treat the devastating paralysis associated with this injury.[1] The functional impairments that such patients with complete quadriplegia or paraplegia endure have sparked tremendous research initiatives in the clinical, neuroscientific, and bioengineering disciplines. This chapter will review the concepts of neuroprotection and axonal regeneration following acute and chronic spinal cord injury (SCI) and describe some of the promising therapies that are being intensely investigated in these fields.

NEUROPROTECTION: PAST AND PRESENT

An evaluation of magnetic resonance imaging (MRI) scans of a completely paralyzed individual who has recently suffered a traumatic SCI will typically reveal that the spinal cord itself is not transected, despite the absence of distal motor and sensory function. Rather, the "primary" zone of SCI that received the brunt of the mechanical forces from the spinal column injury is surrounded by a surrounding zone of "secondary injury" (Fig. 21E.1). The acute pathophysiologic processes, including inflammation, ischemia, lipid peroxidation, excitotoxicity, and programmed cell death (apoptosis), started by the initial injury are thought to further damage the spinal cord.[2] The concept of neuroprotection is based on the premise that interventions instituted soon after injury can attenuate these acute pathophysiologic processes, thus minimizing secondary tissue damage at the injury site. Both human and animal studies have confirmed that small amounts of spared cord tissue at the injury site can often retain significant amounts of distal neurologic function. Therefore, a strong rationale exists for the neuroprotective strategies that might achieve this.[3–8]

Many animal studies have documented improved spinal cord tissue sparing and retention of neurologic function after the administration of treatments that attenuate the previously mentioned pathophysiologic processes, hence substantiating their neuroprotective properties. Nevertheless, it has been remarkably difficult to demonstrate such effective neuroprotection in human studies of SCI. On a large scale, the widespread implementation of protocols for trauma stabilization, immobilization, and resuscitation are thought to be neuroprotective insofar as the past 40 years have seen a decrease in the proportion of complete SCIs, with a corresponding rise in the proportion of

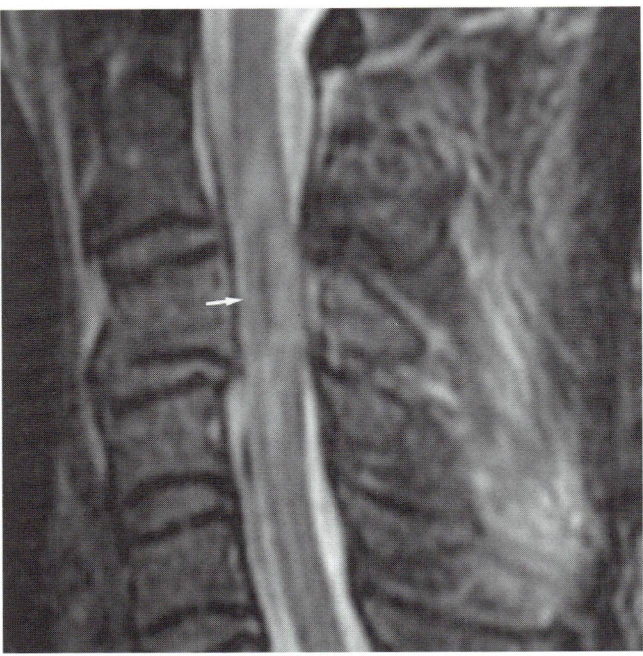

FIGURE 21E.1. The T2-weighted magnetic resonance imaging of this individual demonstrates the area of initial "primary" injury caused by the burst fragment impacting the cord *(arrow)*, and the surrounding zone of edema and inflammation representing areas of "secondary" injury. Neuroprotective strategies aim to reduce this area of secondary injury by attenuating the acute pathophysiologic processes that are initiated by the initial insult.

incomplete injuries.[9] The administration of high-dose methylprednisolone after acute SCIs (ASCIs) was entrenched into standards of practice following the second and third National Acute Spinal Cord Injury Studies (NASCIS).[10,11] However, more recent critiques on the interpretation of these studies have prompted many to advocate steroids as a treatment option only and some to discontinue it altogether.[12–15] Early surgical decompression has anecdotally been reported to promote improved neurologic function, but while this has clear conceptual rationale and is passionately adhered to by many surgeons, strong evidence for its efficacy is lacking.[16] A large, prospective multicenter observational trial, the Surgical Treatment of Acute Spinal Cord Injury Trial (STASCIS), will, in the coming years, likely provide critical data on this important issue.

Given the controversy over the effectiveness of methylprednisolone, substantial efforts are being made to develop more convincingly efficacious, neuroprotective pharmacologic agents. Much attention has been directed recently at drugs that are used for common—and typically unrelated—clinical indications but recently have been found to have neuroprotective effects. These include minocycline, erythropoietin, and atorvastatin (Lipitor).

Minocycline, a tetracycline derivative used for the treatment of acne and chronic periodontitis, has been found to have a number of neuroprotective properties,[17] and has been shown to be neuroprotective in animal models of ischemic stroke,[18,19] Parkinson disease,[20,21] Huntington disease,[22,23] and amyotrophic lateral sclerosis.[24–26] Independent laboratories using a variety of animal injury models have also found minocycline to be neuroprotective.[27–30] These have prompted the initiation of a pilot study in Calgary, Alberta, Canada, to evaluate minocycline in patients with ASCIs.

Erythropoietin is a hormone that is in widespread clinical use for the treatment of anemia in the setting of chemotherapy, chronic renal failure, and autologous blood donation. It has also been discovered to be neuroprotective in animal models of stroke,[31,32] multiple sclerosis,[33] Parkinson disease,[34] myocardial infarction,[35,36] and spinal cord injury.[37–39] The neuroprotective mechanisms of erythropoietin appear to be mediated by different receptor interactions and intracellular signaling pathways than the erythropoietic properties.[40] A small prospective randomized, double-blinded study of human patients with acute stroke found at an early follow-up that erythropoietin led to decreased infarct size and improved neurologic function.[41] A human trial in SCI is likely to be forthcoming.

Atorvastatin, more commonly known as Lipitor, is a member of the statin family of cholesterol-lowering drugs, which have recently been discovered to have significant neuroinflammatory effects.[42] Research into the use of the statins in SCI is still quite early compared to that in minocycline and erythropoietin, but a recent animal study found that atorvastatin administered before SCI resulted in significant tissue sparing and neurologic recovery.[43]

These pharmacologic agents all share the common characteristic of being in widespread clinical use. With a well-recognized safety profile in humans, it is only natural to expect that we will soon have clinical data on their application in human SCI.

AXONAL REGENERATION

The contrast between the potential for axonal regeneration to occur in the injured central nervous system and peripheral nervous system could not be greater. Although we expect transected peripheral nerves to regenerate after primary suture repair, we all recognize that axonal regeneration within the merely contused spinal cord is limited (as reflected by the poor neurologic recovery seen in SCI). Delineating the factors that account for such differences is the focus of much neuroscientific interest. In very simple conceptual terms, the inability of neurons within the central nervous system to regenerate after SCI is related to a limited intrinsic growth propensity and to inhibitory elements within the injured spinal cord that make it a nonpermissive environment.[44] Conversely, neurons of the peripheral nervous system elicit a much greater growth response to axonal injury, and the Schwann cells provide a permissive environment for regenerating axons. Therapies to promote axonal regeneration within the central nervous system, therefore, focus on trying to emulate the success within the peripheral nervous system, either by augmenting the neuron's intrinsic ability to regenerate or attenuating the inhibitory central nervous system environment into which they must regrow.

The administration of neurotrophic factors is a commonly used approach for stimulating axonal growth within the injured central nervous system. Neurotrophic factors (of which there are dozens) are proteins that exert considerable influence on a wide spectrum of processes within the developing and mature nervous system.[45] The process of axonal growth within the central nervous system appears to be considerably more complex than the process of bone growth, and, thus, it is important to realize that although a single commercially available bone morphogenetic protein (e.g., BMP-2 or BMP-7) may by itself promote bone fusion, a single neurotrophic factor by itself is unlikely to elicit all of the necessary biologic changes within the relevant neural and glial cell populations of the spinal cord to promote full neurologic recovery. In combination with strategies to provide a permissive growth environment, the application of various neurotrophic factors has been shown to induce axonal regeneration of central nervous system neurons and functional recovery after SCI in animal models.

One of the mechanisms by which neurotrophic factors augment the intrinsic growth propensity of central nervous system neurons is by elevating intracellular levels of cyclic adenosine monophosphate (cAMP). Investigators have reported that the administration of cAMP analogs can increase the intrinsic regenerative capacity to such an extent as to promote axonal growth even through the inhibitory environment of the injured spinal cord.[46,47] Combining this strategy of elevating intracellular cAMP with cellular substrates such as Schwann cells[4] or embryonic spinal cord tissue[49] that can provide a more permissive environment for axonal regeneration has shown promising results in animal models of SCI. It is widely believed that effective therapies for spinal cord injury in the future will require such a combinatorial approach.

Addressing the other side of the axonal regeneration equation, that is, the nonpermissive environment of the injured spinal cord, is also the subject of tremendous scientific interest. The two major impediments to axonal regeneration in the injured spinal cord are central nervous system myelin and the glial scar; a great deal has been learned about some of the molecular constituents of both that appear to confer this growth inhibition. Within central nervous system myelin, the best characterized inhibitory elements include the protein referred to as Nogo,[50–53] myelin-associated glycoprotein (MAG),[54] and oligodendrocyte-myelin glycoprotein (OMgp).[55] Of interest, these three myelin components may all signal through the same receptor (the Nogo receptor[56]), which raises the potential that therapies interfering with this single receptor and its downstream signaling may effectively mitigate the inhibitory effects of all three molecules.[57]

Within the glial scar, the astrocytes form a physical and biochemical barrier to axonal growth. One of the prominent inhibitory components of this scar is chondroitin sulphate proteoglycans (CSPGs). A potentially promising therapeutic intervention to address the CSPG inhibition to axonal growth is to enzymatically degrade the proteoglycans. Chondroitinase ABC is an enzyme that removes part of the glycosaminoglycan chains from CSPGs, leaving a protein core that is less inhibitory to axonal growth than the intact molecule. Animal studies in which chondroitinase ABC is applied to the SCI site have reported increased axonal growth and functional recovery.[58,59]

Outside of the inhibitory glial scar and central nervous system myelin, one of the obvious impediments to axonal growth across the chronic SCI site is the presence of the cystic cavity that is often established within the spinal cord over time. It is only intuitive that one consider filling this cavity with some form of cellular graft that might serve as a conduit for axonal growth. In this regard, a great deal of work is being done to evaluate cellular substrates that could potentially bridge the SCI site and facilitate the regeneration of axons into the graft and then back out into the spinal cord to synapse with distal targets. As it turns out, achieving axonal growth into such cellular grafts is often far less challenging than persuading the axons to leave and reenter the CNS environment, in part because of the aforementioned central nervous system myelin inhibitors and the glial scar that may become established at the graft–host interface. Leading candidates for such cellular transplantation include Schwann cells and peripheral nerve transplants, olfactory ensheathing cells, and stem cells. Promising results from animal research has prompted preliminary human application of peripheral nerve transplants and olfactory ensheathing cells in a number of international centers outside of North America.[60] Peer-reviewed results of such clinical application hopefully will be forthcoming in the years ahead.

CONCLUSION

The pace at which scientific discovery in spinal cord research is being made and the rapidity with which it is now being put into human practice generates much hope amongst patients, scientists, and clinicians that effective treatments for paralysis are around the corner. Much has yet to be learned, however, about the basic neurobiology of SCI and the mechanisms by which the spinal cord can be protected after injury and then induced to regrow new axons to promote neurologic recovery. The desperation of many patients with spinal cord paralysis for treatments to reverse their devastating paralysis will undoubtedly lead to the temptation to try experimental therapies that may have little biologic rationale, and, in this regard, clinicians will be called on to provide leadership and integrity in the evaluation of these novel technologies.

REFERENCES

1. Adams M, Cavanagh JF. International Campaign for Cures of Spinal Cord Injury Paralysis (ICCP): another step forward for spinal cord injury research. *Spinal Cord* 2004;42:273–280.
2. Kwon BK, Tetzlaff W, Grauer JN, et al. Pathophysiology and pharmacologic treatment of acute spinal cord injury. *Spine J* 2004;4:451–464.
3. Kaelan C, Jacobsen P, Morling P, et al. A quantitative study of motoneurons and cortico-spinal fibers related to function in human spinal cord injury (SCI). *Paraplegia* 1989;27:153.
4. Kakulas BA. The applied neuropathology of human spinal cord injury. *Spinal Cord* 1999;37:79–88.
5. Blight AR. Cellular morphology of chronic spinal cord injury in the cat: analysis of myelinated axons by line-sampling. *Neuroscience* 1983;10:521–543.
6. Eidelberg E, Straehley D, Erspamer R, et al. Relationship between residual hindlimb-assisted locomotion and surviving axons after incomplete spinal cord injuries. *Exp Neurol* 1977;56:312–322.

7. Fehlings MG, Tator CH. The relationships among the severity of spinal cord injury, residual neurological function, axon counts, and counts of retrogradely labeled neurons after experimental spinal cord injury. *Exp Neurol* 1995;132:220–228.
8. Kloos AD, Fisher LC, Detloff MR, et al. Stepwise motor and all-or-none sensory recovery is associated with nonlinear sparing after incremental spinal cord injury in rats. *Exp Neurol* 2005;191:251–265.
9. Tator CH, Duncan EG, Edmonds VE, et al. Changes in epidemiology of acute spinal cord injury from 1947 to 1981. *Surg Neurol* 1993;40:207–215.
10. Bracken MB, Shepard MJ, Collins WF, et al. A randomized, controlled trial of methylprednisolone or naloxone in the treatment of acute spinal-cord injury: results of the Second National Acute Spinal Cord Injury Study. *N Engl J Med* 1990;322:1405–1411.
11. Bracken MB, Shepard MJ, Holford TR, et al. Administration of methylprednisolone for 24 or 48 hours or tirilazad mesylate for 48 hours in the treatment of acute spinal cord injury: results of the Third National Acute Spinal Cord Injury Randomized Controlled Trial. National Acute Spinal Cord Injury Study. *JAMA* 1997;277: 1597–1604.
12. Hurlbert RJ. Methylprednisolone for acute spinal cord injury: an inappropriate standard of care. *J Neurosurg* 2000;93:1–7.
13. Coleman WP, Benzel D, Cahill DW, et al. A critical appraisal of the reporting of the National Acute Spinal Cord Injury Studies (II and III) of methylprednisolone in acute spinal cord injury. *J Spinal Disord* 2000;13:185–199.
14. Short DJ, El Masry WS, Jones PW. High dose methylprednisolone in the management of acute spinal cord injury: a systematic review from a clinical perspective. *Spinal Cord* 2000;38:273–286.
15. Hugenholtz H, Cass DE, Dvorak MF, et al. High-dose methylprednisolone for acute closed spinal cord injury: only a treatment option. *Can J Neurol Sci* 2002;29:227–235.
16. Fehlings MG, Perrin RG. The role and timing of early decompression for cervical spinal cord injury: update with a review of recent clinical evidence. *Injury* 2005;36(suppl 2):S13–S26.
17. Zemke D, Majid A. The potential of minocycline for neuroprotection in human neurologic disease. *Clin Neuropharmacol* 2004;27:293–298.
18. Arvin KL, Han BH, Du Y, et al. Minocycline markedly protects the neonatal brain against hypoxic-ischemic injury. *Ann Neurol* 2002;52:54–61.
19. Wang CX, Yang T, Noor R, et al. Delayed minocycline but not delayed mild hypothermia protects against embolic stroke. *BMC Neurol* 2002;2:2.
20. Wu DC, Jackson-Lewis V, Vila M, et al. Blockade of microglial activation is neuroprotective in the 1-methyl-4-phenyl-1,2,3,6-tetrahydropyridine mouse model of Parkinson disease. *J Neurosci* 2002;22:1763–1771.
21. Du Y, Ma Z, Lin S, et al. Minocycline prevents nigrostriatal dopaminergic neurodegeneration in the MPTP model of Parkinson's disease. *Proc Natl Acad Sci USA* 2001;98:14669–14674.
22. Wang X, Zhu S, Drozda M, et al. Minocycline inhibits caspase-independent and -dependent mitochondrial cell death pathways in models of Huntington's disease. *Proc Natl Acad Sci U S A* 2003;100:10483–10487.
23. Chen M, Ona VO, Li M, et al. Minocycline inhibits caspase-1 and caspase-3 expression and delays mortality in a transgenic mouse model of Huntington disease. *Nat Med* 2000;6:797–801.
24. Kriz J, Nguyen MD, Julien JP. Minocycline slows disease progression in a mouse model of amyotrophic lateral sclerosis. *Neurobiol Dis* 2002;10:268–278.
25. Van Den BL, Tilkin P, Lemmens G, et al. Minocycline delays disease onset and mortality in a transgenic model of ALS. *Neuroreport* 2002;13:1067–1070.
26. Zhu S, Stavrovskaya IG, Drozda M, et al. Minocycline inhibits cytochrome c release and delays progression of amyotrophic lateral sclerosis in mice. *Nature* 2002;417:74–78.
27. Wells JE, Hurlbert RJ, Fehlings MG, et al. Neuroprotection by minocycline facilitates significant recovery from spinal cord injury in mice. *Brain* 2003;126:1628–1637.
28. Lee SM, Yune TY, Kim SJ, et al. Minocycline reduces cell death and improves functional recovery after traumatic spinal cord injury in the rat. *J Neurotrauma* 2003;20:1017–1027.
29. Stirling DP, Khodarahmi K, Liu J, et al. Minocycline treatment reduces delayed oligodendrocyte death, attenuates axonal dieback, and improves functional outcome after spinal cord injury. *J Neurosci* 2004;24:2182–2190.
30. Teng YD, Choi H, Onario RC, et al. Minocycline inhibits contusion-triggered mitochondrial cytochrome c release and mitigates functional deficits after spinal cord injury. *Proc Natl Acad Sci U S A* 2004;101:3071–3076.
31. Brines ML, Ghezzi P, Keenan S, et al. Erythropoietin crosses the blood-brain barrier to protect against experimental brain injury. *Proc Natl Acad Sci U S A* 2000;97:10526–10531.
32. Kumral A, Ozer E, Yilmaz O, et al. Neuroprotective effect of erythropoietin on hypoxic-ischemic brain injury in neonatal rats. *Biol Neonate* 2003;83:224–228.
33. Sattler MB, Merkler D, Maier K, et al. Neuroprotective effects and intracellular signaling pathways of erythropoietin in a rat model of multiple sclerosis. *Cell Death Differ* 2004;11(suppl 2):S181–S192.
34. Genc S, Kuralay F, Genc K, Erythropoietin exerts neuroprotection in 1-methyl-4-phenyl-1,2,3,6-tetrahydropyridine-treated C57/BL mice via increasing nitric oxide production. *Neurosci Lett* 2001;298:139–141.

35. Moon C, Krawczyk M, Ahn D, et al. Erythropoietin reduces myocardial infarction and left ventricular functional decline after coronary artery ligation in rats. *Proc Natl Acad Sci U S A* 2003;100:11612–11617.
36. Calvillo L, Latini R, Kajstura J, et al. Recombinant human erythropoietin protects the myocardium from ischemia-reperfusion injury and promotes beneficial remodeling. *Proc Natl Acad Sci U S A* 2003;100:4802–4806.
37. Celik M, Gokmen N, Erbayraktar S, et al. Erythropoietin prevents motor neuron apoptosis and neurologic disability in experimental spinal cord ischemic injury. *Proc Natl Acad Sci U S A* 2002;99:2258–2263.
38. Gorio A, Gokmen N, Erbayraktar S, et al. Recombinant human erythropoietin counteracts secondary injury and markedly enhances neurological recovery from experimental spinal cord trauma. *Proc Natl Acad Sci U S A* 2002; 99:9450–9455.
39. Kaptanoglu E, Solaroglu I, Okutan O, et al. Erythropoietin exerts neuroprotection after acute spinal cord injury in rats: effect on lipid peroxidation and early ultrastructural findings. *Neurosurg Rev* 2004;27:113–120.
40. Brines M, Grasso G, Fiordaliso F, et al. Erythropoietin mediates tissue protection through an erythropoietin and common beta-subunit heteroreceptor. *Proc Natl Acad Sci USA* 2004;101:14907–14912.
41. Ehrenreich H, Hasselblatt M, Dembowski C, et al. Erythropoietin therapy for acute stroke is both safe and beneficial. *Mol Med* 2002;8:495–505.
42. Stuve O, Youssef S, Steinman L, et al. Statins as potential therapeutic agents in neuroinflammatory disorders. *Curr Opin Neurol* 2003;16:393–401.
43. Pannu R, Barbosa E, Singh AK, et al. Attenuation of acute inflammatory response by atorvastatin after spinal cord injury in rats. *J Neurosci Res* 2005;79:340–350.
44. Plunet W, Kwon BK, Tetzlaff W. Promoting axonal regeneration in the central nervous system by enhancing the cell body response to axotomy. *J Neurosci Res* 2002;68:1–6.
45. Tuszynski MH. Neurotrophic factors. In: Tuszynski MH, Kordower JH, eds. *CNS Regeneration: Basic Science and Clinical Advances.* San Diego: Academic Press, 1999:109–158.
46. Qiu J, Cai D, Dai H, et al. Spinal axon regeneration induced by elevation of cyclic AMP. *Neuron* 2002;34: 895–903.
47. Neumann S, Bradke F, Tessier-Lavigne M, et al. Regeneration of sensory axons within the injured spinal cord induced by intraganglionic cAMP elevation. *Neuron* 2002;34:885–893.
48. Pearse DD, Pereira FC, Marcillo AE, et al. cAMP and Schwann cells promote axonal growth and functional recovery after spinal cord injury. *Nat Med* 2004;10:610–616.
49. Nikulina E, Tidwell JL, Dai HN, et al. The phosphodiesterase inhibitor rolipram delivered after a spinal cord lesion promotes axonal regeneration and functional recovery. *Proc Natl Acad Sci U S A* 2004;101:8786–8790.
50. Chen MS, Huber AB, van der Haar ME, et al. Nogo-A is a myelin-associated neurite outgrowth inhibitor and an antigen for monoclonal antibody IN-1 [see comments]. *Nature* 2000;403:434–439.
51. GrandPre T, Nakamura F, Vartanian T, et al. Identification of the Nogo inhibitor of axon regeneration as a Reticulon protein. *Nature* 2000;403:439–444.
52. Lu P, Yang H, Jones LL, et al. Combinatorial therapy with neurotrophins and cAMP promotes axonal regeneration beyond sites of spinal cord injury. *J Neurosci* 2004;24:6402–6409.
53. Prinjha R, Moore SE, Vinson M, et al. Inhibitor of neurite outgrowth in humans. *Nature* 2000;403:383–384.
54. McKerracher L, David S, Jackson DL, et al. Identification of myelin-associated glycoprotein as a major myelin-derived inhibitor of neurite growth. *Neuron* 1994;13:805–811.
55. Wang KC, Koprivica V, Kim JA, et al. Oligodendrocyte-myelin glycoprotein is a Nogo receptor ligand that inhibits neurite outgrowth. *Nature* 2000;417:941–944.
56. Fournier AE, GrandPre T, Strittmatter SM. Identification of a receptor mediating Nogo-66 inhibition of axonal regeneration. *Nature* 2001;409:341–346.
57. Kwon BK, Borisoff JF, Tetzlaff W. Molecular targets for intervention in spinal cord injury. *Mol Interv* 2002; 2:244–258.
58. Bradbury EJ, Moon LD, Popat RJ, et al. Chondroitinase ABC promotes functional recovery after spinal cord injury. *Nature* 2002;416:636–640.
59. Chau CH, Shum DK, Li H, et al. Chondroitinase ABC enhances axonal regrowth through Schwann cell-seeded guidance channels after spinal cord injury. *FASEB* J 2004;18:194–196.
60. Steeves J, Fawcett J, Tuszynski M. Report of international clinical trials workshop on spinal cord injury February 20–21, 2004, Vancouver, Canada. *Spinal Cord* 2004;42:591–597.

CHAPTER 21F

Spinal Cord Injury and Pathophysiology: Long-Term Outcomes of Spinal Cord Injury and Functional Prognosis

John R. Dimar

INTRODUCTION

The life expectancy of individuals who suffer a spinal cord injury (SCI) has dramatically improved over the past decade.[1,2] Although quadriplegics are less likely to live long, 25% of these individuals live more than 20 years after SCI and 40% are older than 45 years.[2] Consequently, the social and financial ramifications of SCI remain significant. The total cost of all SCIs has risen from U.S. $4 billion annually in 1992[3] to more than $9.7 billion in 2005.[4]

Techniques used to maximize long-term neurologic recovery following SCI continue to be the subject of intense clinical research. Methods to lessen the acute neurologic injury immediately following trauma include emergent neural decompression and spine stabilization, application of hypothermia to the site of SCI, and use of various pharmacologic agents that limit posttraumatic vascular ischemia and modify cellular inflammatory mediators that are believed to worsen neurologic injury.[3,5–10] The uniform clinical application of these techniques remains extremely difficult.[15–17] One of the most beneficial results of this intense focus on SCI has been a significant improvement in the manner in which emergency personnel manage patients with acute SCI. These injuries are now consistently considered an emergency demanding a timely response and immobilization to prevent secondary injury, maximizing the potential for long-term recovery.[11] However, there are still no randomized prospective studies in patients with acute SCI that definitively demonstrate that any specific treatment modality makes a significant difference in long-term clinical outcomes. This chapter focuses on the long-term treatment options currently available to improve the functional outcomes following SCI.

The literature is replete with various experimental methodologies that may offer potential for long-term improvement of neurologic function following SCI.[3,6–9,12–16] Currently, the most efficacious treatment available remains early immobilization and surgical stabilization of the spine. This prevents secondary neurologic injury and allows for aggressive long-term rehabilitation.

The recovery of neurologic function is of paramount importance because just the return of protective sensation may have significant functional ramifications. Because SCIs present with a wide spectrum of neurologic deficits, the strategy for rehabilitation and expected long-term outcomes will differ greatly for each patient. A complete C5-level quadriplegic will have dramatically different rehabilitation potential and treatment regimen compared to a patient with a C7-level complete lesion. Incomplete lesions offer the greatest potential for rehabilitation because they demonstrate significant long-term improvement of function. This is particularly true in younger patients, because older patients may not have the necessary physiologic reserves required following such a life-changing injury.[2]

Patients often face a prolonged, tumultuous recovery after SCI and need a wide variety of psychosocial and physical support during this phase. The quality of the rehabilitation program and aggressiveness of its application can make a significant difference in the restoration of all potential function. A multidisciplinary center specializing in spinal cord rehabilitation is today commonly employed to bring all of the essential areas of expertise such as locomotor training, pain management, bowel and bladder control, spasticity treatment, orthotic and prosthesis use, functional electrical stimulation (FES), and treatment of the anxiety and depression together to provide quality rehabilitation. Finally, the future application of spinal cord regeneration techniques may prove critical to the long-term restoration of neurologic function and subsequent improved outcomes in these patients.

LOCOMOTOR TRAINING

The recovery of walking function remains the most important treatment at this time for SCI. Body weight–supported treadmill training (BWSTT) and FES show great promise to improve locomotor function in patients with incomplete SCI.[18] These training programs are based on the concept that specific neuronal networks termed central pattern generators (CPGs) are responsible for rhythmic lower extremity walking patterns in quadrupeds.[19] The programs are designed to take advantage of these embedded neuronal pathways by reproducing normal walking patterns that, once enhanced, may significantly improve walking speed and endurance. These improvements in ambulation may subsequently be retained for extended periods following the completion of training.[20] Numerous studies have shown that both conventional therapy and BWSTT (Fig. 21F.1), when integrated into a daily training program following an incomplete SCI, can improve walking function.[21–25] These programs have additionally shown a significant increase in gait speed and endurance along with decreased oxygen consumption during training.[20] Many recent studies have reported encouraging results by combining FES with BWSTT over the first 12 weeks.[25,26] An alternative approach to a BWSTT uses a bicycle combined with FES that is applicable for long-term use at home.[15]

Advancements in FES combined with microprocessors have led to the development of implantable or percutaneous stimulation systems that have demonstrated success in enhancing hand function in C5-6 quadriplegics.[27–30] The Parastep system (Sigmedics, Inc., Fairborn, Ohio) has shown usefulness in restoring reciprocal gait via surface electrodes and a microprocessor that allow for ambulation when combined with a rolling walker (Fig. 21F.2). Excellent upper extremity strength, good range of motion of the lower extremities, normal skin, and a thoracic-level lesion are prerequisites.[17] Recently, more elaborate, fully implantable neuroprosthetic systems have successfully restored significant hand and upper arm function in C6 and C7 quadriplegics. The device employs multiple stimulation and sensor electrodes integrated with joint-angle sensors. The only external component is a transmitter and receiver coil that powers and communicates with the implanted components via electromagnetic radiofrequency waves.[30,31]

SPASTICITY MANAGEMENT

Spasticity results in severe impairment of walking, limits extremity positioning and range of motion, interferes with activities of daily living, and may lead to fixed flexion contractures.[27,31,32] Spasticity is more common in incomplete lesions, with an incidence of 67% to 70% by 1 year following SCI. Spasticity is characterized by hyperreflexia, clonus, spasms, and deformities. It is more uncommon in complete lesions and patients who retain significant voluntary motor function.

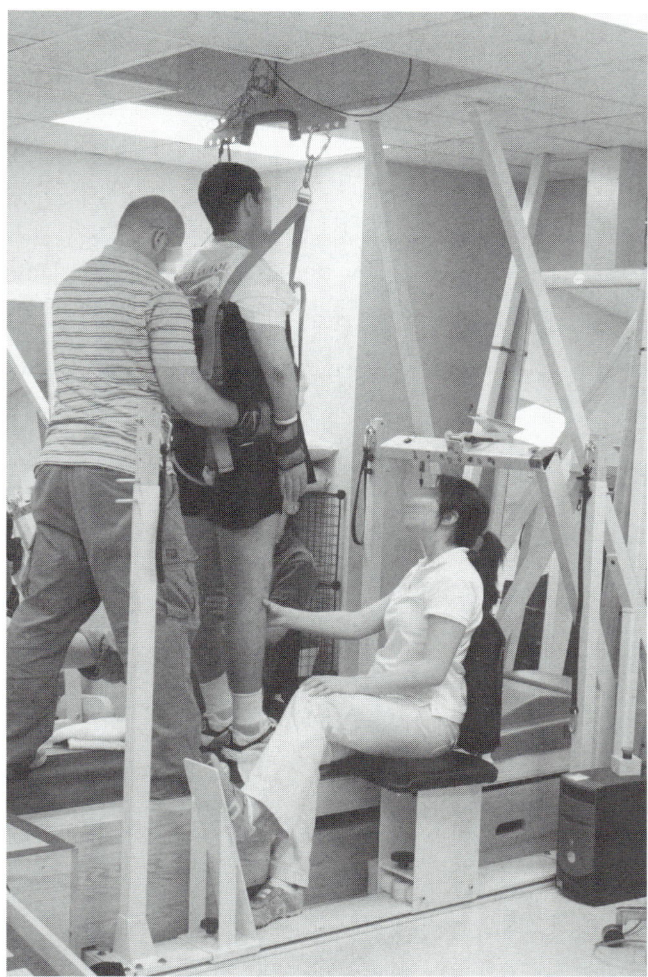

FIGURE 21F.1. Body weight–supporting treadmill training (BWSTT) has shown effectiveness in various studies for improvement of walking function, particularly in an incomplete SCI.

Treatment options include traditional stretching and physical therapy with or without bracing, pharmacologic interventions, and surgical procedures.[31,33] Pharmacologic agents alter the function of neurotransmitters either centrally or peripherally and include oral agents such as baclofen, diazepam, clonidine, dantrolene, tizanidine, gabapentin, injectable agents such as botulinum, and intrathecal agents (via an implantable pump) such as baclofen, which is often used with gabapentin.[27] Surgical interventions that have demonstrated effectiveness in treating spasms include ablation procedures such as rhizotomies and myelotomy or neuromodulation procedures typified by implantable spinal cord stimulators.[27,31]

CHRONIC NEUROGENIC PAIN

The presence of chronic painful sensations following an incomplete SCI remains a significant challenge for successful rehabilitation. These dysesthesias have long been described, with a reported incidence of 60% to 80%. Forty percent are severe enough to affect activities of daily living.[34] Their onset can occur within weeks of the injury and up to 1 year following. Pain is more common in older patients and those with thoracic-level SCIs than with cervical injuries.[35] Aggravating factors include stress, overactivity, weather changes, and spasticity. Rest and medications tend to provide relief. The origin of central neuropathic pain is generally felt to be due to damage to the gray and white matter

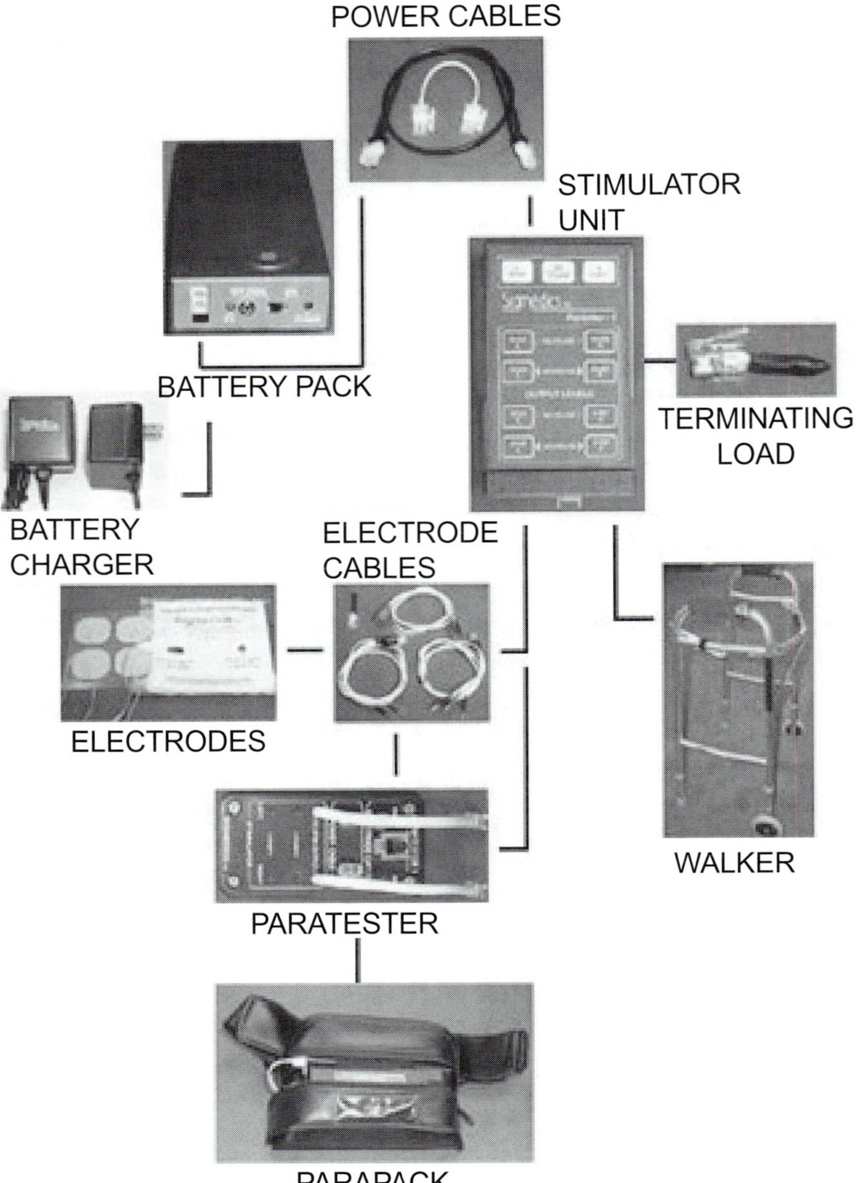

FIGURE 21F.2. The Parastep system and other neuroprosthetic systems have been successful in restoring useful motor function in certain individuals. They generally employ surface or implantable electrodes combined with a microprocessor.

of the spinal cord that produces excitability of spinal neurons similar to that observed in peripheral nerve injuries. Researchers propose the existence of a common central injury cascade that initiates pain following SCI.[36] The theories that explain this phenomenon include an imbalance of the sensory information conveyed by spinal cord sensory tracts, a loss of sensory inhibitory control allowing for spreading of painful sensations, the emergence of a pattern-generating mechanism, and long-term changes in spinal connectivity within the central nervous system termed spinal plasticity.[34–38] Despite the limited effectiveness of pharmacologic agents, they are the primary nonoperative treatment for neuropathic pain. Agents available include antidepressants, anticonvulsants, opioids, clonidine, sodium and potassium channel blockers, baclofen, and gabapentin.[31] Surgical treatment includes dorsal root entry zone ablation,[39] cordotomy,[33] transcutaneous electrical nerve stimulation,[40] spinal cord stimulation,[41] and deep brain stimulation, which has shown poor relief of long-term pain.[42]

NEUROGENIC BOWEL AND BLADDER

SCI results in the alteration of bowel, bladder, and sexual function. Following the resolution of spinal shock, bladder damage has been classified into two types: an upper motor neuron lesion (S1-S2) or a lower motor lesion (S2-S4).[43] A complete upper motor lesion secondary to damage of the spinal cord above the level of the conus results in bladder-sphincter dyssynergia and urinary retention. In this circumstance the bladder contracts reflexively against the unrelaxed, closed bladder neck, resulting in eventual ureteral reflux, which, if left untreated, results in the development of hydronephrosis and urinary infections. Incomplete lesions are different because they have some retained function, resulting in urge incontinence resulting from hyperreflexability of the bladder.[44] The treatment for an upper motor lesion consists of medications, an indwelling catheter, an external catheter, a suprapubic catheter, an implantable FES to aid in emptying, or, if C7 function is present, intermittent catheterization. A lower motor neuron lesion affects the cauda equina and the conus medullaris, interrupting the bladder's reflex arc, resulting in flaccidity and hypocontractility, that is, detrusor areflexia. Treatment consists of intermittent or indwelling catheters. Long-term monitoring of renal function and rapid treatment of a urinary tract infection are critical. Before the availability of antibiotics, renal failure was the leading cause of death (2.8%) in patients with SCI.[2,45]

Gastrointestinal dysfunction is a major physical and psychological problem for individuals who have experienced SCI, especially with a lower motor neuron injury in which anal sphincter tone is lost. Although fecal incontinence is the most troublesome aspect, these patients also experience constipation, diarrhea, reflux, and nausea. Studies have reported that bowel function causes up to 54% of patients with SCI to experience anxiety because of their immobility, the time required for bowel management, and their dependence on others for assistance.[46] Toilet dependency is significantly higher in individuals who are nonambulatory, have cervical injuries, and have more complete injuries. Bowel management programs have shown significant satisfaction rates in improving anxiety in individuals with SCI.[47] These programs generally entail regular fiber intake, specific food avoidance, enemas, suppositories, laxatives, digital or manual stimulation, and manual evacuation. FES also has been shown to improve rectal evacuation, as have surgical treatments, including colostomies and antegrade colonic lavage via an appendicostomy.[46,47]

Sexual dysfunction after SCI is common, with a 75% incidence of impotence in men and a 50% reduction in orgasm rates in women.[44,47,48] Patients with upper motor neuron injuries have short-duration reflex erections up to 92% of the time, whereas those with lower motor neuron injuries have a more difficult time.[49] Treatment modalities for men include pharmacologic agents such as erectile dysfunction drugs, mechanical stimulation, vacuum suction devices, and implantation of surgical devices. Although fertility is generally not a problem in women, male infertility remains a significant problem because of decreased sperm motility, erectile dysfunction, and poor ejaculation ability.[50,51] Ultimately, if pregnancy is desired, there are several methods available to obtain sperm to allow for intrauterine insemination or in vitro fertilization.

PRESSURE ULCERS

Pressure ulcers are a serious, common sequela of SCI as a result of loss of protective sensation. Pressure ulcers are most common on the sacral and ischial tuberosities. Once present, they are a costly and time-consuming problem that results in a serious delay in a patient's recovery. The most effective treatment is prevention, by providing proper wheelchair cushioning such as gel, foam, or air cushions and proper patient education on performing periodic weight shifts to prevent skin ischemia.[27] Once ulcers form, aggressive wound care and protection of the area are critical to allow healing, or inevitably a deep tissue ulcer with potential bony involvement and osteomyelitis will develop, requiring repeated debridements and skin flaps.

ANXIETY AND DEPRESSION

SCI results in a significant change in an individual's activities of daily living and quality of life. As a result, virtually 100% of patients who have sustained SCI will suffer some degree of depression. Another 15% to 45% will experience severe periods of depression, with 25% to 30% even contemplating suicide.[52–54] More recent studies have challenged the historical belief that depression in these individuals is inevitable and is necessary for successful rehabilitation. Different models of depression have proposed that there are two to five stages of psychological recovery that individuals must go through for successful rehabilitation. These models are based on traditional classifications of depression and are in contrast to findings in recent studies that have postulated that although depression is not uncommon in an individual who has experienced SCI, it is not inevitable.[53] Therefore, following such a catastrophic injury, the high incidence of anxiety and depression within this population must be aggressively treated to prevent higher rates of morbidity, longer hospital stays, and less functional improvement during rehabilitation.

SPINAL DEFORMITY

There are numerous late sequelae following SCI that may occur years after the injury. These include problems directly related to the site of the fracture, such as progressive kyphotic deformity resulting from an undetected injury or the development of late kyphosis or scoliosis distal to the neurologic injury.[55] With time, these individuals may develop increasing neck pain, a progressive chin-on-chest deformity, and a potential worsening of the neurologic deficit.[56] Although there is a chance of developing kyphosis following any injury, particularly those treated nonoperatively, there is a significantly enhanced chance of developing kyphosis following an isolated posterior decompression.[57] Additionally, children who suffer a cervical SCI, whether bony or the uncommon (4%) SCI without radiologic abnormality (SCIWORA), have a particularly high risk (96%) for developing a subsequent paralytic spinal deformity if they are rendered quadriplegic (Fig. 21F.3).[58–60] Surgical intervention is clearly indicated if there is progressive neurologic deficit.[56,57] Surgical treatment for deformity is more difficult to elucidate because there are no references that define the degree of cervical kyphosis that is acceptable. However, studies within the thoracic and lumbar spine have identified that kyphosis greater than 30 degrees of angulation is associated with increased pain in the region of kyphosis.[61] Whether the deformity is kyphosis in the cervical spine or a resultant paralytic thoracolumbar scoliosis or kyphosis, early correction of the deformity and stabilization are both technically easier and yield better results than late treatment.[56] Late reconstruction of cervical kyphosis is challenging, often requiring an anterior and posterior procedure, particularly if there is rigidity. However, in the event of a missed injury, unsuccessful closed treatment, pseudarthrosis, or postlaminectomy kyphosis, surgical treatment using osteotomies and rigid internal fixation has yielded excellent results.[57] Thoracolumbar paralytic deformities may need surgical stabilization if the deformity decompensates or interferes with sitting balance.[59,61] Traditional methods used to treat scoliosis and kyphosis are effective, and strong consideration for a long fusion is critical to prevent the subsequent development of adjacent level decompensation.

SYRINGOMYELIA

Posttraumatic cystic myelopathy (PTCM) or syrinx occurs in 0.3% to 3.2% of cases following SCI.[62] A syrinx is an accumulation of cerebrospinal fluid within the spinal cord, resulting in tubular cavitation that follows a traumatic contusion (Fig. 21F.4). The cause of posttraumatic syrinx is con-

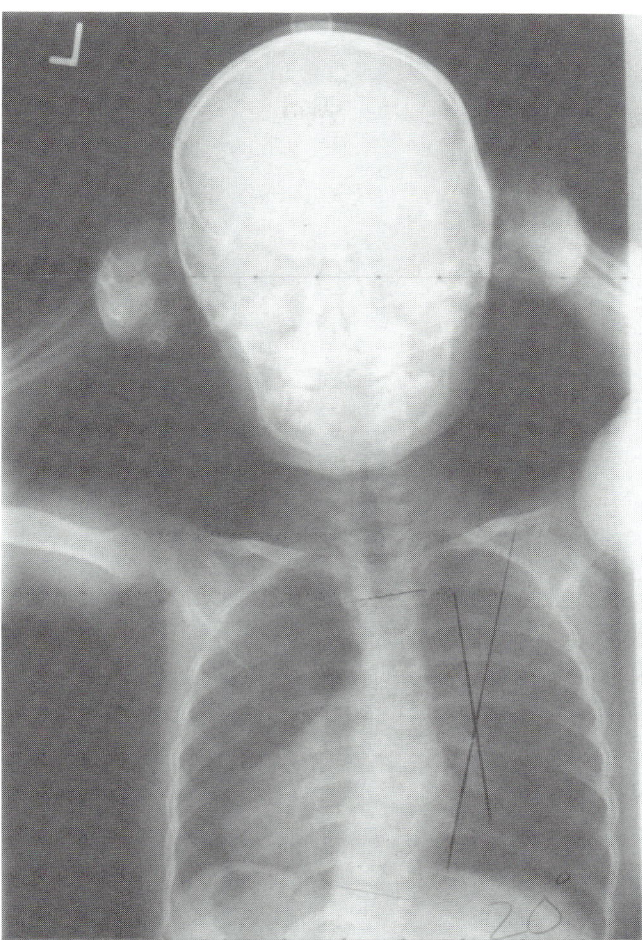

FIGURE 21F.3. Plain anteroposterior radiograph demonstrating a developing paralytic scoliosis in a child. Paralytic scoliosis or kyphosis is common in children following a spinal cord injury, particularly following quadriparesis or after a posterior decompression.

troversial because it does involve disturbances of the normal cerebrospinal fluid flow mechanics and has a unique tendency to extend rostrally.[63] The most common presenting symptom is pain. Ascending sensory level, increasing weakness, increasing spasticity, numbness, and the development of a Horner syndrome are also frequently reported symptoms.[64] Individuals who present with these progressive clinical findings have a 43% chance of having a posttraumatic syrinx.[65] Magnetic resonance imaging (MRI) is the preferred method of imaging, whereas computed tomography and myelography remain useful for certain individuals where MRI fails to fully identify the lesion.[65,66] In addition to a syrinx, the MRI will identify myelomalacia, cord atrophy, cord disruption, and tethering secondary to intradural scarring. The successful treatment of posttraumatic syringomyelia consists of a laminectomy, identification of the syrinx with ultrasonography, untethering if indicated, followed by syringosubarachnoid shunt insertion.[63]

CONCLUSION

SCI remains a devastating injury that leads to dramatic changes in activities of daily living. The level of injury and the degree of completeness appear to be the ultimate predictors of the long-term outcome of an individual suffering such an injury. Currently the most efficacious treatment for SCI is early stabilization to prevent late deformity, followed by a multidisciplinary and aggressive rehabilitation program that addresses all of the problems faced by these individuals. Key aspects of this rehabilitation program should include physical training and mobilization, treatment of depression

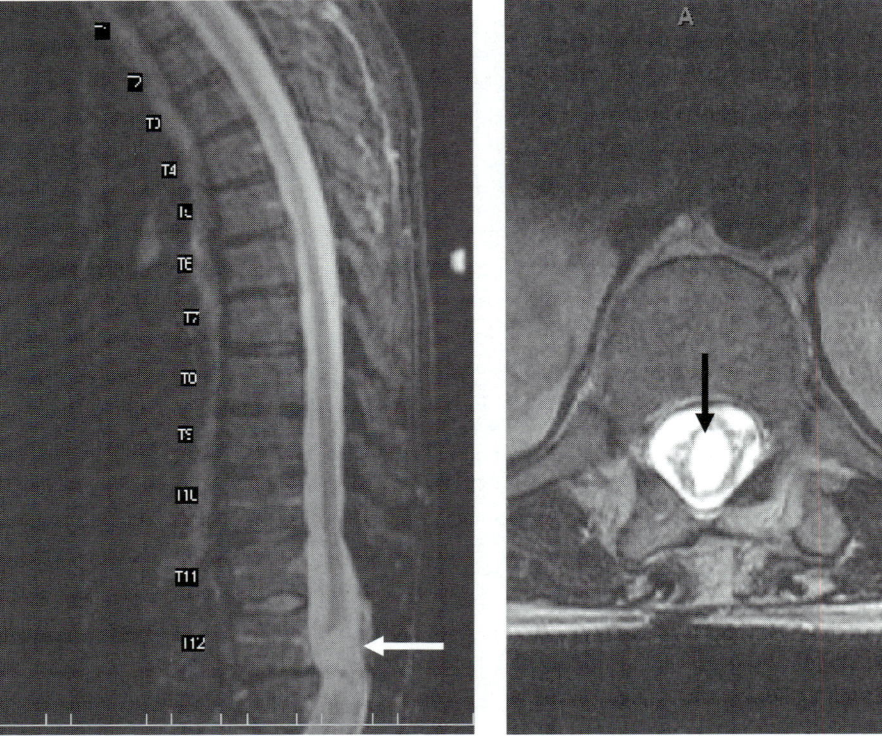

FIGURE 21F.4. Sagittal and axial MRI demonstrating a posttraumatic syrinx within the distal thoracic spinal cord following SCI. The patient presented with increasing numbness and weakness of his lower extremeties.

and anxiety, management of postinjury pain and spasticity, and management of bowel, bladder, and sexual dysfunction. Long-term outcome studies appear to support the efficacy of these combined treatment modalities in improving the lifestyle of these individuals. Additionally, late neurologic and orthopedic complications may occur years later, demonstrating the need for long-term follow-up and treatment. Ultimately, the intense research on spinal cord regeneration may offer the best hope for long-term improvement of functional outcomes in this population.

REFERENCES

1. Becker D, Sadowsky CL, McDonald JW. Restoring function after spinal cord injury. *Neurologist* 2003;9:1–15.
2. Capoor J, Stein AB. Aging with spinal cord injury. *Phys Med Rehabil Clin North Am* 2005;16:129–161.
3. Harvey C, Wilson SE, Greene CG, et al. New estimates of the direct costs of traumatic spinal cord injuries: results of a nationwide survey. *Paraplegia* 1992;30:834–850.
4. National Center for Injury Prevention and Control. Spinal cord injury fact sheet. Available at: http://www.cdc.gov/ncipc/factsheets/scifacts.htm.
5. Dobkin BH, Havton LA. Basic advances and new avenues in therapy of spinal cord injury. *Annu Rev Med* 2004;55:255–282.
6. Bracken MB, Holford TR. Neurological and functional status 1 year after acute spinal cord injury: estimates of functional recovery in National Acute Spinal Cord Injury Study II from results modeled in National Acute Spinal Cord Injury Study III. *J Neurosurg* 2002;96(suppl 3):259–266.
7. Bracken MB, Shepard MJ, Holford TR, et al. Methylprednisolone or tirilazad mesylate administration after acute spinal cord injury: 1-year follow up—results of the Third National Acute Spinal Cord Injury Randomized Controlled Trial. *J Neurosurg* 1998;89:699–706.

8. Dimar JR 2nd, Glassman SD, Raque GH, et al. The influence of spinal canal narrowing and timing of decompression on neurologic recovery after spinal cord contusion in a rat model. *Spine* 1999;24:1623–1633.
9. Dimar JR 2nd, Shields CB, Zhang YP, et al. The role of directly applied hypothermia in spinal cord injury. *Spine* 2000;25:2294–2302.
10. Tator CH, Fehlings MG. Review of the secondary injury theory of acute spinal cord trauma with emphasis on vascular mechanisms. *J Neurosurg* 1991;75:15–26.
11. Geisler FH, Coleman WP, Grieco G, et al. Recruitment and early treatment in a multicenter study of acute spinal cord injury. *Spine* 2001;26(suppl 24):S58–S67.
12. Fehlings MG, Sekhon LH, Tator C. The role and timing of decompression in acute spinal cord injury: what do we know? What should we do? *Spine* 2001:26(suppl 24):S101–S110.
13. Geisler FH, Coleman WP, Grieco G, et al. The Sygen multicenter acute spinal cord injury study. *Spine* 2001; 26(suppl 24):S87–S98.
14. Kishan S, Vives MJ, Reiter MF. Timing of surgery following spinal cord injury. *J Spinal Cord Med* 2005; 28:11–19.
15. McDonald JW, Becker D. Spinal cord injury: promising interventions and realistic goals. *Am J Phys Med Rehabil* 2003;82(suppl 10):S38–S49.
16. Reier PJ. Cellular transplantation strategies for spinal cord injury and translational neurobiology. *NeuroRx* 2004; 1:424–451.
17. Hurlbert RJ, Hamilton MG. Methyprednisone for acute spinal cord injury: 5-year practice reversal. *Can J Neurol Sci* 2008;35(1):41–45.
18. Chaplin E. Functional neuromuscular stimulation for mobility in people with spinal cord injuries: the Parastep I System. *J Spinal Cord Med* 1996;19:99–105.
19. Cazalets JR, Borde M, Clarac F. Localization and organization of the central pattern generator for hindlimb locomotion in newborn rat. *J Neurosci* 1995;15(7 Part 1):4943–4951.
20. Fouad K, Pearson K. Restoring walking after spinal cord injury. *Prog Neurobiol* 2004;73:107–126.
21. Wirz M, Colombo G, Dietz V. Long term effects of locomotor training in spinal humans. *J Neurol Neurosurg Psychiatry* 2001;71:93–96.
22. Dietz V, Harkema SJ. Locomotor activity in spinal cord-injured persons. *J Appl Physiol* 2004;96:1954–1960.
23. Edgerton VR, Leon RD, Harkema SJ, et al. Retraining the injured spinal cord. *J Physiol* 2001;533(Part 1):15–22.
24. Harkema SJ. Neural plasticity after human spinal cord injury: application of locomotor training to the rehabilitation of walking. *Neuroscientist* 2001;7:455–468.
25. Barbeau H, Ladouceur M, Mirbagheri MM, et al. The effect of locomotor training combined with functional electrical stimulation in chronic spinal cord injured subjects: walking and reflex studies. *Brain Res Brain Res Rev* 2002;40:274–291.
26. Postans NJ, Hasler JP, Granat MH, et al. Functional electric stimulation to augment partial weight-bearing supported treadmill training for patients with acute incomplete spinal cord injury: a pilot study. *Arch Phys Med Rehabil* 2004;85:604–610.
27. Kirshblum S. New rehabilitation interventions in spinal cord injury. *J Spinal Cord Med* 2004;27:342–350.
28. Mulcahey MJ, Betz RR, Kozin SH, et al. Implantation of the Freehand System during initial rehabilitation using minimally invasive techniques. *Spinal Cord* 2004;42:146–155.
29. Peckham PH, Keith MW, Kilgore KL, et al. Efficacy of an implanted neuroprosthesis for restoring hand grasp in tetraplegia: a multicenter study. *Arch Phys Med Rehabil* 2001;82:1380–1388.
30. Peckham PH, Kilgore, KL, Keith MW, et al. An advanced neuroprosthesis for restoration of hand and upper arm control using an implantable controller. *J Hand Surg Am* 2002;27:265–276.
31. Burchiel KJ, Hsu FP. Pain and spasticity after spinal cord injury: mechanisms and treatment. *Spine* 2001;26 (suppl 24):S146–S160.
32. Taricco M, Adone R, Pagliacci C, et al. Pharmacological interventions for spasticity following spinal cord injury. *Cochrane Database Syst Rev* 2000;2:CD001131.
33. Barolat G. Surgical management of spasticity and spasms in spinal cord injury: an overview. *J Am Paraplegia Soc* 1988;11:9–13.
34. Yezierski RP. Pain following spinal cord injury: pathophysiology and central mechanisms. *Prog Brain Res* 2000; 129:429–449.
35. Demirel G, Yllmaz H, Gencosmanoglu B, et al. Pain following spinal cord injury. *Spinal Cord* 1998;36:25–28.
36. Yezierski RP. Pain following spinal cord injury: the clinical problem and experimental studies. *Pain* 1996;68: 185–194.
37. Wiesenfeld-Hallin Z, Hao JX, Aldskogius H, et al. Allodynia-like symptoms in rats after spinal cord ischemia: an animal model of central pain. *Prog Pain Res Manage* 1997;4:455–472.
38. Melzack R, Loeser JD. Phantom body pain in paraplegics: evidence for a central "pattern generating mechanism" for pain. *Pain* 1978;4:195–210.
39. Nashold BS Jr, Bullitt E. Dorsal root entry zone lesions to control central pain in paraplegics. *J Neurosurg* 1981;55(3):414–419.

40. Bates JA, Nathan PW. Transcutaneous electrical nerve stimulation for chronic pain. *Anaesthesia* 1980;35(8): 817–822.
41. Cioni B, Meglio M, Pentimalli L, et al. Spinal cord stimulation in the treatment of paraplegic pain. *J Neurosurg* 1995;82:35–39.
42. Kumar K, Toth C, Nath RK. Deep brain stimulation for intractable pain: a 15 year experience *Neurosurgery* 1997; 40:736–746.
43. Rivas DA, Abdill CK, Chancellor MB. Current management of detrusor sphincter dyssynergia. *Top Spinal Cord Injury Rehabil* 1996;1:1–17.
44. Burns AS, Rivas DA, Ditunno JF. The management of neurogenic bladder and sexual dysfunction after spinal cord injury. *Spine* 2001;26:129–136.
45. Donnelly J, Hackler R, Bunts C. Present urologic status of the World War II paraplegic: 25-year follow-up—comparison with status of the 20-year Korean War paraplegic and 5-year Vietnam paraplegic. *J Urol* 1972;108:558–562.
46. Glickman S, Kamm MA. Bowel dysfunction in spinal-cord-injury patients. *Lancet* 1996;347:1651–1653.
47. Kirk PM, King RB, Temple R, et al. Long-term follow-up bowel management after spinal cord injury. *Sci Nursing* 1997;14:56–63.
48. Stone AR. The sexual need of the injured spinal cord patient. *Probl Urol* 1987;3:529–536.
49. Comarr AE. Sexual function among patients with spinal cord injury. *Urol Int* 1970;25:134–168.
50. Ohl DA, McCabe M, Sonksen J, et al. Management of infertility in spinal cord injury. *Top Spinal Cord Inj Rehabil* 1996;1:65–75.
51. Burns AS, Jackson AB. Gynecologic and reproductive issues in women with spinal cord injury. *Phys Med Rehabil Clin North Am* 2001;12:183–199.
52. Kemp BJ, Krause JS. Depression and life satisfaction among people aging with post-polio and spinal cord injury. *Disabil Rehab* 1999;21:241–249.
53. Kennedy P, Rogers A. Anxiety and depression after spinal cord injury: a longitudinal analysis. *Arch Phys Med Rehabil* 2002;81:932–937.
54. Wood-Dauphinee, S, Exner G, and the SCI Consensus Group. Quality of life in patients with spinal cord injury-basic issues, assessment, and recommendations *Restor Neurol Neurosci* 2002;20:135–149.
55. Keene JS. Undetected posttraumatic instability of "stable" thoracolumbar fractures. *J Orthop Trauma* 1988;2: 202–211.
56. Vaccarro AR, Silber JS. Post-traumatic spinal deformity. *Spine* 2001;26:S111–S118.
57. Abumi K, Shono Y. Correction of cervical kyphosis using pedicle screw fixation systems. *Spine* 1999;24:2389–2396.
58. Carreon LY. Pediatric spine fractures: a review of 137 hospital admissions. J *Spinal Disord Tech* 2004;17:447–482.
59. Mayfield JK, Winter RB. Spine deformity subsequent to acquired childhood. *Spinal Cord Injury Am* 1981; 63:1401–1411.
60. Orenstein JB, Klein BL. Age and outcome in pediatric cervical injury: 11-year experience. *Pediatr Emerg Care* 1994;10:132–137.
61. Gertzbein SD. Scoliosis Research Society: Multicenter Spine Fracture Study. *Spine* 1992;17:528–540.
62. Lee TT, Alameda GJ. Outcome after surgical treatment of progressive posttraumatic cystic myelopathy. *J Neurosurg (Spine 2)* 2000;92:149–154.
63. Saremi F, Zee C-S. Syringohydromyelia E-Medicine Specialties Instant Access to Medicine Online Reference.
64. Goetz L, Priebe M. Posttraumatic syringomyelia. E-medicine Specialties Instant Access to Medicine Online Reference. Available at http://emedicine.medscape.com/article/322348-overview. Accessed June 12, 2009.
65. Potter K, Saifuddin A. MRI of chronic spinal cord injury. *Br J Radiol* 2003;76:347–352.
66. Silberstein M, Hennessy O. A comparison between MRI and CT in the investigation of neurological deterioration in longstanding spinal trauma. *Australas Radiol* 1992;36(3):198–203.

CHAPTER 22A

Craniocervical Junction: Occipital Condyle Fractures

Paul K. Kim, Bryan B. Barnes, and Joseph T. Alexander

INTRODUCTION

The traumatic occipital condyle fracture (OCF) was first described by Sir Charles Bell[1] in 1817 on the basis of an autopsy study of a victim from a fall. Conventional radiographic evidence of an OCF in vivo was initially reported in 1962, followed by the first computed tomography (CT) imaging scans of OCF published in 1983.[2] Since then, the improvements in CT technology and the increasing use of CT as a screening modality in trauma patients with routine inclusion of the craniovertebral junction have resulted in more frequent diagnosis and reporting of OCFs. Bloom et al.[3] identified a 16.4% incidence of OCF in a series of 55 patients with blunt craniocervical trauma, whereas older series generally carry lower estimates, ranging from less than 1% to 4% in incidence.[4,5]

The occipital condyles are the prominences of the paired lateral exoccipital segments of the occipital bone below and anterolateral to the foramen magnum. The convex occipital condyle articulate with the concave superior atlantal facets in "cup-shaped" fashion and slope downward from lateral to medial in the coronal plane. The two most important ligamentous structures relative to OCFs and their stability are the tectorial membrane and the alar ligaments (Fig. 22A.1).

The tectorial membrane, essentially a cephalad extension of the posterior longitudinal ligament, is a strong band of longitudinally oriented fibers attached to the dorsal surfaces of the vertebral bodies of C2 and C3, as well as the odontoid process. As it ascends, it widens and attaches to the anterolateral edge of the foramen magnum. The tectorial membrane functions primarily to limit extension, flexion, and vertical translation. Hyperflexion is also checked by contact between the anterior foramen magnum and the odontoid process.

The alar ligaments are paired structures that arise from the dorsolateral aspect of the odontoid process and run obliquely to attach to the inferomedial aspect of the occipital condyles. The alar ligaments function primarily to check lateral flexion and axial rotation. Cadaveric studies have demonstrated that division of the alar ligaments and tectorial membrane results in destabilization of the atlanto-occipital joint, allowing craniocervical dislocation to occur.[2] The paired atlanto-occipital joint capsules are attached above the superior margin of the occipital condyle and caudally to the lateral masses of C1; it is generally felt that the paired atlanto-occipital joint capsules provide poor stability because of their laxity.

The craniocervical junction in children is considered to be less stable than that of the adult because of several factors. Early in life, the plane of articulation of the atlanto-occipital joint is relatively horizontal and the occipital condyles are not deeply seated in the fossa of the superior facet of C1.[6] With maturation, the mass of the condyles increases and they become more deeply situated into the superior facet of C1. This results in a more vertical orientation of the atlanto-occipital joint.

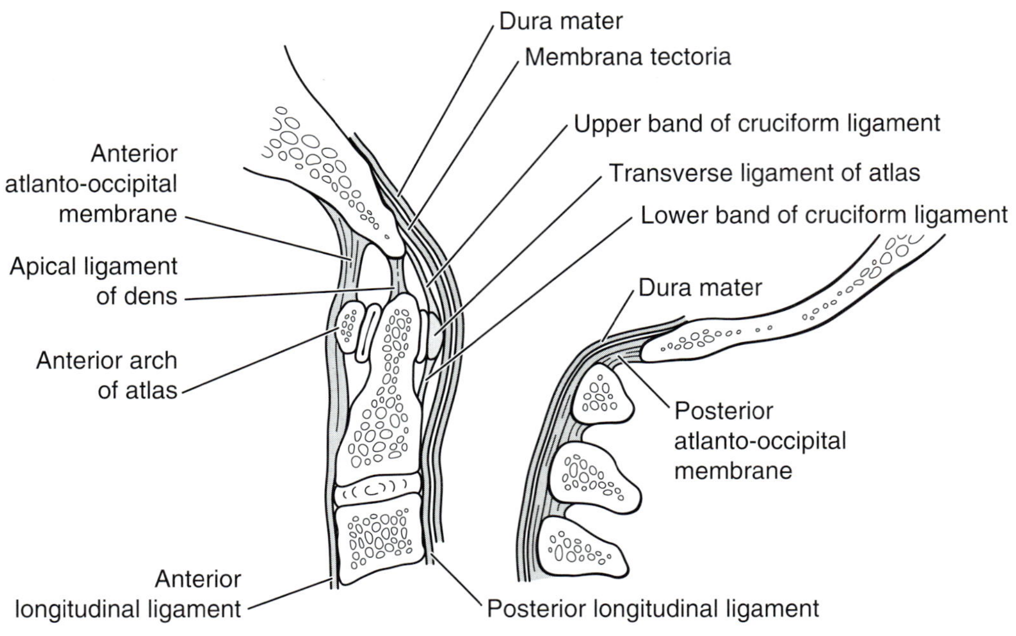

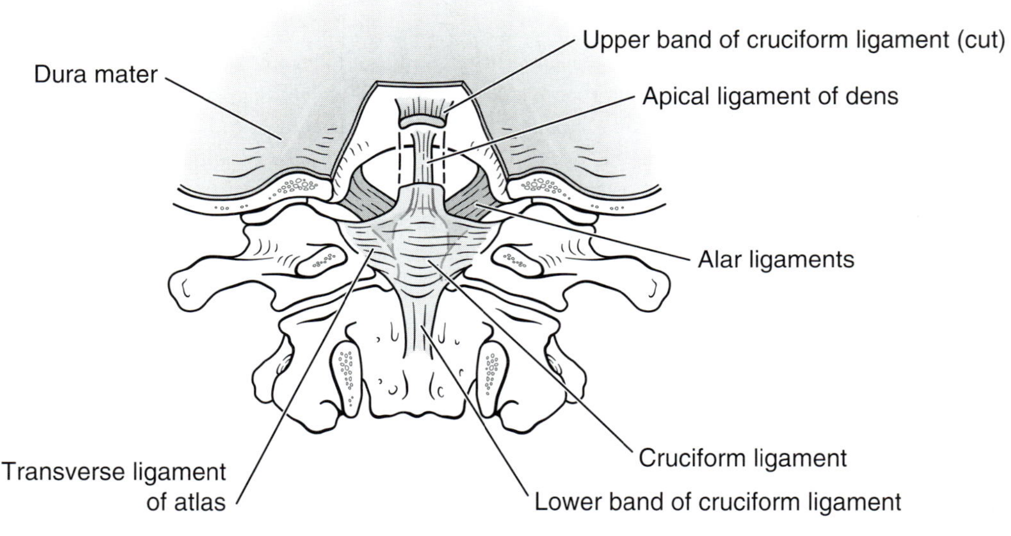

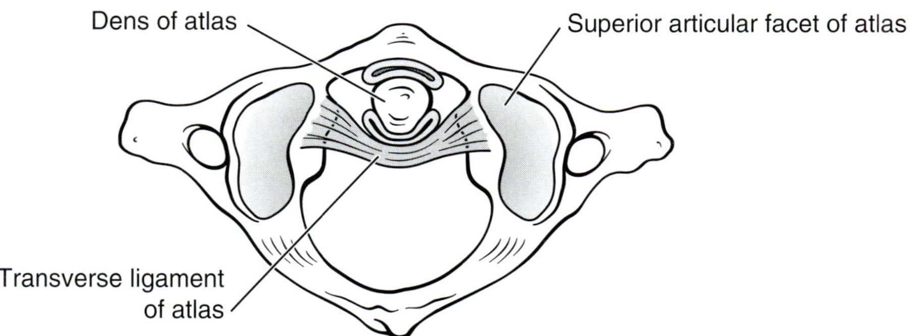

FIGURE 22A.1. The two most important ligamentous structures relative to occipital condyle fractures are the tectorial membrane and the alar ligaments.

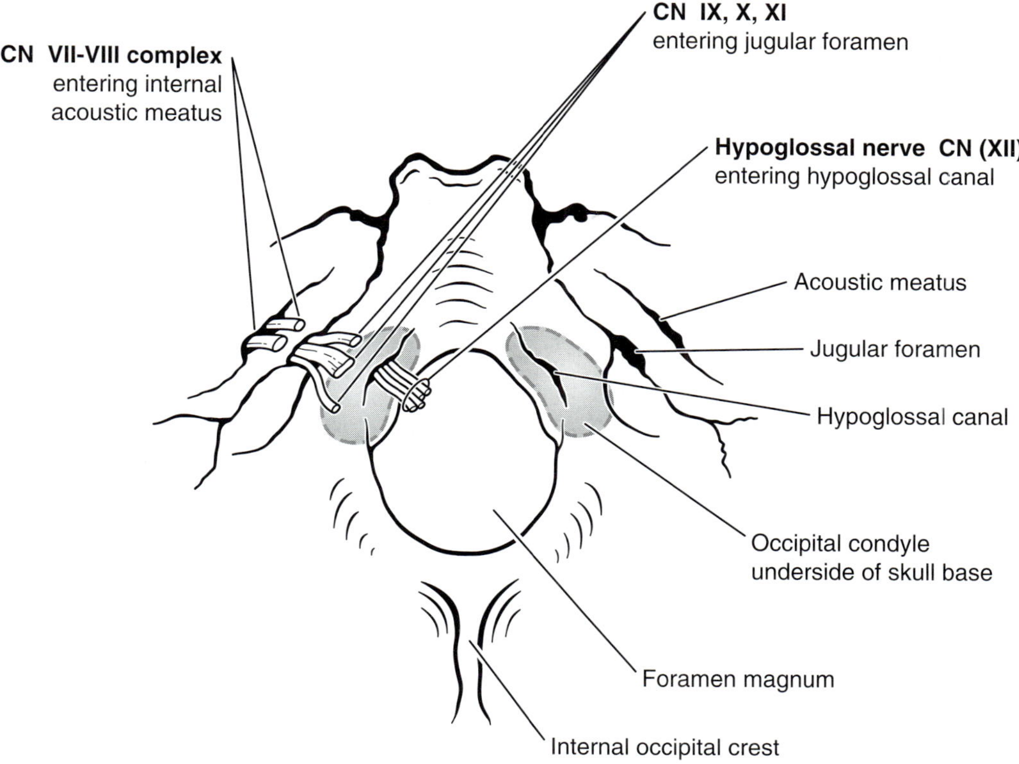

FIGURE 22A.2. Bony anatomic considerations in occipital condyle fracture include the proximity of the hypoglossal canal and jugular foramen to the occipital condyle.

In addition, the ligaments of the craniocervical junction become more developed, contributing to the relative increase of stability of the craniocervical junction in adults.[6]

Bony anatomic considerations in OCF also include the proximity of the hypoglossal canal and jugular foramen to the occipital condyle (Fig. 22A.2). The hypoglossal canal is within the base of the occipital condyle and contains the hypoglossal nerve (cranial nerve XII), a meningeal branch of the ascending pharyngeal artery, and an emissary vein. The jugular foramen is located lateral to the occipital condyle and posterior to the carotid canal and contains cranial nerves IX (glossopharyngeal), X (vagus), and XI (spinal accessory), the inferior petrosal sinus, internal jugular vein, and posterior meningeal artery. Fractures of the occipital condyle may extend to these bony structures, which could result in a palsy of one or more of the lower four cranial nerves.

MECHANISM OF INJURY

OCFs are in general associated with a high-energy craniocervical force generated by blunt trauma. Anderson and Montesano[7] further described an underlying mechanism of rapid deceleration as a cause of OCF in their series. The majority of OCFs occur as a result of motor vehicle collisions, with falls as the second-leading cause. In a recent study of 95 patients identified with OCF, 63% showed CT evidence of diffuse head injury or focal intracranial hematomas.[8] Moreover, 29% of the patients had additional cervical spine fractures or ligamentous or cord injuries. These were localized to the atlantoaxial region in 54% (15 of 28) of the patients, the mid or lower cervical region in 32% (9 of 28) of the patients, and both cervical segments in 14% (4 of 28) of the patients.[7]

CLASSIFICATION

Anderson and Montesano[7] have provided the most definitive classification scheme for OCF. Their classification is based on morphology and mechanism of injury (Fig. 22A.3). Type I OCF is an impacted OCF occurring as a result of an axial loading mechanism of the skull onto the atlas. There are no known factors identifying the likelihood of occurrence of an OCF, atlas fracture, or both in high-energy craniocervical blunt trauma cases with axial loading mechanisms. Whether age, bone

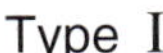

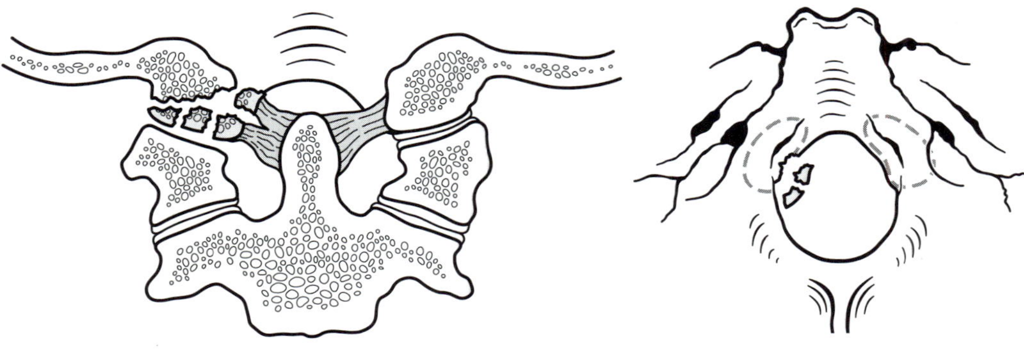

Type II

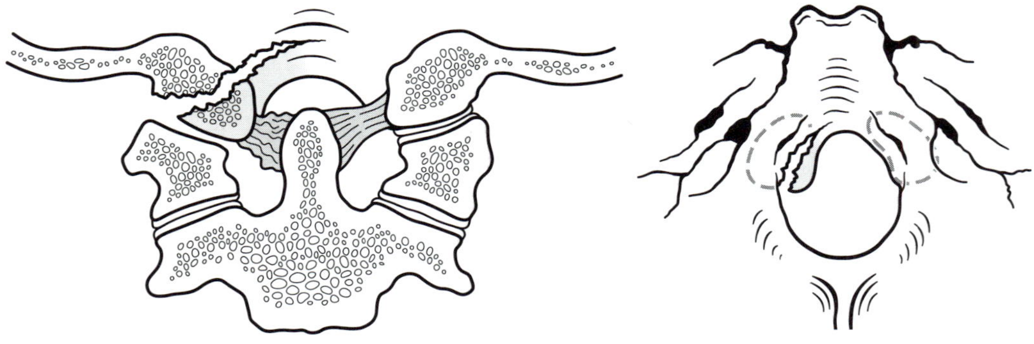

Type III

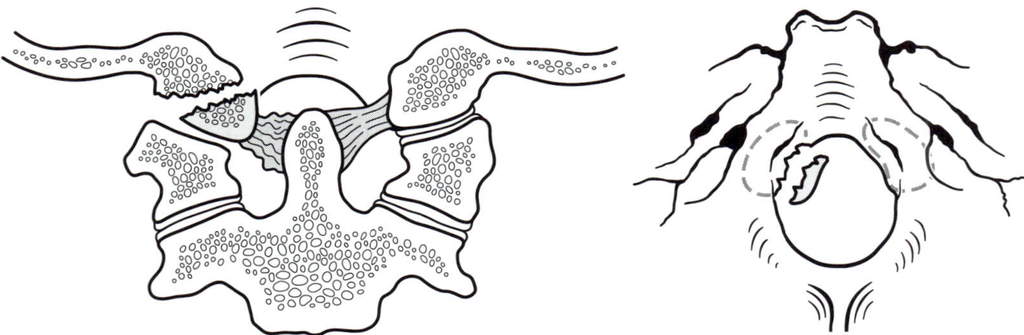

FIGURE 22A.3. Anderson and Montesano classification scheme.

density, or rate of loading play a significant role has not been clearly elucidated. Type I OCF is characterized by a comminuted, nondisplaced fracture with minimal or no displacement of fragments in the foramen magnum. Although the ipsilateral alar ligament may be injured, a type I OCF is considered to be a stable entity because of the integrity of the contralateral alar ligament and tectorial membrane.

Type II OCF is considered to be a basilar skull fracture that extends into the occipital condyle. A fracture line can be seen on CT axial sections of the skull base that exits the occipital condyle and enters the foramen magnum.[7] The mechanism of injury is a direct blow to the skull. There is no injury to the craniocervical ligaments as the tectorial membrane and alar ligaments remain intact, thereby preserving stability unless the fracture fragment is completely disconnected from the occiput.

Type III OCF is an avulsion fracture involving the alar ligaments, resulting in medial displacement of a free fragment from the inferomedial aspect of the occipital condyle into the foramen magnum. The mechanism of injury is forced rotation usually combined with lateral bending. Following occipital condylar avulsion, the contralateral alar ligament and tectorial membrane are stressed and loaded, representing a potentially unstable injury. In any of the fracture types, bilateral OCFs are considered to be unstable, with high likelihood of bilateral ligamentous injury.

Tuli et al.[9] proposed a new classification scheme for the management and treatment of OCF based on the stability of the occiput–C1-C2 junction, reflected by the presence of displacement of the condyle, CT or radiographic evidence of craniocervical instability, and magnetic resonance imaging (MRI) evidence of ligamentous injury. In this system, a type 1 OCF is defined as a nondisplaced fracture and considered to be stable. Type 2 OCFs are classified as displaced fractures that are considered to be either stable without evidence of ligamentous instability (type 2A) or unstable with evidence of ligamentous instability (type 2B). Although this classification scheme was designed to be more useful for clinical decision making and treatment strategy determination, the case example the authors described involved concurrent atlantoaxial instability on MRI of the cervical spine that prompted occipitocervical fusion, rather than atlanto-occipital instability secondary to an isolated OCF.

TREATMENT

INITIAL TREATMENT

Initial treatment should consist of supportive measures to stabilize the patient, including airway protection, ventilatory support, and circulatory support. Evaluation of the patient by a trauma team obviously includes attention to other life-threatening injuries. The presence of a concomitant cervical or thoracic spine fracture with neurologic deficit may warrant the administration of high-dose steroids. Cervical spine immobilization with a rigid cervical collar and log-roll precautions is prudent until the patient's spine can be completely evaluated.

There are few reported cases of cervical traction in the initial management of OCF. In one case, a patient with a type III OCF developed double vision during traction that subsequently resolved with surgical decompression.[10] In another case, a patient who also presented with a type III OCF was managed with cervical traction followed by halo placement, without noted complications. Currently, there are no clear indications for cervical traction in the management of isolated OCF, regardless of type.

The clinical presentation of patients with OCF is highly variable. Many severe neurologic deficits reported in patients with OCF are related to the severity of the associated head injury, rather than the OCF itself. Bloom et al.[3] noted that 4 of 9 patients in their series had significant intracranial injury with reduced Glasgow Coma Scale (GCS) score. However, the GCS score was reported to be normal in 5 of the 9 patients, stressing the fact that OCF should be considered in patients with a normal level of consciousness.

OCF is often seen in association with lower cranial nerve palsies. One study demonstrated that 31% (16 of 51) patients with OCF exhibited lower cranial nerve deficits; of these, 63% (10 of 16) presented initially, whereas 38% (6 of 16) presented in a delayed fashion, days to weeks after the injury.[9] A recent meta-analysis revealed only a 16% incidence of lower cranial nerve deficits in 91 patients.[11] Caroli et al.[12] reported that the hypoglossal nerve was most commonly involved, occurring in 74% of cases. Varying combinations involving cranial nerves IX to XII are also well described with OCF. According to a review of the literature, in 18% of the cases with lower cranial nerve involvement, unilateral palsy of the lower four cranial nerves was demonstrated, a condition referred to as Collet-Sicard syndrome.[12]

Plain radiographs did not depict up to 53% of the cervical spine fractures seen on CT in a recent study.[4] This study indicated that plain films alone are not sensitive in diagnosis of OCF. In one review, 42 of 62 patients diagnosed with OCF on CT had normal radiography studies; moreover, only 2 of 62 (3%) of the patients were identified with OCF on plain radiography.[11] Therefore, CT is regarded as the current standard for establishing the diagnosis of OCF. Many authors recommend that CT be performed as a diagnostic guideline when clinical suspicion is raised by one or more of the following criteria: blunt trauma patients with high-energy craniocervical injuries, altered level of consciousness, occipital pain or tenderness, persistent neck pain or impaired cervical motion, lower cranial nerve paresis, or retropharyngeal or prevertebral soft tissue swelling. Furthermore, it is recommended that CT imaging include thin axial sections with coronal and sagittal reconstructions from the occipital condyles through C2 to adequately evaluate the craniocervical junction.

Although less reliable in detecting OCF, the use of MRI in assessment of ligamentous structures, particularly the tectorial membrane and transverse ligament, is continually increasing. As mentioned previously, Tuli et al.[9] recommended the use of MRI as a diagnostic option to assess the craniocervical ligaments and differentiate stable from unstable OCF. Others have indicated that although MRI may not yield relevant additional diagnostic information concerning OCF, it is the best ancillary diagnostic tool complementing CT for evaluation of associated soft tissue trauma.[2] In addition, MRI remains superior in detection of brainstem and spinal cord compression or injury and confirming occipitoatlantal dissociation.

DEFINITIVE TREATMENT

Currently, there is no Class I evidence to support treatment standards or guidelines in the management of OCF. This is due, in part, to the relatively small number of cases described in the literature, inadequate reported follow-up in many cases, as well as the lack of prospective studies investigating outcome of the different treatment modalities. Of the 91 patients with OCF reviewed in a recent meta-analysis,[11] 23 patients did not receive treatment; 9 of these patients (one type I, one type II, one type III) developed delayed cranial nerve deficits within days to weeks after injury. The deficits resolved or improved in one third of the patients and remained unchanged in another third of the patients. Unfortunately, one third of the outcomes in this group were not reported.

In addition, there were six patients (1 type II, 5 type III) who presented with delayed lower cranial nerve deficits and were subsequently treated with external immobilization. Five of these six patients were managed in a rigid cervical collar for a 6- to 12-week course. Only one of these five patients did not have resolution or improvement of the deficit with collar immobilization; in this patient, deficits related to cranial nerves X to XII developed during treatment in a hard collar. At 1-year follow-up, the patient's cranial X and XI palsies improved, but the hypoglossal palsy persisted.[13]

In the meta-analysis, 44 patients were treated with rigid cervical collar immobilization (8 type I, 8 type II, and 28 type III).[11] Thirteen patients were managed with halo/Minerva immobilization (2 type I, 11 type II). There was no documentation of lower cranial nerve deficits in these treated patients following injury. At least five patients (1 type I, 4 type III) have been reported to have undergone surgical treatment, two of whom underwent surgery for removal of a displaced fracture fragment, with subsequent resolution of lower cranial nerve deficits postoperatively. Two other patients were treated with occipitocervical fusion for concurrent atlanto-occipital dislocation and atlantoaxial instability, respectively.[11]

Given the relatively high rate of delayed cranial nerve palsy in untreated OCF, in addition to the resolution or improvement of neurologic deficits with cervical immobilization noted in several cases, it seems that patients with type III OCF should be treated with external immobilization. Several authors have also suggested that treatment of patients with types I and II OCF may include external immobilization.[11] Although the majority of treated patients have been managed in a hard cervical collar for at least 8 to 12 weeks, the small numbers of reports and the varied management schemes have not reliably identified subgroups of patients who do not require treatment versus those who may require collar immobilization or more rigid halo immobilization.

Most studies have suggested that there is little role for surgical treatment of OCF in patients with a stable craniocervical junction and that conservative treatment is sufficient to promote healing of the fracture and recovery or improvement in all types of isolated OCF. However, surgical decompression with subsequent recovery or improvement of neurologic deficits has been described in a few cases.[13,14] Bozboga et al.[14] and others have proposed that surgical treatment is indicated when neurologic dysfunction resulting from neurovascular compression by a fracture fragment is present.[9,12]

PROGNOSIS

Little has been reported on the long-term outcome and prognosis for OCF. Several studies have demonstrated solid fusion of the fracture site in all patients treated conservatively.[12,15] Unfortunately, long-term morbidity, as a result of factors such as pain and limited range of motion, has not been well reported in many cases. As discussed in the previous section, the overwhelming majority of patients treated with cervical immobilization have demonstrated resolution or improvement of lower cranial nerve palsy and other neurologic deficits. This appears to occur regardless of whether these neurologic deficits occur at the time of injury or present in delayed fashion. It is hypothesized that delayed cranial nerve palsy is most likely caused by the formation of bony callous during the healing process or mobilization of a bone fragment that was not adequately stabilized initially. In many cases, diagnosis is probably delayed because of the difficulty of a complete neurologic assessment in a patient with reduced level of consciousness.

Accurate determination of incidence and prognosis of OCF is difficult because of the broad spectrum of clinical presentation. This patient population ranges from those who are asymptomatic to those whose clinical condition may be masked by concomitant traumatic injuries or death. In fact, some cases of OCF have been described in autopsy series in association with severe intracranial and spinal cord injuries, including occipitocervical dissociation.[16] Lethal brainstem contusion and infarction have been identified on MRI in several cases with isolated OCF, illustrating the potential for a displaced fracture fragment to cause severe neurovascular injury. In spite of this, prognosis for isolated OCF is generally good, with outcome closely tied to recovery or improvement of lower cranial nerve and other neurologic deficits sustained from injury.

COMPLICATIONS

The potential for neurologic injury or death resulting from OCF has been described earlier. Because delayed neurologic deficits may occur as a result of mobilization of an OCF fragment that has not been adequately stabilized, the importance of early diagnosis and treatment of OCF and careful follow-up of asymptomatic patients is emphasized. Clinical suspicion prompting evaluation with CT imaging should include patients with blunt trauma with high-energy craniocervical injuries, altered level of consciousness, occipital pain or tenderness, persistent neck pain or impaired cervical motion, lower cranial nerve paresis, or retropharyngeal or prevertebral soft tissue swelling. Advancements in CT imaging with three-dimensional reconstructions allow for more precise measurement of fracture displacement.

In addition, the increasing use of MRI for diagnosing ligamentous injury may be useful in identifying subgroups of patients who do not require treatment or, conversely, require more rigid halo immobilization rather than collar immobilization. Although a small minority of reported cases have demonstrated no improvement in neurologic deficits with cervical immobilization, neurologic deterioration as a direct result of conservative management is extremely rare.

REFERENCES

1. Bell C. Surgical observations. *Middlesex Hosp J* 1817;4:469–470.
2. Leone A, Cerase A, Colosimo C, et al. Occipital condylar fractures: a review. *Radiology* 2000;216:635–644.
3. Bloom AI, Neeman Z, Slasky BS, et al. Fracture of the occipital condyles and associated craniocervical ligament injury: incidence, CT imaging and complications. *Clin Radiol* 1997;52:198–202.
4. Link TM, Schuierer G, Hufendiek A, et al. Substantial head trauma: value of CT examination of the cervicocranium. *Radiology* 1995;196:741–745.
5. Noble ER, Smoker WR. The forgotten condyle: the appearance, morphology and classification of occipital condyle fractures. *AJNR Am J Neuroradiol* 1996;17:507–513.
6. Gilles FH, Bina M, Sotrel A. Infantile atlantooccipital instability. *Am J Dis Child* 1979;133:30–37.
7. Anderson PA, Montesano PX: Morphology and treatment of occipital condyle fractures. *Spine* 1988;13:731–736.
8. Hanson JA, Deliganis AV, Baxter AB, et al. Radiologic and clinical spectrum of occipital condyle fractures: retrospective review of 107 consecutive fractures in 95 patients. *AJR Am J Roentgenol* 2002;178:1261–1268.
9. Tuli S, Tator CG, Fehlings MG, et al. Occipital condyle fractures. *Neurosurgery* 1997;41:368–377.
10. Wassenberg J, Bartlett RJV. Occipital condyle fractures diagnosed by high-definition CT and coronal reconstructions. *Neuroradiology* 1995;37:370–373.
11. Section on Disorders of the Spine and Peripheral Nerves of the American Association of Neurological Surgeons and the Congress of Neurological Surgeons. "Occipital condyle fractures" in guidelines of the management of acute cervical spine and spinal cord injuries. *Neurosurgery* 2002;50:S114–S119.
12. Caroli E, Rocchi G, Orlando ER, et al. Occipital condyle fractures: report of five cases and literature review. *Eur Spine J* 2005;14:487–492.
13. Bridgeman SA, McNab W. Traumatic occipital condyle fracture, multiple cranial nerve palsies, and torticollis: a case report and review of the literature. *Surg Neurol* 1992;38:152–156.
14. Bozboga M, Unal F, Hepgul K, et al. Fracture of the occipital condyle: case report. *Spine* 1992;17:119–1121.
15. Capuano C, Costagliola C, Shamsaldin M, et al. Occipital condyle fractures: a hidden nosological entity: an experience with 10 cases. *Acta Neurochir (Wien)* 2004;146:779–784.
16. Bucholtz RW, Burkhead WZ, Graham W, et al. Occult cervical spine injuries in fatal traffic accidents. *J Trauma* 1979;19:768–771.

CHAPTER 22B

Craniocervical Junction: Occipitocervical Dissociation

Luis M. Tumialán, Praveen V. Mummaneni, Jeff Pan, and Gerald E. Rodts

INTRODUCTION

Occipitocervical dissociation or dislocation, also referred to as craniocervical dissociation, has been historically thought to be uniformly fatal. Recently, it has become not only a potentially survivable injury but may also have an excellent outcome.[1–8] This has been due primarily to the improvements of emergency management in the field, rigid stabilization of the cervical spine, and rapid transport of injured patients. Furthermore, heightened awareness of this injury has allowed timely diagnosis and intervention. The inherent fatal nature of the severe form of this injury has precluded a true incidence from being obtained, yet authors have speculated that this injury may in fact represent 8% to 19% of all victims following a fatal motor vehicle accident.[9–11] Despite this, occipitocervical dissociation remains a rare traumatic entity in which subtle clinical and radiographic forms may delay diagnosis. These injuries represent a continuum from isolated occipital condyle fractures to complete occipitoatlantal dislocations. Also, the injuries may be unilateral and less commonly bilateral, with the latter being significantly more dangerous.

MECHANISM OF INJURY

The occipitoatlantal and atlantoaxial articulations function biomechanically as a single unit, with the atlas acting as a washer or bushing between the cranium and the axis.[12,13] This relationship facilitates the rotation that occurs especially at C1-C2. These articulations are stabilized by the tectorial ligament, the paired alar ligaments, the cruciate ligament, and the apical dental ligament. Anatomic studies have demonstrated that severing both the alar ligaments and tectorial membrane results in complete occipitocervical dissociation.[14] Disruption of these ligaments usually occurs by shear or distractive forces and causes significant energy to be translated to the victim's craniocervical junction. This most commonly occurs after a high-energy motor vehicle or pedestrian vehicular trauma.[13,15,16]

Neurologic presentations may include flaccid quadriplegia and incomplete spinal cord syndromes, such as Brown-Séquard syndrome. Complete transection at the level of the medulla oblongata or the spinomedullary junction in severe injuries invariably leads to death.

DIAGNOSIS

The craniocervical junction should be always assessed in victims of blunt trauma. However, plain lateral radiographs (in the neutral position) have been shown to have poor reliability. A retrospective review of

79 cases found the diagnosis of this injury was actually possible in 60 of these patients (sensitivity of 76%). Despite this, the diagnosis was made in 45 of the 79 patients (sensitivity of 57%). Thus, the recognition of this injury requires a heightened index of suspicion and rigorous analysis of the radiographs. Prevertebral soft tissue swelling on a lateral cervical radiograph (present in 37 of 41 reported cases, or 90% sensitivity) or subarachnoid hemorrhage on axial head computed tomography (CT) has been associated with occipitocervical dissociation and should prompt further investigation.[17,18]

Analysis of cranial landmarks, such as the basion and opisthion, and their relation to the atlas and dens, can be useful in the diagnosis of occipitocervical dissociation. Wholey and Baker[18] reported that the distance from the occipital basion to the tip of the odontoid is approximately 5 mm in the adult patient and may be as much as 10 mm in the pediatric patient. A displacement of more than 10 mm is considered abnormal and highly suggestive of occipitocervical dissociation. Anterior or posterior translation between the basion and the odontoid should be no greater than 1 mm. Values greater than this suggest instability and possible occipitocervical dissociation. Harris et al.[19] studied the relationship between the dens and basion and the distance between the posterior axial line and the basion. He found that patients with more than 12 mm on either of these measurements were likely to have an occipitocervical dissociation.

Controversy exists regarding the most sensitive and specific method to identify occipitocervical dissociation. Although no radiographic method discussed previously has 100% sensitivity, Harris's rule of 12 appears to be the most reliable measurement to diagnose occipitocervical dissociation. Recent studies have also demonstrated an increase in sensitivity with all of these modalities when these methods are used with CT sagittal reconstruction of the upper cervical spine.[19,20]

Subtle occipitocervical dissociation may be a difficult diagnosis with only plain lateral cervical radiographs. Further investigation with fine-section CT is recommended. Magnetic resonance imaging (MRI) may be used to study the craniocervical ligaments. Specific protocols using fat suppression techniques and frontal plane images may increase the likelihood of imaging the important alar ligaments.[21,22]

On clinical examination, patients may present with an array of neurologic deficits, specifically lower cranial nerve palsies (particularly VI, X, and XII), monoparesis, hemiparesis, quadriparesis, complete and incomplete high cervical cord injury, motor deficits, and cerebellar infarction.[23,24] The presence of any of these findings in the setting of normal plain radiographs warrants additional imaging with CT or MRI to exclude occipitocervical dissociation. Other subtle neurologic findings may include pupillary abnormalities, rotary nystagmus, and ocular bobbing.[24] Approximately 20% of patients with occipitocervical dissociation will have normal neurologic examination findings.

CLASSIFICATION OF INJURIES

Occipitocervical dissociations may be classified based on the relative position of the occiput in relation to the atlas (Fig. 22B.1).[20] Anterior dislocations, the most common, are anterior dislocations of occipital condyles relative to the atlantal lateral masses; similarly, injuries with a posterior dislocation of the condyles are posterior dislocations. Vertical separation or diastasis of the occipital condyles from the atlas are referred to as a longitudinal dissociation. Dislocations may be unilateral or bilateral. Milder injury variants such as subluxations where the normal occipital-atlantal joint congruity is lost are more frequently recognized.

TREATMENT

INITIAL TREATMENT

The initial treatment is to provide immediate reduction and immobilization. Traction should be used with caution because distraction may result in further neurologic and vascular injury.[25] In a retrospective review of 21 patients with occipitocervical dissociation, two patients deteriorated neurologically with traction; in both cases, the deficit improved when traction was removed.

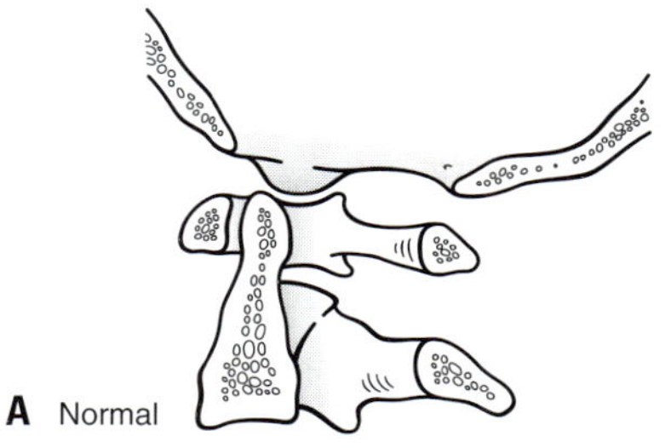

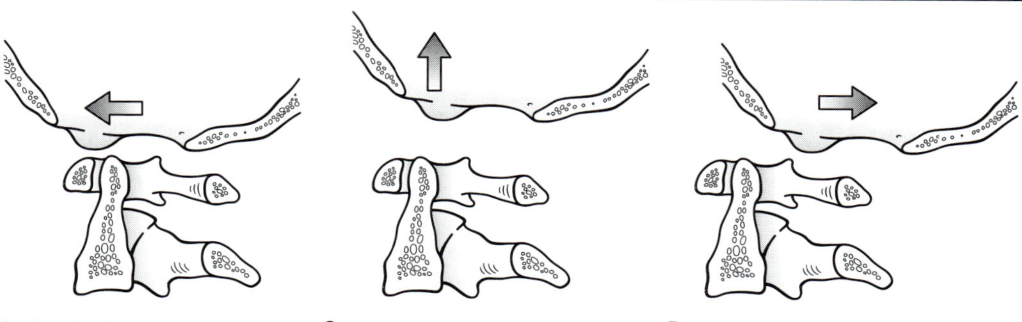

FIGURE 22B.1. The classification of occipital cervical dissociations. **A.** Normal. **B.** Type I anterior displacement of the occiput on the atlas. **C.** Type II longitudinal displacement of the occiput on the atlas. **D.** Type III posterior displacement of the occiput on the atlas.

Reduction is best achieved using the halo vest. Careful orientation of the head relative to the thorax based on initial displacement is used to correct malalignment. The halo vest provides minimal immobilization in unstable upper cervical spines, and displacements may occur. Frequent radiographic confirmations of reduction should be obtained while patients are so immobilized.

DEFINITIVE TREATMENT

Occipitocervical disassociations are associated with significant ligamentous injuries to the alar ligaments and tectorial membrane, which have a poor prognosis. Therefore the majority of cases are best treated with a posterior occipital-to-C2 fusion. Approximately 28% of patients in the literature managed with external immobilization alone either deteriorated neurologically or did not achieve permanent stability of the occipitocervical junction.

The occiput–C1-C2 articulations function as a single unit, with the axis serving as the anchor for the severed ligaments; therefore, the axis must be incorporated into the fusion construct. Hence, occiput-to-C2 fusion is the treatment of choice for this injury, in the absence of additional injury in the subaxial spine.[26]

Patients with occipitocervical dissociation represent an anesthetic and positioning challenge. Awake fiberoptic intubation, somatosensory and brainstem evoked potential monitoring, and positioning under fluoroscopy are recommended to minimize risk for neurologic injury. After general anesthesia is induced, the patient is placed into a three-pin rigid head holder or halo vest and positioned prone. The cervical collar is kept secured on the patient until the head holder is secured to the operating room table and fluoroscopy demonstrates no displacement.

Although wire techniques result in high fusion success, rigid techniques are recommended in patients with occipitocervical dissociation.[27] Children younger than 10 years can be stabilized using a rod-wire technique described by Sontag[28] or technique similar to that used in adults if anatomy is conducive. In adults, screw-plate or newer rod-plate techniques provide sufficient stability to maintain reduction, achieve satisfactory fusion success, and minimize external immobilization requirements.

COMPLICATIONS

Neurologic deterioration is seen commonly in occipitocervical dissociation and is usually secondary to delay in diagnosis. New or evolving neurologic deficits, specifically brainstem findings after immobilization, prompt the concern for vertebral artery dissection. Conventional or CT angiography should be performed to confirm this diagnosis before anticoagulation. Displacement after initial immobilization can occur and should be monitored carefully. The surgical treatment is associated with risk during positioning, intubation, and screw placement.

REFERENCES

1. Gregg S, Kortbeek JB, du Plessis S. Atlanto-occipital dislocation: a case study of survival with partial recovery and review of the literature. *J Trauma* 2005;58:168–171.
2. Shamoun JM, Riddick L, Powell RW. Atlanto-occipital subluxation/dislocation: a "survivable" injury in children. *Am Surg* 1999;65:317–320.
3. Ferrera PC, Bartfield JM. Traumatic atlanto-occipital dislocation: a potentially survivable injury. *Am J Emerg Med* 1996;14:291–296.
4. Yamaguchi N, Ikeda K, Ishise J, et al. Traumatic atlanto-occipital dislocation with long-term survival. *Neurol Med Chir (Tokyo)* 1996;36:36–39.
5. Donahue DJ, Muhlbauer MS, Kaufman RA, et al. Childhood survival of atlantooccipital dislocation: underdiagnosis, recognition, treatment, and review of the literature. *Pediatr Neurosurg* 1994;21:105–111.
6. Hosono N, Yonenobu K, Kawagoe K, et al. Traumatic anterior atlanto-occipital dislocation. A case report with survival. *Spine* 1993;18:786–790.
7. Nischal K, Chumas P, Sparrow O. Prolonged survival after atlanto-occipital dislocation: two case reports and review. *Br J Neurosurg* 1993;7:677–682.
8. Seibert PS, Stridh-Igo P, Whitmore TA, et al. Cranio-cervical stabilization of traumatic atlanto-occipital dislocation with minimal resultant neurological deficit. *Acta Neurochir (Wien)* 2005;147:435–442; discussion 442.
9. Bucholz RW, Burkhead WZ. The pathological anatomy of fatal atlanto-occipital dislocations. *J Bone Joint Surg Am* 1979;61:248–250.
10. Gossman W, June RA, Wallace D. Fatal atlanto-occipital dislocation secondary to airbag deployment. *Am J Emerg Med* 1999;17:741–742.
11. Kondo T, Saito K, Nishigami J, et al. Fatal injuries of the brain stem and/or upper cervical spinal cord in traffic accidents: nine autopsy cases. *Sci Justice* 1995;35:197–201.
12. American Society of Pediatric Neurosurgeons. Section of Pediatric Neurosurgery of the A.A.N.S. *Pediatric Neurosurgery: Surgery of the Developing Nervous System.* 4th ed. Philadephia, Pennsylvania: W.B. Saunders Company, 2001.
13. White AA 3rd, Panjabi MM. The clinical biomechanics of the occipitoatlantoaxial complex. *Orthop Clin North Am* 1978;9:867–878.
14. Vaccaro AR, ed. *Fractures of the Cervical, Thoracic and Lumbar Spine.* New York, NY: Marcel Dekker, Inc., 2003.
15. Lee C, Woodring JH, Goldstein SJ, et al. Evaluation of traumatic atlantooccipital dislocations. *AJNR Am J Neuroradiol* 1987;8:19–26.
16. Tepper SL, Fligner CL, Reay DT. Atlanto-occipital disarticulation. Accident characteristics. *Am J Forensic Med Pathol* 1990;11:193–197.
17. Diagnosis and management of traumatic atlanto-occipital dislocation injuries. *Neurosurgery* 2002;50:S105–13.
18. Brinkman W, Cohen W, Manning T. Posterior fossa subarachnoid hemorrhage due to an atlantooccipital dislocation. *AJR Am J Roentgenol* 2003;180:1476.
19. Dziurzynski K, Anderson PA, Bean DB, et al. A blinded assessment of radiographic criteria for atlanto-occipital dislocation. *Spine* 2005;30:1427–1432.
20. Traynelis VC, Marano GD, Dunker RO, et al. Traumatic atlanto-occipital dislocation. Case report. *J Neurosurg* 1986;65:863–870.
21. Przybylski GJ, Clyde BL, Fitz CR. Craniocervical junction subarachnoid hemorrhage associated with atlanto-occipital dislocation. *Spine* 1996;21:1761–1768.
22. Chaljub G, Singh H, Gunito FC Jr, et al. Traumatic atlanto-occipital dislocation: MRI and CT. *Neuroradiology* 2001;43:41–44.

23. Isaeff SD, Siegel A. Brain scintigraphy of cerebellar infarction secondary to atlanto-occipital dislocation. *Clin Nucl Med* 2000;25:1031–1032.
24. Harty JA, Sparkes J, McCormack D, et al. Recognition of progressive atlanto-occipital dislocation (by a changing neurologic status and clinical deformity). *J Orthop Trauma* 2003;17:299–302.
25. Labbe JL, Leclair O, Duparc B. Traumatic atlanto-occipital dislocation with survival in children. *J Pediatr Orthop B* 2001;10:319–327.
26. Hosalkar HS, Cain EL, Horn D, et al. Traumatic atlanto-occipital dislocation in children. *J Bone Joint Surg Am* 2005;87:2480–2488.
27. Vaccaro AR, Cook CM, McCullen G, et al. Cervical trauma: rationale for selecting the appropriate fusion technique. *Orthop Clin North Am* 1998;29:745–754.
28. McDonnell D, Harrison S. Posterior atlantoaxial fusion: indications and techniques. In Hitchon P, Traynelis V, Rengachary S, eds. *Techniques in Spinal Fusion and Stabilization.* New York, NY: Thieme, 1995:92–106.

CHAPTER 23A

Atlas Injuries: Atlas Fractures

Neal G. Haynes, Troy D. Gust, and Paul M. Arnold

INTRODUCTION

Fractures of the atlas (C1) account for 2% to 13% of cervical spine fractures and just over 1% of all spine fractures. Approximately 21% of patients with an atlas fracture will also have an associated head injury, and 5% to 53% will have an associated axis or other cervical spine injury.[1–6] The overwhelming majority of these fractures are a result of motor vehicle collisions and motorcycle collisions, although falls, assaults, and auto-pedestrian and bicycle accidents are also responsible for some of these injuries.

The anatomy of the atlas is unique in that it is highly susceptible to injury because of its location between the more massive occipital condyles and the lateral masses of C2. Additionally, the thinness of the posterior ring makes it more susceptible to fracture than the posterior elements at other levels, although cadaveric studies show a mean tensile strength of 2280 N.[7] This increased susceptibility to injury is counterbalanced by the fact that isolated atlas fractures rarely cause neurologic compromise. This is generally believed to be due to the unusually large transverse and sagittal diameter of the spinal canal at this level and to the sloping nature of the articular facets, which tend to force the lateral masses outward rather than inward following compression-type injuries (Fig. 23A.1).

There are six basic patterns of atlas fractures, each based on the force vectors responsible for the injury, as well as patient neck position at the time of impact.

The first and most well known is the Jefferson fracture, first described by Sir Geoffrey Jefferson in 1920. This type of fracture is classically described as a four-point fracture of the atlas, with two fractures through the anterior ring, two fractures through the posterior ring, and spreading of the lateral masses; however, three-part and two-part fractures are also generally referred to as Jefferson fractures (Fig. 23A.2). In fact, in Jefferson's original paper, only 3 of the 25 fractures in his literature review and none of the 4 fractures he described were four-part fractures.[8] Jefferson is also credited with the description of the mechanism of injury, which he described as direct vertical compression of the atlas between the occipital condyles and the lateral masses of the axis with the neck in a neutral position. This causes a fracture of the posterior and anterior rings at their thinnest areas, the area of attachment to the lateral masses. The downward-directed vector, coupled with the outwardly sloping shape of the articular facets, forces the lateral masses outward and away from the spinal cord. For this reason, and because of the large transverse and sagittal diameter of the spinal canal at this level, Jefferson fractures rarely are associated with spinal cord injury. Jefferson fractures are of two types, stable and unstable, with the latter having a disrupted transverse ligament. For reliable patients with nondisplaced fractures, a soft or hard collar is usually sufficient to ensure fracture healing.[9,10] For displaced fractures with more than 7 mm of displacement of the lateral masses, a hard collar, or sterno-occipito-mandibular immobilizer (SOMI) brace, should suffice; a halo vest should be considered if the patient is considered to be unreliable.[9,10]

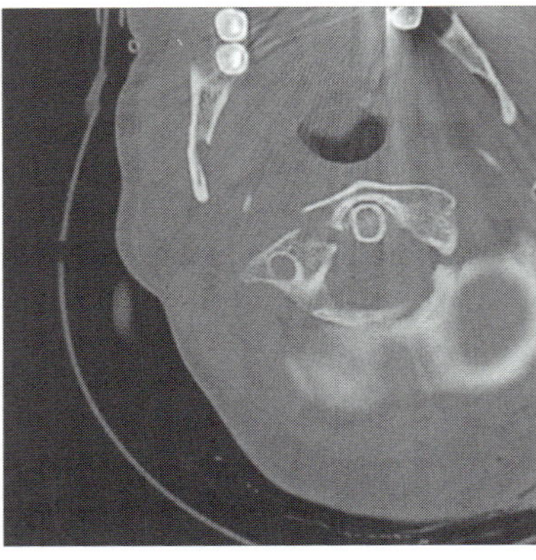

FIGURE 23A.1. Axial CT scan of C1 fracture. Note the widened spinal canal.

A second fracture pattern of the axis consists of an isolated anterior ring fracture (Fig. 23A.3). This is believed to be caused by axial loading with the neck in flexion, trapping just the anterior ring between the occipital condyles and the lateral masses of the axis and sparing the posterior ring.[9,11] Because the posterior ring remains intact, there is no spreading of the lateral masses. These fractures are usually nondisplaced and are normally not associated with neurologic deficits. This fracture is considered to be stable and can be treated with either a soft or hard collar.[12]

A third fracture pattern of the axis is an isolated posterior ring fracture, believed to be caused by axial loading with hyperextension forces (Fig. 23A.4). This causes the posterior ring to fracture at its thinnest point near the grooves of the vertebral artery. This spares the anterior ring, and, thus, there is no spread of the lateral masses. These fractures may or may not be displaced and usually are not associated with neurologic deficits. These fractures are difficult to differentiate from congenital anomalies without computed tomography (CT). As an isolated injury, these fractures are considered to be stable and also can be treated with either a hard or soft cervical collar for comfort.[9,12]

A fourth fracture pattern is a lateral mass fracture caused by axial loading with lateral bending of the cervical spine. If there is less than 2 mm displacement of the lateral mass and the fracture is not in conjunction with an axis fracture, these fractures can be treated with a soft or hard cervical collar. If the displacement is greater than 2 mm or if there is an associated axis fracture, this injury is unstable and may require recumbent traction, a halo vest, or posterior atlantoaxial or occipitoaxial stabilization and fusion.[9]

A fifth and very rare fracture pattern is a transverse fracture of the anterior arch (Fig. 23A.5), which is actually an avulsion of the superior attachment of the longus colli muscles. As an isolated injury, it is considered to be stable and can be treated with a soft or hard collar.

A sixth fracture pattern involves only the transverse process (Fig. 23A.6). Although usually benign, a fracture in this area (as well as the posterior ring) may cause thrombosis, dissection, or disruption of the vertebral artery.[9,13] Immediate sequelae from dissection of a dominate vertebral artery include cerebellar and brainstem infarction and vertebrobasilar insufficiency. Delayed sequelae such as cortical blindness, quadriplegia, and dural arteriovenous fistulas, although rare, have been reported in the literature.[14,15] CT or magnetic resonance angiography is useful in clarifying injury to the vertebral arteries.

Cervical spine fractures are notoriously difficult to diagnose with plain radiographs alone. Diaz et al.[6] found that five-view cervical spine films failed to diagnose 47.2% of C1-C3 fractures that were subsequently imaged by CT. In the same study, no C1-C3 fractures were missed by CT (Fig. 23A.7). In the obtunded trauma patient or in patients with persistent neck pain and negative plain films, it is important to obtain a CT scan with reconstruction of the cervical spine to rule out an occult upper cervical spine fracture.

Initial treatment of atlas fracture involves determining the extent of the trauma, as well as surveying the spine for other injuries. This may include radiographs with flexion-extension views to assess

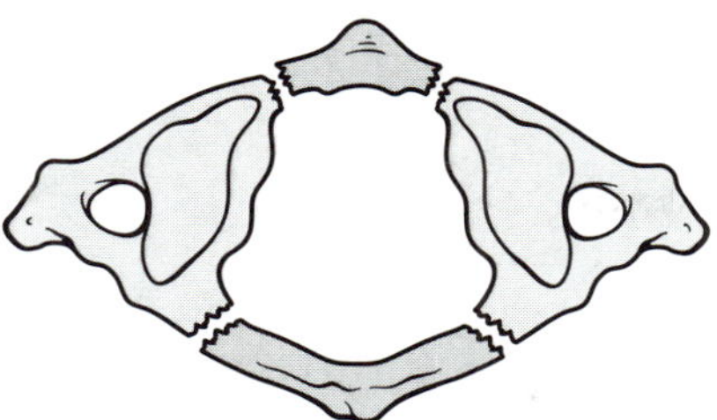

FIGURE 23A.2. Classic Jefferson fracture with evidence of fracture at four points.

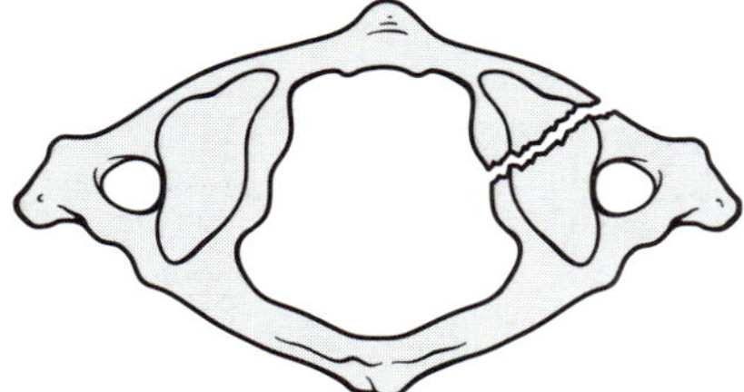

FIGURE 23A.3. Lateral mass fracture.

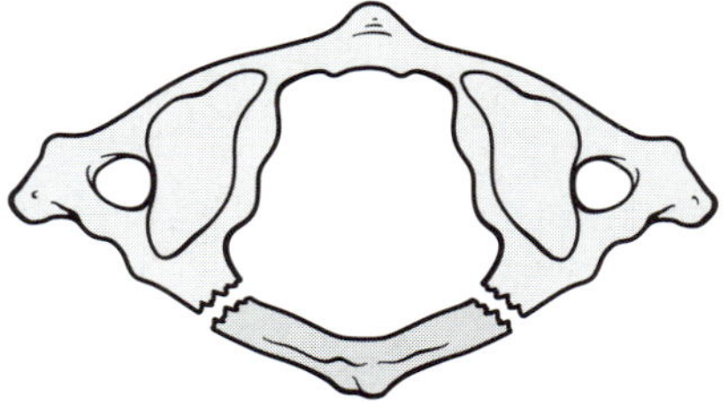

FIGURE 23A.4. Isolated posterior ring fracture.

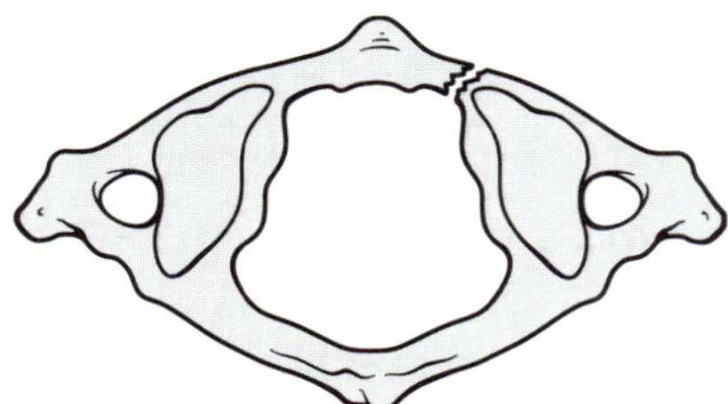

FIGURE 23A.5. Anterior ring fracture.

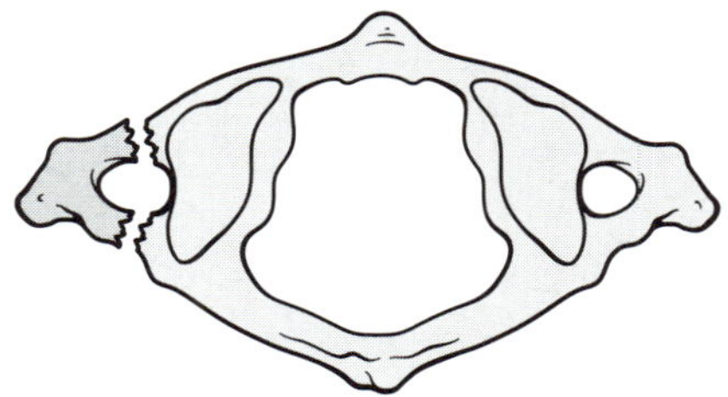

FIGURE 23A.6. Fracture of the transverse process.

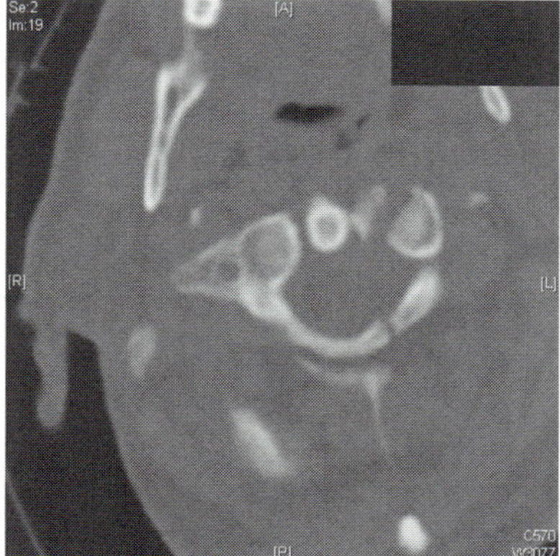

FIGURE 23A.7. Axial CT scan shows C1 fracture.

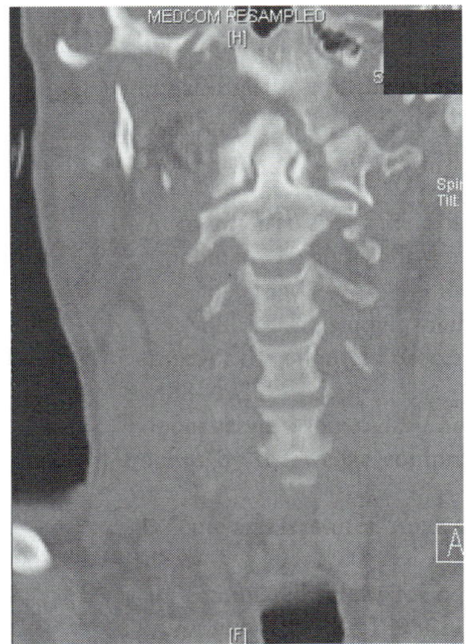

FIGURE 23A.8. Coronal reformatted CT. Note the lateral displacement of the C1 lateral mass.

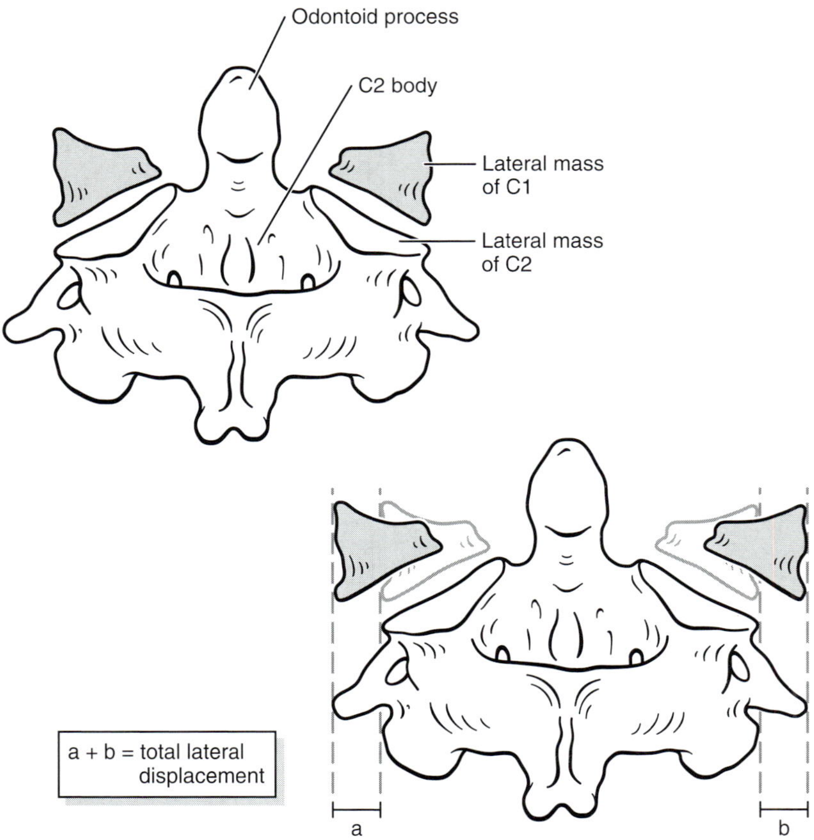

FIGURE 23A.9. Determination of stability of C1 fracture. If a + b ≥7 mm, then the transverse ligament is injured and the fracture is considered unstable.

occult instability; reformatted three-dimensional CT scans to evaluate the injury in multiple planes (Fig. 23A.8); and magnetic resonance imaging (MRI) to evaluate soft tissue and ligamentous damage.

As noted earlier, most patients with isolated C1 fractures do not sustain neurologic injury; these patients can generally be treated with a rigid collar, SOMI brace, or, occasionally, a halo vest. If there is 7 mm or greater displacement of the lateral masses of C1, that is, the transverse ligament is disrupted, healing may or may not occur with halo vest immobilization. Dynamic imaging studies should be obtained at the conclusion of immobilization to assess for any residual cervical instability. Midtransverse ligament injuries are extremely unstable and may be treated primarily with occipitocervical fusion or atlantoaxial fusion in the setting of a displaced atlas fracture (Fig. 23A.9). Treatment of C1 injuries found in conjunction with other spine fractures are generally dictated by those other injuries.

For displacement of the two lateral masses of a total 7 mm or greater (Fig. 23A.9) with an obvious transverse ligamentous avulsion from the medial tubercle of the atlas,[9,10] a cervical orthosis should be employed for a minimum of 8 weeks with a CT of the cervical spine at that time to evaluate healing of the fracture. An additional 8 weeks of immobilization may be required. Some of these fractures may heal by fibrous union without ossification and are considered to be stable. In a series of 32 patients with isolated C1 fractures, Spence et al.[10] found no case of isolated C1 injury that required surgical stabilization or fusion, with all cases successfully treated by immobilization for a mean of 12 weeks. There have been reported cases of cranial nerve injuries following Jefferson fractures as a result of a compression injury to CN IX, X, XI, and XII as they pass between the displaced lateral mass and the styloid process.[13,16]

Complications associated with C1 fractures include injury to the vertebral arteries or lower cranial nerves. Late complications include undiagnosed unstable injuries, which may require surgical stabilization and fusion.

The prognosis for C1 fractures is generally good. These bony injuries usually heal within 3 months, with resolution of the associated neck pain. No further treatment will be necessary if ligamentous disruption and neurologic deficits are absent.

REFERENCES

1. Betz RR, Gelman AJ, DeFilipp GJ, et al. Magnetic resonance imaging (MRI) in the evaluation of spinal cord injured children and adolescents. *Paraplegia* 1987;25:92–99.
2. Brattstrom H, Granholm L. Atlanto-axial fusion in rheumatoid arthritis: a new method of fixation with wire and bone cement. *Acta Orthop Scand* 1976;47619–628.
3. Hadley MN, Dickman CA, Browner CM, et al. Acute traumatic atlas fractures: management and long term outcome. *Neurosurgery* 1988;23:31–35.
4. Fowler JL, Sandhu A, Fraser RD. A review of fractures of the atlas vertebra. *J Spinal Disord* 1990;3:19–24.
5. Sherk HH, Nicholson JT. Fractures of the atlas. *J Bone Joint Surg Am* 1970;52:1017–1024.
6. Diaz JJ Jr, Gilman C, Morris JA, et al. Are five-view plain films of the cervical spine unreliable? A prospective evaluation in blunt trauma patients with altered mental status. *J Trauma* 2003;55:658–663, discussion 663–664.
7. Beckner MA, Heggeness MH, Doherty BJ. A biomechanical study of Jefferson fractures. *Spine* 1998;23:1832–1836.
8. Jefferson G. Fracture of the atlas vertebrae: report of 4 cases and a review of those previously recorded. *Br J Surg* 1920;7:407–422.
9. Scharen S, Jeanneret B. [Atlas fractures]. *Orthopade* 1999;28:385–393.
10. Spence KF Jr, Decker S, Sell KW. Bursting atlantal fracture associated with rupture of the transverse ligament. *J Bone Joint Surg Am* 1970;52:543–549.
11. Bohlman HH, Ducker TD. Spine trauma in adults. In: Herkowitz HM, Garfin SR, Balderston RA, et al., eds. *The Spine*. 4th ed. Philadelphia: WB Saunders, 1999:888–1003.
12. Sonntag VK, Hadley MN. Nonoperative management of cervical spine injuries. *Clin Neurosurg* 1988;34:630–649.
13. Connolly B, Turner C, DeVine J, et al. Jefferson fracture resulting in Collet-Sicard syndrome. *Spine* 2000;25:395–398.
14. Vaccaro AR, Urban WC, Aiken RD. Delayed cortical blindness and recurrent quadriplegia after cervical trauma. *J Spinal Disord* 1998;11:535–539.
15. Vankan Y, Demaerel P, Heye S, et al. Dural arteriovenous fistula as a late complication of upper cervical spine fracture: case report. *J Neurosurg* 2004;100(suppl 4 Spine):382–384.
16. Zielinski CJ, Gunther SF, Deeb Z. Cranial-nerve palsies complicating Jefferson fracture: a case report. *J Bone Joint Surg Am* 1982;64:1382–1384.

CHAPTER 23B

Atlas Injuries: Transverse Ligament Injury

Neel Anand and Tooraj Gravori

INTRODUCTION

Transverse ligament injuries are usually more common in the elderly and, though rare, can be of significant consequence. They can also be easily missed and a high degree of suspicion is necessary to properly evaluate these patients. The mechanism of injury and appropriate imaging studies are critical in addressing this injury.

MECHANISM OF INJURY

Ruptures of the transverse ligament most frequently occur in the older population as a result of hyperflexion of the neck by impact to the back of the neck on falling. Traumatic rupture of the transverse ligament is rare in children because of the synchondrosis of the C2 dens.[1,2]

Injury of the transverse ligament can be anatomically divided into three types: (a) rupture within the substance of the ligament itself, (b) avulsion of the ligament from the lateral mass of C1, and (c) avulsion of the lateral mass at the site of ligamentous insertion (bony fragment attached to the ligament) creating a functionally incompetent transverse ligament.

Patients with transverse ligament injury can present with significant instability compressing the immediately neighboring neuronal structures, including the spinal cord and medulla. The ring of the atlas expands to approximately 3 cm. The width of the spinal cord and the odontoid process are approximately 1 cm each. Based on Steel's rule of thirds, there is a margin of 1 cm for safe pathologic displacement.[3] Injuries causing severe displacement of the spine at this level may potentially damage the centers for cardiac and respiratory control. Such injuries are often incompatible with survival. Less significant instability can present as a mild neuronal deficit such as myelopathy, occipital pain and numbness (stretching of C2 nerve), or pure upper cervical pain. Mild instability may produce compression on the vertebral arteries, causing nausea, vomiting, or visual disturbances. C1-C2 displacement as a result of a ruptured transverse ligament accompanied by an intact odontoid (nonfractured, not atrophic) process may result in significant thecal sac compression of the spinal cord or medulla.[4]

The evaluation of the transverse ligament is initially performed using plain radiographs of the cervical spine that include lateral and open mouth views. An increased atlantodens interval (ADI), more evident on flexion cervical view,[1,5] displacement of the atlas over the axis,[3] presence of bony fragments within the spinal canal on an open mouth view, or evidence of soft tissue injury anterior to the upper cervical spine should raise the examiner's suspicion for an injury to the upper cervical spine, especially the transverse ligament. These imaging modalities rely on bony displacement as an indicator of transverse ligament injury. Therefore, further examination with computed tomography (CT) and or magnetic resonance imaging (MRI) can be performed to confirm and further delineate potential injury to the ligament, surrounding bony structures, and neuronal elements. MRI is the modality of choice for direct and reliable examination of the transverse ligament.[6,7]

The odontoid process and its related ligamentous structures provide the primary stabilizing strength of the atlantoaxial articulation.[8] The transverse ligament, a major component of the cruciate ligamentous complex, plays an important role in maintaining atlantoaxial stability.[6,9] It prevents anterior subluxation of C1 on C2 in anatomically intact specimens. Integrity of this ligament is required for stability even after a healed atlantoaxial fracture.[5,6,9] Following rupture of the transverse ligament, the alar ligament is inadequate in preventing significant C1 on C2 displacement.[1] Greene et al.[10] reported three cases of type II fractures that had documented transverse ligamentous injury demonstrated by MRI. All three required surgical fusion after delayed atlantoaxial instability, odontoid fracture nonunion, and acute instability.[10]

An intact transverse ligament allows approximately a maximum ADI of 3 mm in adults and 5 mm in children. Experimentally produced transverse ligament insufficiency with intact alar and apical ligaments allowed a maximal translation of 5 mm, as shown by Fielding et al.[1] However, if the alar ligament and the tectorial membrane are disrupted, displacement of more than 7 mm is observed.

In burst fractures of C1, the transverse ligament ruptures secondary to the tension created between the displaced lateral masses of the atlas (apical and alar ligaments remain intact). Spence et al.[3] demonstrated that combined displacement of 7 mm or more occurs only with disruption of the transverse ligament.

CLASSIFICATION

Transverse ligament disruption may occur in isolation or in association with other upper cervical injuries (Fig. 23B.1). There are well-known classification systems of odontoid fractures as well as C1-C2 displacement with or without associated transverse ligamentous injury.[11] Fielding and Hawkins[11] suggested a four-part classification scheme for C1-C2 displacement. Type I is simple rotatory displacement with an intact transverse ligament. Type II injuries involve anterior displacement of C1 on C2 of 3 to 5 mm, with one lateral mass serving as a pivot point and a deficiency of the transverse ligament. Type III injuries involve more than 5 mm of anterior displacement of both C1 and C2 articulations. Type IV injuries involve the posterior displacement of C1 on C2. Types III and IV are thought to be highly unstable.

Injury to the transverse ligament is best described by the classification of Dickman et al.[12] This system is unique because previous studies had depended entirely on plain radiographs to identify a transverse ligament injury. Using thin-section CT or MRI, Dickman et al.[12] classified disruptions of the midsubstance of the ligament as type I injuries and avulsion of the ligament from the C1 lateral mass as type II injuries.

TREATMENT

INITIAL TREATMENT

Advancement in our understanding of the anatomic structure and dynamic function of the transverse ligament has led to great discussion about acceptable treatment techniques. Detailed visualization of the ligament and the surrounding bony structures is of utmost importance. Assessment of the ADI and accompanying surrounding injuries provides a basis for treatment recommendations.

Nonoperative management with immobilization is the first line of treatment for transverse ligamentous avulsion injuries. Immobilization may be with a hard cervical collar or halo brace. Midsubstance disruption of the transverse ligament is extremely unstable, and surgical intervention is recommended.

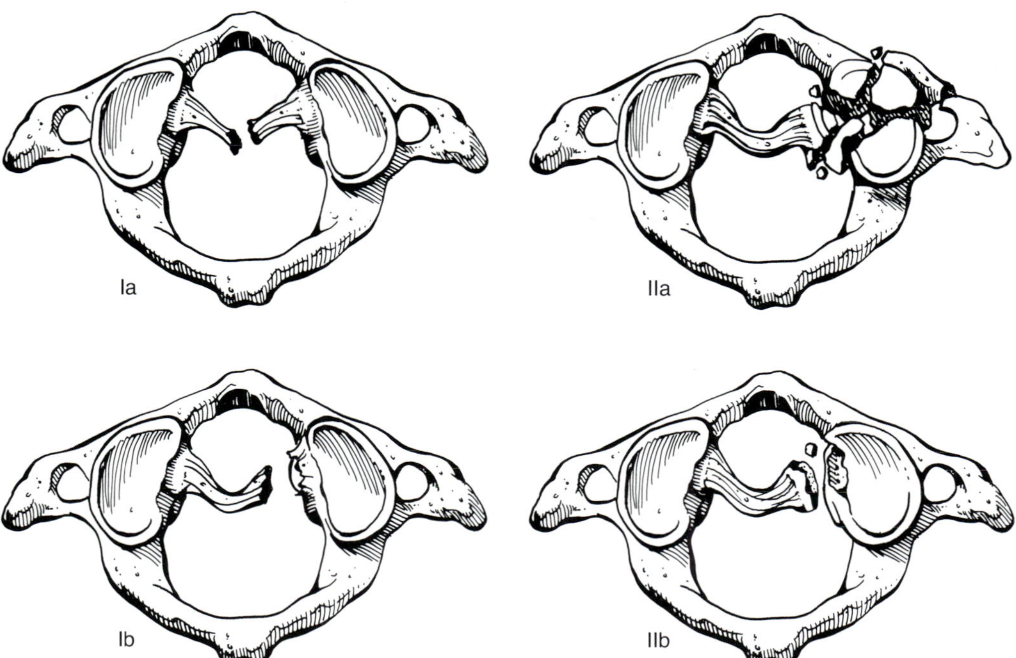

FIGURE 23B.1. Classification of injuries to the transverse atlantal ligament. Type I injuries disrupt the ligament substance in its midportion (Ia) or at its periosteal insertion (Ib). Type II injuries disconnect the tubercle for insertion of the transverse ligament from the C1 lateral mass involving a comminuted C1 lateral mass (IIa) or avulsing the tubercle from an intact lateral mass (IIb). (Reprinted with permission from Barrow Neurological Institute.)

In the setting of an avulsion injury, treatment depends on the degree of initial displacement and identification of any coexistent fractures. If the ADI is less than 5 mm in a neurologically intact patient, collar immobilization is sufficient initially. For an ADI greater than 5 mm, nonsurgical treatment, including halo immobilization, has generally yielded poor results except in selected cases of C1 bony avulsion. In the study by Dickman et al.,[12] none of the type I injuries healed spontaneously and all required arthrodesis. Of type II injuries, 74% healed with immobilization.[13]

Surrounding soft tissues, including blood vessels and bony structures, also are at risk at the time of trauma. Therefore, the initial evaluation and treatment should include a complete survey of the brain, vertebral arteries, posteroinferior cerebellar arteries, and lower cranial nerves. Conventional angiography or magnetic resonance angiography is recommended for the diagnosis of vertebral artery injury.

DEFINITIVE TREATMENT

External Immobilization

In cases in which a cervical collar or halo is used for immobilization, close monitoring of the clinical examination and cervical alignment is indicated. Depending on the degree of spinal realignment, age of the patient, and quality of the bone, a period of 6 weeks to 3 months of immobilization is reasonable to allow healing. Further instability at the end of this period is treated with surgical fusion.

Surgical Options

The goals of surgery are to protect the spinal cord, stabilize the spinal column, decompress neural tissue, and reduce any spinal deformity. Surgical stabilization is indicated in cases in which the transverse ligament is interrupted within its length, as well as when external immobilization fails. Postsurgical follow-up is critical to monitor hardware competency and ensure proper fusion.

Surgical stabilization consists of a C1-C2 fusion. Techniques vary from sublaminar wiring techniques such as Brooks or Gallie, to Halifax clamps, or transarticular C1-C2 screw fixation. Recently, C1 lateral mass screws and C2 pedicle screws have been used to immobilize this segment. In situations of associated injuries, extending the fusion cephalad or caudad may be necessary. The method of fusion depends on the degree of instability, the quality of bone, and the experience of the surgeon.

PROGNOSIS

The prognosis for surgically treated patients depends on preoperative medical and neurologic status and the quality of internal fixation.

COMPLICATIONS

Complications relating to injury of the transverse ligament depend on the existence of associated injuries and the degree of dislocation and presence or absence of a neural deficit. With C1-C2 instability, the tip of the odontoid can migrate posteriorly, as well as superiorly, causing acute injury to the brainstem and spinal cord. Resulting complications may include brainstem and spinal cord injury.

Damage to the vertebral arteries and sometimes the posteroinferior cerebellar arteries may result in posterior fossa stroke or transient ischemic attacks (the PICA syndrome).

Complications associated with surgery are directly related to implant insertion and the morbidity related to anesthesia and the surgical procedure.

REFERENCES

1. Fielding JW, Cochran G Van B, et al. Tears of the transverse ligament of the atlas: a clinical and biomechanical study. *J Bone Joint Surg Am* 1974;56:1683–1691.
2. Pennecot GF, Leonard P, Peyrot Des Gachons S, et al. Traumatic ligamentous instability of the cervical spine in children. *J Pediatr Orthop* 1984;4:339–345.
3. Spence KF Jr, Decker S, Sell KW. Bursting atlantal fracture associated with rupture of the transverse ligament. *J Bone Joint Surg Am* 1970;52:543–549.
4. Watson-Jones R. *Fractures and Joint Injuries.* Vol. 2. 4th ed. Baltimore: Williams and Wilkins, 1955:190.
5. Steel HH. Anatomical and mechanical considerations of atlanto-axial articulations. *J Bone Joint Surg Am* 1968;50:1481–1482.
6. Dickman CA, Mamourian A, Sonntag VKH, et al. Magnetic resonance imaging of the transverse atlantal ligament for the evaluation of atlantoaxial instability. *J Neurosurg* 1991;75:221–227.
7. Mamourian AC, Dickman CA, Wallace R, et al. Magnetic resonance appearance of the transverse ligament: an in vitro and in vivo anatomical and imaging study. *BNI Q* 1994;10:27–30.
8. Anderson LD, Clark CR. Fractures of the odontoid process of the axis. In: The Cervical Spine Research Society Editorial Committee, ed. *The Cervical Spine.* Philadelphia: JB Lippincott, 1989:325–343.
9. Lipson SJ. Fractures of the atlas associated with fractures of the odontoid process and transverse ligament ruptures. *J Bone Joint Surg Am* 1977;59:940–943.
10. Green KA, Dickman CA, Marciano FF, et al. Transverse atlantal ligament disruption associated with odontoid fractures. *Spine* 1994;19;2307–2314.
11. Fielding JW, Hawkins RJ. Atlanto-axial rotatory fixation (fixed rotatory subluxation of the atlanto-axial joint). *J Bone Joint Surg Am* 1977;59:37–44.
12. Dickman CA, Greene KA, Sonntag VK. Injuries involving the transverse atlantal ligament: classification and treatment guidelines based upon experience with 20 injuries. *Neurosurgery* 1996;38:44–50.

CHAPTER 23C

Atlas Injuries: Atlantoaxial Subluxation/Dissociation

Sanjay S. Dhall, Regis W. Haid Jr., and Praveen V. Mummaneni

INTRODUCTION

The articulation between the atlas and axis is complex, and the bony and cartilaginous articulations of the lateral facet joints allow for a wide range of motion. This articulation is unique from the remaining spinal column most notably because it contains the dens, which is the projection from C2 that lies within C1 and behind its anterior arch. There is little inherent bony stability except to resist posterior translation. Strong complex ligaments give this joint its stability, yet it maintains a wide range of motion.[1] As a result, bony and especially soft tissue injuries, whether by trauma, congenital anomaly, or degenerative disease, can lead to instability and catastrophic neurologic injury.[2] Similarly, nontraumatic cases of atlantoaxial instability often present in children with a variety of syndromes, such as Down and Klippel-Feil, and in patients of all ages with rheumatoid arthritis. Since the first description of atlantoaxial instability in 1966, a variety of classification schemes have been proposed and continue to guide the surgical and conservative management of these injuries.[3] The surgical options have also evolved and expanded to include cable fixation with bone graft, transarticular screw fixation, and atlantolateral mass screw fixation with C2 screw fixation.[4,5]

BIOMECHANICS

The occipitoatlantoaxial complex functions as a single unit that allows movement of the head on the spine. This complex is unique because the segmental structures between the occiput and atlas and between the atlas and axis do not provide significant stability. Instead, a majority of the stability of the occipitoatlantoaxial complex is derived from the internal ligaments and muscles directly between the occiput and C2. Cadaveric studies have revealed that the tectorial membrane is critical to occipitoatlantoaxial stability.[6,7] As a well-developed continuation of the posterior longitudinal ligament, it straps the body of C2 firmly to the clivus and anterior rim of the foramen magnum. Sectioning of the tectorial membrane alone led to instability with flexion, extension, and distraction in the occipitoatlantoaxial complex.[7] The alar ligament spans from the dens tip on each side passing relatively transversely to attach to the tubercules on the medial aspect of the lateral masses of the atlas. This stout ligament controls rotation of both the occipitoatlantal and the atlantoaxial joints. Furthermore, they are the most important stabilizers to prevent occipitoatlantal dislocation and are secondary restraints to anterior atlantoaxial subluxation.

PATIENT EVALUATION CLASSIFICATION

White and Panjabi[1] describe five patterns of dislocation of the atlantoaxial complex. Two types are translational dislocations and three are rotatory subluxations. Translation includes anterior dislocation, which often results from fracture of the dens or disruption of the transverse ligament. Anterior dislocation may also occur in cases of a dysplastic or aplastic odontoid process. Posterior translation is less common and results from fracture of the anterior arch of the atlas, an odontoid fracture, or dysplasia/aplasia of the dens.[1]

Rotatory dislocations may be unilateral anterior, unilateral posterior, and combined anteroposterior atlantoaxial displacement. Unilateral anterior dislocation, the most common of these, involves movement of one of the C1 lateral masses anterior to the ipsilateral lateral mass of C2 with the contralateral facet joint remaining intact. In addition to disruption of the ipsilateral C1-C2 facet joint capsule, this is often associated with odontoid and or transverse ligament injury.

In contrast, in unilateral posterior dislocation, a fractured or dysplastic odontoid process or fractured anterior ring of the atlas allows one of the C1 lateral masses to rotate posterior to the ipsilateral C2 lateral mass, again maintaining the integrity of the contralateral C1-C2 facet joint.

Finally, combined unilateral anterior and posterior C1-C2 dislocations are the consequence of twisting of C1 on C2 with the dens as the axis of rotation. This leads to anterior disruption of the facet on one side and posterior disruption on the other. In this case, the dens, transverse ligament, and tectorial membrane remain intact.

Other classification systems of atlantoaxial instability have been proposed. Chapman and Mirza[8] described three categories of traumatic atlantoaxial injuries. Category A is rotatory displacement in the axial plane; category B is injuries that are translationally unstable in the sagittal plane and result from compromise of the transverse atlantal ligament; and category C includes vertical atlantoaxial dissociation.

Category A, rotatory displacement, is described using the system of Fielding and Hawkins. Type I rotatory subluxation involves rotation without translation. Type II involves unilateral lateral mass subluxation of 3 to 5 mm. Type III is unilateral subluxation of greater than 5 mm. There may be anterior translation of the contralateral C1-C2 articulation with this subtype. Finally, type IV involves posterior displacement of C1 on C2.[9–11]

Category B, translational atlantoaxial instability, typically results from violation of the transverse ligament (Fig. 23C.1). As a result, these are unstable injuries. Dickman et al.[12] separated these injuries

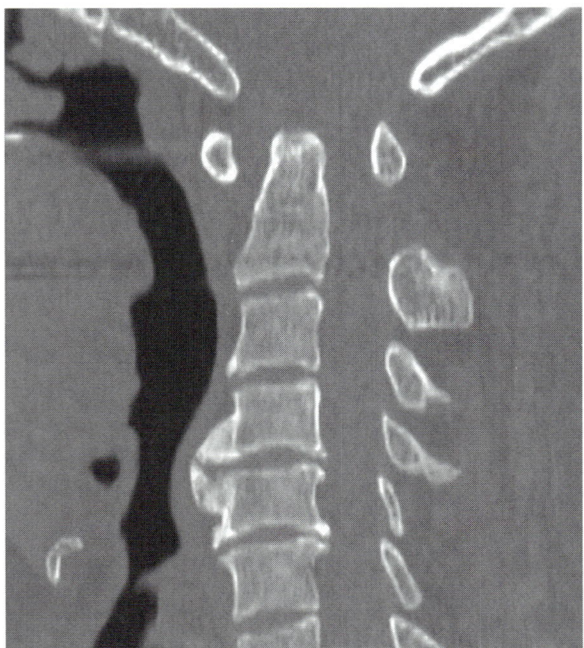

FIGURE 23C.1. Computed tomography sagittal reconstruction demonstrating translational atlantoaxial instability with anterior translation of the atlas relative to the dens. This is indicative of the transverse ligament.

further into type I and type II based on the source of the ligamentous incompetence. Type I injuries disrupt the transverse ligament in its midportion (IA) or at its periosteal insertion (IB). Type II injuries involve comminuted lateral mass fractures that disconnect the ligament (IIA) or avulsion of the bony tubercle from the lateral mass (IIB). The clinical significance of this classification scheme lies in that Dickman et al. observed that type I injuries did not heal and required internal fixation as compared to type II injuries, which had a 74% success rate of healing with rigid external orthosis.[12,13]

Category C is comprised of atlantoaxial injuries that involve vertical distraction forces. Among atlantoaxial dislocation injuries, vertical distraction is particularly uncommon, and its description in the literature is limited to case reports. On autopsy, injuries to the tectorial membrane and alar ligaments are present, indicating combined occipitocervical and atlantoaxial instability. It is likely that a majority of these injuries result in death.[14] The authors of this chapter treated a 7-year-old girl with this type of injury with resultant complete quadriplegia. This child, ejected in a motor vehicle accident, suffered cardiac arrest at the scene and resultant anoxic brain injury. Despite these devastating injuries, the patient, who underwent occiput to C2 fusion, went on to make significant neurologic recovery, including ambulation and near normal motor strength of the upper extremities.

TREATMENT

INITIAL TREATMENT

The primary treatment goals for patients with atlantoaxial dislocation are relief of neural compression and elimination of instability. Often, before definitive surgical treatment can be pursued, an attempt must be made to realign the osseous anatomy and relieve the neural compression. This can often be achieved with traction; however, it is contraindicated in some cases of complex rotary subluxations and all cases of occipitoatlantoaxial dislocations. Alternatively, reduction can be performed with application of the halo vest. If reduction is not achieved, manipulation of the head position relative to the thorax can be performed until reduction is achieved.

When using traction, the authors recommend that patients be carefully monitored to ensure frequent neurologic examinations, pulse oximetry, and respiratory function. Typically, traction is applied via a halo ring or tongs with a starting weight of 5 to 7 lb. This can be gradually increased to a maximum of 5 to 10 lb per level over the span of 36 hours. In most patients, mild extension is applied with traction to achieve neutral position. Caution must be taken as excessive traction may lead to vertebral distraction and vertebral artery injury. Dickinson et al.[15] reported a patient who had a brainstem stroke secondary to vertebral artery dissection thought to be from traction for treatment of basilar impression.

Children with rotatory subluxation may also be treated with halter traction and sedation. Once reduction has been achieved, the patient should be immobilized for 3 months in a halo or Guilford brace. In cases of rotatory subluxation for longer than 3 months, halo-vest traction is recommended for 3 months.[16]

DEFINITIVE TREATMENT

Many factors are important to consider when choosing definitive treatment. These include which ligamentous structures are injured, patient age, body habitus, and type of lesion. In children, rotary subluxation reduced early may have attempted nonoperative treatment. Rotatory subluxation that recurs after halo-vest traction or is long-standing should be treated with traction to achieve maximal reduction. This should be followed by surgical arthrodesis typically of C1 and C2. A lateral approach to the dislocated joints may be selected and allows for identification and preservation of the vertebral artery while also accommodating both ventral and dorsal access to the dislocated joint. Typically, soft tissue interposition is noted, explaining the failure of nonoperative reduction. Open reduction is supplemented with bone graft insertion into the joint followed by halo immobilization and/or instrumentation to fixate C1-C2 (Fig. 23C.2).

The majority of patients with atlantoaxial instability should be treated with posterior C1-C2 fusion. Several wire techniques may be useful in young children, such as the Gallie[5] and Brooks'

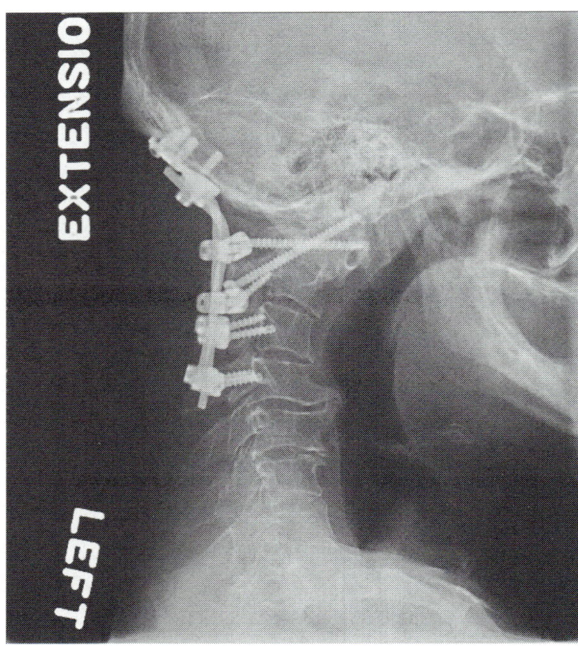

FIGURE 23C.2. Postoperative lateral image of occiptocervical (occiput-C4) fusion to manage the translational atlantoaxial instability illustrated in Figure 23C.1.

fusions. These generally require postoperative immobilization using a halo vest. More rigid techniques are the Magerl C1-C2 transarticular screw fixation and C1 lateral mass–C2 pedicle screws as popularized by Harms. These are exacting techniques that provide high fusion rates and excellent stability but have increased incidence of neurovascular complications. Details of the surgical techniques are discussed in Chapter 16.

C1-C2 DISSOCIATION RISK FACTORS

TRAUMATIC RISK FACTORS

In the setting of trauma, factors that predispose to atlantoaxial instability in children include disproportionately large cranial mass and underdeveloped neck musculature. This leads to greater bending of the cervical spine under flexion and extension forces. This is exacerbated by greater elasticity of the interspinous and posterior joint capsules that results in hypermobility. Children are the most frequent patient population to suffer from traumatic C1-C2 subluxation and dissociation.

NONTRAUMATIC RISK FACTORS

Nontraumatic atlantoaxial instability may result from aplasia or hypoplasia of the odontoid process, insufficiency of the transverse ligament, or assimilation of the atlas. Syndromes associated with atlantoaxial instability include Down syndrome, Klippel-Feil syndrome, Morquio syndrome, osteogenesis imperfecta, neurofibromatosis, congenital scoliosis, and a variety of skeletal dysplasias.[17] The atlantoaxial joint is the most mobile segment in the vertebral column and consequently has the least inherent stability. The odontoid process, emanating from the body of the axis and secured against the anterior ring of C1 by the transverse ligament, functions as a brace against hyperextension. However, in cases of flexion, migration of the dens into the central canal and the spinal cord is prevented only by a ligamentous structure. As a result, violation of the transverse ligament can result in impingement of the spinal cord by an otherwise intact odontoid process.

Down Syndrome

Although the incidence of radiographic atlantoaxial instability in patients with Down syndrome has been reported to be as high as 14% to 24%, the incidence of symptomatic atlantoaxial instability in these patients is thought to be less than 1%.[18] Reported symptoms include neck pain, cervical deformity, cervicomedullary compression resulting in neurologic impairment, and even sudden death.[19]

This instability in patients with Down syndrome is usually attributable to ligamentous instability; however, many of these patients also may have osseous abnormalities at the craniovertebral junction. These include os odontoideum, hypoplastic odontoid process, and abnormal ossification of the arch of C1. Os odontoideum in this patient population is felt to correlate with instability of the atlantoaxial complex and often indicates surgical fixation.[18]

Rheumatoid Arthritis

In the setting of rheumatoid arthritis, the multitude of synovial joints in the cervical spine predisposes the cervical spine to significant pathology. The most frequent problem in patients with rheumatoid arthritis is atlantoaxial subluxation. These patients may also suffer from cranial settling or rheumatoid granulation tissue at C2 causing cord compression.

Atlantoaxial subluxation results from loss of tensile strength and stretching of the transverse ligament. This laxity of the ligaments and softening of bone results in horizontal or anteroposterior translation, as well as rotary luxation of the atlas and axis vertebrae.[20]

PROGNOSIS

The true incidence of traumatic atlantoaxial dissociation is unknown, but it is probably extremely rare, at least among survivors. A majority of victims die before receiving medical care. This injury mostly occurs in children aged 0 to 9 years who are the victims of high-speed auto-pedestrian accidents. Those children who survive the initial injury tend to present with either severe head injury exacerbated by anoxic encephalopathy or only minor neck pain, subtle signs of myelopathy, or C2 hypesthesia or hypoesthesia. In fact, some cases are not initially diagnosed at all. As a result, long-term survivors of this injury rarely have severe myelopathy, perhaps because of the dichotomy in this patient population.[6]

COMPLICATIONS

NEUROLOGIC

Although reports of spinal cord injury associated with atlantoaxial fusion are uncommon, they have been reported. Such risk is minimized with proper preoperative planning, including thin-cut computed tomography and intraoperative use of fluoroscopic guidance.

VASCULAR

In the setting of internal fixation of atlantoaxial instability, one of the most feared complications is vertebral artery injury, especially resulting from the placement of C1-C2 transarticular screws. Although some patients may compensate with collateral flow from the contralateral vertebral artery, there is risk for brainstem or cerebellar stroke. The option of vascular bypass in the case of vertebral artery injury depends highly on the availability at the institution. It is recommended that if vertebral artery injury occurs during screw placement, the surgeon should complete placement of the screw to tamponade bleeding on that side; however, to avoid the risk for bilateral vertebral artery injury, the contralateral screw should not be placed. The patient should then undergo an angiogram and possible embolization of the injured vertebral artery.[21]

PSEUDARTHROSIS

Other more frequent complications of atlantoaxial fixation surgery include pseudarthrosis and persistent instability. These complications are very difficult to manage and can be limited by placement of transarticular screws or atlantolateral mass screws with C2 pars screws in the appropriate setting with adequate bone graft and the use of postoperative rigid immobilization.[22–24]

CONCLUSION

Instability of the atlantoaxial complex, whether congenital or resulting from trauma or degenerative processes, is a difficult surgical problem, often with grave neurologic consequences. It can be managed successfully, however, with prompt recognition in susceptible populations, immediate immobilization, and surgical management when indicated.

REFERENCES

1. White AA, Panjabi MM. The clinical biomechanics of the occipitoatlantoaxial complex. *Orthop Clin North Am* 1978;9:867–878.
2. Yoganandan N, Maiman D, Pintar F, et al. Cervical spine injuries from motor vehicle accidents. *J Clin Eng* 1990;15:505–513.
3. Dzenitis AJ. Spontaneous atlanto-axial dislocation in a mongoloid child with spinal cord compression: case report. *J Neurosurg* 1966;25:458–460.
4. Fiore AJ, Haid RW, Rodts GE, et al. Atlantal lateral mass screws for posterior spinal reconstruction: technical note and case series. *Neurosurg Focus* 2002;12:E5.
5. Gallie WE. Fractures and dislocations of the cervical spine. *Am J Surg* 1939;46:495–499.
6. Davis D, Bohlman H, Walker AE, et al. The pathological findings in fatal craniospinal injuries. *J Neurosurg* 1971;34:603–613.
7. Maiman D, Yoganandan N. Biomechanics of cervical spine trauma. *Clin Neurosurg* 1990;37:543–570.
8. Chapman JR, Mirza SK. Fractures of the upper cervical spine. In: Bucholz RW, Heckman JD, eds. *Rockwood and Green's Fractures in Adults.* Philadelphia: Lippincott Williams and Wilkins, 2001:1333–1334.
9. Fielding JW, Hawkins RJ, Ratzan S. Fusion for atlantoaxial instability. *J Bone Joint Surg Am* 1987;58:429.
10. Fielding JW, Francis WR, Hawkins RJ. Atlantoaxial rotary deformity. *Semin Spine Surg* 1991;3:33–38.
11. Fielding JW, Hawkins RJ, Hensinger RN, et al. Atlantoaxial rotary deformities. *Orthop Clin North Am* 1978;9: 955–967.
12. Dickman CA, Greene KA, Sonntag VK. Injuries involving the transverse atlantal ligament: classification and treatment guidelines based upon experience with 39 injuries. *Neurosurgery* 1996;38:44–50.
13. Dickman CA, Sonntag VK. Posterior C1-C2 transarticular screw fixation for atlantoaxial arthrodesis. *Neurosurgery* 1998;43:275–280, discussion 280–281.
14. Weiner BK, Brower RS. Traumatic vertical atlantoaxial instability in a case of atlanto-occipital coalition. *Spine* 1997;22:1033–1035.
15. Dickinson LD, Tuite GF, Colon GP, et al. Vertebral artery dissection related to basilar impression: case report. *Neurosurgery* 1995;36:835–838.
16. Subach BR, McLaughlin MR, Albright AL, et al. Current management of pediatric rotatory subluxation. *Spine* 1998;23:2174–2179.
17. Holzgreve W, Grope H, Von Figwrak E. Morquio syndrome: clinical findings in 11 patients with mucopolysaccharidosis type IVA and two with mucopolysaccharidosis type IVP. *Hum Genet* 1981;57:360–365.
18. Nader-Sepahi A, Casey AT, Hayward R, et al. Symptomatic atlantoaxial instability in Down syndrome. *J Neurosurg* 2005;103(suppl 3):231–237.
19. Pueschel SM, Herndon JH, Gelch MM, et al. Symptomatic atlantoaxial subluxation in persons with Down syndrome. *J Pediatr Orthop* 1984;4:682–688.
20. Sonntag VK, Vollmer DG. Spine: degenerative disease. In: Winn HR, ed. *Youmans Neurological Surgery.* 5th ed. Philadelphia: Elsevier.
21. Vender JR, Rekito AJ, Harrison SJ, et al. The evolution of posterior cervical and occipitocervical fusion and instrumentation. *Neurosurg Focus* 2004;16:E9.
22. Grob D, Dvorak J, Panjabi M, et al. Posterior occipitocervical fusion: a preliminary report of a new technique. *Spine* 1991;16(suppl 3):S17–S24.
23. Hadley MN, Zabramski JM, Browner CM, et al. Pediatric spinal trauma: review of 122 cases of spinal cord and vertebral column injuries. *J Neurosurg* 1988;68:18–24.
24. Mitchell TC, Sadasivan KK, Ogden AL, et al. Biomechanical study of atlantoaxial arthrodesis: transarticular screw fixation versus modified Brooks posterior wiring. *J Orthop Trauma* 1999;13:483–489.

CHAPTER 24A

C2 Fractures: C2 Body Fractures

Ignacio Madrazo, Carlos Zamorano, and Eduardo Magallón

INTRODUCTION

The C2 vertebral body is the region of the vertebra that lies below the odontoid process and between the pars interarticularis bilaterally. C2 body fractures are not rare, accounting for approximately 10% of all upper cervical spinal fractures. They are associated with a high incidence of concomitant subaxial cervical spine injury. Sagitally oriented fractures are associated with severe head injury because of the mechanism of injury responsible for this injury pattern. The majority of these fractures heal well with immobilization.

ANATOMY

The C2 vertebral body is the region of the vertebra that lies below the odontoid process and between the pars interarticularis bilaterally (Figs. 24A.1 and 24A.2). The C2 pedicle is located more ventrally and medially than the pedicles at lower cervical spine levels. Consequently, it forms a posterolateral extension of the vertebral body, connecting it with its superior articulating process (lateral mass). The pars interarticularis of C2 has a more horizontal orientation than this structure at more caudal spinal levels. This affects the way in which an axial load is transmitted through the upper cervical spine and the type of injury sustained when the load limit is exceeded.[1]

INCIDENCE

Fractures of the C2 body are not rare and represent a significant proportion of upper cervical spine fractures. The University of New Mexico Hospital statistics noted an incidence of 10% of all upper cervical spine fractures.[2] In this registry, 208 patients were identified with an upper cervical spine fracture, and 21 (9.7%) of these were noted to have a C2 body fracture. Greene et al.[3] reported on 340 axis fractures, and Burke and Harris[4] reported on 165 axis fractures in which 13.0% were classified as extension teardrop and 6.0% were classified as hyperextension dislocations. None of these authors classified these fractures specifically as C2 body fractures, but they drew attention to the fact that nonodontoid, nonhangman C2 fractures are more common than previously recognized.

MECHANISM OF INJURY

Benzel et al.[1] reported 15 cases of vertical C2 body fractures in which the mechanism of injury was firmly postulated. This information was determined through (a) identification of the point of injury impact on clinical examination, (b) evaluation of soft tissue changes on computed tomography (CT) and magnetic resonance imaging (MRI), (c) provided history of the mechanism of injury, and

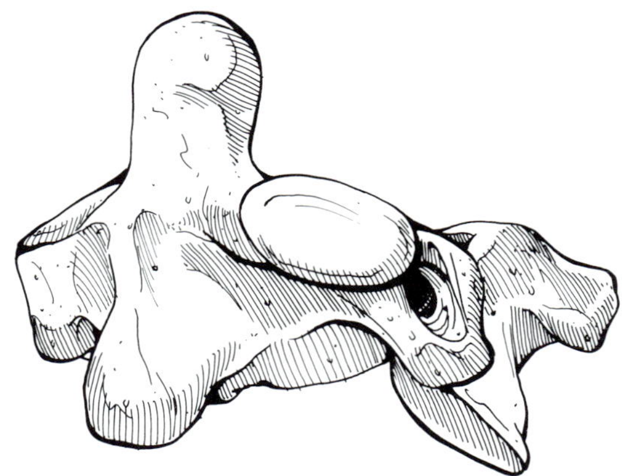

FIGURE 24A.1. The C2 pedicle is located more ventrally and medially than the pedicles at lower cervical spinal levels. In consequence, it forms a posterolateral extension of the vertebral body, connecting it with its superior articulating process (lateral mass). The pars interarticularis of C2 has a more horizontal orientation than this structure at more caudal spinal levels. This affects the way in which an axial load is transmitted through the upper cervical spine and the type of injury sustained when the load limit is exceeded.[1] (Courtesy of Hospital Ángeles del Pedregal.)

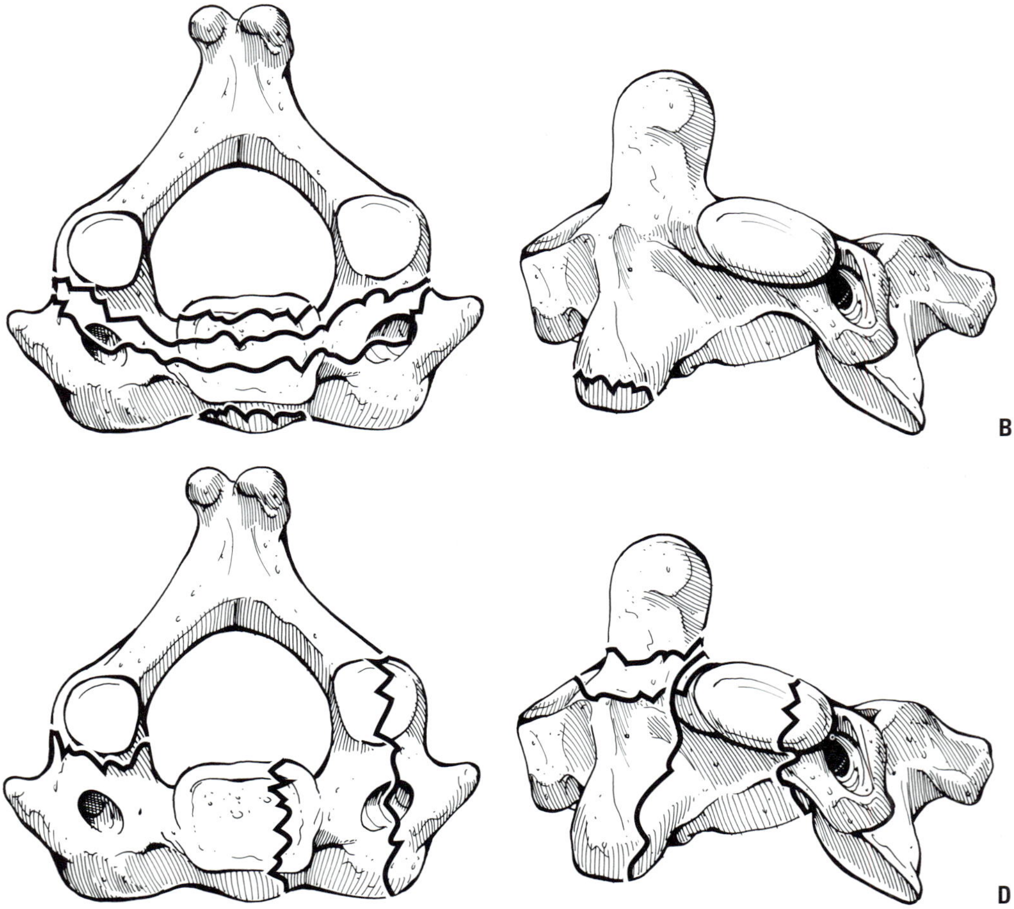

A

B

C

D

FIGURE 24A.2. Four views of the C2 vertebral body depicting fracture locations. **A.** Caudal view of type I C2 body fracture locations. **B.** An anterior oblique view depicting an anterior teardrop. Type II C2 body fractures, the type III C2 body fracture, fractures through the pars interarticularis, and the dens fracture on a caudal view and an anterior oblique view **(D).** (Adapted from Benzel EC, Hart B, Ball P, et al. Fractures of the C-2 vertebral body. *J Neurosurg* 1994; 81:206–212, with permission.)

TABLE 24A.1 Fractures of the C2 Vertebral Body and Mechanisms of Injury

Type I: Coronally oriented vertical
Mechanisms of injury
Capital extension with slight[5] axial load
Axial load with slight capital extension
Axial load with slight capital flexion
Capital flexion with distraction
Variants: Extension teardrop and hyperextension dislocation
Capital extension and hyperextension
Type II: Sagittally oriented vertical
Isolated axial load
Variant: Lateral vertical
Significant axial load with lateral component
Type III: Horizontal rostral
Dorsal-to-ventral oriented blow to the head

(d) available spinal imaging (plain radiographs, CT, and MRI) of the C2 body fracture and surrounding soft tissues.

Based on this information, the fractures were grouped according to the mechanism of injury and type of fracture observed. Vertical C2 body fractures were divided into those that were coronally oriented (type I, 12 patients) and those that were sagitally oriented (type II, 3 patients) (Table 24A.1).

CORONALLY ORIENTED VERTICAL C2 BODY FRACTURE (TYPE I)

Coronally oriented C2 fractures may occur through four possible mechanisms, as discussed in the following sections.[1]

Extension with Axial Load

Extension with axial load occurs with less head extension than that associated with traumatic spondylolisthesis of the axis. The fracture line travels through the posterior C2 vertebral body instead of the pars interarticularis of C2. This has been termed an atypical traumatic spondylolisthesis of the axis by Burke and Harris[4] and Effendi et al.[5] and an unusual type of hangman fracture by Marotta et al.[6] However, it is neither atypical nor particularly unusual and is not a spondylolisthesis of the axis. This fracture is characterized by a dorsally positioned vertical C2 body fracture.

Hyperextension with Axial Load

A force vector applied to the high forehead region results in the application of an axial load and a head hyperextension force to the upper cervical spine. The C2 vertebral body may fail in a similar location to that described above, but because of the direction and magnitude of the applied force, it results in a distraction disruption of the intervertebral disc of C2-C3. This causes an opening of the anterior disc interspace and a teardrop avulsion fracture of the anterior inferior aspect of the C2 vertebral body. The vertically oriented axial load causes a significant compression of the C2-C3 disc interspace. This is also associated with a shearing mechanism applied in the anteroposterior plane of the vertebral body. Three distinct imaging patterns are seen with this fracture mechanism: (a) an anterior teardrop component (most commonly associated with a significant axial load component), (b) posterior element fractures, and (c) fractures involving the foramina transversarium. The first two reflect the hyperextension component of the mechanism of injury, and the latter is a manifestation of the lateral extension of a C2 body fracture. These mechanisms of injury can also result in an arch fracture of C1. The abutment of the posterior arch of C1 onto the posterior elements of C2 or the occiput may cause an isolated disruption of the posterior arch of C1 bilaterally at the junction of the posterior arch with the lateral masses, as opposed to a burst fracture of C1.

Flexion-Axial Load

The application of a dorsally applied force vector with an axial load component to the calvaria may result in opening the dorsal aspect of the C2-C3 disc interspace, translating the ventral component of the C2 complex forward on C3 with tearing of the anterior longitudinal ligament, thus causing an accompanying posterior C2 body fracture. Because the C2-C3 disc interspace is slanted ventrally and caudally, this orientation is nearly in line with the applied force vector. This results in a translational deformation of C2 forward on C3. The bony boundaries of the foramina transversarium are often fractured.

Flexion-Distraction

If a capital flexion injury is combined with a distraction component, usually caused by deceleration over a fulcrum (e.g., the shoulder harness of a seat belt), a flexion-distraction force complex occurs. This results in a bending moment arising around the ventral caudal aspect of C2, leading to an opening of the disc interspace dorsally, maintenance or exaggeration of disc space height, and preservation of anterior soft tissue integrity unless excessive distraction results in anterior longitudinal ligament disruption. This fracture is virtually identical in appearance to one caused by the previously described mechanism of injury.

SAGITALLY ORIENTED VERTICAL C2 BODY FRACTURE (TYPE II)

The sagitally oriented C2 body fracture is caused by axial loading to the point of failure. An axial load applied to the vertex of the calvaria may result in several injury types. If other spinal elements do not fail first (resulting in a Jefferson fracture or a subaxial cervical spine burst fracture), the load applied to the articular pillars of C2 may result in a comminuted burst fracture of the C2 body with a sagitally oriented vertical fracture line. Because of the sagital nature of the fracture line, this injury is best visualized on an anteroposterior plain radiogaphic view.

When an axial load is applied to the calvarium, the lateral masses of C2 accept the load. No structural support exists immediately below the superior articulating process of C2; thus, a fracture line may occur through the vertebral body junction with the pedicles, resulting in a burst-type injury. The C2 body fails in the region of the pedicle's junction with the vertebral body. Because the posterior wall of the C2 vertebral body is thrust into the spinal canal as a result of the predominant axial load applied, it is similar in appearance to the burst fracture as defined.

A lateral variant of the type II C2 body fracture can occur if there is a slight lateral orientation of the applied force vector. This fracture variant is oriented vertically through the lamina, facets, and foramina transversarium.

HORIZONTAL ROSTRAL C2 BODY FRACTURE (TYPE III)

The previously defined type III odontoid process fracture of Anderson and D'Alonzo[7] is not actually an odontoid process fracture but a horizontal rostral C2 body fracture. Its mechanism of injury has previously been described as resulting from a dorsal blow to the head.[8]

CLASSIFICATION

Based on the information discussed previously, Benzel et al.[1] proposed a classification system based on a series of 15 C2 body fractures, as follows:

Type I: Vertical, coronally oriented
Type II: Vertical, sagitally oriented
Type II: Transverse, axially oriented

The type I fracture was considered by Starr and Eismont[9] to be an atypical traumatic spondylolisthesis of the axis or by Marotta et al.[6] to be an atypical hangman fracture.

TREATMENT

INITIAL TREATMENT

External immobilization is recommended for treatment of isolated fractures of the axis body. In a review of the literature conducted for the development of the Guidelines for Management of Acute Cervical Spinal Injuries,[10] there was no Class I or Class II medical evidence addressing the management of traumatic fractures of the axis body. All articles reviewed contain Class III evidence that supports the use of external immobilization as the initial treatment strategy.

DEFINITIVE TREATMENT

The experience of most surgeons in the treatment of vertical C2 body fractures is anecdotal based on isolated experiences, case reports,[6,11–15] or small patient series often included as a subset of axis fractures.[9,16,17] The largest series was reported by Fujimura et al.[16] and included 31 cases of C2 body fractures classified into four types: (a) avulsion, (b) transverse, (c) burst, and (c) saggital oriented fractures. Twenty of the lesions were considered isolated, and 11 were considered combined: 3 atlas, 3 dens, 7 hangman, and 2 C3 fractures. The avulsion fracture described by these authors is similar to the type I injury described by Benzel and colleagues.[2] In this variant of a type I coronally oriented C2 body fracture, the fracture involves the anteroinferior portion of the C2 body and probably represents an avulsion fracture at the insertion of the anterior longitudinal ligament. Of the nine avulsion fractures treated by Fujimura et al.,[16] all healed by nonoperative means (Philadelphia collar or a halo vest). Korres et al.[17] also described good results with nonoperative management for these fractures in a report on 14 patients with a mean follow-up of 8.5 years. Of the 17 saggital fractures, 15 were treated nonoperatively with a Philadelphia collar or halo vest. The remaining two patients had an associated type III dens fracture and underwent transoral atlantoaxial fusions. In spite of the reported surgical management of these fractures,[6,9,14] the vast majority may be treated successfully with nonoperative treatment.

These fractures usually have a benign natural history because the upper cervical spinal canal is more capacious than the lower cervical canal, providing a greater degree of safety regarding spinal cord injury than observed in the subaxial cervical spine. As a general rule, vertical C2 body fractures do not compromise the spinal canal. Coronally oriented type I fractures are often minimally displaced. However, unlike a hangman fracture, the spinal cord is not necessarily decompressed by the anteroposterior widening of the canal. This fact was demonstrated by Starr and Eismont[9] in a report on six cases of atypical hangman fractures identical to the type I C2 coronal body fracture, of which two were associated with significant subluxation, angulation, and spinal cord injury. These authors thought that the fracture pattern actually places the patient at risk for spinal cord injury because of the incomplete disruption of the ring of C2, without the provision of spinal cord decompression. Four other neurologically intact patients in their series with the same fracture pattern demonstrated much less translation and angulation.

Sagitally oriented type II fractures do not usually displace significantly. They are often associated with severe brain injury. This association is related to the cranially applied force vector and the significant kinetic energy required to produce such a fracture. The kinetic energy is thus imparted to the head and brain.

Osteologically, vertical C2 body fractures often are not displaced significantly and are not comminuted. Both of these factors help optimize the chance of a successful fracture healing. Greene et al.[3] reported a 1.6% nonunion rate in the management of 61 miscellaneous axis fractures. On the contrary, Fujimura et al.[16] reported an association with chronic neck pain and degeneration of the atlantoaxial joint with significantly displaced type II fractures. These authors reported that 8 of 17 patients with saggital fractures eventually required atlantoaxial fusion for treatment of chronic neck pain. These series suggest that type I and type II vertical C2 body fractures may be treated conservatively by bracing.

Given the small number of patients reported in the literature, recommendations regarding a specific device for external immobilization cannot be made with certainty. The use of three orthotic devices has been described in the management of these injuries. This reflects an evolution of management corresponding to increasing experience with managing these fractures. Initially, all C2 body fractures were managed with a Minerva jacket by Benzel.[1] One patient treated with a halo had a combined C1-C2 injury. As experience with the treatment of these fractures was gained, cases with minimal displacement of the fracture fragments were eventually managed with a hard cervical collar. By now, the choice of orthosis remains with the good judgment of the treating physician.

Halo immobilization is preferred by some authors for most type I and type II C2 body fractures, particularly when they occur in combination with a C1 fracture.[18] Available medical evidence (Class III) suggests that a variety of external orthoses are effective treatment options.[3] Follow-up is essential to verify that bony union and stability have been achieved.

COMPLICATIONS AND PROGNOSIS

In the 21 patients treated by German et al.[2] with a vertical C2 body fracture, three died during the treatment period. The remainder had radiographic evidence of fusion at the time of their last follow-up. Documentation of fusion consisted of plain flexion-extension radiographs (18 cases), with (3 cases) or without (15 cases) CT. Of the patients who died during the treatment period, two of the deaths were related to brain trauma. The third case was an elderly patient who died of aspiration pneumonia before a follow-up evaluation was performed. In the surviving 18 patients, treatment consisted of external immobilization with a Minerva jacket (13 cases [72%]), a cervical collar (4 cases [22%]), or halo vest followed by a Minerva jacket (1 case [6%]). The latter patient had an associated C1 fracture. The average length of treatment for type I and type II fractures was 3.4 ± 1.2 months and 3.75 ± 1.5 months, respectively. The average length of follow-up for type I and type II fractures was 7.1 ± 6.6 months and 5.0 ± 1.4 months, respectively. All 18 surviving patients were followed until symptoms (e.g., neck pain) resolved and radiographic evidence of a stable fusion was demonstrated.

CONCLUSION

C2 body fractures are not rare, accounting for approximately 10% of all upper cervical spinal fractures. They are associated with a high incidence (approximately one third) of concomitant subaxial cervical spine injury.

Sagitally oriented fractures are associated with severe head injury because of the mechanism of injury responsible for this injury pattern (axial loading). The majority of these fractures heal well with immobilization.

REFERENCES

1. Benzel EC, Hart B, Ball P, et al. Fractures of the C-2 vertebral body. *J Neurosurg* 1994;81:206–212.
2. German JW, Hart BL, Benzel EC. Nonoperative management of vertical C2 body fractures. *Neurosurgery* 2005;56:516–521.

3. Greene KA, Dickman CA, Marciano FF, et al. Acute axis fractures: analysis of management and outcome in 340 cases. *Spine* 1997;22:1843–1852.
4. Burke JT, Harris JH Jr. Acute injuries of the axis vertebra. *Skeletal Radiol* 1989;18:335–346.
5. Effendi B, Roy D, Cornish B, et al. Fractures of the ring of the axis: a classification based on the analyisis of 131 cases. *J Bone Joint Surg Br* 1981;63:319–327.
6. Marotta TR, White L, ter Brugge KG, et al. An unusual type of hangman's fracture. *Neurosurgery* 1990;26:848–851.
7. Anderson LD, D'Alonzo RT. Fractures of the odontoid process of the axis. *J Bone Joint Surg Am* 1974;56: 1663–1674.
8. Mouradian WH, Fietti VG Jr, Cochran GVB, et al. Fractures of the odontoid: a laboratory and clinical study of mechanisms. *Orthop Clin North Am* 1978;9:985–1001.
9. Starr JK, Eismont FJ. Atypical hangman's fracture. *Spine* 1993;18:1954–1957.
10. Guidelines for management of acute cervical spinal injuries. *Neurosurgery* 2002;50(suppl):S125–S139.
11. Bohay D, Gosselin RA, Contreras DM. The vertical axis fracture: a report on three cases. *J Orthop Trauma* 1992;6:416–419.
12. Iizuka H, Shimusu T, Hasegawa W, et al. Fractures of the posterior part of the body and unilateral spinous process of the axis: a case report. *Spine* 2001;26:E528–E530.
13. Lozano-Requena JA, Pina-Medina A, Aracil-Silvestre J, et al. Sagittal fracture of the second cervical vertebral body. *Int Orthop* 1994:18:114–115.
14. Rainov NG, Heidecke V, Burkert W. Coronally oriented vertical fracture of the axis body: surgical treatment of a rare condition. *Minim Invasive Neurosurg* 2004;41:93–96.
15. Vialle R, Schmider L, Levassor N, et al. Extension tear-drop nfracture of the axis: a surgically treated case. *Rev Chir Orthop Reparatrice Appar Mot* 2004;90:152–155.
16. Fujimura Y, Nishi Y, Kobayashi K. Classification and treatment of axis body fractures. *J Orthop Trauma* 1996;10:536–540.
17. Korres DS, Zoubos AB, Kavadias K, et al. The "tear drop" (or avulsed) fracture of the anterior inferior angle of the axis. *Eur Spine J* 1994;3:151–154.
18. German JW, Hart BL, Benzel EC. Nonoperative management of vertical C2 body fractures (see Hadley MN. Comments). *Neurosurgery* 2005;56:516–521.

CHAPTER 24B

C2 Fractures: Odontoid

Nazih Assaad and Lali H. S. Sekhon

INTRODUCTION

Odontoid fractures occur in young and elderly patients and can present with management dilemmas. Potential spinal cord injury, instability, and pseudoarthrosis are not uncommon associations of these fractures and surgical management can be challenging to due bony variations and local neurovascular structures. These fractures account for 9%–15% of all fractures. In the elderly, they are associated with falls. In the younger patient, high velocity trauma is the association. Hypertension or hyperflexion are the common mechanisms of injury. Treatment ranges from immobilization in a collar or halo vest or surgical management with either anterior or posterior approaches. The peculiarity of the C1-C2 anatomy, adjacent structures, demographics of patients affected, and difficulty of some surgical approaches makes the management of odontoid fractures both challenging and still controversial.

EMBRYOLOGY

Somites and sclerotomes are numbered from rostral to caudal, either directly numerically or segmentally (occipital, cervical, etc.). There are four occipital and eight cervical sclerotomes. Therefore, sclerotome 1 corresponds with occipital sclerotome 1 (O1 sclerotome), sclerotome 5 corresponds with cervical sclerotome 1 (C1 sclerotome), etc. Sclerotomes 5 to 7 (C1 to C3) form three centra designated X (tip of dens), Y (base of dens), and Z (centrum of axis) (Fig. 24B.1). During development, an intervertebral disc transiently exists between Y and Z. Rudiments occasionally may be seen in the adult.

The axis has five primary and two secondary ossification centers (Fig. 24B.2). Two primary centers compose the vertebral arch, one the centrum and two the dens. The bilateral primary ossification centers of the dens appear at 6 months gestation and unite before birth. Even at this time they are still cleft at the apex by cartilage that forms the tip of the odontoid. The two secondary ossification centers develop at the apex of the dens (5 to 8 years of age) and below the body of the axis (puberty). The tip of the dens is usually ossified and fused with the conical mass by 12 years of age.

The apical ligament and the odontoid tip are thought to be derived from the centrum of the proatlas (fourth occipital sclerotome).

The two primary ossification centers of the dens are separated from the centrum by a subdental synchondrosis. This had been thought to disappear by adolescence. However, histomorphometric data suggest that this synchondrosis may persist to some degree in up to 87% of individuals. This has clinical significance in regard to development of type II odontoid fractures and the formation of pseudarthrosis at the base of the dens.

Developmental anomalies of the odontoid are not uncommon and may result in atlantoaxial instability. If this apical center fails to fuse with the dens, an ossiculum terminale persistens is formed.

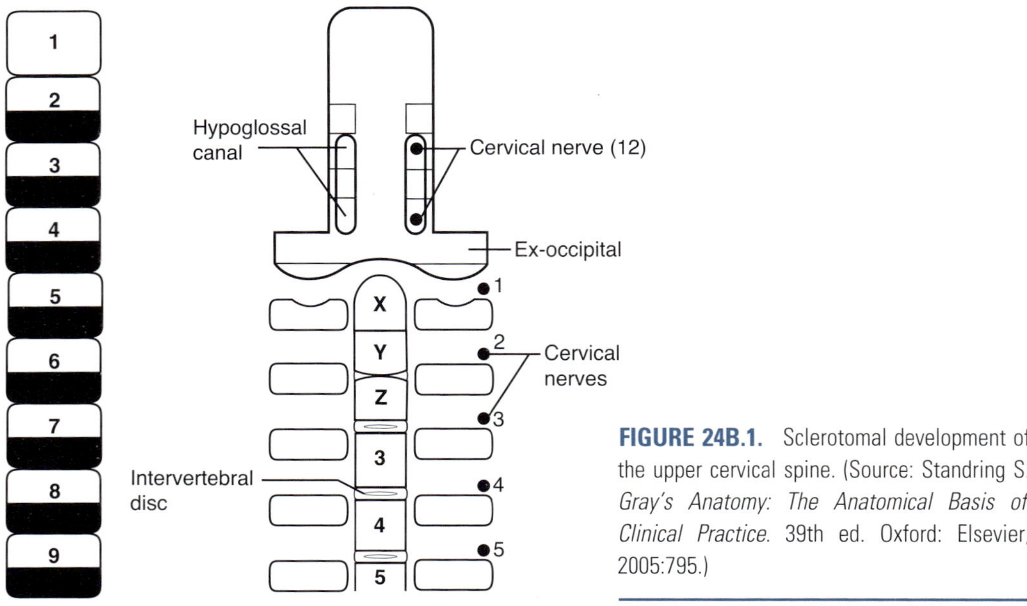

FIGURE 24B.1. Sclerotomal development of the upper cervical spine. (Source: Standring S. *Gray's Anatomy: The Anatomical Basis of Clinical Practice.* 39th ed. Oxford: Elsevier, 2005:795.)

Other anomalies include aplasia and hypoplasia of the dens. The etiology of an os odontoideum is debated between this congenital cause and an acquired cause related to unrecognized trauma.

BONY ANATOMY OF THE ODONTOID

The adult odontoid is conical in shape and projects superiorly from the body of the axis. As it projects, it may be tilted up to 14 degrees posteriorly but can occasionally be tilted slightly anteriorly. Lateral tilting can be up to 10 degrees. The mean height of the dens is about 14.4 mm, with a standard deviation of 1.6 mm. It is higher in men than in women. Its diameter is smallest at the level where the transverse ligament passes, at which point the posterior surface is grooved to accommodate the ligament. The dens lies within the ring of the atlas; often quoted is Steele's rule of thirds, which states that at the level of the atlas and viewed from the lateral aspect, the dens, subarachnoid space, and spinal cord each occupy one third of the total anteroposterior diameter of the canal.

On the anterior surface of the dens, there is an ovoid facet that articulates with the anterior arch of the atlas. Laterally are also found articular facets at the junction of the body and the neural arch.

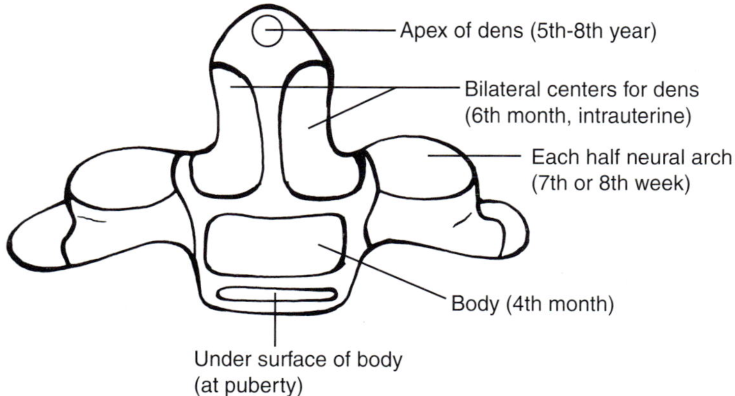

FIGURE 24B.2. Ossification centers for the axis vertebra. (Source: Standring S. *Gray's Anatomy: The Anatomical Basis of Clinical Practice.* 39th ed. Oxford: Elsevier, 2005:745.)

These articulate with the lateral masses of the atlas. At the apex and base of the dens are found numerous nutrient foramina that admit the rich arterial plexus supplying it. Anteriorly the lower border is triangular in shape and projects downward, attaching the anterior longitudinal ligament while posteriorly the lower border attaches the posterior longitudinal ligament and the tectorial membrane.

In a detailed account of the anatomy and pathology of the aging spine, Prescher[1] found that in the aging odontoid, degenerative changes take place at the median atlantoaxial joint, partly dislocating the anterior articular facet in a cranial direction. This leads to a groove in the anterior apex of the dens as a result of bony addition and has been termed a crowned dens, peridental aureole, and arthrotic coulisse of the dens. This is accompanied by cystic changes and trabeculations on the posterior dens. Parts of this may break away and be mistaken for ossicles or fractures. This crowning of the dens is a different entity again from calcification or ossification of the ligaments of the dens.

LIGAMENTOUS ANATOMY

The ligamentous attachments of the odontoid consist of the cruciform, apical, and alar ligaments (Fig. 24B.3). The cruciform ligament lies behind the odontoid and immediately anterior to and in contact with the tectorial membrane. It consists of two bands of fibers, namely the transverse and longitu-

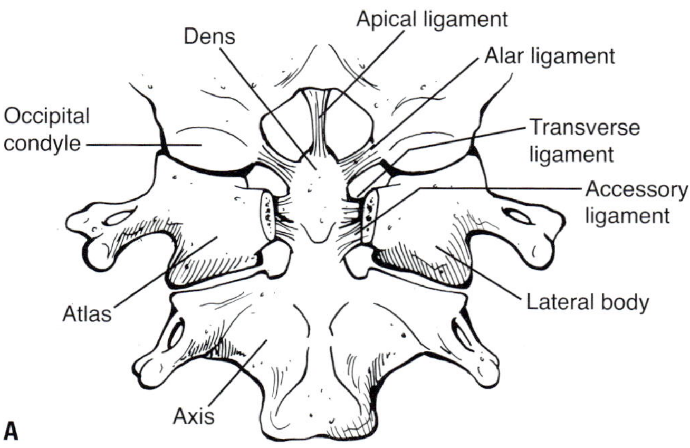

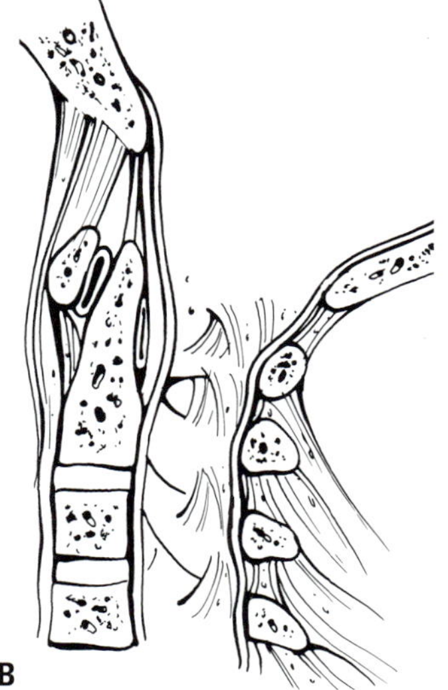

FIGURE 24B.3. A. Ligamentous attachments of the C1-C2 complex. **B.** Sagittal sketch of the complex arrangement of ligaments between the odontoid, occiput, and C1 arch. The apical ligaments at the top of the odontoid may play a factor in pulling fracture fragments apart once a fracture occurs, leading to potential pseudoarthritis. (Image A from Clarke CR, Ducker TB, Dvorak J, et al. *The Cervical Spine.* 3rd ed. Philadelphia: Lippincott Raven, 1998: 419, Figure 29-4; image B from Tubbs RS, Grabb P, Spooner A, et al. The apical ligament: anatomy and functional significance. *J Neurosurg (Spine 2)* 2000;92: 197–200, Figure 2.)

dinal ligaments. The transverse ligament is attached to the tubercles of the lateral masses of the atlas on both sides and serves to prevent posterior displacement of the dens into the vertebral canal during head motion or, put another way, holds the dens forward against the posterior surface of the anterior arch of the atlas. The longitudinal fibers are attached to the body of the axis and the foramen magnum. There is a synovial bursa between the cruciform ligament and the dens. Projecting from the odontoid and, therefore, anterior to the upper longitudinal fibers of the cruciform ligament, is the midline apical ligament with the alar ligaments on either side. The apical (middle odontoid or suspensory) ligament joins the apex of the dens with the foramen magnum (basion). This ligament is absent in 20% of cadavers and is considered to be a vestigial structure, a fibrous remnant of the notochord. It is thought not to contribute significantly to craniocervical stability. The alar (Mauchart's) ligaments fan out from the dens on both sides of the apical ligament and attach to the margins of the foramen magnum and occasionally to the atlas. These are strong ligaments that limit rotation of the head. The anterior atlanto-occipital membrane lies immediately in front of the apical and alar ligaments.

The anterior longitudinal ligament attaches anteriorly to the dens, and the posterior longitudinal ligament and the tectorial membrane attach posteriorly.

ARTERIAL SUPPLY

The odontoid is supplied mainly by branches from the vertebral arteries, with some contributions from the external carotid arteries (Fig. 24B.4). The vertebral arterial branches gain access to the odontoid via the C2-3 intervertebral foramen. There are paired longitudinal anterior and posterior branches that penetrate the base and apex of the dens. The anterior arteries are supplemented by the external carotid artery via the muscular branches of longus colli, as well as small branches via the odontoid apical ligaments. There are contributions from the ascending pharyngeal arteries, which gain access via the occipital condyles. An arterial arcade is formed at the apex of the dens.

The arterial supply of the odontoid has been implicated as a reason for poor union after fractures. However, the work of Schatzker et al.[2] and Althoff[3] has demonstrated this arterial supply from below and above; as described, this makes it unlikely that devascularization of the odontoid is the only cause of nonunion as there are alternate routes of supply; however, a potential watershed may exist between these two networks that may play a role.

VARIATIONS IN VERTEBRAL ARTERY ANATOMY IN THE ATLANTOAXIAL REGION

It should be noted that uncommonly there are important variations in the vertebral artery in the vicinity of the axis. These variations have implications for safe screw placement. It is recognized that in some patients the vertebral arteries may be ectatic and so may lie partly in the planned screw trajectories. Additionally, however, rarer variations exist, as documented by Tokuda et al.[4] These include the artery passing through the C1-C2 intervertebral foramen without passing through the foramen transversarium of C1; duplication of the artery after it leaves the C2 foramen transversarium, with one vessel running the usual course and the other running through the C1-C2 intervertebral foramen, the two vessels then reuniting; and early take-off of the posterior inferior cerebellar artery between C1 and C2. There are other variations, and these should be sought radiologically and identified preoperatively.

CLASSIFICATION OF ODONTOID FRACTURES

The most widely accepted classification is that proposed by Anderson and D'Alonzo[5] in 1974 (Fig. 24B.5). This is a three-tiered classification system that is simple to apply and is clinically useful in determining management of these fractures. Type I fractures are through the tip of the dens. The least common of odontoid fractures, they are, essentially, avulsion fractures of the alar and apical ligaments. Type II fractures occur through the base of the dens. They are the most common type

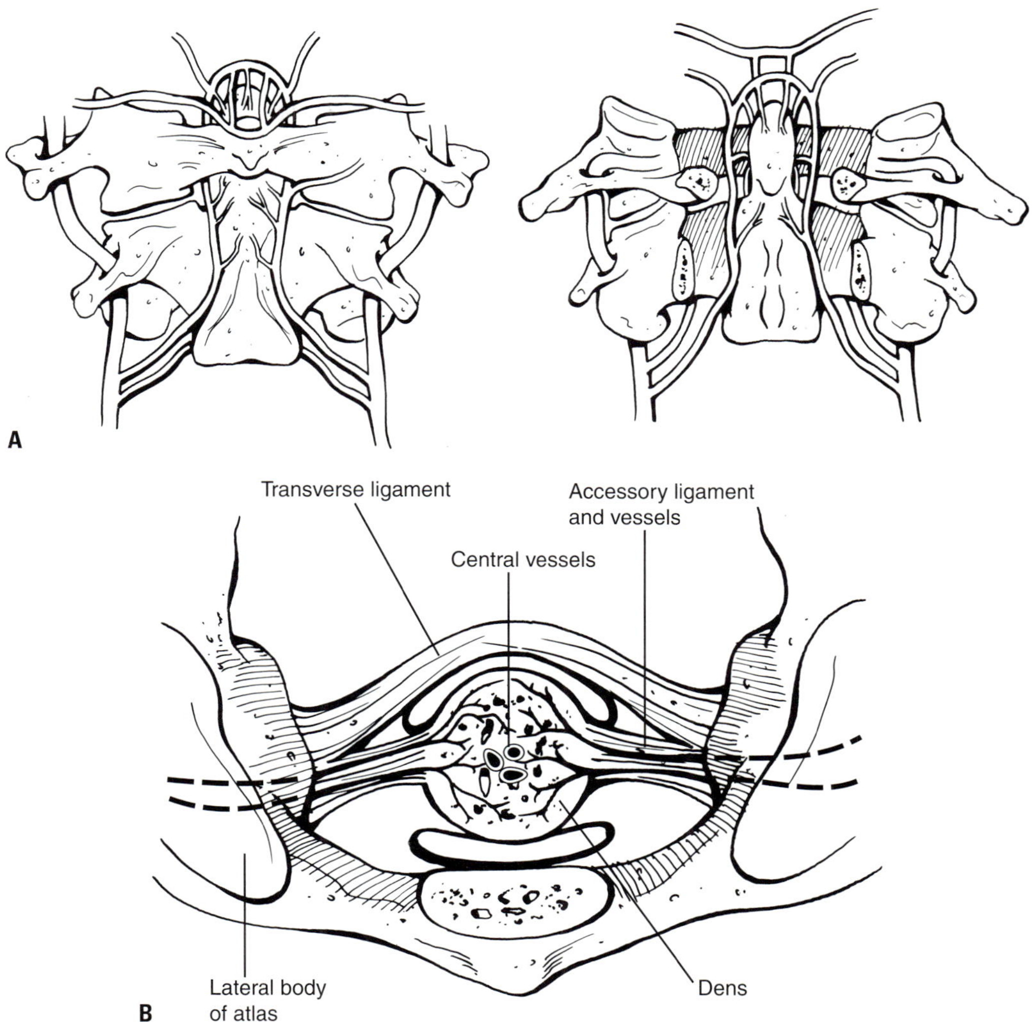

FIGURE 24B.4. A. The complex blood supply to the odontoid is shown. Branches enter the odontoid both apically and caudally with a watershed at the neck of the odontoid, one possible factor for pseudoarthrosis. **B.** The blood supply of the odontoid in axial section showing vessels crossing with the alar ligaments. Disruption of these ligaments would mean potential devascularization contributing to instability propagating potential nonunion. (Image A from Clarke CR, Ducker TB, Dvorak J, et al. *The Cervical Spine.* 3rd ed. Philadelphia: Lippincott-Raven, 1998:419, Figure 29-4B; image B from Clarke CR, Ducker TB, Dvorak J, et al. *The Cervical Spine.* 3rd ed. Philadelphia: Lippincott-Raven, 1998:418, Figure 29-3A,B.)

of odontoid fracture. The high rate of persistence of the subdental synchondrosis (87% in cadaver specimens) may have some bearing on the development and healing of these fractures. In 1988, Hadley et al.[6] proposed a type IIA subgroup for those type II fractures in which there was comminution of the fracture fragments. Type III odontoid fractures are those in which the fracture line extends from the odontoid to involve the body of the axis. These are, essentially, C2 body fractures.

The Anderson and D'Alonzo classification overlaps with Benzel's classification of C2 body fractures inasmuch as type III fractures within each system describe the same entity. Types I and II of the Benzel classification are vertical fractures of the C2 body and do not involve the odontoid.

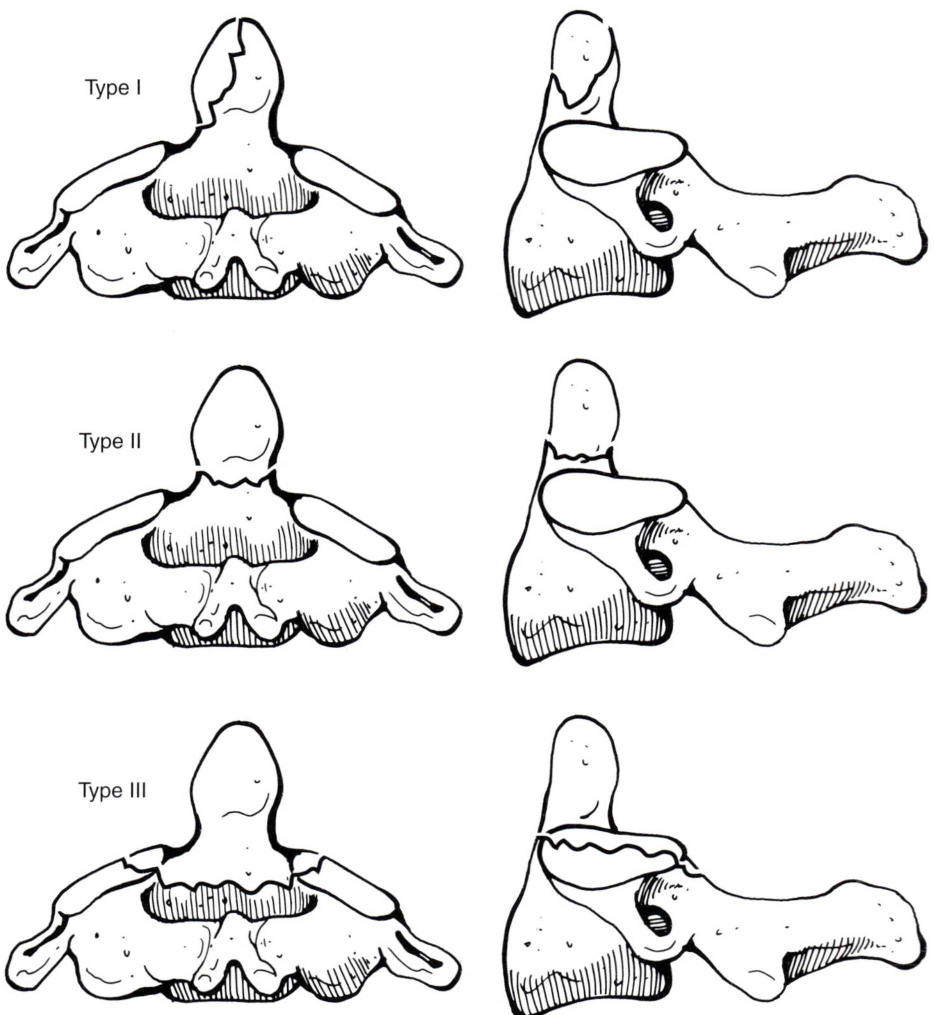

FIGURE 24B.5. The classification system of odontoid fractures proposed by Anderson and D'Alonzo. (Image from Frymoyer JW, Ducker TB, Hadler NM, et al. *The Adult Spine: Principles and Practice.* 2nd ed. Philadelphia: Lippincott-Raven, 1997:1262, Figure 13.)

In 2005, Grauer et al.[7] proposed a modification to the Anderson and D'Alonzo system (Fig. 24B.6). They pointed out the difficulty in distinguishing some type II and shallow type III fractures and so proposed that type II fractures be redefined as those in which the fracture was through the base of the dens, irrespective of how far they extended into the body of C2 as long as the superior articular facets of C2 were spared. Type III fractures would then be redefined as odontoid fractures extending into the C2 body and the C2 superior facet. The other issue addressed was the different patterns of type II fractures and how these are managed differently. They thus proposed subdividing the type II fractures according to their morphology to take this into consideration. Type IIA were nondisplaced fractures for which they recommended external immobilization; type IIB were anterosuperior to posteroinferior and displaced transverse fractures for which they recommended anterior screw fixation; type IIC were anteroinferior to posterosuperior or comminuted fractures for which posterior atlantoaxial fusion was recommended. The method of fixation was predicated on the quality of bone to ensure adequate screw fixation. This classification has yet to be validated.

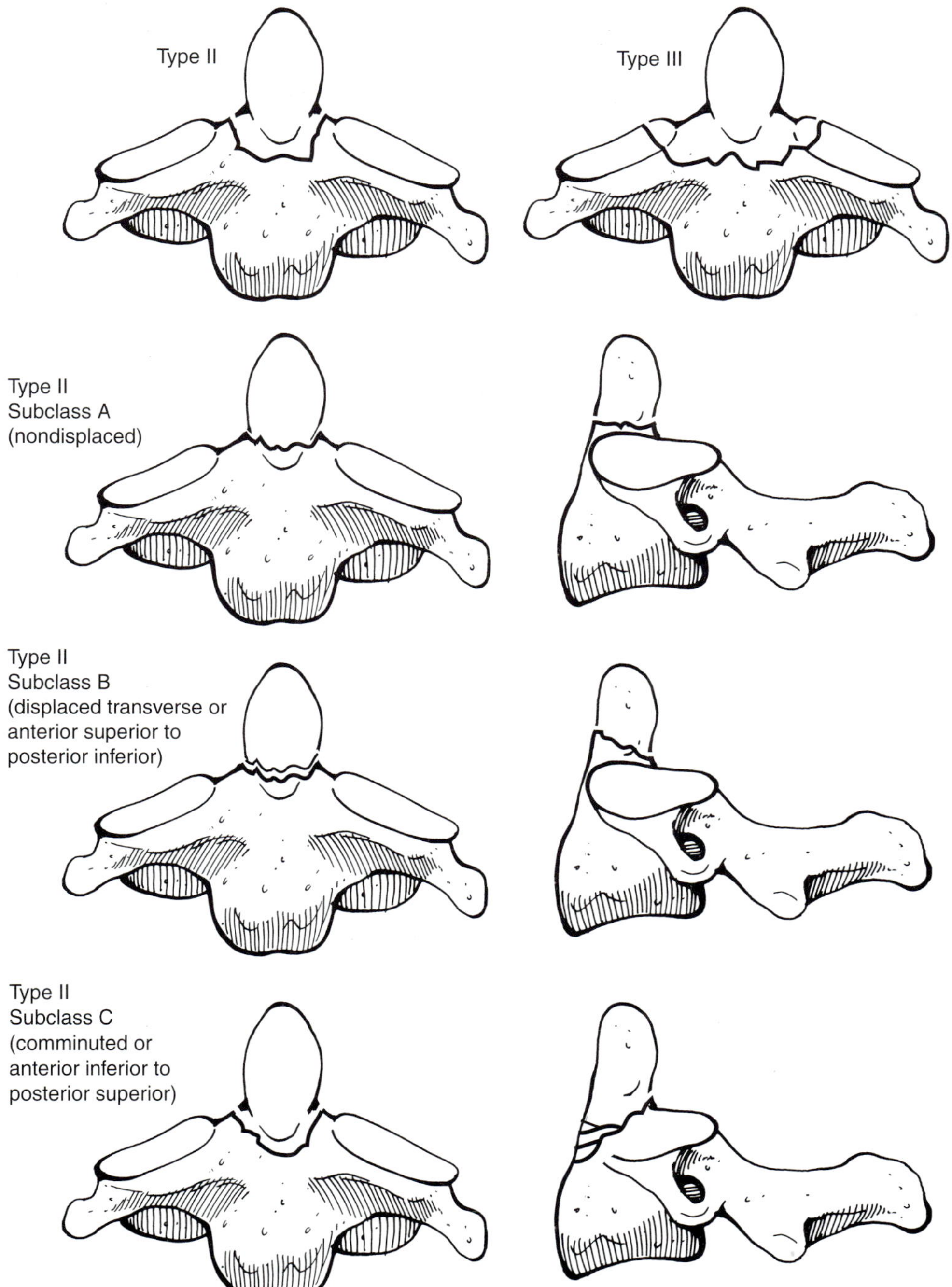

FIGURE 24B.6. Classification system of odontoid fractures advocated by Grauer et al. (Images from Grauer JN, Shafi B, Hilibrand AS, et al. Proposal of a modified, treatment-oriented classification of odontoid fractures. *Spine J* 2005;5:123–129, with permission.)

ODONTOID FRACTURE BIOMECHANICS

The exact mechanisms responsible for the various patterns of odontoid fractures have been a matter of debate. They are the result of high-energy trauma in most cases, although the injury may be more trivial in elderly patients. In most series these fractures occur most commonly as a result of motor vehicle collisions or falls, but the directions of loading resulting in fracture are not yet completely resolved. Based on a study of postmortem radiographs, it was hypothesized that these fractures were due to hyperextension, but the issue proved to be more complex than this. In a cadaveric study, Althoff[3] demonstrated that the direction of the force affected the way the dens fractured. It was shown that as the direction of the vector of the impact force moved from the sagittal plane laterally, the dens fractured more superiorly; that is, an anterior force caused a type III fracture, lateral loading a type I fracture, and an oblique force a type II fracture. However, in a study by Mouradian et al.,[8] a lateral load produced predominantly type II fractures.

A more recent study by Puttlitz et al.[9] used finite element modeling based on human cadavers to apply force loads and measure intraosseous stresses leading to different fractures. It was found that type I fractures resulted when head extension was coupled with lateral shear or compression and type II fractures resulted when axial rotation and lateral shear were applied. The model did not account for type III fractures.

A study of the microarchitecture of the axis by Amling et al.[10] showed that there was 55% less trabecular bone in the base of the odontoid than in the body of the axis and the odontoid process itself. The thickness of the cortical bone was also less in the odontoid base than the odontoid process. It was concluded that the microarchitecture of the odontoid gives its base a predilection for fracture. This would seem to be consistent with the clinical situation in which type II fractures are indeed the most frequent.

TREATMENT OF ODONTOID FRACTURES

There are a wide variety of treatment options available for these fractures. The multicenter study by Clark and White[11] definitively demonstrated that the union rate of odontoid fractures with no treatment is zero, so that, be it nonsurgical or surgical, some form of treatment is required. Nonsurgical treatment options include different types of orthoses for external immobilization, such as a rigid cervical collar, halo immobilization, sterno-occipito-mandibular immobilizer (SOMI) brace, Minerva jacket, etc. Surgical treatments include anterior odontoid screw fixation, posterior cervical fusion, and transarticular screw fixation techniques. Decision making in the management of these fractures takes into account several factors, including fracture type, displacement and angulation of the odontoid, association with atlas fractures, associated ligamentous injuries, patient age, and other patient factors, such as coexisting Down syndrome, rheumatoid arthritis, etc. However, there are not sufficient evidence-based data to develop treatment standards at this time.

TYPE I

Type I odontoid fractures are thought by many authors to be due to avulsions of the alar ligaments. They are so rare that meaningful data on stability and treatment are not available. These fractures were generally considered stable. However, Scott et al.[12] reported a case of a type I fracture associated with atlanto-occipital and atlantoaxial dislocation leading to death. They proposed that the fracture was a manifestation of the atlantoaxial instability and that type I fractures were rare in isolation and likely not to be stable. The issue of stability of these fractures remains controversial.

These fractures have a high rate of bony fusion approaching 100%. Such rates have been reported with rigid cervical collar immobilization, as well as halo immobilization. If coexistent ligamentous injury is suspected, surgical intervention should be considered in the form of a posterior C1-C2 fusion.[13–15]

TYPE II

These fractures are usually unstable and have a high rate of nonunion. Authors have suggested reasons for the high rate of nonunion, implicating factors such as vascular compromise, poor bone quality, and a persisting subdental synchondrosis. However, given that the fusion rate is zero when no immobilization is used but increases even with rigid collar immobilization, it is most likely that the reason most contributory to the high rate of nonunion is poor immobilization, although other factors may also play a role.

The healing rate with rigid cervical collar immobilization is approximately 53%. With 6 to 12 weeks of halo immobilization, the rate increases to approximately 65% to 75%. If initial halo immobilization fails, consideration may be given to a longer period of immobilization, and approximately one third of these patients will go on to fusion. The remainder of the failed halo unions require surgical fusion, which may be undertaken when the initial halo immobilization fails in any case. Halo immobilization is associated with significant morbidity, particularly in the elderly, and age may be a relative contraindication to its use.

A very important factor in the likelihood of nonunion is the degree of displacement of the fractured odontoid at the time of immobilization. Hadley et al.[6] showed a nonunion rate of 67% when the dens was displaced 6 mm or more as opposed to 26% when it was displaced less than 6 mm. This finding has also been confirmed by other authors. This failure to heal is independent of age, direction of the displacement, and the presence of a neurologic deficit.

Fractures that are at high risk for nonunion, such as significantly displaced fractures or those that have failed external immobilization, should be considered for surgical treatment for internal fixation. The options for surgery broadly fall into anterior and posterior procedures (Fig. 24B.7).

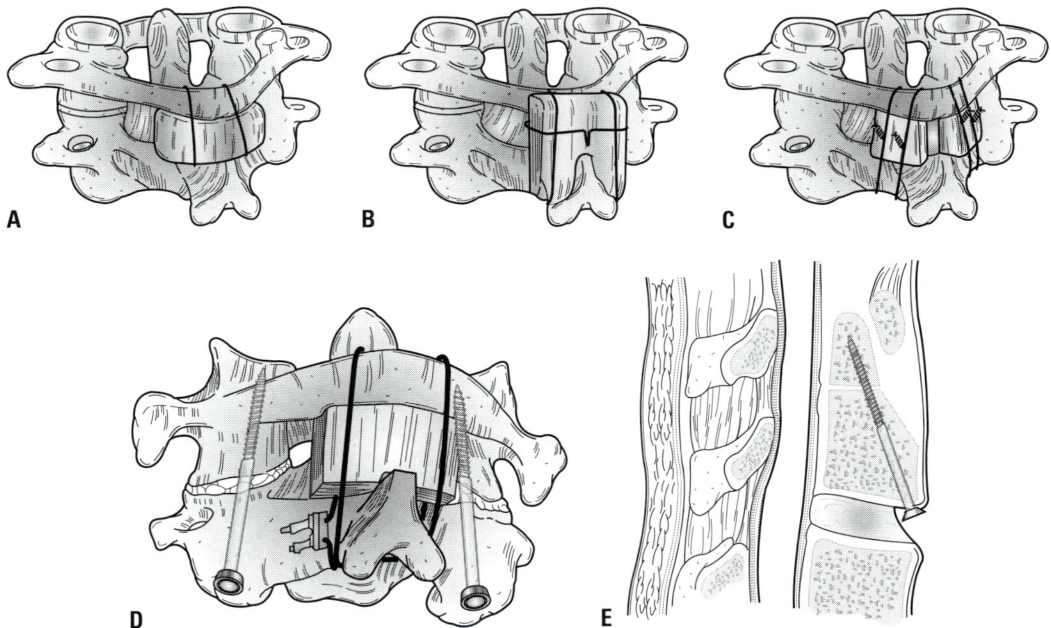

FIGURE 24B.7. The commonly used posterior and anterior surgical methods of management of odontoid fracture. The Sonntag technique **(A)** uses a single sublaminar C1 loop. The Gallie fusion **(B)** has the graft placed dorsal to the arch of the atlas. The Brooks and Jenkins fusion **(C)** uses wedge compression with two grafts and two sublaminar wires/cables beneath the arches of C1 and C2. Combining a posterior graft/loop construct with transarticular screws **(D)** gives added stability and three-point fixation. Finally, anterior odontoid screw placement **(E)** can be used for type II fractures with no C1-C2 instability. (Images from Menezes AH, Sonntag VKH. *Principles of Spinal Surgery*. Vol. 2. New York: McGraw-Hill, 1996;878, 881, with permission.)

Posterior cervical fixation in the form of a C1-C2 fusion has the advantage of a high fusion rate, but the cost is loss of rotatory motion because approximately 50% of cervical spine rotation takes place at the C1-C2 level. The fusion rate of the operative site approaches 100% and is 35% to 87% at the fracture site. There are several techniques described, including wiring of the C1-C2 (e.g., Sonntag, Gallie, Brooks methods) and the use of lateral mass screws into C1. If the C1 arch or C2 lamina is fractured, wiring techniques cannot be used there. In this situation, screw-rod constructs between C1 and C2 can be used or an occiput to C2 fusion considered. Patients who undergo posterior C1-C2 fixation may still require halo immobilization postoperatively to reduce rotation until fusion has taken place. The use of bilateral C1-C2 transarticular screw fixation prevents this rotation and so reduces the need for postoperative halo immobilization. A reasonable alternative to this is C1 lateral mass screw fixation combined with C2 pars or pedicle screws, obviating the need for C2 transarticular screws. The C1-C2 joint can be directly exposed, decorticated, and packed with bone.

Anterior cervical fixation has the advantage of preserving rotation as well as having a surgical approach that is familiar to most spine surgeons. The key to the surgery and the challenging aspect of it is the screw placement, which requires biplanar intraoperative fluoroscopy. A single or double screw technique is used; there is no significant difference in fusion rates. The use of lag screws ensures the distal fracture fragment firmly apposes the proximal fragment. The anterior fixation technique is contraindicated in patients with disruption of the transverse ligament demonstrated on MRI or those in whom the fracture line extends obliquely posterosuperiorly to anteroinferiorly in the sagittal plane. Suspected C1-C2 instability should counsel against use of this technique. Fusion rates range from 88% to 96% with anterior fixation. However, the rate declines precipitously when the procedure is delayed beyond 6 months to approximately 25%. This may be due to the development of a fibrous union that impedes bony fusion. Newer constructs using bioresorbable implants may gain more widespread use in the future.

TYPE III

Type III fractures, like type I, have a high rate of bony union, thought largely to be the result of the presence of cancellous bone at the fracture line. Even with only a rigid cervical collar the rate 50% to 65%. With 8 to 14 weeks of halo immobilization, the rate increases to 84% to 100%. Thus, external immobilization is considered the treatment of first choice for these fractures. If the fracture configuration is such that there is significant displacement or obvious associated ligamentous injury, surgery should instead be considered. Posterior cervical fixation is the procedure most used as outlined previously in the discussion about type II fractures. The fusion rate for type III fractures posteriorly approaches 100%. Again, bilateral transarticular screw fixation may be incorporated to minimize the need for postoperative halo immobilization. Anterior screw fixation may also be used in a similar fashion to type II fractures.

TREATMENT OF COMBINED ODONTOID AND ATLAS FRACTURES

Several patterns of axis fractures are associated with atlas injuries, as outlined by Dickman et al.[16] It was found that approximately 16% of axis fractures were associated with an atlas injury. The spectrum of C1 fractures includes posterior unilateral, multiple arch fractures, as well as lateral mass fractures. When atlantoaxial displacement was less than 6 mm, external immobilization (e.g., halo) was used and a 95% fusion rate achieved. In patients with significant (i.e., greater than 6 mm) atlantoaxial displacement or in whom external immobilization had failed, posterior cervical fixation was used in the form of a C1-C2 fusion. There was a 100% fusion rate with this method. As noted previously, in the presence of a C1 arch fracture, wiring techniques may not be possible, so C1-C2 transarticular screw, use of C1 lateral mass screws–C2 pars/pedicle screws, or occiput/C2 fusions should be considered. Patients who have an injury to the transverse ligaments as documented on MRI should be considered for early surgical intervention rather than external immobilization.

TREATMENT OF ODONTOID FRACTURES IN THE ELDERLY

This remains a controversial issue in the management of odontoid fractures, and there are data expounding both for and against surgical treatment in this age group. The main arguments for surgical fixation relate to the issues of the poor tolerance of patients over 75 years of age to external immobilization. Fusion rates with external immobilization in the elderly have been reported to be as low as 23% in type II fractures. These low rates can be argued on the grounds that many of these odontoid fractures are not diagnosed early. In addition, the point is raised that healing by fibrous union without radiologic bony fusion may indeed be an acceptable outcome because it can provide stability and protection from neurologic injury. There have been reports of nonunions progressing to late-onset myelopathy, but the true incidence of this is unknown and remains controversial. In a large series looking at the treatment of type II fractures in all ages, displacement greater than 6 mm was found to be a major determining factor on fusion rates independent of age. In yet another series, age greater than 50 years was the major factor determining poor nonunion, with no significant contribution by degree of displacement in patients with type II fractures treated with halo immobilization.

On the other hand, a high rate of fusion, on the order of 86%, has been shown in type II fractures in patients over 65 years of age treated with posterior fixation. In this study, low fusion rates were found with anterior screw fixation and external immobilization.[17] However, the fusion rate in patients older than 65 years treated with anterior screw fixation has also been reported to be as high as 85%. By nature of the presence of comorbidities at this age, there is a certain degree of morbidity and mortality associated with surgery; this figure has been reported to be as high as 28%. However, it should be noted that up to a 26% mortality has been reported in elderly patients treated with external immobilization alone. These are high mortality rates, but even more so when one considers that the mechanism of injury in elderly patients is more likely due to simple falls rather than high-energy trauma with other associated injuries, as is more the case in younger patients. Morbidity and mortality are generally attributable to bed rest and immobilization.

Overall, the management of elderly patients with odontoid fractures remains a contentious issue. Cases should be considered on an individual basis, taking into account factors such as type of fracture, degree of displacement, association with other fractures or ligamentous injury, patient's level of function before the injury, and medical comorbidities.

TREATMENT OF ODONTOID FRACTURES IN CHILDREN

The subdental (neurocentral) synchondrosis usually fuses by adolescence. In children in whom it has yet to fuse, high-energy trauma may lead to odontoid epiphysiolysis through this synchondrosis. In most cases, children with odontoid fractures may be managed with external immobilization, most commonly with halo immobilization, even for odontoid epiphysiolysis, in which there is an 80% fusion rate. Most series report their rate of surgical intervention at 3% to 20% in the paediatric group. These are patients in whom closed reduction could not be initially achieved or later maintained with external fixation. The majority of procedures were posterior C1-C2 fixations, although anterior odontoid screw fixation has also been used with good outcomes.

REFERENCES

1. Prescher A. Anatomy and pathology of the aging spine. *Eur J Radiol* 1998;27(3):181–195.
2. Schatzker J, Rorabeck CH, Waddell JP. Non-union of the odontoid process. An experimental investigation. *Clin Orthop Relat Res* 1975;108:127–137.
3. Althoff B, Goldie IF. The arterial supply of the odontoid process of the axis. *Acta Orthop Scand* 1977;48(6):622–629.
4. Tokuda K, Miyasaka K, Abe H, et al. Anomalous atlantoaxial portions of vertebral and posterior inferior cerebellar arteries. *Neuroradiology* 1985;27(5):410–413.
5. Anderson LD, D'Alonzo RT. Fractures of the odontoid process of the axis. *J Bone Joint Surg Am* 1974;56: 1663–1674.
6. Hadley MN, Browner CM, Liu SS, et al. New subtype of acute odontoid fractures (type IIA). *Neurosurgery* 1988; 22(1 Pt 1):67–71

7. Grauer JN, Shafi B, Hilibrand AS, et al. Proposal of a modified, treatment-oriented classification of odontoid fractures. *Spine J* 2005;5(2):123–129.
8. Mouradian WH, Fietti VG Jr, Cochran GV, et al. Fractures of the odontoid: a laboratory and clinical study of mechanisms. *Orthop Clin North Am* 1978;9(4):985–1001.
9. Puttlitz CM, Goel VK, Traynelis VC, et al. A finite element investigation of upper cervical instrumentation. *Spine* 2001;26(22):2449–2455.
10. Amling M, Hahn M, Wening VJ, et al. The microarchitecture of the axis as the predisposing factor for fracture of the base of the odontoid process. A histomorphometric analysis of twenty-two autopsy specimens. *J Bone Joint Surg Am* 1994;76(12):1840–1846.
11. Clark CR, White AA III. Fractures of the dens: a multicenter study. *J Bone Joint Surg Am* 1985;67:1340–1348.
12. Scott EW, Haid RW Jr, Peace D. Type I fractures of the odontoid process: implications for atlanto-occipital instability. Case report. *J Neurosurg* 1990;72(3):488–492.
13. Gallie WE. Fractures and dislocations of the upper cervical spine. *Am J Surg* 1939;46:495–499.
14. Brooks AL, Jenkins EB. Atlanto-axial arthrodesis by the wedge compression method. *J Bone Joint Surg Am* 1978;60:279–284.
15. Greene KA, Dickman CA, Marciano FF, et al. Acute axis fractures. Analysis of management and outcome in 340 consecutive cases. *Spine* 1997;22(16):1843–1852.
16. Dickman CA, Foley KT, Sonntag VKH, et al. Cannulated screws for odontoid screw fixation and atlantoaxial transarticular screw fixation: technical note. *J Neurosurg* 1995;83:1095–1100.

CHAPTER 24C

C2 Fractures: Os Odontoideum

Ajit A. Krishnaney and Iain H. Kalfas

INTRODUCTION

Os odontoideum was first described by Giacomini in 1886. It is defined as an independent bony ossicle rostral to the C2 vertebral body in the position of the odontoid process. The ossicle has smooth cortical margins and is separated from a hypoplastic dens by a horizontal gap of variable width. Typically, the gap between the os odontoideum and the remnant of the odontoid process is above the level of the superior facet of C2. This creates a potential for incompetence of the transverse ligament with subsequent atlantoaxial instability (Fig. 24C.1).[1]

Although the definition of this rare anomaly is uniform throughout the literature, there is debate about the etiology, with evidence for congenital, vascular, and traumatic causes. Regardless of the etiology, the condition can result in significant spinal instability and compression of neural structures. Early diagnosis and management of os odontoideum is directed at preventing these sequelae.

MECHANISM OF INJURY

The two leading theories for the cause of os odontoideum promote a congenital origin or an acquired anomaly. Embryologically, C2 is formed from the proatlas (apex), C1 (dens), and C2 (body) sclerotomes. Failure of any of these to fuse can result in the anomaly.[2] Proponents of the congenital theory cite numerous cases of the anomaly with no identifiable history of cervical trauma. Os odontoideum has also been associated with other congenital cervical anomalies and has been seen in monozygotic twins.[3–5]

The more widely accepted theory is that os odontoideum is acquired. This theory postulates that a minor cervical injury during infancy leads to an undetected bony or ligamentous injury. Fielding et al.[6] noted that most patients describe a significant episode of trauma before the diagnosis of os odontoideum. Following a fracture through the base of the odontoid, a separation of the bone fragments occurs as a result of contracture of apical ligaments attached to the superior margin of the odontoid process. The ossicle continues to receive a blood supply through an arcade of vessels traveling through the apical, alar, and accessory ligaments. However, the separation of the inferior margin of the ossicle from the body of the axis creates a vascular watershed zone at the site of the fracture. This tenuous blood supply results in poor healing of the fracture, increasing the potential for nonunion.[7] The fact that nonunion occurs in as many as 62% of type II odontoid fractures lends further support to this theory.[8]

CLASSIFICATION

Plain cervical spine radiographs are usually sufficient to make the diagnosis of os odontoideum.[9] The ossicle typically presents as a rounded or oval mass that is circumferentially corticated and positioned above the vertebral body of C2. The rostral margin of the C2 vertebral body also has a cortical

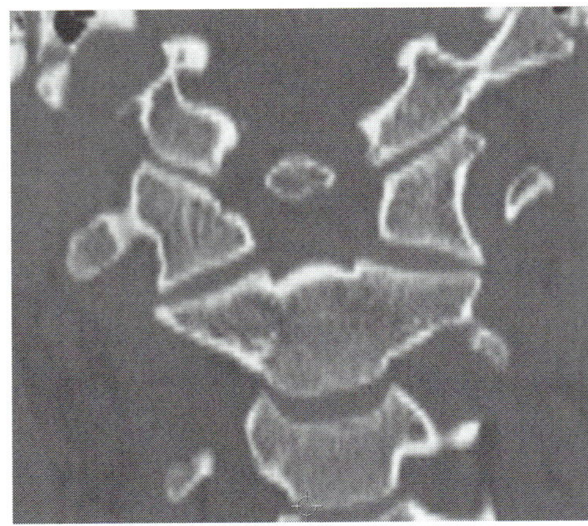
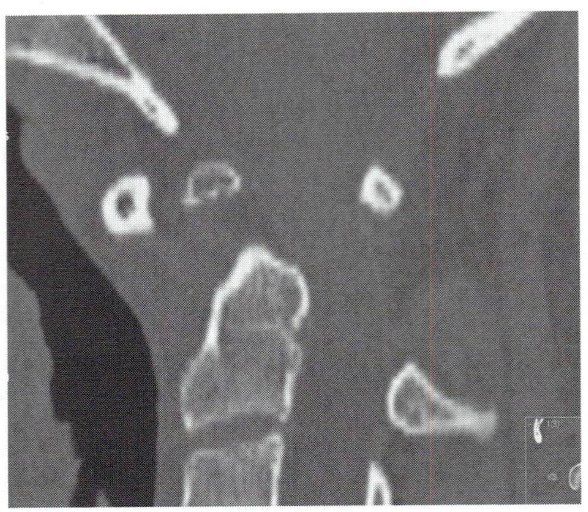

FIGURE 24C.1. Coronal **(A)** and sagittal **(B)** computed tomography reconstructions of an orthotopic os odontoideum illustrating ventral subluxation of the ossicle-C1 complex on C2 causing posterior compression of the neural elements.

margin. In most cases a pronounced horizontal gap exists between the body of C2 and the ossicle. Conversely, with acute odontoid fractures the gap is typically narrow and irregular and can extend into the body of C2. Sclerotic margins adjacent to the fracture line are not present.[1] In children younger than 5 years of age, the normal epiphyseal line may be confused with the presence of an os odontoideum or a fracture.

Based on the radiographic appearance, there are two types of os odontoideum: orthotopic and dystopic.[6] With the orthotopic type, the ossicle lies in the location of the normal dens and moves with the axis and the ventral arch of C1. This type is often associated with an intact cruciate ligament (Fig. 24C.1).[1,10]

With the dystopic type, the ossicle is located near the basion and is often fused to the clivus. The anterior arch of C1 is hypertrophied, and the posterior arch is hypoplastic. Dystopic os odontoideum has a greater likelihood of causing neurologic compromise than the orthotopic variant.[6,11] This can occur as a result of the spinal cord being compressed by the posterior arch of C1 during flexion and by the mobile ossicle during extension.[10] In cases of chronic subluxation, dense granulation tissue may form behind the ossicle, creating compression of the ventral cervicomedullary region.

Although the diagnosis can usually be established with plain radiographs, several other imaging studies can assist in developing a management plan. Dynamic cervical flexion-extension radiographs can be used to determine the amount of abnormal motion between C1 and C2. Approximately 67% of individuals with os odontoideum will have anterior instability, with the os odontoideum subluxating ventrally in relation to the body of the axis. Less than 15% of individuals with the anomaly will have posterior instability, in which the ossicle moves dorsally into the canal with cervical extension. The remaining individuals with os odontoideum (18%) will have minimal or no abnormal motion on dynamic films.[6,11]

Magnetic resonance imaging (MRI) or computed tomography (CT) following myelography are helpful in determining the presence and degree of spinal cord compression. MRI with the patient's neck in both flexed and extended positions can be extremely useful. Yamashita et al.[12] found that although the degree of myelopathy did correlate with the degree of cord compression on MRI, it did not correlate with the distance of C1-C2 subluxation on flexion-extension radiograph. However, several authors have reported that a spinal canal anteroposterior diameter of less than 13 mm on plain radiography does predict the presence of myelopathy.[11,13,14]

TREATMENT

INITIAL TREATMENT

Patients with os odontoideum can present with a wide range of clinical signs and symptoms. In some patients, the abnormality appears as an incidental finding on radiographs taken for other reasons. In others, neck pain prompts the radiographic studies that demonstrate the lesion. These patients may also present with any combination of headache, neck stiffness, neck weakness, dizziness, and torticollis.[2,15] Patients with atlantoaxial instability and spinal cord encroachment may present with signs and symptoms of myelopathy. The myelopathic signs and symptoms may be intermittent, static, or progressive. If atlantoaxial instability is present, compression of the adjacent vertebral arteries may occur, resulting in signs and symptoms of vertebrobasilar insufficiency.

Because many of the presenting signs and symptoms of symptomatic os odontoideum can also result from a variety of other causes, the diagnosis is usually not considered until imaging of the cervical spine is performed.[15]

The management of patients with os odontoideum is determined by the degree of both the clinical and radiographic findings. These patients may present in any of the following categories: asymptomatic with no radiographic signs of instability, asymptomatic with radiographic instability, local symptoms (e.g., neck pain) without radiographic instability, local symptoms with radiographic instability, and patients with myelopathy or other neurologic injury. Patients with myelopathy can be further classified as those with transient (traumatic), stable, or progressive myelopathy.[6,15]

The goals of managing patients with os odontoideum are to prevent neurologic injury, ensure stability of C1-C2, and alleviate local symptoms. Management is complicated by the fact that the natural history of the anomaly has not been fully understood. There are multiple case series in the literature suggesting a benign natural history in asymptomatic patients.[2,13] However, several examples of sudden spinal cord injury related to minor trauma have also been reported.[16]

Because of the lack of consistently reliable predictors of outcome, a variety of treatment paradigms have been promoted. In patients who are relatively asymptomatic and have no signs of myelopathy or radiographic evidence of instability or spinal canal compromise, a conservative approach with intermittent updating of cervical radiographs is a reasonable approach. These patients are typically advised to avoid contact sports and activities that can generate rapid acceleration forces at the craniovertebral junction, such as diving, parachuting, and roller coaster riding.

DEFINITIVE TREATMENT

Proposed indications for surgical stabilization have included the simple presence of the anomaly, os odontoideum in association with cervical pain, and os odontoideum in association with neurologic deficit or atlantoaxial instability.[2,6,13,15]

Prophylactic stabilization in the asymptomatic individual may be indicated in younger patients with active lifestyles because they may be at higher risk for future neurologic deterioration. In patients who present with neck pain that is position and activity related, surgical stabilization is relatively indicated. The improvement of the pain while at rest or in a cervical collar is a reasonably good predictor for the potential success of C1-C2 arthrodesis.

Patients who have evidence of myelopathy or atlantoaxial instability require surgical stabilization. It is critical to determine not only the presence of neural compression but also the reducibility of this finding. If persistent compressive pathology is present, a period of cervical traction may be indicated. If the compression can be reduced by preoperative or intraoperative cervical traction, a posterior atlantoaxial stabilization procedure may be sufficient. However, as with other long-standing deformities of the craniovertebral junction, several days of traction may be required to achieve proper realignment and relief of the neural compression. If the compressive pathology is not reducible, a decompressive procedure, either through a posterior or anterior transoral approach, may be required in addition to the stabilization procedure.

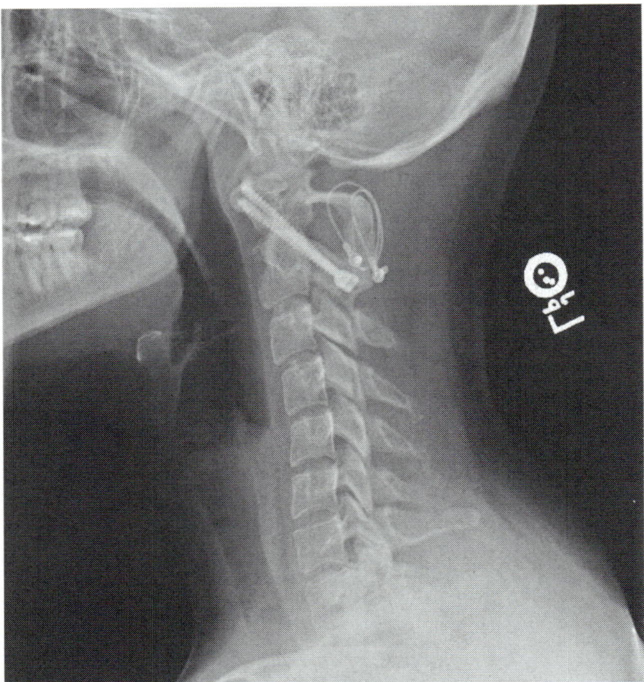

FIGURE 24C.2. Postoperative lateral plain radiograph of C1-C2 arthrodesis using a posterior wiring technique supplemented with transarticular screw fixation.

Most patients with os odontoideum and cervical instability can be managed by atlantoaxial stabilization. Inclusion of the occiput is rarely required, although it may be considered in cases with a significantly deficient posterior arch of C1 or with posterior neural compression necessitating a C1 laminectomy.

The technique options for atlantoaxial stabilization include several variations of wire/cable and bone grafting methods. Typically, iliac crest autograft is the preferred grafting material for this procedure. Any of these arthrodesis techniques may be supplemented with a screw fixation construct employing either transarticular screws passed across the C1-C2 facet joints or separate screws placed into both C1 lateral masses and across both C2 pedicles (Fig. 24C.2). The addition of screw fixation provides immediate internal immobilization of the arthrodesis site, increasing the likelihood of achieving a successful fusion.[17]

COMPLICATIONS

Complications associated with the management of os odontoideum can occur as a result of either conservative or surgical treatment. In patients managed expectantly, the most common complication is development or progression of a neurologic deficit. Close monitoring of asymptomatic patients along with early intervention in cases of progressive instability may help reduce the risk for this complication.

The most common complications associated with surgical management of os odontoideum include pseudarthrosis, failure of the internal fixation device, and neurologic or vascular injury, typically resulting from misplacement of fixation screws. The risk for these complications can usually be prevented by obtaining adequate preoperative imaging, the development of a biomechanically sound construct design, the preferential use of autograft bone, and the use of meticulous surgical technique.

CONCLUSION

Os odontoideum is a relatively rare anomaly of the atlantoaxial complex. It may have either a traumatic or congenital cause. It is best managed on an individualized basis, depending on the presence of spinal instability or neural compression. Although many patients are managed with surgery to stabilize the atlantoaxial complex, asymptomatic patients without spinal instability can be managed conservatively with interval radiographic assessment of the anomaly.

REFERENCES

1. Menezes AH, Ryken TC. Craniovertebral junction abnormalities. In: Weinstein SL, ed. *The Pediatric Spine: Principles and Practice.* Philadelphia: Lippincott-Raven, 1994:307–321.
2. Dai LY, Yuan W, Ni B, et al. Os odontoideum: etiology, diagnosis and management. *Surg Neurol* 2000;53:106–109.
3. Sherk HH, Dawoud S. Congenital os odontoideum with Klippel-Feil anomaly and fatal atlantoaxial instability. *Spine* 1981;6:42–45.
4. Kirlew KA, Hathout GM, Reiter SD, et al. Os odontoideum in identical twins: perspectives on etiology. *Skeletal Radiol* 1993;22:525–527.
5. Verska JM, Anderson PA. Os odontoideum: a case report of one identical twin. *Spine* 1997;22:706–709.
6. Fielding JW, Hensinger RN, Hawkins RJ. Os odontoideum. *J Bone Joint Surg Am* 1980;62:376–383.
7. Alp MS, Crockard HA. Late complication of undetected odontoid fracture in children. *Br Med J* 1990;300: 319–320.
8. Schatzker J, Rorabeck DH, Waddell JP. Fractures of the dens (odontoid process): an analysis of 37 cases. *J Bone Joint Surg Br* 1971;53:392–405.
9. Lowry DW, Pollack IF, Clyde B, et al. Upper cervical spine fusion in the pediatric population. *J Neurosurg* 1997;87:671–676.
10. Menezes AH. Os odontoideum: pathogenesis, dynamics and management. In: Marlin AE, ed. *Concepts in Pediatric Neurosurgery.* Basel: Karger, 1995:133–145.
11. Shirasaki N, Okada K, Oka S, et al. Os odontoideum with posterior atlantoaxial instability. *Spine* 1991;16:706–715.
12. Yamashita Y, Takahashi M, Sakamoto Y, et al. Atlanto axial subluxation: radiography and magnetic resonance imaging correlated to myelopathy. *Acta Radiol* 1989;30:135–140.
13. Spierings EL, Braakman R. The management of os odontoideum: analysis of 37 cases. *J Bone Joint Surg Br* 1982; 64:422–428.
14. Watanabe M, Toyama Y, Fujimura Y. Atlantoaxial instability in os odontoideum with myelopathy. *Spine* 1996; 21:1435–1439.
15. Anonymous. Os odontoideum. *Neurosurgery* 2002;50(suppl):S148–S155.
16. Menezes AH, Ryken TC. Craniocervical abnormalities in Down's syndrome. *Pediatr Neurosurg* 1992;18:24–33.
17. Dickman CA, Sonntag VKH. Posterior C1-C2 transarticular screw fixation for atlantoaxial arthrodesis. *Neurosurgery* 1998;43:275–281.

CHAPTER 24D

C2 Fractures: Hangman Fracture—Traumatic Spondylolisthesis of the Axis

F. Cumhur Öner

INTRODUCTION

The basic architecture of the vertebral bodies is essentially the same throughout the spine except in the cranial and caudal extremes. In the upper cervical spine, the first two vertebrae have evolved into a radically different body configuration to form a unique junctional relationship with the cranium. This unique occipitocervical junction, consisting of the occipital condyles, atlas, and atlantoaxial articulation, is capable of extreme rotation especially between C1 and C2. This is achieved by the relationship of the anterior ring of C1 to the C2 dens and the absence of an intervertebral disc space, replaced by motion through the C1-C2 and dens-C1 articulations, resulting in motion parallel to the base of the skull. However, the connection of upper cervical vertebrae to the subaxial spine is somewhat different than the subaxial facet articulations. The C2 body is connected to the facet of C3 through an elongated pedicle-isthmus complex. The motion planes of the superior and inferior articular processes of C2 are thus separated to a greater extent than those of the subaxial vertebrae and have a considerable offset between them. The motion plane of the C1-C2 joint is ventral, whereas the C2-C3 joint is dorsal to the spinal canal. This connection is further weakened by the vertebral artery penetrating the axis just at the base of the pedicles (Fig. 24D.1).

This unique anatomic characteristic makes the C2-C3 articulation vulnerable to an "isthmic failure." Although a stress fracture type of isthmic failure, such as the common lumbar spondylolysis, is unknown at this region, probably because of the relatively small weights carried through this junction, traumatic failure of this connection is a well-known phenomenon. Why this traumatic spondylolysis of the axis, usually associated with some degree of spondylolisthesis, is called the hangman fracture has a curious origin. Killing people by hanging, euphemistically referred to as "judicial" hanging, has been common practice throughout history. One common observation of these judicial hangings was that sometimes the person died suddenly and apparently without much suffering. Usually this form of death ended in a distasteful strangulation during lasting 10 to 20 minutes. To overcome this "inhumane" treatment, the enlightened French of the 18th century came up with the "scientific" solution of the guillotine. However, being a French invention, this could not be accepted by the British, so they went on with their discussion of "sound and humane" hanging. The first discussion in the medical literature on the hangman type injury was by Reverend S. Houghton in 1866. This discussion was further carried on by British and American anatomists, surgeons, and jail physicians until the 1920s. One possible explanation was that a violent dissociation of the lamina of the

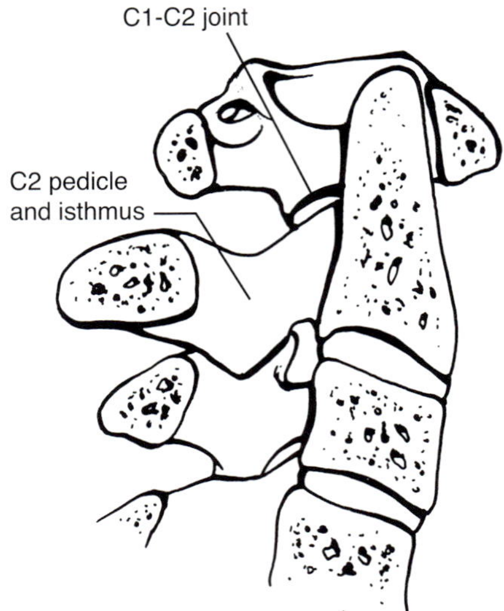

FIGURE 24D.1. The atlantoaxial complex lacks a true facet joint. Instead, part of the disc area is transformed into a joint. This causes a big offset and a sharp angle between the motion planes of C1-C2 and C2-C3 joints. Note also the elongated isthmus of C2 and the foramen of the vertebral artery along the base of this isthmus/pedicle.

axis followed by dislocation at the C2-C3 junction would cause a sudden and painless death. Many recommendations were developed to achieve that. Although it is unclear how similar these "humane judicial injuries" are to the traumatic spondylolysis, which we encounter today, this name has commonly been used in the surgical literature for the traumatic spondylolisthesis of the axis.

With the invention of high-speed transportation, this type of fracture has become a common result of violent hyperextension and hyperflexion forces associated with deceleration injuries. Typically today these injuries are caused by motor vehicle collisions, diving, or falls from a height and are frequently associated with head injuries. Although the real incidence is unknown, in the largest series of cervical injuries in the literature, the traumatic spondylolisthesis of the axis comprised around 4% of all cervical fractures. The real incidence of neurologic involvement is also unknown because significant injury at this level is usually fatal. The incidence of spinal cord or nerve root injury in the surviving patients has been reported in 6% to 57% of the cases.

CLASSIFICATION

The most commonly used classification is the Effendi classification modified by Levine and Edwards. This scheme is based on the morphology and the presumed mechanism of injury and the measured amount of angulation and translation between C2 and C3. The majority of these injuries are caused by flexion–axial loading–extension forces. The order of these forces together with force coupling caused by the different motion planes of the two articulations of the axis are believed to explain the variations in different patterns. One special and uncommon type, though, may be predominantly caused by distractive forces.

TYPE 1

The type 1 fracture is through the isthmus just posterior to the body, and the fracture line is predominantly vertical (Fig. 24D.2). On the initial radiograph there is no angulation and less than 3 mm of translation. These injuries are believed to be caused by hyperextension and axial loading. There is no injury to the disc or ligaments.

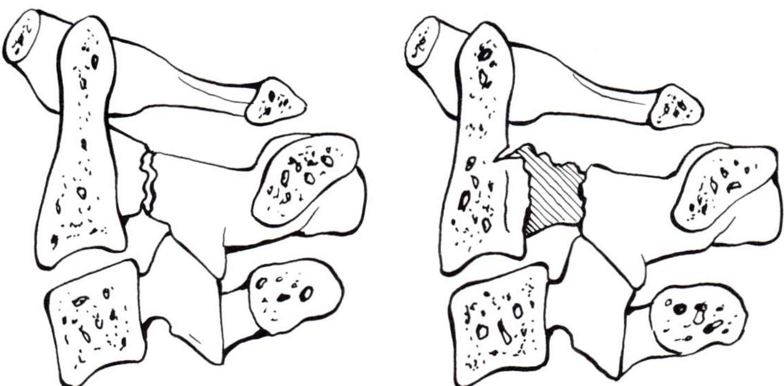

FIGURE 24D.2. Type 1 and type 1A fractures.

Type 1A

Type 1A fracture is also termed the atypical hangman fracture. The fracture lines of the left and right isthmus are not parallel, and therefore, they may not be easily visible on radiographs. They are thought to be caused by forces of hyperextension combined with lateral bending. On computed tomography (CT), one of the fracture lines can be seen running obliquely into the vertebral body, often through the foramen of the vertebral artery.

TYPE 2

Type 2 injuries show significant angulation and more than 3 mm of translation (Fig. 24D.3). The fracture lines are similar to those in type 1 and are predominantly vertical. It is generally believed that this type is caused by a combination of hyperextension and axial loading leading to a type 1 injury followed by a flexion force. This flexion force in the presence of type 1 fracture causes the disruption of the disc where the anterior longitudinal ligament is stripped off together with a crushed anterosuperior corner of the C3 endplate.

Type 2A

This is an uncommon but potentially confusing injury type. There is little or no translation but a significant angulation. The direction of the fracture line is oblique, running from anteroinferior to

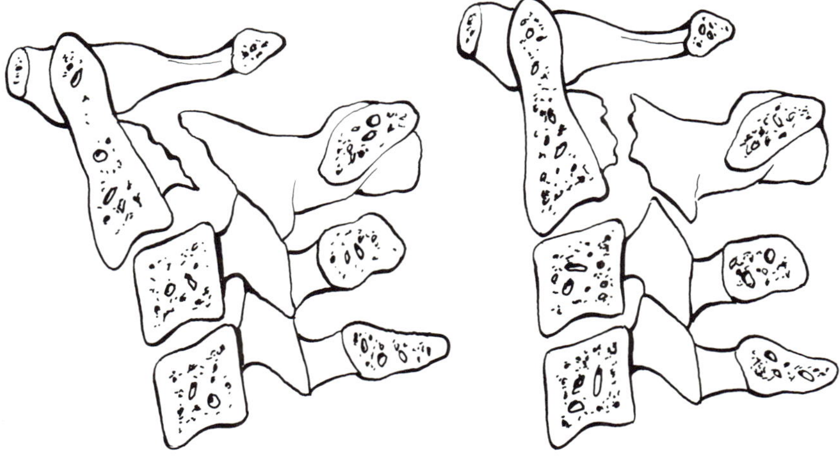

FIGURE 24D.3. Type 2 and type 2A fractures.

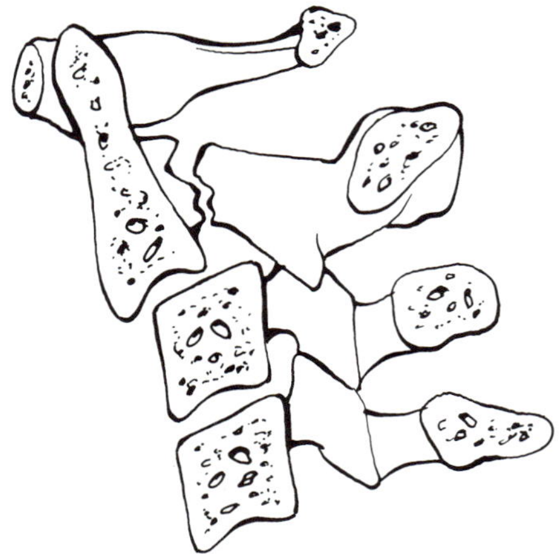

FIGURE 24D.4. Type 3 fracture.

posterosuperior. This injury is a result of flexion-distraction forces. The isthmus fails in tension as a result of hyperflexion forces causing a rupture of the disc from posterior to anterior. There is no crushing of the C3 endplate and the anterior longitudinal ligament is intact.

TYPE 3

Type 3 fractures may occur in a several configurations. The most common form is a type 1 fracture in combination with bilateral dislocation of C2-C3 facet joints (Fig. 24D.4). Another potential pattern is a unilateral facet dislocation and contralateral isthmus fracture. The mechanism is unclear. It has been suggested that these result from a flexion injury causing the facet dislocation followed by a hyperextension force causing the fracture. The neural arch in this type of injury has become a free-floating fragment with disruption of the Posterior Ligamentory Complex (PLC) between C2-C3, as well as the bony connection to the body of the axis.

Other injuries to the C2-C3 segments are also possible without a fracture of the axis isthmus but with a similar traumatic spondylolisthesis such as bilateral C2 laminar fractures or bilateral C2 facet fractures.

DIAGNOSIS

Although the majority of these injuries are easily discernable on standard trauma radiographs, some types such as type 1A can be missed (Fig. 24D.5).

All patients with significant head injury should be examined with a high degree of suspicion. CT scans with sagittal reformatting provide an excellent imaging of these injuries. Some type 2 injuries, however, can be spontaneously reduced and can be seen as type 1 injuries, especially if there is no or insignificant C3 endplate fracture. Although for this type of injury flexion-extension radiographs have been suggested, this should be definitely postponed in the presence of distracting injury or subdued consciousness. If there is any doubt about the type of injury or if there is a neurologic deficit, magnetic resonance imaging (MRI) should be obtained. Small reports in the literature show that ligamentary injuries associated with hangman fractures can be visualized on MRI.

TREATMENT

The majority of the patients can be treated with cervical immobilization with good results. Type 1 and 1A fractures can be successfully treated with a semirigid collar for 12 weeks and usually reach bony union without significant deformity. Left untreated, type 2 injuries could potentially result in substantial deformity (Fig. 24D.6).

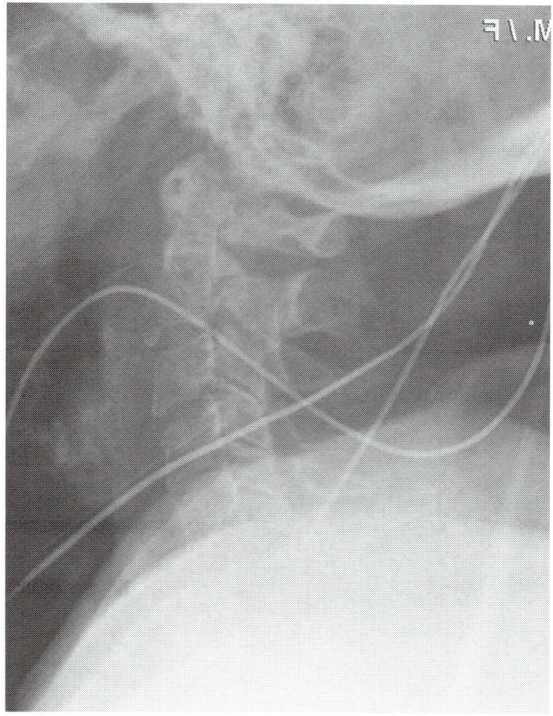

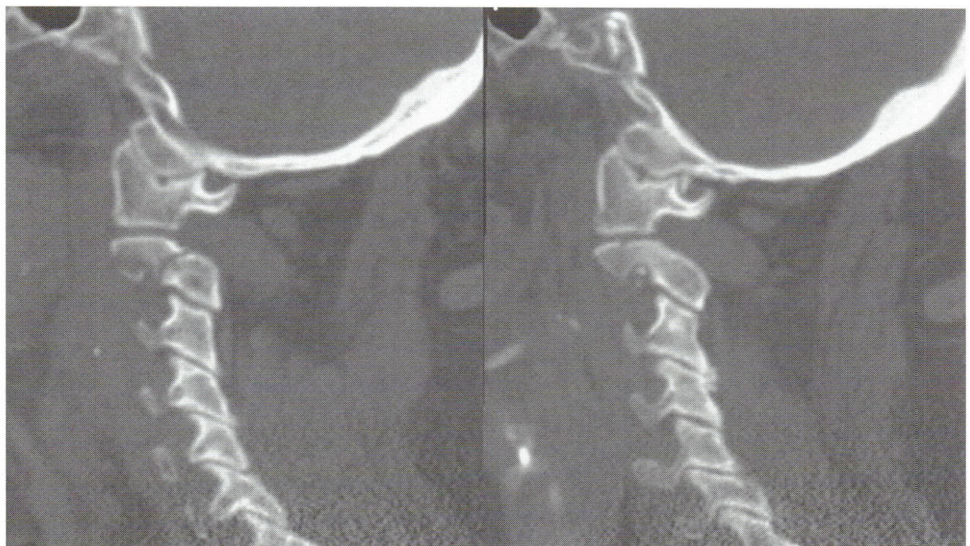

FIGURE 24D.5. Type 1A fractures can be easily missed on radiographs. Note the asymmetric fracture lines on computed tomography.

If the fracture heals in considerable angulation, this may cause compensatory hyperextension in the lower cervical spine with consequent degenerative disease. The best treatment for type 2 injuries is halo traction in extension to achieve reduction followed by halo-vest immobilization for 12 weeks. Traction for an average of 2 to 5 days is usually sufficient for a good reduction. Radiographs after the initial traction should be obtained to make sure that there is no distraction as a result of an unsuspected ligamentary injury. If the injury is type 2A, traction should be avoided because it may

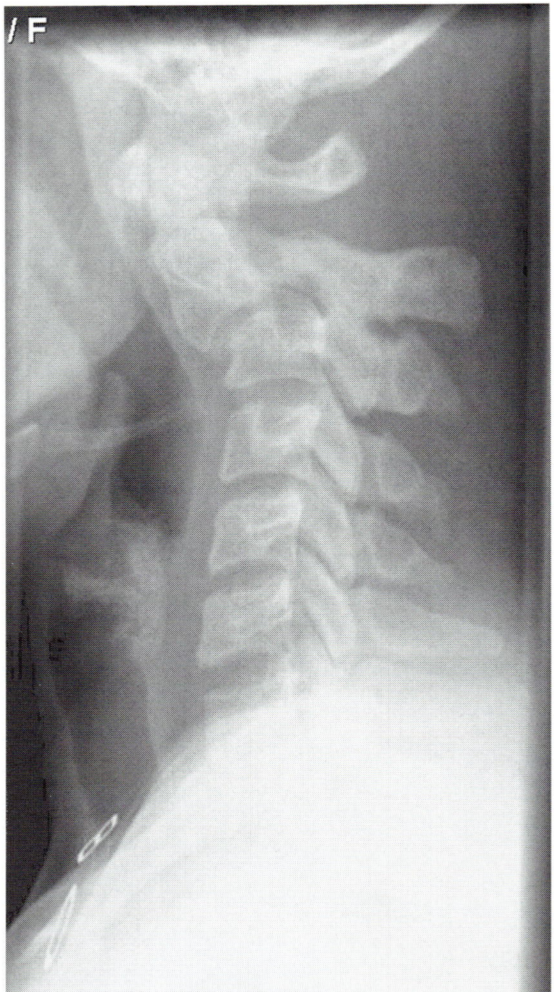

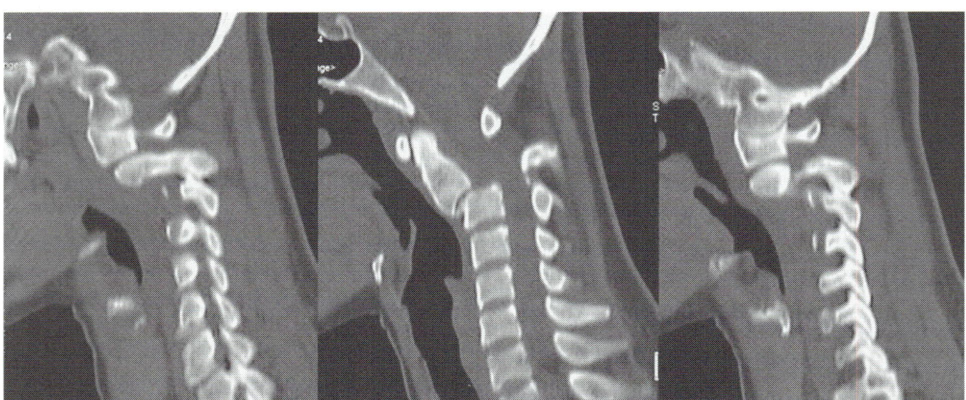

FIGURE 24D.6. This untreated type 2 fracture led to a serious kyphosis. Note the elongated isthmus and the spontaneous anterior C2-C3 fusion.

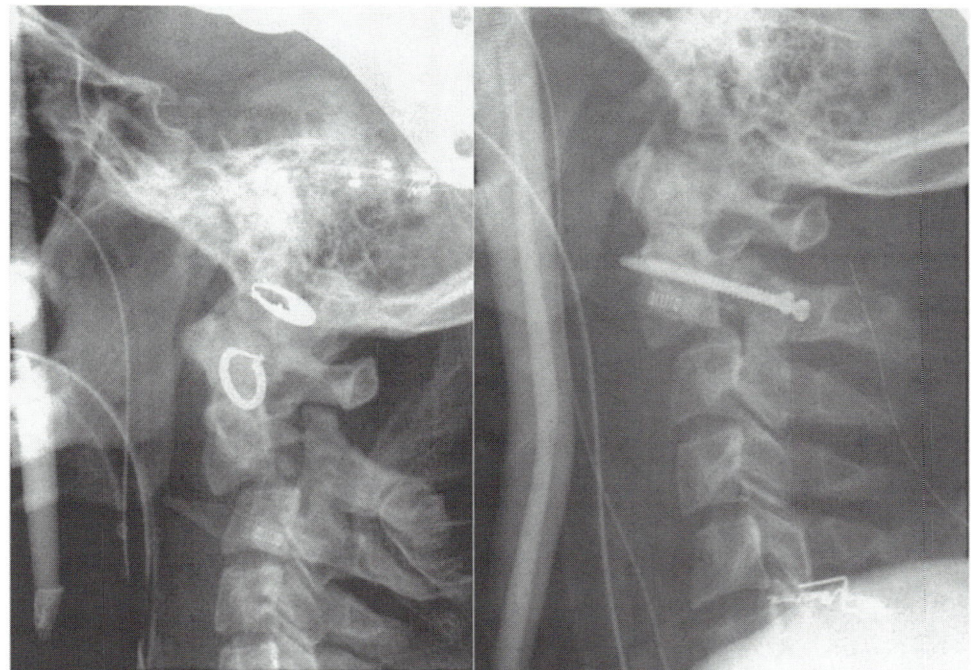

FIGURE 24D.7. Open reduction with internal fixation with lag screw technique for type 2 fracture with a high degree of kyphosis.

cause increasing angulation. Angulation of more than 12 degrees has been associated with loss of reduction, and extended traction is necessary to maintain alignment or surgery may be considered. Type 2 injuries can be treated surgically either by an anterior C2-C3 fusion or posterior screw fixation. Anterior fusion at this level is associated with a high incidence of approach-related complications. Posterior open reduction and screw fixation is an effective method of kyphosis correction in injuries with high-degree angulation (Fig. 24D.7).

This is technically demanding and should be performed by only experienced surgeons because of the danger of vertebral artery injury. The entry point for the screw is a couple of millimeters proximal to the usual entry point for transarticular C1-C2 screw, and the drill direction is more horizontal. The patient can be treated postoperatively with a semirigid collar for 6 weeks. There is no consensus in the literature on the indication for surgery for type 2 injuries. Type 3 injuries are usually not amenable to closed reduction and should be treated by open reduction and posterior C1-C3 fusion or pedicle screw fixation of C2, as described, connected with a rod to lateral mass screws at C3 along with fusion. In this way, fusion of C1-C2 with significant loss of rotation can be avoided. MRI is recommended before surgery to exclude a traumatic Hernia Nucleus Pulposi (HNP).

SUGGESTED READINGS

Levine AM. Traumatic spondylolisthesis of the axis: "Hangman's fracture." In: The Cervical Spine Research Society Editorial Committee, ed. *The Cervical Spine.* 3rd ed. Philadelphia: Lippincott-Raven, 1998;429–448.

Guidelines for management of acute cervical spine injuries. *Neurosurgery* 2002;50(suppl 3):S7–S17.

Vaccaro AR, Madigan L, Bauerle WB, et al. Early halo immobilization of displaced traumatic spondylolisthesis of the axis. *Spine* 2002;27:2229–2233.

CHAPTER 25A

Subaxial Injuries: Flexion-Compression Injuries

John C. France

INTRODUCTION

Flexion compression injuries are the result of an axial load to the top of the head that then results in a flexion moment; thus, there is a combination of compression across the anterior elements of the spine and distraction through the posterior structures. This is the classic injury that results from diving head first into shallow water but can be seen in falls from height and motor vehicle accidents when the occupant's head strikes the windshield. It is important to recognize this fracture pattern since it is often highly unstable and the risk of immediate as well as late neurological deficit is substantial. In this chapter, we hope to clarify the mechanism and fracture pattern, define the factors that influence treatment, and offer a rational for treatment.

MECHANISM OF INJURY

Flexion-compression injuries in the cervical spine are commonly called teardrop fractures or quadrangular fractures. This nomenclature has often been a source of confusion because the term teardrop is used in reference to two distinctly different fractures, with different mechanisms of injury (Fig. 25A.1). The first is usually a benign injury that can be managed with a rigid collar and seldom has long-term consequences. It has an extension mechanism and is radiographically identified by a small fleck of bone from the anterior-inferior aspect of a vertebral body. Anatomically, the bony fragment is an avulsion of the anular attachment. In the other the piece of bone is pulled from the corner of the vertebral body by the anulus. The second injury is much more ominous and thus requires more aggressive treatment. It has the flexion-compression mechanism that is the focus of this chapter. Radiographically, it similarly has a bony fragment separated from the anterior-inferior corner of the vertebral body but differs in that the bony fragment is a larger chunk of bone. This piece of bone is essentially pushed off the vertebral body as the upper part of the spine is flexed and axially loaded into the lower vertebrae (Fig. 25A.2). Other radiographic characteristics that can be identified include kyphosis, retrolisthesis of the upper vertebrae, and often lack of facet congruity.[1] In addition, the axial images on computed tomography (CT) demonstrate the coronal fracture line associated with the anterior fracture fragment and a characteristic sagittal split[2,3] (Fig. 25A.3).

The name of the fracture (flexion-compression) is based on the mechanism of injury. This type of fracture is often the pattern seen on diving injuries,[4] but is also seen with football spear tackling injuries,[5] falls from height, auto collisions, or other high-speed events in which the patient is catapulted into a stationary object head first. For this specific pattern of injury to occur, there must be an axially oriented load compressing the cephalad vertebrae into the caudal vertebrae, with the neck

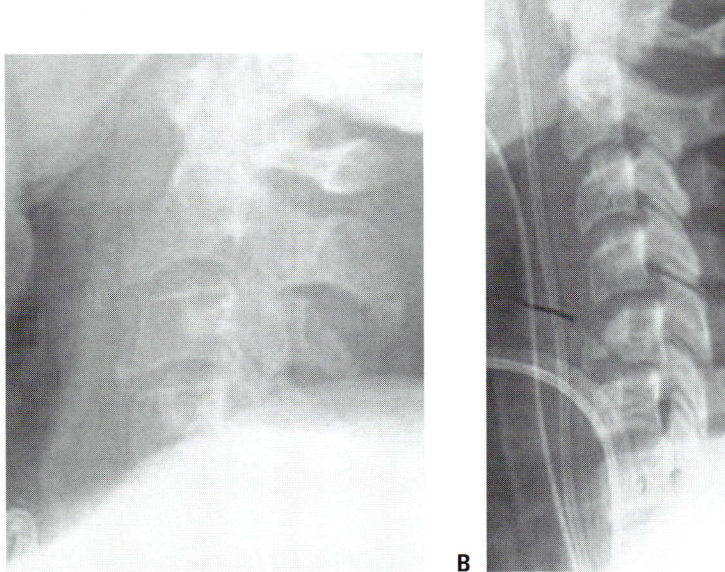

FIGURE 25A.1. An extension-type "teardrop" fracture **(A)** is generally considered a benign injury compared to the flexion-compression "teardrop" fracture **(B)**. Note that the bony fragment off the anterior-inferior margin of the vertebral body is a small chip in **A** versus the larger chunk of bone in **B**.

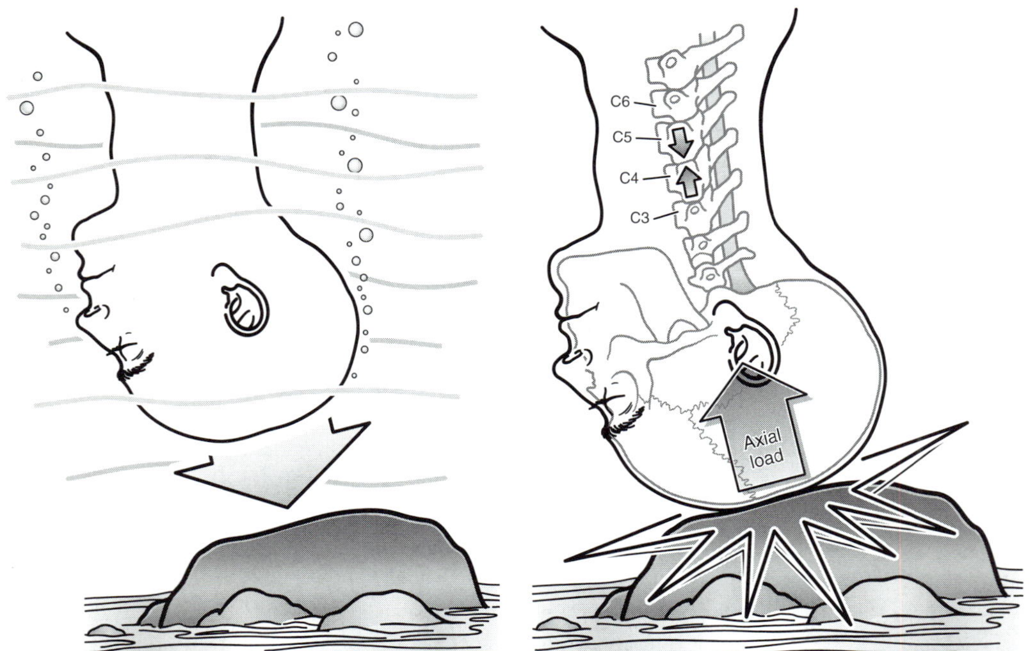

FIGURE 25A.2. The sequence of drawings **A** through **C** represent the mechanism of injury for a typical flexion-compression injury that creates the classic fracture pattern illustrated in **C**. (*continued*)

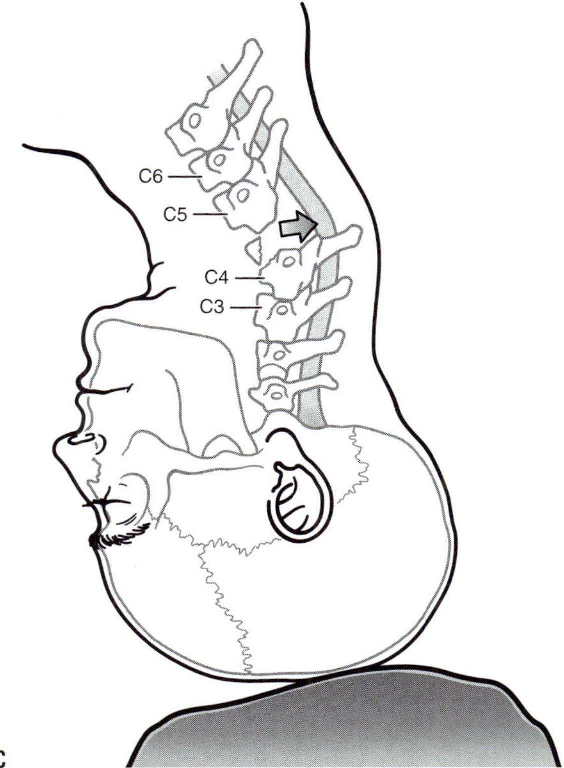

FIGURE 25A.2. *(Continued)*

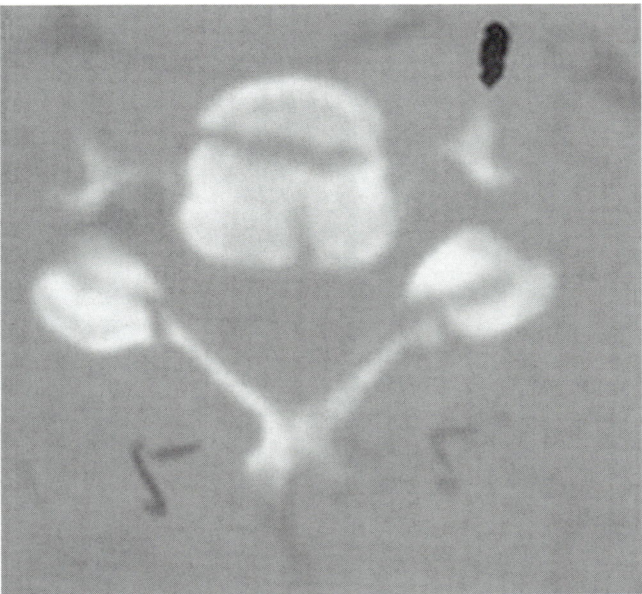

FIGURE 25A.3. The classic axial computed tomography image with a coronal fracture plain from the avulsed fragment anteriorly and the sagittal split within the posterior half of the vertebral body.

simultaneously being forced into flexion. It is the axial load that breaks off the anterior bony fragment, and as the neck is forced into flexion, the posterior inferior corner of the cephalad vertebrae is forced backward into the spinal canal and the facets suffer a hyperflexion injury. The greater the amount of energy imparted on the spine, the more posterior disruption is noted, which plays an important role in treatment decisions that will be discussed later.

Because these injuries are often the result of high-energy trauma and the posterior-inferior corner of the cephalad vertebrae is forced into the spinal canal, there is a high incidence of associated spinal cord injury. Thus, it is a pattern of injury that must be understood and identified to minimize new or additional neurologic injury.

CLASSIFICATION

The first question to be answered in classifying this fracture is the neurologic status. Is the patient neurologically intact or is there a concomitant neurologic injury? If a spinal cord injury exists, is it complete or incomplete? Typically, those patients with a spinal cord injury can immediately be assumed to have an unstable fracture pattern that will ultimately warrant surgical stabilization.

The second question is the status of the posterior elements. As the magnitude of force increases for this injury, the neck is forced into more flexion and then posterior disruption tends to increase. In the neurologically intact patient, it is generally the extent of posterior disruption that dictates whether or not surgical stabilization is necessary. In addition, in those patients deemed appropriate for surgical stabilization, the degree of posterior disruption plays a key role determining the approach to stabilization. The question that needs to be addressed is whether stability can be achieved with an anterior or posterior approach alone or a combined anterior-posterior approach is necessary.

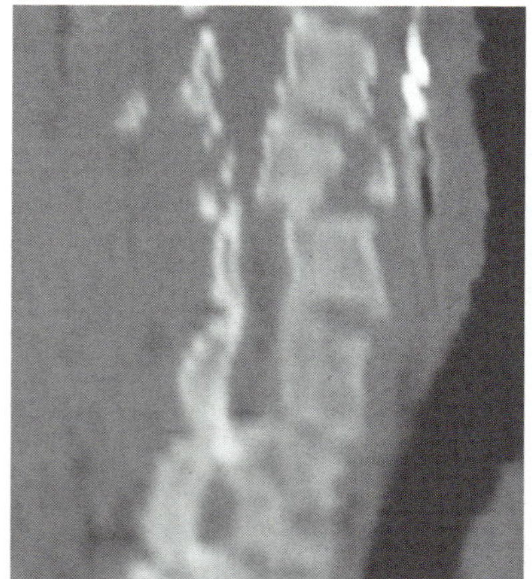

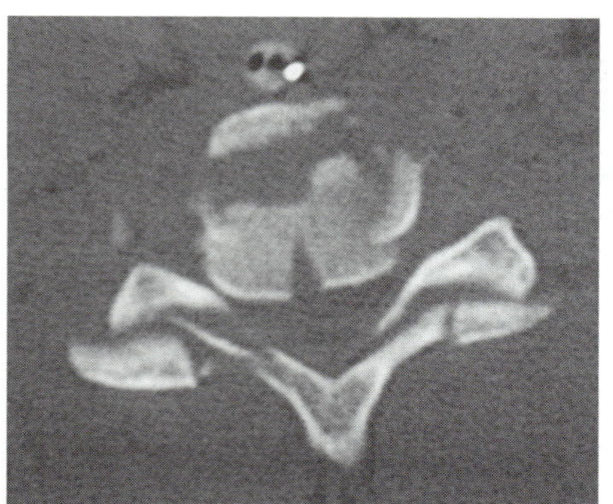

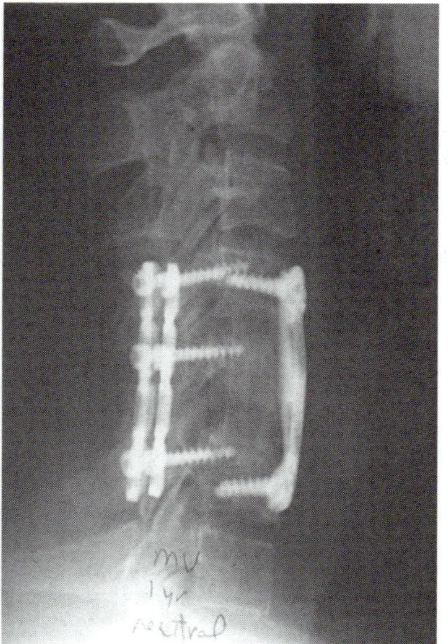

FIGURE 25A.4. A severe compression-flexion injury (CFS5) with posterior destruction that would likely require anterior and posterior stabilization. A sagittal **(A)** and axial **(B)** computed tomography scan showing the posterior destruction and a lateral radiograph of the fixation **(C)**.

The mechanistic classification of Allen and Ferguson[6] subdivides flexion-compression injuries into five stages to clarify the progression of injury severity. This grading system is based on radiographic characteristics that imply mechanism. Compression flexion stage 1 (CFS1) is manifested by simple blunting of the anterosuperior aspect of the vertebral body. Compression flexion stage 2 (CFS2) involves some loss of height of the anterior vertebral body, with injury extending into the inferior endplate, but lacks a clear fracture line through the body. Compression flexion stage 3 (CFS3) includes the more classic oblique fracture from the anterior wall of the vertebral body into the inferior endplate, which has long been considered the hallmark of the teardrop fracture. Compression flexion stage 4 (CFS4) begins to involve greater destruction of the posterior tension band structures allowing mild (<3 mm) displacement of the inferior-posterior corner of the vertebral body into the neural canal. Lastly, compression flexion stage 5 (CFS5) includes greater destruction of the posterior elements with further compromise of the neural canal (Fig. 25A.4). No study exists that attempts to use this severity subclassification as a guide to treatment, but as treatment options are discussed, one can envision the need to impart greater stability to the spine as the severity increases from CFS1 to CFS5.

TREATMENT

INITIAL TREATMENT

The first step in treatment of this injury is early identification and recognition of it as a dangerous fracture pattern with great potential for neurologic disaster. Quite often the overall alignment of the spine on the initial lateral radiograph is close to anatomic because the patient is supine, allowing the neck to extend, and there is no longer an axial load, thus reversing the mechanism of injury, which in turn reduces the fracture. The subtle retrolisthesis and the size of the bony fragment are the keys to identification pending further imaging. Once the injury is identified, rigid immobilization and strict cervical precautions should be maintained to protect the underlying neurologic elements. There is frequently an associated spinal cord injury that should be recognized, and appropriate pharmacologic and other measures should be taken to minimize further cord damage, as outlined in earlier chapters. Usually these fractures are reasonably aligned with patient in the supine position, and this maintains a patent spinal canal. If a significant retrolisthesis persists in that position, cervical traction via Gardner-Wells tongs can be applied to improve the reduction. This should be done with caution and radiographic vigilance to avoid overdistraction at the level of injury because of the posterior ligamentous injury. The majority of these fractures will ultimately be treated operatively. The type of temporary stabilization used until that procedure may vary depending on the degree of instability for the individual fracture and the duration of time until that planned procedure. For example, if a patient is going to be taken directly to the operating room, the initial stabilization can be a rigid collar and sandbags. If a longer delay is expected, either halo immobilization or cervical traction should be considered. The degree of immobilization is usually dictated by the degree of posterior element disruption. In the event that the definitive treatment is going to be nonoperative, one should proceed without delay in applying the appropriate form of external immobilization.

An important part of initial treatment is the radiographic imaging. CT is indicated in all of these fractures to aid in fracture identification and in characterization of the bony injury. In addition to the typical coronal and sagittal fracture lines discussed earlier, one can assess the degree of posterior fracture in the facets, lateral masses, and spinous processes, which offers clues to the degree of instability. Ligamentous injury can be implied by gapping or incongruity of the facet joints. Coronal and sagittal reconstructions should be included as part of routine CT imaging. The role of magnetic resonance imaging (MRI) is less clearly defined. The soft tissues such as ligaments, discs, and spinal cord are much better visualized and can offer guidance in determining instability, any ongoing source of cord compression, and neurologic prognosis. Assessment of the posterior ligamentous complex is well

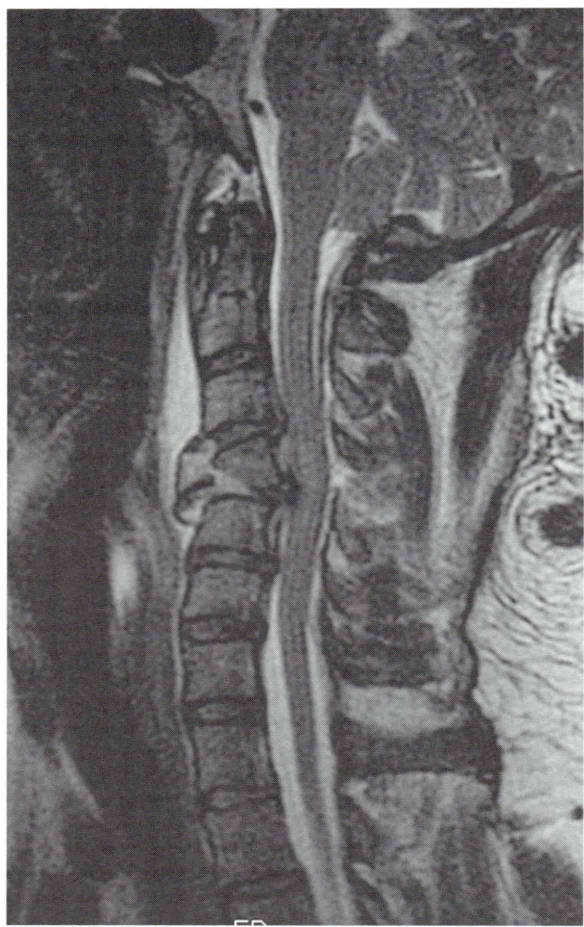

FIGURE 25A.5. A sagittal T2-weighted magnetic resonance imaging image of a flexion-compression injury showing disruption of the posterior ligamentous complex.

visualized on MRI, and this information may aid in deciding on the extent of stabilization that will be required (Fig. 25A.5). However, many of the changes seen on MRI are difficult to specifically associate with pathoanatomy and the extent of associated instability. It could also have implications in direction of surgical approach (anterior or posterior) if a unidirectional procedure is planned.

DEFINITIVE TREATMENT

The majority of flexion-compression fractures are considered unstable and benefit from surgical stabilization. Essentially, all patients with a spinal cord injury are managed surgically, leaving only the neurologically intact patients to be considered for nonoperative treatment. It is wise to start with the premise that surgical stabilization is usually indicated, even in neurologically intact patients, and work cautiously backward from there when considering someone for nonoperative management. Few modern studies exist that directly compare surgical stabilization to nonoperative treatment. Fisher et al.[7] included patients with and without neurologic deficit. Nonoperative treatment was halo vest immobilization, and operative treatment was anterior cervical strut fusion with plating. In that study the surgical group had better restoration and maintenance of sagittal alignment, but they were unable to demonstrate any significant clinical differences. The influence on neurologic outcome was not analyzed. Koivikko et al.[8] also compared nonoperative and operative treatment but included burst fractures with the flexion-compression teardrop fractures. They also demonstrated better restoration and maintenance of alignment with surgical treatment, as well as improved neurologic recovery on Frankel grading.

In the neurologically intact patient, it is the posterior injury that determines stability. In that group of patients, nonoperative treatment can be considered if the posterior elements remain intact from a bony and ligamentous standpoint, and an anatomic sagittal alignment is maintained, such as Allen-Ferguson CFS1 and CFS2. The CT scan may offer enough information if there is clear posterior injury. If the CT lacks sufficient evidence to make this determination, MRI should be used for further assessment. If, based on these studies, the fracture is deemed to have adequate stability, nonoperative treatment consists of external immobilization with a Minerva brace or halo vest depending on the stability, associated injuries, patient desires, and anticipated compliance. Immobilization should create an extension moment and should be maintained for 12 weeks. At that time, flexion-extension lateral radiographs are used to ensure stability. The patient should be counseled on neurologic symptoms and to avoid any activities that would risk further injury, then reassessed with lateral flexion-extension radiographs approximately 1 month later.

In patients who remain neurologically intact, the degree of skeletal instability determines the need for surgical stabilization. Unfortunately, stability is not an all or none determination but is instead a continuum. The Allen-Ferguson classification attempts to subclassify flexion-compression injuries, as noted earlier. The key factor in determining the degree of instability for this fracture pattern tends to be the posterior elements. The greater the ligamentous injury and facet damage, the greater is the degree of instability. If the facets remain congruent and no posterior element fracture exists, nonoperative treatment can be considered, as outlined above. If the posterior elements are disrupted through the bone or ligaments, then operative treatment is warranted. These are more likely CFS3 and perhaps some CFS4 subtypes. With neurologically intact patients, surgical stabilization can usually be done unidirectionally (anterior or posterior). It is uncommon in flexion-compression injuries without a neurologic deficit to have instability sufficiently severe to require a combined anterior-posterior approach. Unidirectional anterior or posterior fixation have both been described. Because the mechanism of injury is in part an axial load and the fracture occurs through the vertebral body, the spinal column loses the ability to resist further axial load. Therefore, it makes biomechanical sense to bolster the anterior column of the spine with a strut graft reestablishing axial support.[9] This is accomplished through an anterior approach and is the author's preferred approach (Fig. 25A.6).[10,11]

If a patient has a neurologic deficit, operative treatment is recommended to decrease any persistent cord compression, protect the cord from recurrent damage, and achieve biomechanical stability. Because a neurologic deficit exists, the primary goal of surgery is decompression. Because cord compression is located anteriorly, the primary direction of decompression is via an anterior approach. If, after decompression, adequate stability can be achieved through the same anterior approach, the entire surgical procedure is done anteriorly alone, like in the CFS3 or CFS4 subtype. As discussed previously, it is the amount of injury to the posterior elements that dictates whether or not additional posterior stabilization is warranted, such as in the CFS5 subtype (Fig. 25A.7). There is no hard and fast rule to determine whether an additional posterior procedure is necessary, leaving this decision as a judgment call. One goal of the procedure should be to avoid the need for postoperative external immobilization in anything more than a rigid collar. Thus, the surgeon must be satisfied that the degree of stability achieved during the procedure will be adequate to limit the need for aggressive external immobilization (more than a rigid collar).

There are some key points that can be used to aid in the decision regarding the need for an additional posterior procedure. If the facets are intact or have only minor fractures and can be locked or overlapped enough to protect against shear forces, an anterior procedure alone may be enough. The assessment of facet integrity can be done preoperatively on the CT scan. Both the superior facet of the caudal vertebra and the inferior facet of the cephalad vertebra must be scrutinized for fracture to determine if enough of the bony anatomy remains to recreate a bony buttress against shear forces. In addition, one has to be careful to avoid over distraction intraoperatively that would also limit the ability of the superior facet to buttress the inferior facet. Reestablishing lordosis is also critical because any residual kyphosis also diminishes the bony contact between facets. (Fig. 25A.8).

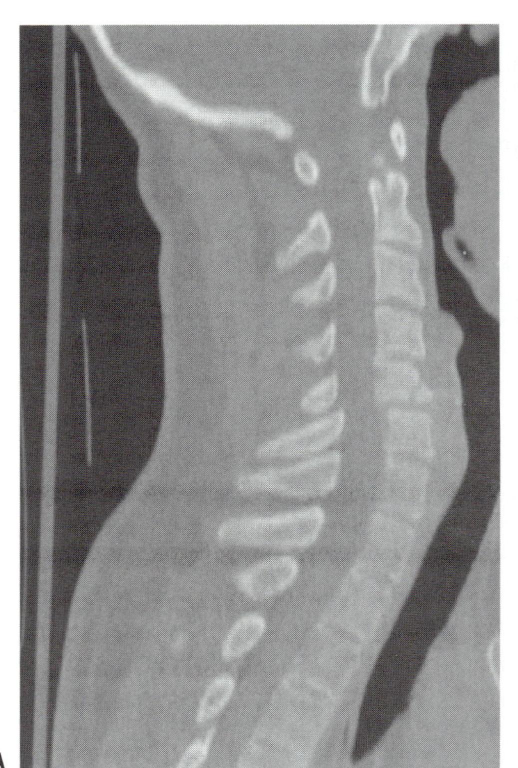

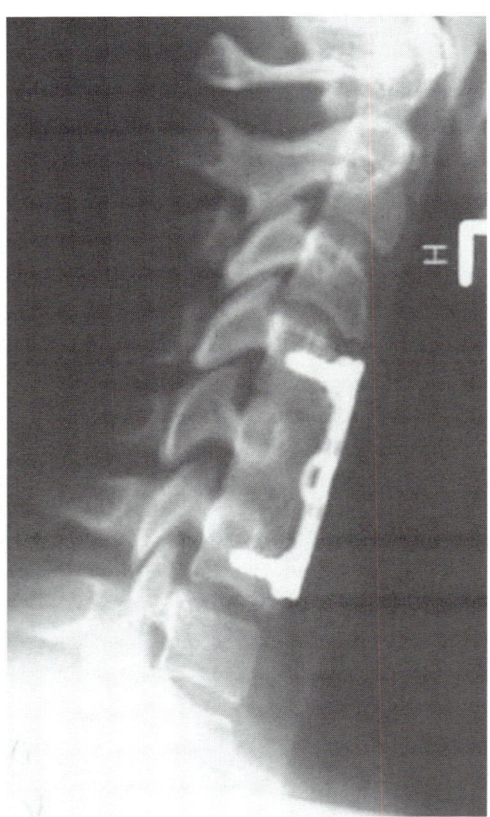

FIGURE 25A.6. A sagittal computed tomography reconstruction of a flexion-compression injury with minimal posterior disruption **(A)** and typical anterior reconstruction after corpectomy on late follow-up **(B)**.

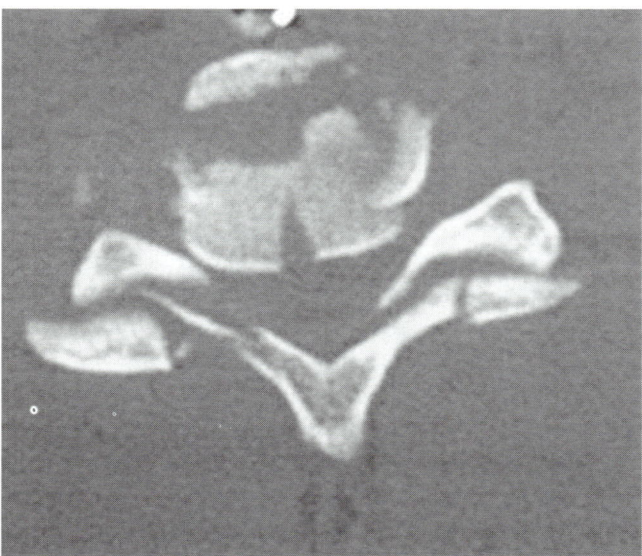

FIGURE 25A.7. Axial computed tomography demonstrating significant posterior destruction that would likely warrant anteroposterior fixation.

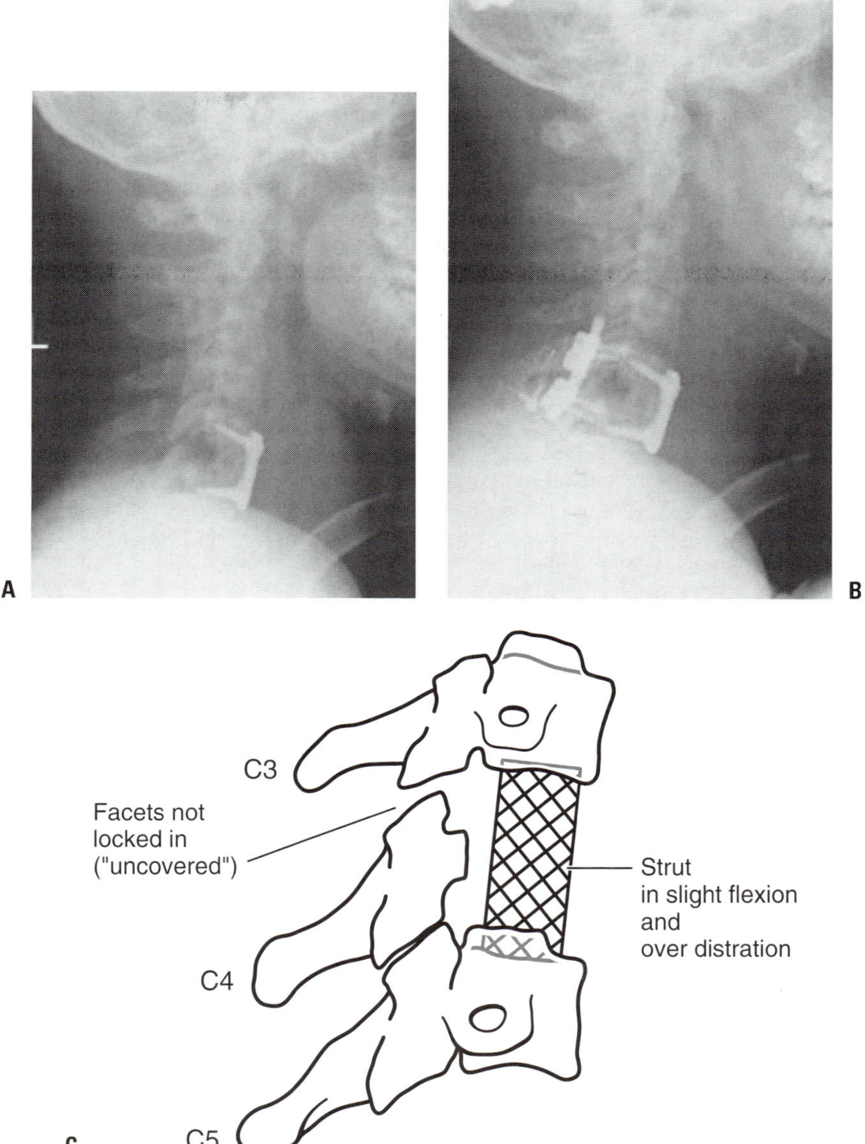

FIGURE 25A.8. **A.** Over-distraction was used anteriorly, and the facets do not have adequate overlap or contact to prevent loss of fixation. There will be a tendency for this construct to fail as the cephalad vertebrae translates forward on the caudal one. If recognized, an additional posterior stabilization is required **(B)**. This is illustrated diagrammatically in **(C)**.

At the present time there are several options for anterior struts, including autologous iliac crest or fibula, allograft iliac crest or fibula, and a variety of metallic cages. These would then be supported with anterior plate fixation. If an additional posterior procedure is deemed necessary, lateral mass fixation is the treatment of choice, using autologous iliac crest graft for fusion. The iliac crest graft could be obtained anteriorly if one has chosen an autologous anterior iliac strut or obtained posteriorly if allograft was used for the anterior part of the procedure. Bone graft substitutes are currently playing a larger role and may one day replace iliac crest for posterior cervical fusion. It would be a rare circumstance in which a laminectomy would be necessary as part of the posterior procedure. Such a circumstance might be the presence of an associated lamina fracture indenting the posterior cord.

PROGNOSIS

The prognosis of these fractures is largely dictated by the neurologic deficit. Unfortunately there is a relatively high incidence of complete spinal cord injury with these fractures. If no neurologic deficit exists, the long-term prognosis is based on the skeletal injury. In those patients lucky enough to require only external immobilization as the definitive means of treatment, the prognosis is based on the damage to the adjacent discs, direct injury to the articular surface of the facets, indirect injury to the facets via persistent incongruity from residual malalignment, and residual kyphosis. At the time of this writing there is a paucity of long-term results that clearly define residual pain and dysfunction issues.

COMPLICATIONS

Complications unique to the treatment of cervical flexion-compression injuries are generally related to the instability of this fracture pattern and would be manifested by loss of alignment. If nonoperative treatment is chosen, serial radiographic follow-up is used to assess for loss of alignment that would need to be salvaged with surgical intervention. Radiographs should be obtained in the hospital after the patient has been mobilized, then weekly for the first 2 weeks to rule out displacement. If alignment is maintained for the first 2 weeks, subsequent films can be obtained at 6 and 12 weeks, at which time the collar can be removed.

In those patients initially managed by surgical stabilization, a postoperative film is used to verify that satisfactory alignment has been achieved. Also, the postoperative films should be carefully assessed for clues that might predict subsequent loss of fixation. This includes overdistraction of facets, residual kyphosis, and poor screw placement. If these radiographic features are identified in a patient who had an isolated anterior approach, consideration should be given for supplementing this with posterior instrumentation before loss of fixation occurs. In those patients with satisfactory postoperative alignment, the next films are obtained at 2, 6, and 12 weeks.

When surgical stabilization is needed, at least a two-level fusion is required. Although the loss of clinical range of motion is usually minimal, some patients suffer persistent cervical stiffness. This may be related to soft tissue injury in the surrounding musculature or perhaps psychosocial issues such as fear of reinjury. In addition, the possibility of adjacent segment degeneration exists, as it would in any two-level fusion.

The remainder of possible complications are related to the neurologic injury or are similar to those in any patient undergoing cervical surgery and are beyond the scope of this chapter.

REFERENCES

1. Kim KS, Chen HH, Russell EJ, et al. Flexion teardrop fracture of the cervical spine: radiographic characteristics. *AJR Am J Roentgenol* 1989;152:319–326.
2. Favero KJ, Van Peteghem PK. The quadrangular fragment fracture: roentgenographic features and treatment protocol. *Clin Orthop Relat Res* 1989;239:40–46.
3. Lee C, Kim KS, Rogers LF. Sagittal fracture of the cervical vertebral body. *AJR Am J Roentgenol* 1982;139:55–60.
4. Aito S, D'Andrea M, Werhagen L. Spinal cord injuries due to diving accidents. *Spinal Cord* 2005;43:109–116.
5. Torg JS, Pavlov H, O'Neill MJ, et al. The axial load teardrop fracture: a biomechanical, clinical and roentgenographic analysis. *Am J Sports Med* 1991;19:355–364.
6. Allen BL Jr, Ferguson RL, Lehmann TR, et al. A mechanistic classification of closed, indirect fractures and dislocations of the lower cervical spine. *Spine* 1982;7:1–27.
7. Fisher CG. Dvorak MF, Leith J, et al. Comparison of outcomes for unstable lower cervical flexion teardrop fractures managed with halo thoracic vest versus anterior corpectomy and plating. *Spine* 2002;27:160–166.
8. Koivikko MP, Myllynen P, Karjalainen M, et al. Conservative and operative treatment in cervical burst fractures. *Arch Orthop Trauma Surg* 2000;120:448–451.
9. Traynelis VC, Donaher PA, Roach RM, et al. Biomechanical comparison of anterior Caspar plate and three-level posterior fixation techniques in a human cadaveric model. *J Neurosurg* 1993;79:96–103.
10. Cabanela ME, Ebersold MJ. Anterior plate stabilization for bursting teardrop fractures of the cervical spine. *Spine* 1988;13:888–891.
11. de Oliveira JC. Anterior plate fixation of traumatic lesions of the lower cervical spine. *Spine* 1987;12:324–329.

CHAPTER 25B

Subaxial Injuries: Vertical Compression Injuries

Brian Walsh and Vincent Traynelis

INTRODUCTION

There have been many attempts at classification schemes for spinal fractures, but few have been universally accepted.[1–6] In the classification scheme proposed by Allen et al.[1] subaxial cervical spinal injuries are considered separately from those of the upper cervical spine. A single vector force acting on the spine can cause predictable patterns of injury that are dependent on the magnitude and initial direction of the force and the position of the spine at initial impact. Allen et al.[1] made the following hypotheses as they constructed this injury classification scheme:

1. Forces producing injury are considered as major or minor injury vectors.
2. Injury vectors can be deduced from radiographs.
3. The magnitude of vectors determines injury severity.
4. Similar injury vectors yield similar injuries.
5. A spectrum of injury exists within each mechanism of injury from mild to severe.

The terms compression and distraction refer to the predominant direction of force in the Y-axis causing the most obvious damage to the motion segment. Tension or shear is the stress causing ligament failure in distraction, because ligaments do not fail in compression.[7] Rotation is considered a local force, not a major injury vector in this scheme.

Vertical compression fractures in this scheme arise from an axial force acting on a straight cervical spine. Other classification systems often refer to these fractures as burst fractures. Severe neurologic injuries, including both incomplete and complete spinal injury, are associated with this family of fractures.

BIOMECHANICS

Vertical compression fractures in the lower cervical spine arise from an axially directed force acting on a straight spine with no flexion or extension present. A diving accident is a prototypical case for this group. The force applied to the head is transmitted via the occipital condyles to a straight cervical spine, with the vector traveling down the center of the vertebral body. Forces of sufficient magnitude will cause failure of the spinal elements, resulting in a Jefferson fracture in the upper cervical spine or a burst fracture in the subaxial cervical spine.

Maiman et al.[8] have shown that immediate preinjury neck alignment strongly influences the resultant cervical spine injury. A straightened cervical spine dissipates forces less efficiently, resulting in injury at lower force levels than occur in a curved spine.[9] Another factor affecting injury is differential stiffness along the spine, with the midcervical spine being stiffer than the lower cervical region.[10]

The individual components of the cervical spine have different failure characteristics. This partially explains how force applied from varying directions to the spine can result in distinct injury groupings depending on the components stressed to failure.

The vertebral bodies are composed of both a hard, brittle cortical shell and a spongy cancellous center. C6 is structurally the stiffest vertebral body in the subaxial spine. Studies show that the structural integrity of all of the cervical vertebrae begins to diminish after 40 years of age.[7] The stiff outer anulus of the intervertebral disc accounts for the majority of disc stiffness. In vitro studies have shown that axial loading alone will not result in disc disruption.[11] Axial compression produces stiffening of the intervertebral disc. If the force is great enough, the disc may be driven in a pistonlike fashion into the endplate, causing a vertebral body fracture. The main nonosseous determinants of cervical spinal stability are the anterior longitudinal ligament, the posterior longitudinal ligament, and the disc. Ligaments fail by ripping and tearing under shear forces, but they do not fail not under compression.

CLASSIFICATION OF VERTICAL COMPRESSION FRACTURES

A vertical compressive force can create cervical fractures. Depending on the magnitude of force, the possible injuries range from a minimal posterior body wall fracture to extensive vertebral body comminution and posterior element disruption. The most frequent posterior column injury associated with vertical compressive forces is a posterior arch fracture. The injury to the vertebral body may be so severe that there is spinal cord impingement. Vertical compression fractures have been classified into the following three types according to severity:

VC stage 1 (VCS1):
    One endplate fracture consisting of a cupping deformity

VC stage 2 (VCS2):
    Same vertebral body with both endplates fractured and showing cupping deformities

VC stage 3 (VCS3):
    Vertebral body fracture with comminution and fragmentation with displacement of the fracture pieces

In severe cases, posterior ligamentous disruption occurs. Some consider the teardrop fracture as described by Schneider and Kahn[12] to be a variant belonging in this subgroup. Allen et al.[1] feel that the fracture as described has elements of compression-flexion and vertical compression and most closely approximates injuries in a separate (CFS5) group. In general, ligamentous structures are usually intact in vertical compression injuries, and it is the bone fractures that are most significant in this subset.[13]

INITIAL EVALUATION

Spinal injuries can cause excitement and anxiety for all concerned. Strict adherence to trauma protocols with their systematic approach ensures the greatest chance for clinical success. Maintenance of an adequate airway, ventilation, and blood pressure is paramount. The cervical spine is immobilized while the clinical and radiologic assessments are performed. The imaging studies should include at a minimum anteroposterior, lateral, and open mouth odontoid cervical radiographs. Some advocate helical computed tomography (CT) scanning as the initial procedure of choice[14–16] (Fig. 25B.1). CT scanning is more sensitive than plain radiography because it has a 99% to 100% sensitivity in diagnosing cervical fractures.[14,17] CT scanning can be performed 50% faster as well.[16] Grogan et al.[18] showed that overall hospital costs are lessened by using CT over plain films. Given cost concerns and computer reformatting abilities, this will likely largely replace plain films in patients with severe trauma.

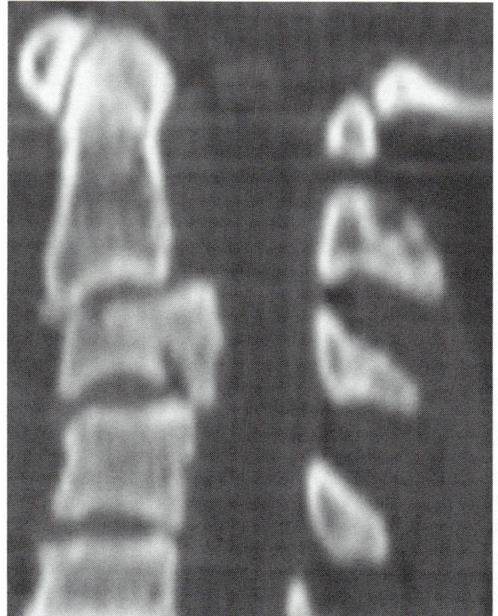
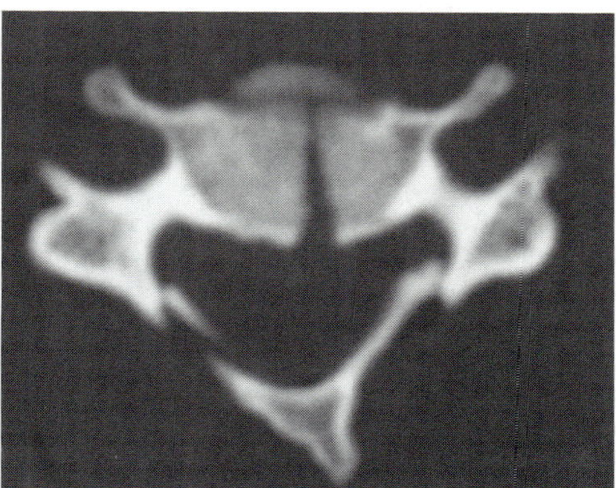

FIGURE 25B.1. **A.** Sagittal MRI scan of a C3 burst fracture. **B.** Axial computed tomography image of a C3 burst fracture.

Magnetic resonance imaging (MRI) scanning is indicated in select cases based on positive radiographic results or clinical suspicion of soft tissue, ligamentous, or spinal cord injury (Fig. 25B.2). Disk abnormalities and nerve root impingement are best seen on MRI, as well as frank spinal cord injury, showing edema and hematoma within the cord parenchyma. Acute ligamentous tears are best seen within the first few days after injury.[19,20]

TREATMENT

Early closed reduction of a fracture-dislocation with restoration of normal spinal alignment is an initial goal, after life-threatening problems are controlled. Fortunately, the incidence of neurologic deterioration after closed reduction is quite rare.[21] This is despite up to a 50% chance of a concurrent disc disruption seen on MRI.[22,23] Initial MRI scanning may be more meaningful in the 20% of patients who fail closed reduction, usually as a result of significant anatomic deformity. Cervical traction is well described, yet there remains controversy concerning specific initial and final weight application. Ongoing neurologic assessment should occur in parallel with weight application. Once reduction is achieved, it should be maintained up to the time of surgical correction or placement of an orthosis. Most patients with a vertical compressive injury have reasonable sagittal alignment. Traction may be helpful in providing stability and in moving bone fragments out of the spinal canal by means of ligamentotaxis.

Multiple opinions exist as to the optimal definitive management of vertical compression fractures and the teardrop variant. The ultimate goals of treatment are to attain normal cervical alignment, provide for ongoing dynamic stability, and ensure neurologic decompression. The means to achieve these ends, including the role of surgery, its timing, and operative approaches, all remain controversial.

NONOPERATIVE TREATMENT

Absent posterior element damage, placement of a halo or Minerva device may be sufficient. Ducker et al.[24] recommended 4 weeks of traction followed by 8 weeks in a halo orthosis. Chan et al.[25] and Cheshire[26] prefer 12 weeks of halo vest placement. In one patient series, 80% of these injuries

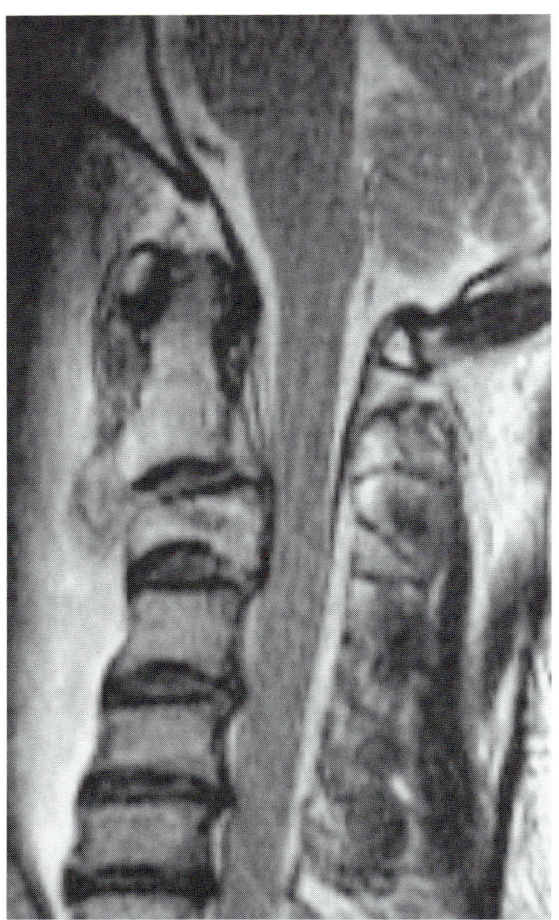

FIGURE 25B.2. Sagittal reconstruction of a computed tomography scan demonstrating a C3 burst fracture.

spontaneously healed.[27] There is approximately a 10% to 15% chance of delayed instability, usually a kyphosis, when nonoperative therapy is used.[28]

SURGICAL TREATMENT

Surgery has a role in the treatment of this injury subset. When the spinal cord is compromised from bone fragments in patients with incomplete spinal cord lesions, surgery should be strongly considered because several studies have shown neurologic improvement after decompression and stabilization.[24,29–34] An inability to achieve or maintain reduction, severe kyphotic angulation, and vertebral body injury involving more than 40% loss of height are other possible indications for surgery.

An anterior approach for corpectomy and grafting has advantages for this fracture pattern. Intraoperative positioning is easier, and traction can be maintained. The hazards of positioning and ventilating a prone patient are avoided. The exposure is relatively atraumatic and less painful than the posterior approach. Bone fragments causing impingement can be removed under direct vision and the decompression immediately assessed. Bone graft material is under compression and encased by a well-vascularized bed, both of which promote the development of a solid arthrodesis. Traynelis et al.[35] reported that bicortical anterior plating is usually biomechanically sufficient in this injury subset, and this type of stabilization has been clinically successful.[36] Modern unicortical plating systems have demonstrated equivalent long-term outcomes. Should a posterior procedure be necessary, it is safe to perform it in the same setting as the anterior approach. Circumferential instrumentation provides a much stiffer construct with a higher rate of fusion over an anterior approach alone.[37]

COMPLICATIONS AND OUTCOMES

Patients with vertical compression fractures are at risk for the usual types of complications that may occur in all patients suffering from a cervical spinal fracture. These include, but are not limited to, infections, deep venous thrombosis, pulmonary embolism, neurologic deficits, spinal deformity, and chronic neck pain. The outcome is directly related to the patient's neurologic condition at presentation. Patients with little or no neurologic deficit usually enjoy a fairly complete recovery, whereas those with significant impairment often retain at least some degree of neurologic dysfunction.

REFERENCES

1. Allen BL Jr, Ferguson RL, Lehmann TR, et al. A mechanistic classification of closed, indirect fractures and dislocations of the lower cervical spine. *Spine* 1982;7:1–27.
2. Babcock JL. Cervical spine injuries: diagnosis and classification. *Arch Surg* 1976;111:646–651.
3. Beatson TR. Fractures and dislocations of the cervical spine. *J Bone Joint Surg Br* 1963;45:21–35.
4. Gehweiler JA Jr, Clark WM, Schaaf RE, et al. Cervical spine trauma: the common combined conditions. *Radiology* 1979;130:77–86.
5. Harris JH Jr, Edeiken-Monroe B, Kopaniky DR. A practical classification of acute cervical spine injuries. *Orthop Clin North Am* 1986;17:15–30.
6. Whitley JE, Forsyth HF. The classification of cervical spine injuries. *Am J Roentgenol Radium Ther Nucl Med* 1960;83:633–644.
7. White AA III, Panjabi MM. *Clinical Biomechanics of the Spine.* 2nd ed. Philadelphia: Lippincott Williams & Wilkins, 1990.
8. Maiman DJ, Yoganandan N, Pintar FA. Preinjury cervical alignment affecting spinal trauma. *J Neurosurg (Spine 1)* 2002;97:57–62.
9. Oktenoglu T, Ozer AF, Ferrara LA, et al. Effects of cervical spine posture on axial loading bearing ability: a biochemical study. *J Neurosurg (Spine 1)* 2001;94:108–114.
10. Shea M, Edwards WT, White AA, et al. Variations of stiffness and strength along the human cervical spine. *J Biomech* 1991;24:95–107.
11. Adams MA, Hutton WC. Prolapsed intervertebral disc: a hyperflexion injury. 1981 Volvo Award in Basic Science. *Spine* 1982;7:184–191.
12. Schneider RC, Kahn EA. Chronic neurological sequelae of acute trauma to the spine and spinal cord. I: The significance of acute-flexion or "tear-drop" fracture-dislocation of the cervical spine. *J Bone Joint Surg Am* 1956; 38:985–997.
13. Rah AD, Errico TJ. Classification of lower cervical fractures and dislocations. In: The Cervical Spine Research Society Editorial Committee, eds. *The Cervical Spine.* 3rd ed. Philadelphia: Lippincott-Raven, 1998:449–456.
14. Brown CV, Antevil JL, Sise MJ, et al. Spiral computed tomography for the diagnosis of cervical, thoracic, and lumbar spine fractures: its time has come. *J Trauma* 2005;58:890–896.
15. Burke DC, Berryman D. The place of closed manipulation in the management of flexion-rotation dislocations of the cervical spine. *J Bone Joint Surg Br* 1971;53:165–182.
16. Daffner RH. Helical CT of the cervical spine for trauma patients: a time study. *AJR Am J Roentgenol* 2001;177: 677–679.
17. Widder S, Doig C, Burrowes P, et al. Prospective evaluation of computed tomographic scanning for the spinal clearance of obtunded trauma patients: preliminary results. *J Trauma* 2004;56:1179–1184.
18. Grogan EL, Morris JA Jr, Dittus RS, et al. Cervical spine evaluation in urban trauma centers: lowering institutional costs and complications through helical CT scan. *J Am Coll Surg* 2005;200:160–165.
19. Horn EM, Lekovic GP, Feiz-Erfan I, et al. Cervical magnetic resonance imaging abnormalities not predictive of cervical spine instability in traumatically injured patients. *J Neurosurg (Spine 1)* 2004;1:39–42.
20. Ullrich CG. Magnetic resonance imaging of the cervical spine and spinal cord. In: The Cervical Spine Research Society Editorial Committee, eds. *The Cervical Spine.* 3rd ed. Philadelphia: Lippincott-Raven, 1998:271–286.
21. Grant GA, Mirza SK, Chapman JR, et al. Risk of early closed reduction in cervical spine subluxation injuries. *J Neurosurg (Spine 1)* 1999;90:13–18.
22. Hadley MN, Walters BC, Grabb PA, et al. Guidelines for the management of acute cervical spine and spinal cord injuries. *Neurosurgery* 2002;50(suppl 3):S44–S50.
23. Harrington JF, Likavec MJ, Smith AS. Disc herniation in cervical fracture subluxation. *Neurosurgery* 1991;29: 374–379.
24. Ducker TB, Bellegarrigue R, Salcman M, et al. Timing of operative care in cervical spinal cord injury. *Spine* 1984;9:525–531.

25. Chan RC, Schweigel JF, Thompson GB. Halo-thoracic brace immobilization in 188 patients with acute cervical spine injuries. *J Neurosurg* 1983;58:508–515.
26. Cheshire DJ. The stability of the cervical spine following the conservative treatment of fractures and fracture-dislocations. *Paraplegia* 1969;7:193–203.
27. White AA, Southwick WO, Panjabi MM. Clinical instability in the lower cervical spine: a review of past and current concepts. *Spine* 1976;1:15–27.
28. Glaser JA, Whitehill R, Stamp WG, et al. Complications associated with the halo-vest: a review of 245 cases. *J Neurosurg* 1986;65:762–769.
29. Benzel EC, Larson SJ. Recovery of nerve root function after complete quadriplegia from cervical spine fractures. *Neurosurgery* 1986;19:809–812.
30. Benzel EC, Larson SJ. Functional recovery after decompressive spine operation for cervical spine fractures. *Neurosurgery* 1987;20:742–746.
31. Fehlings MG, Tator CH. An evidence-based review of decompressive surgery in acute spinal cord injury: rationale, indications, and timing based on experimental and clinical studies. *J Neurosurg (Spine 1)* 1999;91:1–11.
32. Koivikko MP, Myllynen P, Karjalainen M, et al. Conservative and operative treatment in cervical burst fractures. *Arch Orthop Trauma Surg* 2000;120:448–451.
33. Levi L, Wolf A, Rigamonti D, et al. Anterior decompression in cervical spine trauma: does the timing of surgery affect the outcome? *Neurosurgery* 1991;29:216–222.
34. Maiman DJ, Larson SJ, Benzel EC. Neurological improvement associated with late decompression of the thoracolumbar spinal cord. *Neurosurgery* 1984;14:302–307.
35. Traynelis VC, Donaher PA, Roach RM, et al. Biomechanical comparison of anterior Caspar plate and three-level posterior fixation techniques in a human cadaveric model. *J Neurosurg* 1993;79:96–103.
36. Aebi M, Benzel EC. Cervical spine burst fractures. In: The Cervical Spine Research Society Editorial Committee, eds. *The Cervical Spine*. 3rd ed. Philadelphia:
37. Schultz KD Jr, McLaughlin MR, Haid RW Jr, et al. Single-stage anterior-posterior decompression and stabilization for complex cervical spine disorders. *J Neurosurg (Spine 2)* 2000;93:214–221.

CHAPTER 25C

Subaxial Injuries: Distractive Flexion Injuries

Bizhan N.M.N. Aarabi, Karl M. Schweitzer Jr., and Alexander R. Vaccaro

INTRODUCTION

Despite numerous clinical[1–10] and experimental[11–22] studies, precise recommended management of traumatic cervical spine and spinal cord injuries remains elusive. Part of the difficulty is lack of Class I evidence supporting the effectiveness of therapeutic modalities, whether surgical or nonoperative.[2,7,8,23–30] Distractive flexion injuries of the cervical spine, as described in the Allen and Ferguson mechanistic classification of lower cervical spine fractures, have been studied and intensely debated.[31–37] Urgent reduction and timely fixation of lower cervical spine distractive flexion injuries is recommended at this time by the Guidelines for the Management of Acute Cervical Spine and Spinal Cord Injuries.[38]

MECHANISM OF INJURY

Translation of kinetic energy into major and minor injury vectors centered on a transitional axis ventral to the cervical spine results in a continuum of injuries coined by Allen et al.[31] as distractive flexion injuries. On the Ducker/McAfee/Allen clock face, the load path ranges from 9:00 to 11:30 (Fig. 25C.1).[31,39] In addition to flexion and distraction, rotational injury forces are of paramount significance in producing unilateral and bilateral locked facets.[40,41] Progressive disruption of the posterior ligamentous complex (PLC), including the facet capsule, ligamentum flavum, posterior annulus, posterior longitudinal ligaments, and anterior longitudinal ligament is characteristic of the distractive flexion phylogeny.[31,40–44] Although fractures of the articulating processes, laminae, or endplate of the caudal vertebral body may occasionally be noticed, these injuries characteristically involve ligamentous disruption that determines the degree of instability (Fig. 25C.2).[31,39,43] The resultant loss of ligamentous integrity and poor capacity for healing is the main reason behind loss of closed reduction and fusion failures following management of such injuries.[5,45–48]

CLASSIFICATION

The Distractive Flexion phylogeny is a descriptive and mechanistic classification introduced by Allen et al.,[31] based on their experience with 165 patients with lower cervical spine injuries. This classification is functionally prognostic and valuable in guiding treatment. In this scheme, the anatomic damage to a motion segment is based on four stages of injury. As the stages in this phylogeny increase, so does the degree of damage to the osteoligamentous complex and spinal cord. From 2003 to 2005, 35 patients with distractive flexion injury and neurologic deficit were admitted to the

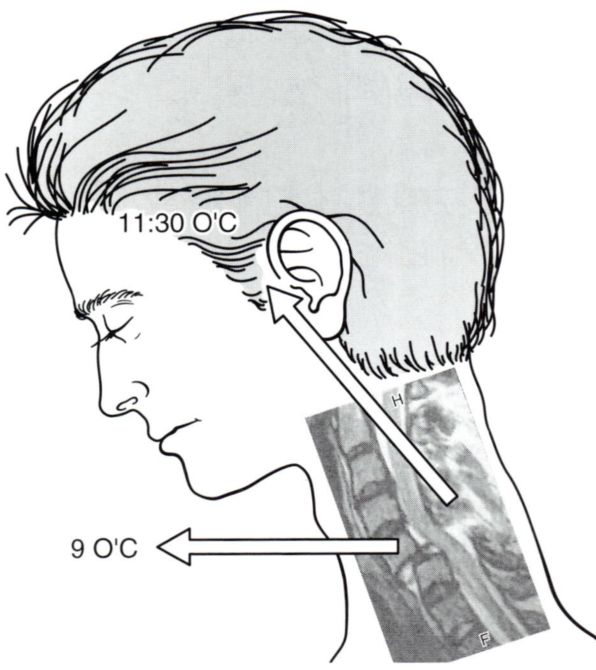

FIGURE 25C.1. Schematic representation of distractive flexion phylogeny, with translation of kinetic energy into injury vectors with propagating forces along 9:00 to 11:30 of the Ducker/Ferguson/Allen clock face.

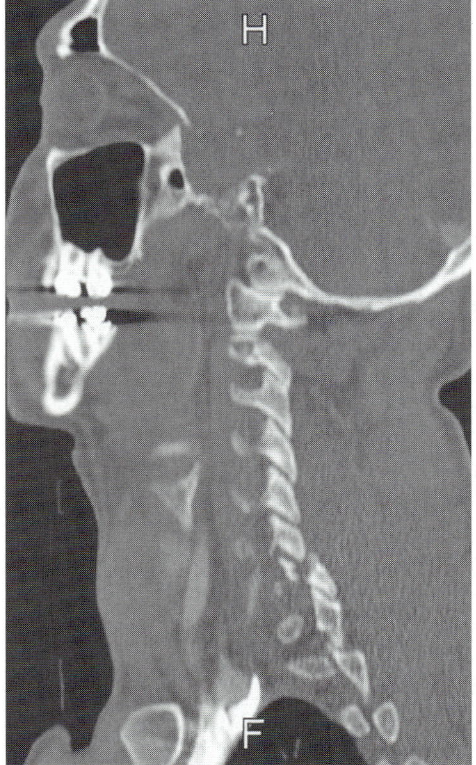

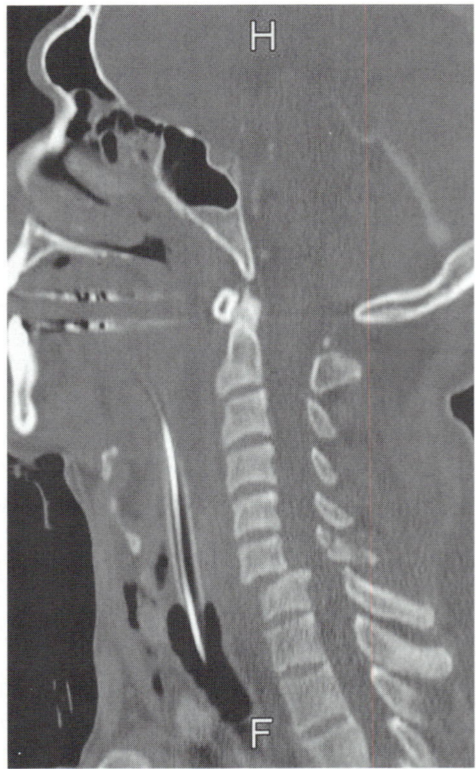

FIGURE 25C.2. **A.** Reformatted sagittal computed tomography views of the cervical spine from a 30-year-old man after a motor vehicle collision, with C6-C7 distractive flexion stage 3 injury and brittle fracture of the C7 superior articulating process on the left side. **B.** Reformatted midsagittal computed tomography views of the cervical spine from the patient described in Figure 25C.2A indicating rounding of the anterior superior aspect of the endplate of C7. *(continued)*

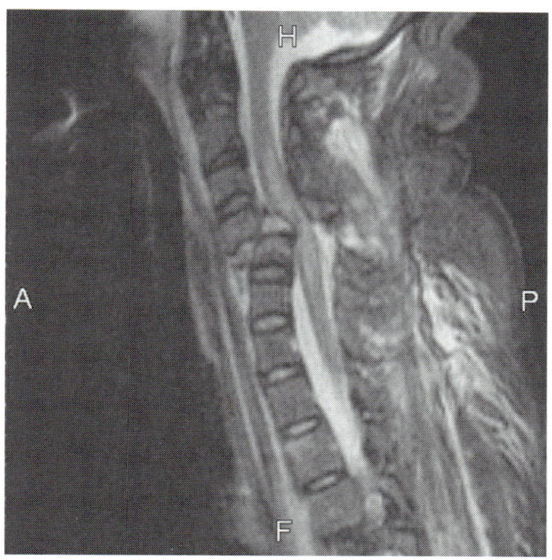

FIGURE 25C.2. *(continued)* **C.** Reformatted cervical spine magnetic resonance imaging (STIR views) from a 36-year-old man after a motor vehicle collision, with a C4-C5 distractive flexion stage 4 injury and C4 quadriplegia, indicating complete disruption of the posterior ligamentous complex, ligamentum flavum, posterior longitudinal ligament, annulus, and anterior longitudinal ligament.

Shock Trauma Center in Baltimore. In this group of patients the proportion of American Spinal Injury Association (ASIA) A patients increased from 0 to 80% as the severity of injury increased from stage 1 to stage 4 (Fig. 25C.3). Using the Schaefer et al.[49] prognostic classification of admission magnetic resonance imaging, a rough correlation between phylogenetic stages and magnetic resonance imaging (MRI) evidence of parenchymal cord damage was noted (Figs. 25C.4 and 25C.5).

DISTRACTIVE FLEXION STAGE 1

Also known as a flexion sprain, distraction flexion stage 1 (DFS1) is the least severe form of distractive flexion phylogeny and the most likely to be missed. The injury force and direction damages the

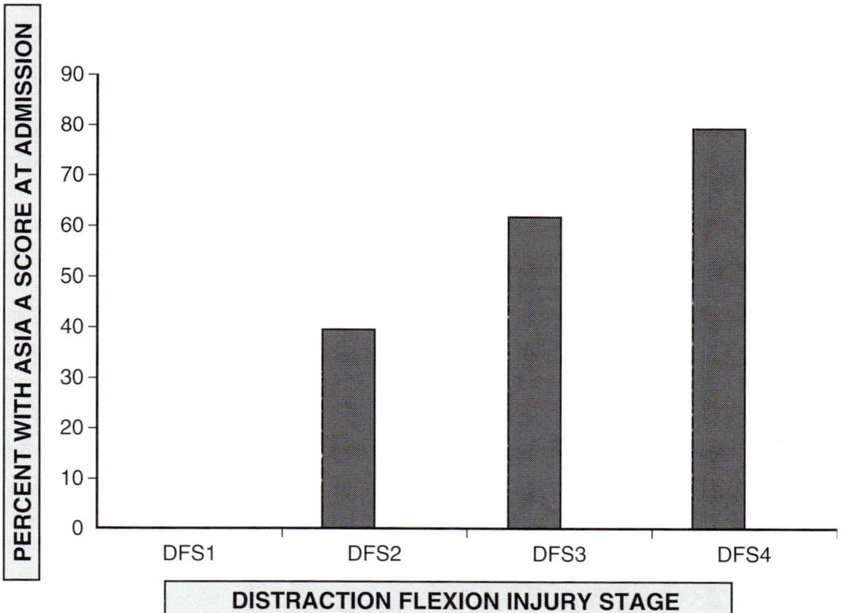

FIGURE 25C.3. Graph of 35 patients with distractive flexion injury seen over 36 months at the Shock Trauma Center in Baltimore indicating progressive increase in the incidence of ASIA A patients from 0 to 80% as the severity of injury increases from distractive flexion stage 1 injury to stage 4.

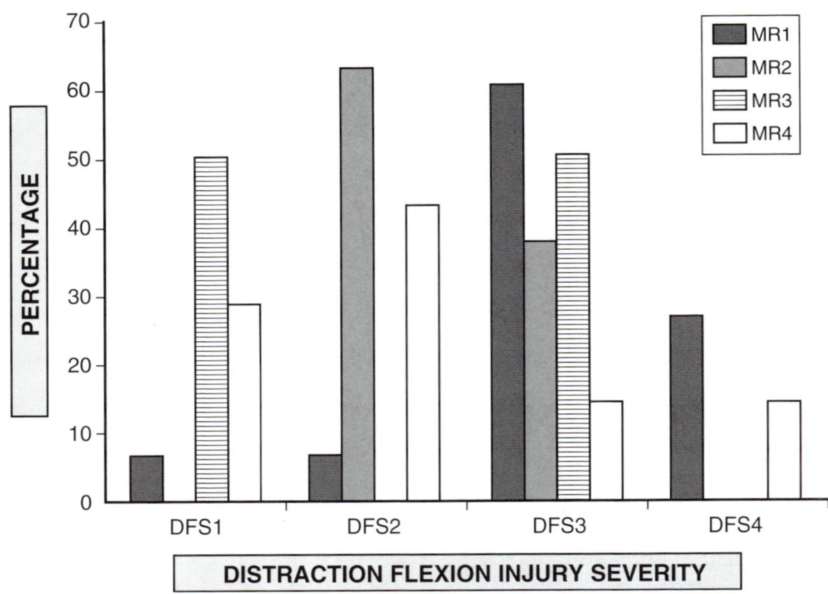

FIGURE 25C.4. Graph reflecting increase in magnetic resonance grade as distractive flexion injury stage severity increases.

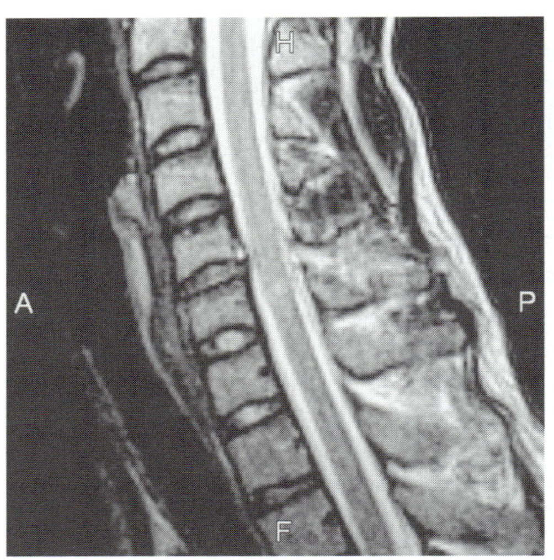

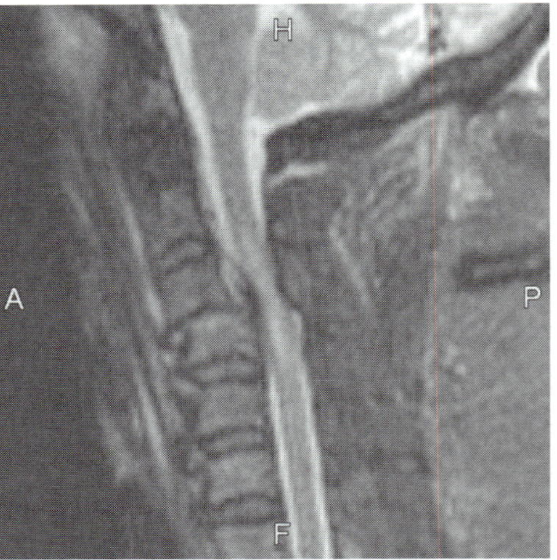

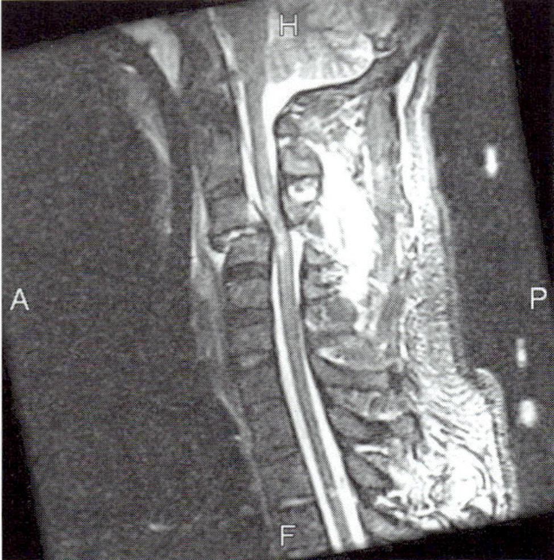

FIGURE 25C.5. **A.** Cervical T2-weighted magnetic resonance imaging (MRI) scans (type III) from a 21-year-old man after a motor vehicle collision (MVC), with a distraction flexion stage 1 injury. The patient complained of severe dysesthesias of his hands associated with slight bilateral grip weakness. MRI views indicate high signal change below the level of injury, with a diameter of less than one vertebral segment. **B.** Cervical T2-weighted MRI images (type II) from a 39-year-old woman after an MVC, with a distractive flexion injury stage 2 at C3-C4 and quadriplegia at C4. MRI views indicated high signal change at the zone of injury, more than one vertebral segment cranially. **C.** Cervical T2-weighted MRI images (type I) from a 27-year-old man after an MVC, with a distractive flexion injury stage 3 at C3-C4 and C4 quadriplegia. MRI views indicated high signal change at the zone of injury, with hemorrhage inside the spinal cord.

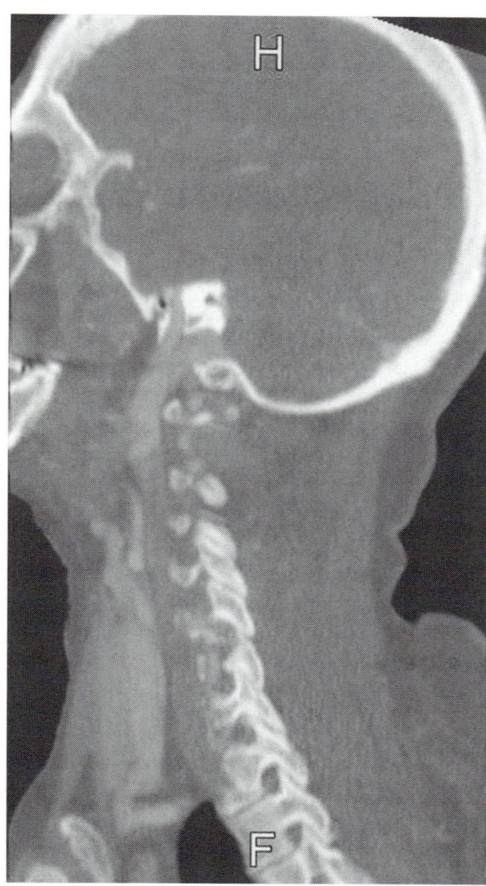

FIGURE 25C.6. Reformatted sagittal computed tomography views of the cervical spine from a 57-year-old after a motor vehicle collision, with C5-C6 distractive flexion stage 1 injury and central cord syndrome. She had an ASIA motor score of 88.

PLC and facet capsule but fail to dislocate the facet joints. On the lateral plain radiograph, spinous processes of the involved segment diverge and the facet capsule is clearly torn.[31,39,43] Four of 35 patients seen at the Shock Trauma Center had stage 1 injury: three had a mild central cord syndrome (ASIA motor 88 to 98) and one had a C6 radiculopathy. All injuries were at C5-C6; in two patients there was an associated articular process fracture, and one patient had an associated herniated disc. MRI findings in two patients were normal, one patient had a small area of high signal on short tau inversion recovery (STIR) T2-weighted sagittal images (Fig. 25C.5A), and one patient had a high signal on STIR T2-weighted sagittal images with a small amount of cord hemorrhage (type I) (Fig. 25C.6).[49]

DISTRACTIVE FLEXION STAGE 2

The injury vector in distractive flexion stage 2 (DFS2) involves a rotational moment to dislocate one facet joint.[40,41,44] Besides injury to the PLC and facet capsule, there is injury to the ligamentum flavum and less than 25% translation of the rostral vertebral body over the caudal vertebral body (Fig. 25C.7). This injury is more commonly known as a unilateral facet dislocation. In the literature review by Andreshak et al.[50] that included 308 patients with unilateral locked facets, complete spinal cord injury (SCI) was noted in 15% of the patients, radiculopathy in 37%, and incomplete SCI in 22%; 25% of the patients had normal neurologic findings. Ten patients in our series had a DFS2 injury associated with a neurologic deficit. Four patients had a complete and three an incomplete SCI, and three patients had a radiculopathy. MRI demonstrated high signal changes over more than one vertebral segment in five patients (type II), changes over one segment in one patient, and normal findings in three patients. One patient did not have admission MRI.

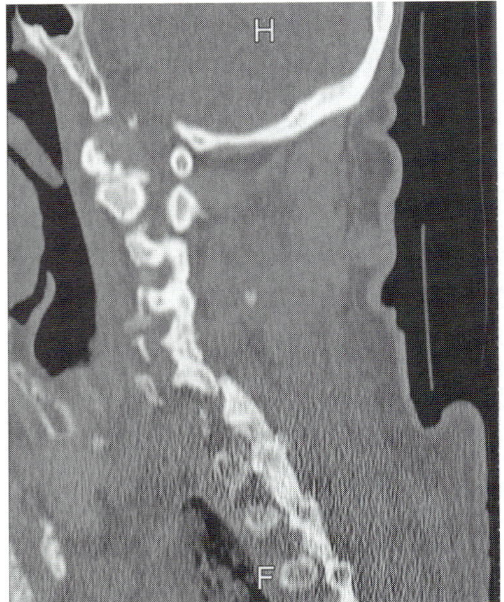

A

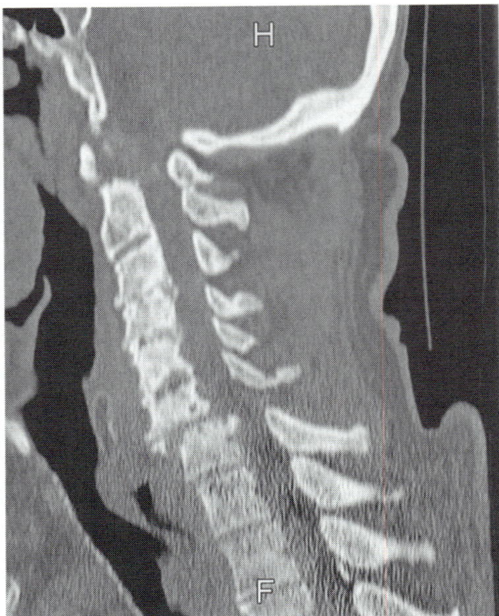

B

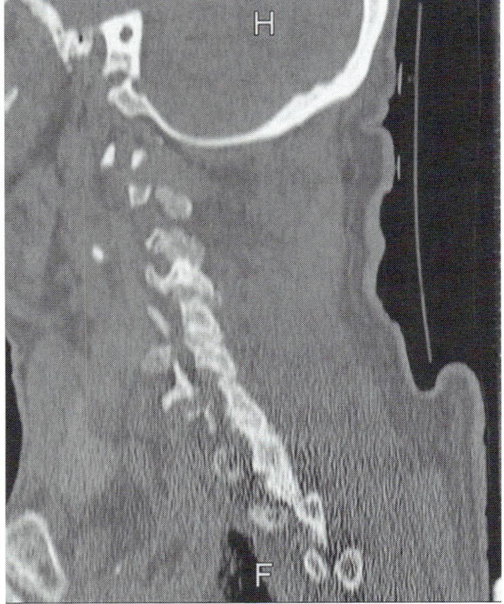

C

FIGURE 25C.7. Reformatted sagittal computed tomography views of the cervical spine from a 93-year-old man after an accidental fall, with C6-C7 distractive flexion stage 2 injury and central cord syndrome. He had an ASIA motor score of 83. There is subluxation of C6-C7 facet joint on the left side.

DISTRACTIVE FLEXION STAGE 3

In distractive flexion stage 3 (DFS3), there is a bilateral facet dislocation with close to 50% listhesis of the superior vertebra over the caudal vertebra (Fig. 25C.8). There is disruption of the PLC, facet joint, ligamentum flavum, and disc annulus. Clinical studies and cadaveric research have demonstrated the presence of severe instability in this group of patients.[31,37,44,51] Of the 16 patients in this group seen at the Shock Trauma Center, 10 were ASIA A, 2 were ASIA B, 2 were ASIA D, and 2 were ASIA E (one upper extremity monoparesis and one a mild central cord syndrome). MRI findings of injury using the Schaefer et al.[49,52] prognostic classification system were read as type I in 9 patients, type II in 3 patients, type III in 1 patient, and normal in 1 patient. MRI was not performed in two patients.

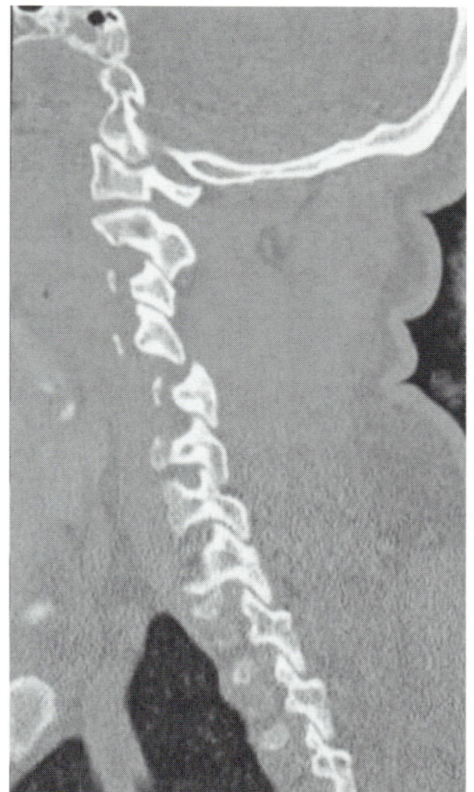
A

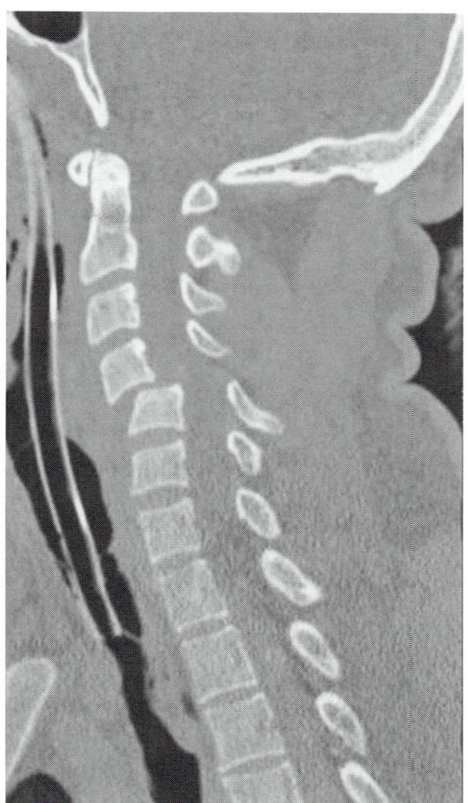
B

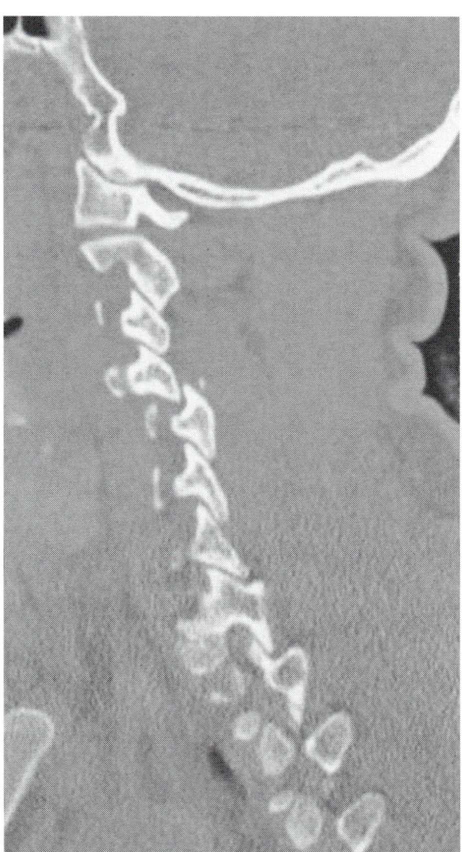
C

FIGURE 25C.8. Reformatted sagittal computed tomography views of cervical spine from a 33-year-old man after an accidental fall, with C4-C5 distractive flexion stage 3 injury and quadriplegia at C5. He had an ASIA motor score of 4.

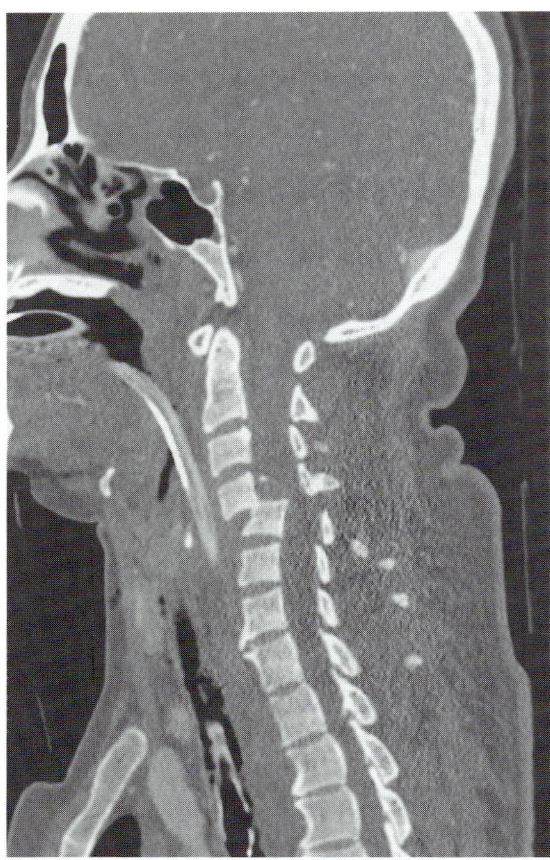

FIGURE 25C.9. Reformatted sagittal computed tomography views of cervical spine from a 36-year-old man after a motor vehicle collision, with C4-C5 distractive flexion stage 4 injury and complete quadriplegia. He had C4 sensory level.

DISTRACTIVE FLEXION STAGE 4

Distractive flexion stage 4 (DFS4) is also known as a floating vertebra. Patients in this category have damage to the PLL and ALL. Almost 100% of the rostral vertebral body is translated over the caudal vertebral body.[31,43] Clinically, in the Shock Trauma series of five patients with DFS4, four had a complete SCI and one was neurologically intact except for severe neck pain and bilateral shoulder paresthesias (Fig. 25C.9).

TREATMENT

A universal objective in distractive flexion injuries is the urgent acquisition of spinal realignment and therefore direct or indirect decompression of the spinal cord with the secondary goal of spinal stability and prevention of future deformity, pain, loss of reduction, and further spinal cord damage.[38,53–65] Initial radiographic assessment may not fully define the extent of three-column instability in DFS1 and DFS2 injuries. Case reports have cited the failure of halo-vest stabilization in distraction flexion injuries, as well as single-stage (anterior or posterior) stabilization of higher stages of distractive flexion injures. Therefore, many surgeons recommend a combined surgical approach in cases with obvious disruption of both anterior and posterior supporting ligamentous structures.[5,33,45,46,50,66–75]

INITIAL AND DEFINITIVE TREATMENT OF PATIENTS WITH DISTRACTIVE FLEXION STAGE 1

DFS1 is characterized by injury to the PLC and facet capsule of the involved vertebral segment. These patients may complain of pain and tenderness over the injury site. In unconscious, uncooperative, or intoxicated patients, it may be necessary to rely primarily on the MRI STIR images to detect injury to the PLC. A DFS1 injury may become evident on delayed dynamic flexion-extension radiographs.[53,60,76] If one considers an orthosis for definitive management of these patients, a lateral radiograph should be obtained before discharge to ensure reduction. Flexion-extension radiographs are performed at the conclusion of bracing to rule out subacute instability.[77] Indications for surgical intervention are failure of nonoperative treatment, presence of a neurologic injury, or intractable pain. Both anterior and posterior approaches appear successful. All four patients with a DFS1 injury seen at the Shock Trauma Center underwent an arthrodesis and internal fusion. This was performed anteriorly in three patients and with a combined approach in one patient.

INITIAL AND DEFINITIVE TREATMENT OF PATIENTS WITH DISTRACTIVE FLEXION STAGE 2

Patients with DFS2 injuries should undergo a timely traction or open reduction of the unilateral facet dislocation to minimize the potential for further injury displacement and neurologic injury.[78–81] A delay in traction reduction to perform MRI to rule out a herniated disc is not supported by the current literature.[82–87] Traction may not be successful in all cases.[88–91] In the series by Rizzolo et al.[92] of 131 patients, traction was successful in 86% of the patients. Following reduction, halo-vest immobilization or fusion may prevent vertebral redisplacement.[45,47,48,67,72,93–98] Inadequate evidence is available to make any conclusion on which treatment is best. In general, patients with comminution, neurologic injury, or who lose reduction are treated surgically. In injuries that fail to reduce with traction, MRI is performed, followed by either a posterior open reduction and internal fixation (ORIF), an anterior decompression and fusion followed by a posterior open reduction, or an anterior decompression and reduction followed by a fusion procedure.[43] Of the 10 patients admitted to the Shock Trauma Center with a DFS2 injury, all underwent acute reduction with closed skeletal traction. One patient died, one underwent a posterior arthrodesis, four underwent an anterior cervical discectomy and allograft arthrodesis and plating, and five underwent a combined anterior and posterior arthrodesis and internal fixation.

INITIAL AND DEFINITIVE TREATMENT OF PATIENTS WITH DISTRACTIVE FLEXION STAGES 3 AND 4

Urgent closed or open reduction of these high-grade injuries is recommended according to the Guidelines for the Management of Acute Cervical Spine and Spinal Cord Injuries.[38] Because of significant ligamentous injury in DFS3 and DFS4 injuries with resultant three-column instability, a posterior or anteroposterior short segment fusion and fixation is recommended. An alternative treatment that is gaining in popularity is immediate anterior open reduction and fusion with a plate. Although reduction in acute settings can be easily accomplished, delays in getting patients to surgery may prolong the time of dislocation, theoretically worsening neurologic injury. Of the 21 patients in this category treated at the Shock Trauma Center, 15 underwent a combined approach, 1 underwent an anterior only procedure, and 3 underwent a posterior only fusion (Fig. 25C.10). Surgery was not performed in two patients. One had a cerebellar stroke, and one had severe hemodynamic instability. Both patients died soon after their acute admission.

PROGNOSIS AND COMPLICATIONS FOLLOWING DISTRACTIVE FLEXION INJURIES

FUNCTIONAL OUTCOME

The mechanistic classification of distractive flexion phylogeny proposed by Allen and Ferguson[31] is predictive of immediate functional loss, prognostic for long-term disability, and helpful in guiding clinical management. Unless misdiagnosed, DFS1 or "flexion sprain" injuries should not cause any significant immediate physical disability. In the original paper by Allen et al.,[31] 12 of 61

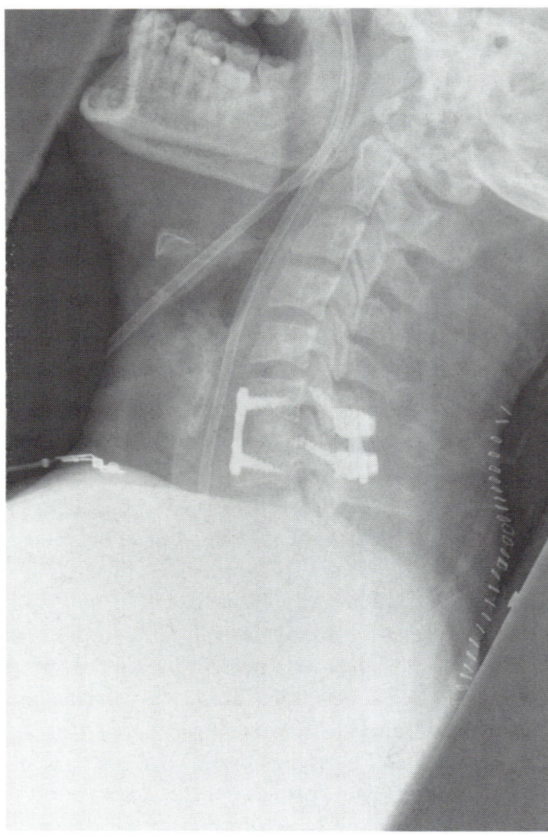

FIGURE 25C.10. Postoperative lateral plain radiograph view of cervical spine from a 23-year-old man after a motor vehicle collision, with C6-C7 distractive flexion stage 4 injury and complete quadriplegia. He had an ASIA motor score of 20. Following traction reduction, the patient had a one-stage anteroposterior short segment fusion of C6 and C7 vertebrae. He was kept in a hard collar for 3 months. In general, patients with comminution, neurologic injury, or who have a loss of reduction are treated surgically.

patients had a DFS1 injury, of whom only 4 had neurologic findings (2 radiculopathy and 2 central cord syndrome). The majority of patients with a suspected DFS1 injury and a normal neurologic examination may be managed with an orthosis, followed in an outpatient facility, and subsequently assessed for worsening neck pain, the onset of a neurologic deficit, or a spinal (kyphotic) deformity.[77] Progression of instability mandates consideration for surgical intervention.

Despite significant advances in our understanding of the pathophysiology and recovery of function following SCI,[11,16,17,99–105] translation of experimental studies into practice guidelines in DFS3 and DFS4 has not been that successful.[8,38,65,67] There is, however, significant Class III evidence that early traction-reduction may improve functional recovery,[24,89,90,107–109] and there is further evidence that early decompression and stabilization may improve functional outcome following spinal cord injury.[3,19,20,107,110–117]

SKELETAL OUTCOME

Since the introduction of skeletal traction by Crutchfield[88] and the adoption of specific methods of safely reducing facet dislocations,[42,118,119] there has been a gradual change of attitude toward immediate closed skeletal reduction followed by surgical stabilization.[66,67,120,121] Recent evidence indicates that internal fixation of fractures and dislocations of the lower cervical spine may be superior to halo-vest fixation.[5,45–48,69,122] This is in part due to significant progress in surgical technology and the poor long-term skeletal results of external orthoses such as the halo vest. These poor results include loss of reduction, kyphotic deformity, unexpected recurrence of pain, and the onset of new neurologic deficits.[74,75,95,123] Whether the anterior or posterior approach or a combination of both is best for managing distractive flexion injuries remains to be proved by prospective studies.[37,72,75,92,96,97,123,124]

COMPLICATIONS

COMPLICATIONS RELATED TO INJURY

Systemic Complications

Systemic complications include neurogenic shock, hypothermia, pulmonary insufficiency, risk for gastrointestinal bleeding, urinary tract infection, decubiti, deep vein thrombosis, and venous thromboembolism in patients with distractive flexion injury, similar to those reported in all patients with spinal cord injury.[125–136]

Vascular Complications

Patients with distractive flexion phylogeny are prone to vertebral artery intimal damage, dissection, pseudoaneurysm formation, or complete occlusion. CT angiography or magnetic resonance angiography in this group of patients may be indicated. Of 61 patients with cervical spine injury who were studied with magnetic resonance angiography, 12 had vertebral artery injury; of these, 10 had distractive flexion or compression flexion phylogenies.[137–139] The significance of injuries to the vertebral arteries in asymptomatic patients is unknown.

Chronic Complications

Autonomic dysreflexia, neuropathic pain, and posttraumatic syrinx formation are rare but potential complications, the cause of which is not fully understood.[140–143]

MANAGEMENT COMPLICATIONS

Traction reduction, especially in heavily sedated and anesthetized patients, and surgical intervention have been described as causes of neurologic deterioration.[144] In 1987 Marshall et al.[144] reported neurologic worsening in 14 of 283 patients with spinal cord injury. Neurologic worsening occurred in 4 of 134 operative patients, 3 of 60 patients undergoing traction, 2 of 68 patients during application of a halo vest, 2 of 56 patients while being turned on a Stryker frame, and 1 of 57 patients while in a Rotorest bed.[144] Acute disc herniation, overdistraction, edema spread, and mechanical compression have all been mentioned as possible causes of neurologic deterioration.[82–85,87,108,145–148]

Skeletal Complications

Loss of reduction, subacute and chronic instability, progressive or new neurologic deficit, kyphotic deformity, and instrumentation failure are complications that occur with external or internal fixation of distractive flexion injuries. The incidence of these complications seems to be lower with internal fixation as compared to halo-vest immobilization or postural reduction and bed rest.[5,25,33,46–48,69,74,93,95,122–124,150–154]

CONCLUSION

Distractive flexion injuries are common entities and frequently result in spinal cord and nerve root injury. The injuries result from tensile forces created in the posterior ligamentous complex and then propagating from a posterior to anterior direction. The severity ranges from sprain of the posterior ligaments to complete disruption of all spinal ligaments. Small amounts of rotation can create unilateral facet dislocations. Treatment recommendations include early reduction. Definitive treatment for milder DFS1 is nonoperative, although failures are common. Similarly a DFS2 lesion in neurologically intact patients can be treated in a halo vest, although those with fractures may fail secondary to redislocation. In these cases, either an anterior or posterior approach can be performed. The more severe DFS3 and DFS4 are treated surgically by either an anterior or posterior approach or in some cases by a combined approach.

REFERENCES

1. Anderson PA, Bohlman HH. Anterior decompression and arthrodesis of the cervical spine: long-term motor improvement. II: Improvement in complete traumatic quadriplegia. *J Bone Joint Surg Am* 1992;74:683–692.
2. Benzel EC, Larson SJ. Functional recovery after decompressive spine operation for cervical spine fractures. *Neurosurgery* 1987;20:742–746.
3. Bohlman HH, Anderson PA. Anterior decompression and arthrodesis of the cervical spine: long-term motor improvement. I: Improvement in incomplete traumatic quadriparesis. *J Bone Joint Surg Am* 1992;74:671–682.
4. Bracken MB, Collins WF, Freeman DF, et al. Efficacy of methylprednisolone in acute spinal cord injury. *JAMA* 1984;251:45–52.
5. Bucci MN, Dauser RC, Maynard FA, et al. Management of post-traumatic cervical spine instability: operative fusion versus halo vest immobilization—analysis of 49 cases. *J Trauma* 1988;28:1001–1006.
6. Duh MS, Shepard MJ, Wilberger JE, et al. The effectiveness of surgery on the treatment of acute spinal cord injury and its relation to pharmacological treatment. *Neurosurgery* 1994;35:240–248.
7. Fehlings MG, Sekhon LH, Tator C. The role and timing of decompression in acute spinal cord injury: what do we know? What should we do? *Spine* 26(suppl 24):S101–S110.
8. Fehlings MG, Tator CH. An evidence-based review of decompressive surgery in acute spinal cord injury: rationale, indications, and timing based on experimental and clinical studies. *J Neurosurg* 1999;91:1–11.
9. Schlegel J, Bayley J, Yuan H, et al. Timing of surgical decompression and fixation of acute spinal fractures. *J Orthop Trauma* 1996;10:323–330.
10. Tator CH, Fehlings MG, Thorpe K, et al. Current use and timing of spinal surgery for management of acute spinal surgery for management of acute spinal cord injury in North America: results of a retrospective multicenter study. *J Neurosurg* 1999;91(suppl 1):12–18.
11. Anderson TE, Stokes BT. Experimental models for spinal cord injury research: physical and physiological considerations. *J Neurotrauma* 1992;9(suppl 1):S135–S142.
12. Baffour R, Achanta K, Kaufman J, et al. Synergistic effect of basic fibroblast growth factor and methylprednisolone on neurological function after experimental spinal cord injury. *J Neurosurg* 1995;83:105–110.
13. Balentine JD, Greene WB. Ultrastructural pathology of nerve fibers in calcium-induced myelopathy. *J Neuropathol Exp Neurol* 1984;43:500–510.
14. Bregman BS, Diener PS, McAtee M, et al. Intervention strategies to enhance anatomical plasticity and recovery of function after spinal cord injury. *Adv Neurol* 1997;72:257–275.
15. Bregman BS, Kunkel-Bagden E, Schnell L, et al. Recovery from spinal cord injury mediated by antibodies to neurite growth inhibitors. *Nature* 1995;378:498–501.
16. Carlson GD, Gorden CD, Nakazowa S, et al. Perfusion-limited recovery of evoked potential function after spinal cord injury. *Spine* 2000;25:1218–1226.
17. Carlson GD, Minato Y, Okada A, et al. Early time-dependent decompression for spinal cord injury: vascular mechanisms of recovery. *J Neurotrauma* 1997;14:951–962.
18. Carlson GD, Warden KE, Barbeau JM, et al. Viscoelastic relaxation and regional blood flow response to spinal cord compression and decompression. *Spine* 1997;22:1285–1291.
19. Dolan EJ, Tator CH, Endrenyi L. The value of decompression for acute experimental spinal cord compression injury. *J Neurosurg* 1980;53:749–755.
20. Guha A, Tator CH, Endrenyi L, et al. Decompression of the spinal cord improves recovery after acute experimental spinal cord compression injury. *Paraplegia* 1987;25:324–339.
21. Kobrine AI, Evans DE, Rizzoli HV. Experimental acute balloon compression of the spinal cord: factors affecting disappearance and return of the spinal evoked response. *J Neurosurg* 1979;51:841–845.
22. Teng YD, Mocchetti I, Taveira-DaSilva AM, et al. Basic fibroblast growth factor increases long-term survival of spinal motor neurons and improves respiratory function after experimental spinal cord injury. *J Neurosci* 1999; 19:7037–7047.
23. Bohlman HH, Eismont FJ. Surgical techniques of anterior decompression and fusion for spinal cord injuries. *Clin Orthop* 1981;154:57–67.
24. Brunette DD, Rockswold GL. Neurologic recovery following rapid spinal realignment for complete cervical spinal cord injury. *J Trauma* 1987;27:445–447.
25. Donovan WH, Kopaniky D, Stolzmann E, et al. The neurological and skeletal outcome in patients with closed cervical spinal cord injury. *J Neurosurg* 1987;66:690–694.
26. Kiwerski JE. Early anterior decompression and fusion for crush fractures of cervical vertebrae. *Int Orthop* 1993;17:166–168.
27. Levi L, Wolf A, Rigamonti D, et al. Anterior decompression in cervical spine trauma: does the timing of surgery affect the outcome? *Neurosurgery* 1991;29:216–222.
28. Rosenfeld JF, Vaccaro AR, Albert TJ, et al. The benefits of early decompression in cervical spinal cord injury. *Am J Orthop* 1998;27:23–28.
29. Tator CH, Fehlings M. Review of clinical trials of neuroprotection in acute spinal cord injury. *Neurosurg Focus* 1999;6:1–14.

30. Zeidman SM, Ling GS, Ducker TB, et al. Clinical applications of pharmacologic therapies for spinal cord injury. *J Spinal Disord* 1996;9:367–380.
31. Allen BL Jr, Ferguson RL, Lehmann TR, et al. A mechanistic classification of closed, indirect fractures and dislocations of the lower cervical spine. *Spine* 1982;7:1–27.
32. Argenson C, Lovet J, Sanouiller JL, et al. Traumatic rotatory displacement of the lower cervical spine. *Spine* 1988;13:767–773.
33. Hadley MN, Fitzpatrick BC, Sonntag VK, et al. Facet fracture-dislocation injuries of the cervical spine. *Neurosurgery* 1992;30:661–666.
34. Lukhele M. Fractures of the vertebral lamina associated with unifacet and bifacet cervical spine dislocations. *S Afr Med J* 1994;32:112–114.
35. Mahale YJ, Silver JR. Progressive paralysis after bilateral facet dislocation of the cervical spine. *J Bone Joint Surg Br* 1992;74:219–223.
36. Paeslack V, Frankel H, Michaelis L. Closed injuries of the cervical spine and spinal cord: results of conservative treatment of flexion fractures and flexion rotation fracture dislocation of the cervical spine with tetraplegia. *Proc Veterans Adm Spinal Cord Inj Conf* 1973;19:39–42.
37. Sonntag VK. Management of bilateral locked facets of the cervical spine. *Neurosurgery* 1981;8:150–152.
38. Hadley MN, Walters BC, Grabb PA, et al. Guidelines for the management of acute cervical spine and spinal cord injuries. *Neurosurgery* 2002;50;S1–S199.
39. McAfee PC. Cervical spine trauma. In: Frymoyer JW, ed. *The Adult Spine: Principles and Practice.* New York: Raven Press, 1991:1063–1106.
40. Holdsworth FH. Fractures, common dislocations, fractures-dislocations of the spine. *J Bone Joint Surg Br* 1963; 45:6–26.
41. Roaf R. A study of the mechanics of spinal surgery. *J Bone Joint Surg Br* 1960;42:810–823.
42. Cheshire DJ. The stability of the cervical spine following the conservative treatment of fractures and fracture-dislocations. *Paraplegia* 1969;7:193–203.
43. Dekutoski M, Cohen-Gadol AA. Distractive flexion cervical spine injuries: a clinical spectrum. In: Vaccaro AR, ed. *Fractures of the Cervical, Thoracic, and Lumbar Spine.* New York: Marcel Dekker, 2003:191–205.
44. McLain RF, Aretakis A, Moseley TA, et al. Sub-axial cervical dissociation: anatomic and biomechanical principles of stabilization. *Spine* 1994;19:653–659.
45. Beyer CA, Cabanela ME, Berquist TH. Unilateral facet dislocations and fracture-dislocations of the cervical spine. *J Bone Joint Surg Br* 1991;73:977–981.
46. Bucholz RD, Cheung KC. Halo vest versus spinal fusion for cervical injury: evidence from an outcome study. *J Neurosurg* 1989;70:884–892.
47. Sears W, Fazl M. Prediction of stability of cervical spine fracture managed in the halo vest and indications for surgical intervention. *J Neurosurg* 1990;72:426–432.
48. Whitehill R, Richman JA, Glaser JA. Failure of immobilization of the cervical spine by the halo vest: a report of five cases. *J Bone Joint Surg Am* 1986;68:326–332.
49. Schaefer DM, Flanders AE, Osterholm JL, et al. Prognostic significance of magnetic resonance imaging in the acute phase of cervical spine injury. *J Neurosurg* 1992;76:218–223.
50. Andreshak JL, Dekutoski MB. Management of unilateral facet dislocations: a review of the literature. *Orthopedics* 1997;20:917–926.
51. Zdeblick TA, Abitbol JJ, Kunz DN, et al. Cervical stability after sequential capsule resection. *Spine* 1993;18: 2005–2008.
52. Schaefer DM, Flanders A, Northrup BE, et al. Magnetic resonance imaging of acute cervical spine trauma. *Spine* 1989;14:1090–1095.
53. Ajani AE, Cooper DJ, Scheinkestel CD, et al. Optimal assessment of cervical spine trauma in critically ill patients: a prospective evaluation. *Anaesth Intensive Care* 1999;26:487–491.
54. Alexander RH, Proctor HJ. *Advanced Trauma Life Support (ATLS) Program for Physicians: 1993 Instructor Manual.* Chicago: American College of Surgeons, 1993.
55. Banit DM, Grau G, Fisher JR. Evaluation of the acute cervical spine: a management algorithm. *J Trauma* 2000; 49:450–456.
56. Berne JD, Velmahos GC, El-Tawil Q, et al. Value of complete cervical helical computed tomographic scanning in identifying cervical spine injury in the unevaluable blunt trauma patient with multiple injuries: a prospective study. *J Trauma* 1999;47:896–902.
57. Blackmore CC, Emerson SS, Mann FA, et al. Cervical spine imaging in patients with trauma: determination of fracture risk to optimize use. *Radiology* 1999;211:759–765.
58. Chiu WC, Haan JM, Cushing BM, et al. Ligamentous injuries of the cervical spine in unreliable blunt trauma patients: incidence, evaluation, and outcome. *J Trauma* 2001;50:457–463.
59. Freemyer B, Knopp R, Piche J, et al. Comparison of five-view and three-view cervical spine series in the evaluation of patients with cervical trauma. *Ann Emerg Med* 1989;18:818–821.
60. Lewis LM, Docherty M, Ruoff BE, et al. Flexion-extension views in the evaluation of cervical-spine injuries. *Ann Emerg Med* 1991;20:117–121.

61. MacDonald RL, Schwartz ML, Mirich D, et al. Diagnosis of cervical spine injury in motor vehicle crash victims: how many X-rays are enough? *J Trauma* 1990;30:392–397.
62. Sees DW, Rodriguez Cruz LR, Flaherty SF, et al. The use of bedside fluoroscopy to evaluate the cervical spine in obtunded trauma patients. *J Trauma* 1998;45:768–771.
63. Tehranzadeh J, Bonk RT, Ansari A, et al. Efficacy of limited CT for nonvisualized lower cervical spine in patients with blunt trauma. *Skeletal Radiol* 1994;23:349–352.
64. Bracken MB, Shepard MJ, Collins WF, et al. A randomized, controlled trial of methylprednisolone or naloxone in the treatment of acute spinal-cord injury: results of the Second National Acute Spinal Cord Injury Study. *N Engl J Med* 1990;322:1405–1411.
65. Bracken MB, Shepard MJ, Holford TR, et al. Administration of methylprednisolone for 24 or 48 hours or tirilazad mesylate for 48 hours in the treatment of acute spinal cord injury: results of the Third National Acute Spinal Cord Injury Randomized Controlled Trial. National Acute Spinal Cord Injury Study. *JAMA* 1997;277:1597–1604.
66. Chan RC, Schweigel JF, Thompson GB. Halo-thoracic brace immobilization in 188 patients with acute cervical spine injuries. *J Neurosurg* 1983;58:508–515.
67. Cooper PR, Maravilla KR, Sklar FH: Halo immobilization of cervical spine fractures: indications and results. *J Neurosurg* 1979;50:603–610.
68. Cybulski GR, Douglas RA, Meyer PR Jr, et al. Complications in three-column cervical spine injuries requiring anterior-posterior stabilization. *Spine* 1992;17:253–256.
69. Glaser JA, Whitehill R, Stamp WG, et al. Complications associated with the halo-vest: a review of 245 cases. *J Neurosurg* 1986;65:762–769.
70. Goffin J, Plets C, Van den Bergh R. Anterior cervical fusion and osteosynthetic stabilization according to Caspar: a prospective study of 41 patients with fractures and/or dislocations of the cervical spine. *Neurosurgery* 1989;25: 865–871.
71. Lemons VR, Wagner FC Jr. Stabilization of subaxial cervical spinal injuries. *Surg Neurol* 1993;39:511–518.
72. Nazarian SM, Louis RP. Posterior internal fixation with screw plates in traumatic lesions of the cervical spine. *Spine* 1991;16:S64–S71.
73. Ripa DR, Kowall MG, Meyer PR Jr, et al. Series of ninety-two traumatic cervical spine injuries stabilized with anterior ASIF plate fusion technique. *Spine* 1991;16:S46–S55.
74. Roy-Camille R, Saillant G, Laville C, et al. Treatment of lower cervical spinal injuries: C3 to C7. *Spine* 1992;17: S442–S446.
75. Shapiro SA. Management of unilateral locked facet of the cervical spine. *Neurosurgery* 1993;33:832–837.
76. Bolinger B, Shartz M, Marion D. Bedside fluoroscopic flexion and extension cervical spine radiographs for clearance of the cervical spine in comatose trauma patients. *J Trauma* 2004;56:132–136.
77. Herkowitz HN, Rothman RH. Subacute instability of the cervical spine. *Spine* 1984;9:348–357.
78. Anderson DK. Chemical and cellular mediators in spinal cord injury. *J Neurotrauma* 1991;9:143–145.
79. Carlson SL, Parrish ME, Springer JE, et al. Acute inflammatory response in spinal cord following impact injury. *Exp Neurol* 1998;151:77–88.
80. Tator CH, Fehlings MG. Review of the secondary injury theory of acute spinal cord trauma with emphasis on vascular mechanisms. *J Neurosurg* 1992;75:15–26.
81. Young W. Secondary injury mechanisms in acute spinal cord injury. *J Emerg Med* 1993;11:13–22.
82. Doran SE, Papadopoulos SM, Ducker TB, et al. Magnetic resonance imaging documentation of coexistent traumatic locked facets of the cervical spine and disc herniation. *J Neurosurg* 1993;79:341–345.
83. Eismont FJ, Arena MJ, Green BA. Extrusion of an intervertebral disc associated with traumatic subluxation or dislocation of cervical facets: case report. *J Bone Joint Surg Am* 1991;73:1555–1560.
84. Grant GA, Mirza SK, Chapman JR, et al. Risk of early closed reduction in cervical spine subluxation injuries. *J Neurosurg* 1999;90(suppl 1):13–18.
85. Harrington JF, Likavec MJ, Smith AS. Disc herniation in cervical fracture subluxation. *Neurosurgery* 1991;29: 374–379.
86. Rizzolo SJ, Piazza MR, Cotler JM, et al. Intervertebral disc injury complicating cervical spine trauma. *Spine* 1991;16(suppl 6):S187–S189.
87. Vaccaro AR, Falatyn SP, Flanders AE, et al. Magnetic resonance evaluation of the intervertebral disc, spinal ligaments, and spinal cord before and after closed traction-reduction of cervical spine dislocations. *Spine* 1999;24: 1210–1217.
88. Crutchfield W. Skeletal traction in treatment of injuries to the cervical spine. *JAMA* 1954;155:29–32.
89. Lee AS, MacLean JC, Newton DA. Rapid traction for reduction of cervical spine dislocations. *J Bone Joint Surg Br* 1994;76:352–356.
90. Star AM, Jones AA, Cotler JM, et al. Immediate closed reduction of cervical spine dislocations using traction. *Spine* 1990;15:1068–1072.
91. Walton G. A new method of reducing dislocation of cervical vertebrae. *J Nerv Ment Dis* 1893;20:609.
92. Rizzolo SJ, Vaccaro AR, Cotler JM. Cervical spine trauma. *Spine* 1994;19:2288–2298.

93. Aebi M, Zuber K, Marchesi D. Treatment of cervical spine injuries with anterior plating: indications, techniques, and results. *Spine* 1991;16:S38–S45.
94. Aldrich EF, Crow WN, Weber PB, et al. Use of MR imaging-compatible Halifax interlaminar clamps for posterior cervical fusion. *J Neurosurgery* 1991;74:185–189.
95. Benzel EC, Kesterson L. Posterior cervical interspinous compression wiring and fusion for mid to low cervical spinal injuries. *J Neurosurg* 1989;70:893–899.
96. Fehlings MG, Cooper PR, Errico TJ. Posterior plates in the management of cervical instability: long-term results in 44 patients. *J Neurosurg* 1994;81:341–349.
97. Feldborg Nielsen C, Annertz M, Persson L, et al. Fusion or stabilization alone for acute distractive flexion injuries in the mid to lower cervical spine? *Eur Spine J* 1997;6:197–202.
98. Lifeso RM, Colucci MA. Anterior fusion for rotationally unstable cervical spine fractures. *Spine* 2000;25: 2028–2034.
99. Carlson G, Gorden C, Wada E, et al. Vascular re-perfusion and neural preservation after spinal cord injury. *J Neurotrauma* 1998;15:860.
100. de la Torre JC. Spinal cord injury: review of basic and applied research. *Spine* 1981;6:315–335.
101. Joshi M, Fehlings MG. Development and characterization of a novel, graded model of clip compressive spinal cord injury in the mouse: II. Quantitative neuroanatomical assessment and analysis of the relationships between axonal tracts, residual tissue, and locomotor recovery. *J Neurotrauma* 2002;19:191–203.
102. Nashmi R, Fehlings MG. Changes in axonal physiology and morphology after chronic compressive injury of the rat thoracic spinal cord. *Neuroscience* 2001;104:235–251.
103. Nashmi R, Fehlings MG. Mechanisms of axonal dysfunction after spinal cord injury: with an emphasis on the role of voltage-gated potassium channels. *Brain Res Rev* 2001;38:165–191.
104. Schwartz G, Fehlings MG. Evaluation of the neuroprotective effects of sodium channel blockers after spinal cord injury: improved behavioral and neuroanatomical recovery with riluzole. *J Neurosurg* 2001;94(suppl 2):245–256.
105. Stokes BT. Experimental spinal cord injury: a dynamic and verifiable injury device. *J Neurotrauma* 1992; 9:129–131.
106. Aebi M, Mohler J, Zach GA, et al. Indication, surgical technique and results of 100 surgically-treated fractures and fracture-dislocation of the cervical spine. *Clin Orthop* 1986;203:244–257.
107. Burke DC, Berryman D. The place of closed manipulation in the management of flexion-rotation dislocations of the cervical spine. *J Bone Joint Surg Br* 1971;53:165–182.
108. Dall DM. Injuries of the cervical spine. II. Does anatomical reduction of the bony injuries improve the prognosis for spinal cord recovery? *S Afr Med J* 1972;46:1083–1090.
109. Hadley MN, Argires PJ. The acute/emergent management of vertebral column fracture dislocation injuries. In: *Neurological Emergencies.* Park Ridge, Ill: American Association of Neurological Surgeons, 1992;661–666.
110. Fehlings MG, Perrin RG. The role and timing of early decompression for cervical spinal cord injury: update with a review of recent clinical evidence. *Injury* 2005;2:B13–B26.
111. La Rosa G, Conti A, Cardali S, et al. Does early decompression improve neurological outcome of spinal cord injured patients? Appraisal of the literature using a meta-analytical approach. *Spinal Cord* 2004;42:503–512.
112. Maiman DJ, Barolat G, Larson SJ. Management of bilateral locked facets of the cervical spine. *Neurosurgery* 1986;18:542–547.
113. Maynard FM, Reynolds GG, Fountain S, et al. Neurological prognosis after traumatic quadriplegia: three-year experience of California Regional Spinal Cord Injury Care System. *J Neurosurg* 1970;50:611–616.
114. Papadopoulos SM, Selden NR, Quint DJ, et al. Immediate spinal cord decompression for cervical spinal cord injury: feasibility and outcome. *J Trauma* 2002;52:323–332.
115. Pollard ME, Apple DF. Factors associated with improved neurologic outcomes in patients with incomplete tetraplegia. *Spine* 2003;28:33–39.
116. Tator CH, Duncan EG, Edmonds VE, et al. Comparison of surgical and conservative management in 208 patients with acute spinal cord injury. *Can J Neurol Sci* 1987;14:60–69.
117. Vaccaro AR, Daughtery RJ, Sheehan TP, et al. Neurologic outcome of early versus later surgery for cervical spinal cord injury. *Spine* 1997;22:2609–2613.
118. Burke DC, Tiong TS. Stability of the cervical spine after conservative treatment. *Paraplegia* 1975;13:191–202.
119. Frankel HL, Hancock DO, Hyslop G, et al. The value of postural reduction in the initial management of closed injuries of the spine with paraplegia and tetraplegia. I. *Paraplegia* 1969;7:179–192.
120. Della Torre P, Rinonapoli E. Halo-cast treatment of fractures and dislocations of the cervical spine. *Int Orthop* 1992;16:227–231.
121. Ersmark H, Kalen R. A consecutive series of 64 halo-vest-treated cervical spine injuries. *Arch Orthop Trauma Surg* 1986;105:243–246.
122. O'Brien PJ, Schweigel JF, Thompson WJ. Dislocations of the lower cervical spine. *J Trauma* 1982;22:710–714.
123. Cahill DW, Bellegarrigue R, Ducker TB. Bilateral facet to spinous process fusion: a new technique for posterior spinal fusion after trauma. *Neurosurgery* 1983;13:1–4.

124. Shapiro S, Snyder W, Kaufman K, et al. Outcome of 51 cases of unilateral locked cervical facets: interspinous braided cable for lateral mass plate fusion compared with interspinous wire and facet wiring with iliac crest. *J Neurosurg* 1999;91:19–24.
125. Cahill DW, Rechtine GR. Acute complications of spinal cord injury. In: Narayan RK, Wilberger JE, Povlishock JT, eds. *Neurotrauma*. New York: McGraw-Hill, 1996:1229–1236.
126. Chen Y, Devivo MJ, Jackson AB. Pressure ulcer prevalence in people with spinal cord injury: age-period-duration effects. *Arch Phys Med Rehab* 2005;86:1208–1213.
127. Como JJ, Sutton ER, McCunn M, et al. Characterizing the need for mechanical ventilation following cervical spinal cord injury with neurologic deficit. *J Trauma* 2005;59:912–916.
128. Epstein N, Hood DC, Ransohoff J. Gastrointestinal bleeding in patients with spinal cord trauma. *J Neurosurg* 1981;54:16–20.
129. Frisbie JH. Breathing and the support of blood pressure after spinal cord injury. *Spinal Cord* 2005;43:406–407.
130. Green D. Diagnosis, prevalence, and management of thromboembolism in patients with spinal cord injury. *J Spinal Cord Med* 2004;26:329–334.
131. Harrop JS, Sharan AD, Scheid EH Jr, et al. Tracheostomy placement in patients with complete cervical spinal cord injuries: American Spinal Injury Association Grade A. *J Neurosurg* 2004;100(suppl Spine 1):20–23.
132. Knudson MM, Ikossi DG. Venous thromboembolism after trauma. *Curr Opin Crit Care* 2004;10:539–548.
133. Linares HA, Mawson AR, Suarez E, et al. Association between pressure sores and immobilization in the immediate post injury period. *Clin Ortho* 1987;10:517–573.
134. Neville AL, Crookes P Velmahos GC, et al. Esophageal dysfunction in cervical spinal cord injury: a potentially important mechanism of aspiration. *J Trauma* 2005;59:905–911.
135. Porth SC. Recognition and management of respiratory dysfunction in children with tetraplegia. *J Spinal Cord Med Suppl* 2004;1:S75–S79.
136. Stawicki SP, Grossman MD, Cipolla J, et al. Deep venous thrombosis and pulmonary embolism in trauma patients: an overstatement of the problem? *Am Surg* 2005;71:387–391.
137. Giacobetti FB, Vaccaro AR, Bos-Giacobetti MA, et al. Vertebral artery occlusion associated with cervical spine trauma: a prospective analysis. *Spine* 1997;22:188–192.
138. Vaccaro AR, Klein GR, Flanders AE, Long-term evaluation of vertebral artery injuries following cervical spine trauma using magnetic resonance angiography. *Spine* 1998;23:789–794.
139. Weller SJ, Rossitch E Jr, Malek AM. Detection of vertebral artery injury after cervical spine trauma using magnetic resonance angiography. *J Trauma* 1999;46:660–666. 1999.
140. Fleischman S, Shah P. Autonomic dysreflexia: an unusual radiologic complication. *Diagn Radiol* 1977;124: 695–697.
141. Hida K, Iwasaki Y, Imamura H, et al. Posttraumatic syringomyelia: its characteristic magnetic resonance imaging findings and surgical management. *Neurosurgery* 1994;35:886–891.
142. McKinley W, Meade MA, Kirshblum S, et al. Outcomes of early surgical management versus late or no surgical intervention after acute spinal cord injury. *Arch Phys Med Rehabil* 2004;85:1818–1825.
143. Weaver LC, Verghese P, Bruce JC, et al. Autonomic dysreflexia and primary afferent sprouting after clip-compression injury of the rat spinal cord. *J Neurotrauma* 2001;18:1107–1119.
144. Marshall LF, Knowlton S, Garfin SR, et al. Deterioration following spinal cord injury: a multicenter study. *J Neurosurg* 1987;66:400–404.
145. Brooke WS. Complete transverse cervical myelitis caused by traumatic herniation of an ossified nucleus pulposus. *JAMA* 1944;125:117–120.
146. Farmer J, Vaccaro A, Albert TJ, et al. Neurologic deterioration after spinal cord injury. *J Spinal Disord* 1998;11:192–196.
147. Mahale YJ, Silver JR, Henderson NJ. Neurological complications of the reduction of cervical spine dislocations. *J Bone Joint Surg Br* 1993;75:403–409.
148. Olerud C, Johnsson H Jr. Compression of the cervical spinal cord after reduction of fracture dislocations: report of 2 cases. *Acta Orthop Scand* 1991;62:599–601.
149. Campagnolo DI, Esquieres RE, Kopacz KJ. Effect of timing of stabilization on length of stay and medical complications following spinal cord injury. *J Spinal Cord Med* 1997;20:331–334.
150. Kishan S, Vives MJ, Reiter MF. Timing of surgery following spinal cord injury. *J Spinal Cord Med* 2005;28:11–19.
151. McAfee PC, Bohlman HH. One-stage anterior cervical decompression and posterior stabilization with circumferential arthrodesis: a study of twenty-four patients who had a traumatic or a neoplastic lesion. *J Bone Joint Surg Am* 1989;71:78–88.
152. Mirza SK, Krengel WF 3rd, Chapman JR, et al. Early versus delayed surgery for acute cervical spinal cord injury. *Clin Orthop* 1999;359:104–114.
153. Ordonez BJ, Benzel EC, Naderi S, et al. Cervical facet dislocation: techniques for ventral reduction and stabilization. *J Neurosurg* 2000;92:18–23.
154. Ostl OL, Fraser RD, Griffiths ER. Reduction and stabilisation of cervical dislocations: an analysis of 167 cases. *J Bone Joint Surg Br* 1989;71:275–282.

CHAPTER 25D

Subaxial Injuries: Extension-Distraction Injuries

D. Greg Anderson and Chadi Tannoury

INTRODUCTION

Cervical spinal column injuries, from various traumatic mechanisms, remain a major source of morbidity and mortality. In particular, patients sustaining significant injuries to the cervical spinal cord continue to have suboptimal clinical outcomes in many cases. Fortunately, the modern trauma system in the United States, which promotes early spinal immobilization and transfer to tertiary care facilities, has decreased the rate of patients with complete as opposed to incomplete spinal cord lesions. In recent years, advancements in spinal imaging and surgical technique have provided spine surgeons with better methods of treatment for patients with traumatic injuries to the cervical spinal column.

In 1982, Allen et al.[1] proposed a comprehensive, mechanistic classification for cervical spine trauma. In their scheme, cervical spine fractures were grouped into phylogenies on the basis of the presumed injury mechanism. Within each mechanistic phylogeny, a spectrum of stages was used to classify injuries according to the severity of the disruption. Although this classification system was proposed empirically by examining injury radiographs, without proof of the specific biomechanical cause of each disruption, it has proven useful to clinicians over time and has improved the ability of spine surgeons to communicate regarding commonly seen injury patterns. In addition, this classification has been used to guide treatment of particular injuries by defining the location of anatomic disruption.

In this chapter we will discuss the extension-distraction injury pattern in the cervical spine. Our discussion will include the demographics, classification, diagnostic workup, treatment, and outcome of this relatively uncommon cervical spine injury.

DEMOGRAPHICS AND CLASSIFICATION

The extension-distraction (or distraction-extension) injury pattern is one of the more common patterns seen in older patients and is also common in patients with stiff cervical spines as a result of ankylosing spondylitis or diffuse idiopathic skeletal hyperostosis (DISH). This injury is caused by traumatic hyperextension of the cervical spine (Fig. 25D.1), leading to tensile failure of the anterior aspect of the spinal column.[1] With increasing severity of injury, the disruption extends from the anterior to the posterior elements of the cervical segment (Fig. 25D.2).

Extension-distraction injuries are much more commonly seen in stiff or spondylotic spines than in normal spines. This injury pattern results from stress concentration by the noncompliant spine to the injury level, rather than stress dissipation by motion at multiple levels in a normal, compliant

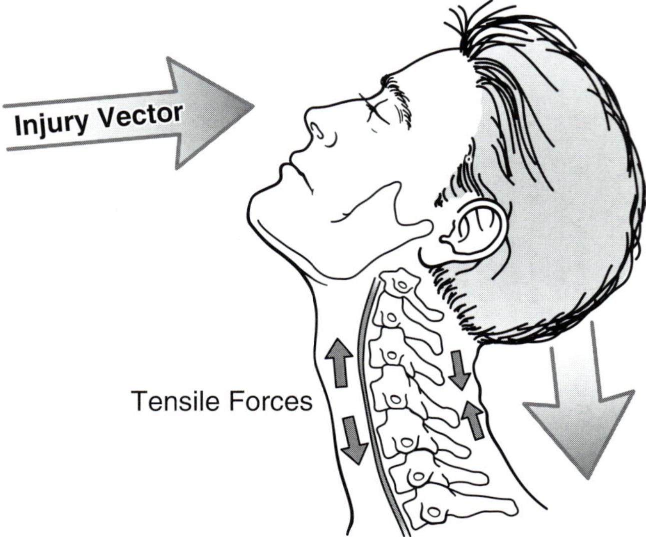

FIGURE 25D.1. A schematic illustration of the extension-distraction injury mechanism of the cervical spine.

spine. Because stiff and spondylotic spines are vulnerable to the extension-distraction injury pattern, these injuries are commonly encountered in the elderly population, as well as those with ankylosing spondylitis and DISH. In addition, this same patient population is at risk for falls, which are a common injury mechanism leading to extension-distraction injury.

The path of the disruption often traverses the disc space, making the injury relatively difficult to detect on plain lateral radiograph of the cervical spine. Even highly unstable injuries may spontaneously

EXTENSION-DISTRACTION

Anterior longitudinal ligament

Stage 1

Stage 2

FIGURE 25D.2. A schematic illustration of extension-distraction injury stages 1 and 2.

realign in a cervical collar or with the neck in flexion at the time radiographs are obtained. For this reason, the treating physician must have a high index of suspicion when evaluating a patient with a suggestive injury mechanism and significant neck pain. Subtle clues to watch for with this injury pattern include fracture through an anterior osteophyte, anterior soft tissue swelling, or widening of the anterior aspect of the disc compared to the posterior disc or adjacent levels. When plain films are not diagnostic, advanced imaging studies such as magnetic resonance imaging (MRI) are often helpful. MRI may demonstrate increased signal in the involved disc space on T2-weighted images or demonstrate disruption of the anterior portion of the disc and anterior longitudinal ligament (ALL). Late, missed injuries may demonstrate reactive changes at the involved disc space several weeks after the injury or manifest signs of instability on flexion-extension images.

According to Allen et al.,[1] the extension-distraction injury pattern includes two stages (stages 1 and 2) on the basis of injury severity. In a stage 1 extension-distraction injury, the ALL and disc space are disrupted. The injury may also include avulsion fractures through the vertebral body or along the margin of the anterior disc space. On plain radiographs, the hallmark of the injury is widening of the anterior disc space; however, significant retrolisthesis of the upper vertebral body is not present in a stage 1 injury. Most commonly, patients with a stage 1 extension-distraction injury are neurologically intact or demonstrate an incomplete spinal cord injury (SCI) (e.g., central cord injury).

In the stage 2 injury, a more significant disruption of the spinal column exists allowing posterior subluxation (retrolisthesis) of the superior vertebral body. A stage 2 injury is recognized by the presence of more than 2 mm of retrolisthesis of the superior vertebral body on the plain lateral radiograph. Because of the involvement of the spinal canal with this injury pattern, the risk for a significant neurologic injury is increased. Stage 2 extension-distraction injuries include some disruption of the posterior ligamentous complex, in particular the facet capsules, which is necessary to allow the retrolisthesis to occur.

The type of degree of neurologic injury varies significantly among those sustaining extension-distraction injuries. Patients with severe preexisting cervical spinal stenosis resulting from advanced spondylosis are at high risk for SCI, as are those with ankylosing spondylitis and DISH. According to Taylor,[2] during a hyperextension injury, the posteroinferior margin of the cephalad vertebra compresses the anterior aspect of the cord against the lamina and ligamentum flavum of the caudal vertebra, resulting in cord trauma. Clinically, central cord syndromes are most commonly seen with more minor degrees of trauma, although patients with severe anterior cord syndromes and even complete cord injuries are occasionally encountered with stage 2 injuries.

TREATMENT

Patients with either stage 1 or 2 extension-distraction injuries are generally considered candidates for surgical stabilization. Because of the unstable nature of these injuries, surgery provides the best method to prevent vertebral displacement and neural injury. Some patients with severe medical comorbidities may not be good candidates for surgical treatment. In such cases, halo-vest or rigid cervical orthosis immobilization may be considered, although displacement or incomplete healing remains a risk with nonoperative treatment.

Patients with stage 1 injuries who are acceptable candidates for surgical treatment are most commonly treated with anterior discectomy and fusion using rigid anterior cervical plating. Such a construct restores the disrupted anterior tension band and allows long-term stability through the fusion of the anterior column.

Stage 2 injuries can be more difficult to manage. Reduction of the retrolisthesis of the upper cervical body can be difficult to achieve from an anterior approach. In cases in which significant malalignment is present, a posterior procedure will allow realignment of the spinal column. This can then be followed by an anterior discectomy and fusion using anterior plating to reconstruct the disrupted anterior column. Vaccaro et al.[3] suggested such an approach, using an initial posterior approach to realign the spine, followed by anterior grafting and plating. Alternative strategies, including corpectomy of the superior vertebral body to obtain adequate decompression of the spinal cord with a circumferential stabilization procedure, have been recommended by some authors, especially in the setting of preexisting cervical canal stenosis at the site of the injury. A disadvantage of this technique is that a corpectomy increases the degree of instability at the site of injury and thus circumferential instrumentation should be included.

OUTCOME

The long-term outcome of extension-distraction injuries depends to a large degree on the neurologic status of the patient following the injury. Stable reconstruction of the spinal column is achievable with modern instrumentation and fusion techniques. However, significant neurologic injury may result in severe functional consequences that are not repairable at the current time. Because extension-distraction injuries often occur in patients who are elderly or afflicted with ankylosing spondylitis, medical comorbidities also play a significant role in their overall outcome.

REFERENCES

1. Allen BL Jr, Ferguson RL, Lehmann TR, et al. A mechanistic classification of closed, indirect fractures and dislocations of the lower cervical spine. *Spine* 1982;7:1–27.
2. Taylor AR. The mechanism of injury to the spinal cord in the neck without damage to vertebral column. *J Bone Joint Surg Br* 1951;33:543–547.
3. Vaccaro AR, Klein GR, Thaller JB, et al. Distraction extension injuries of the cervical spine. *J Spinal Disord* 2001;14:193–200.

CHAPTER 25E

Subaxial Injuries: Lateral Compression Injuries

Carl N. Graf and David Schwartz

INTRODUCTION

Traditionally, injuries to the cervical spine have been attributed to hyperflexion- and hyperextension-type mechanisms. In the 1960s, Roaf and Holdsworth proposed that rotational and compressive forces were also dominant in these injuries. Since then, there has been a relative lack of information concerning lateral flexion injuries in the literature. Allen and Ferguson[1] developed a classification system to describe cervical spine injuries based on the mechanism of the injury. The mechanism was determined by the posture of the head and neck at the time of injury, as well as the location and direction of force. The Allen and Ferguson classification describes injuries as compressive flexion, vertical compression, distractive flexion, compressive extension, distractive extension, and, as described in this chapter, lateral flexion. Of Allen and Ferguson's 165 cases, only 5 were included in the lateral flexion category, making it the one with the least frequent injuries in their study. Thus, there are relatively limited reports in the literature of lateral flexion injuries. Of these five patients, four were men and one was a woman. The average age was 22.8 years. In this series, only one patient sustained a spinal cord injury (SCI). This patient's injury was classified as a lateral flexion stage 2 pattern and a complete neurologic injury. The remaining four were all lateral flexion type 1 patterns, and all were neurologically intact. In another series of lateral flexion injuries, Roaf[2] reported on five cases. All had a neurologic deficit, either a SCI or a brachial plexus injury.

MECHANISM OF INJURY AND CLASSIFICATION

The mechanism of this injury consists of lateral compression of the vertebral body, disc, uncovertebral joints, and posterior elements. The incidence of neurologic deficit is variable in these types of injuries.[3,4] There is an association with injuries of the brachial plexus. These injuries are commonly referred to as "burners" or "stingers" and are often seen in contact sports such as football. Cervical orthoses are now commonly placed to help prevent lateral flexion and hyperextension neck movements and thus avoid these types of injuries (Fig. 25E.1).[5]

As previously noted, the classification of lateral flexion injuries was developed by Ferguson and Allen. This classification further divided the lateral flexion injury group into two stages. A stage 1 injury consists of an asymmetric compression fracture of the vertebral body plus a vertebral arch fracture on the ipsilateral side without displacement on an anteroposterior radiographic view. The asymmetric compression injury may involve an articular process or uncovertebral joint.

The lateral flexion stage 2 injury has two components. The first is a unilateral compression fracture of the vertebral body, such as that seen in the lateral flexion stage 1 injury. The second is either a

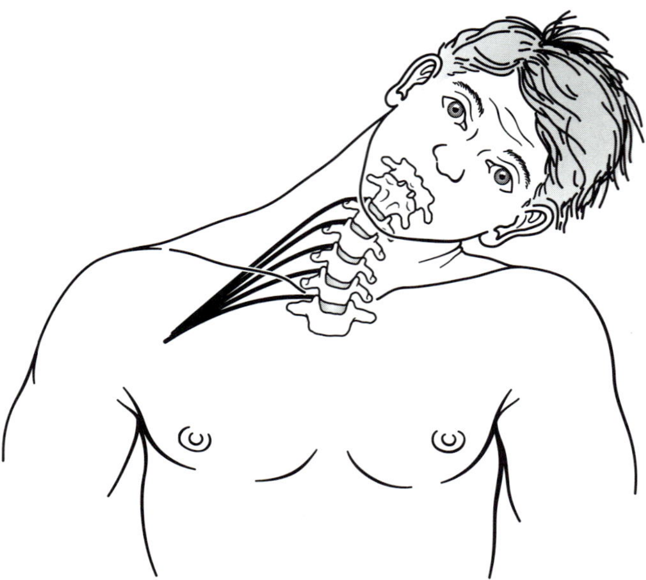

FIGURE 25E.1. Representation of stretched brachial plexis during violent lateral flexion of head.

displaced fracture of the posterior arch, ipsilateral to the lateral vertebral body compression fracture, or a contralateral ligamentous injury. The fracture lines of the displaced fragment of the arch are often through the lamina or facet joint and the pedicle. The contralateral ligamentous injury is easily seen on the anteroposterior radiograph as a separation of the contralateral facet joint articulation.

In both stages the vertebral body experiences a rotational moment. This results in a primary compressive force between the vertebral bodies on the side contralateral to the side in which the force is applied. Additionally there is a secondary minor distractive force on the side ipsilateral to where the force to the head is applied. In the stage 2 injury, these combined forces result in either fracture and displacement of the ipsilateral posterior arch or a separation of the ipsilateral joint under distractive forces. This is in addition to the compression fracture of the vertebral body (Fig. 25E.2).

DIAGNOSIS

These injuries are initially diagnosed with plain radiographs. However, without close scrutiny, they may be missed. One may see a sagittally oriented fracture of the lateral mass on lateral cervical spine radiographs, although this may be difficult to identify. On the anteroposterior radiographs an asymmetric compression of one side of the vertebral body may be noted. This should lead to further investigation. Although oblique radiographs may be helpful, currently computed tomography (CT) is the study of choice. The CT study should include thin cuts, as well as both sagittal and coronal reconstructions. With these studies the type of injury should be discernable. Additionally, CT will help determine the stability of the injury, leading to treatment recommendations. In the lateral flexion stage 2 fracture, it is important to determine the competency of the facet joints. Both the displaced facet joint and the distracted facet joint should be considered unstable. Magnetic resonance imaging (MRI) is also valuable in delineating the presence of soft tissue and ligamentous injuries and the integrity of the spinal cord.

TREATMENT

INITIAL TREATMENT

It is important to note that these injuries are usually secondary to great force, and other concomitant spinal or brachial plexus injuries may exist. According to the protocol for any spine fracture, a full

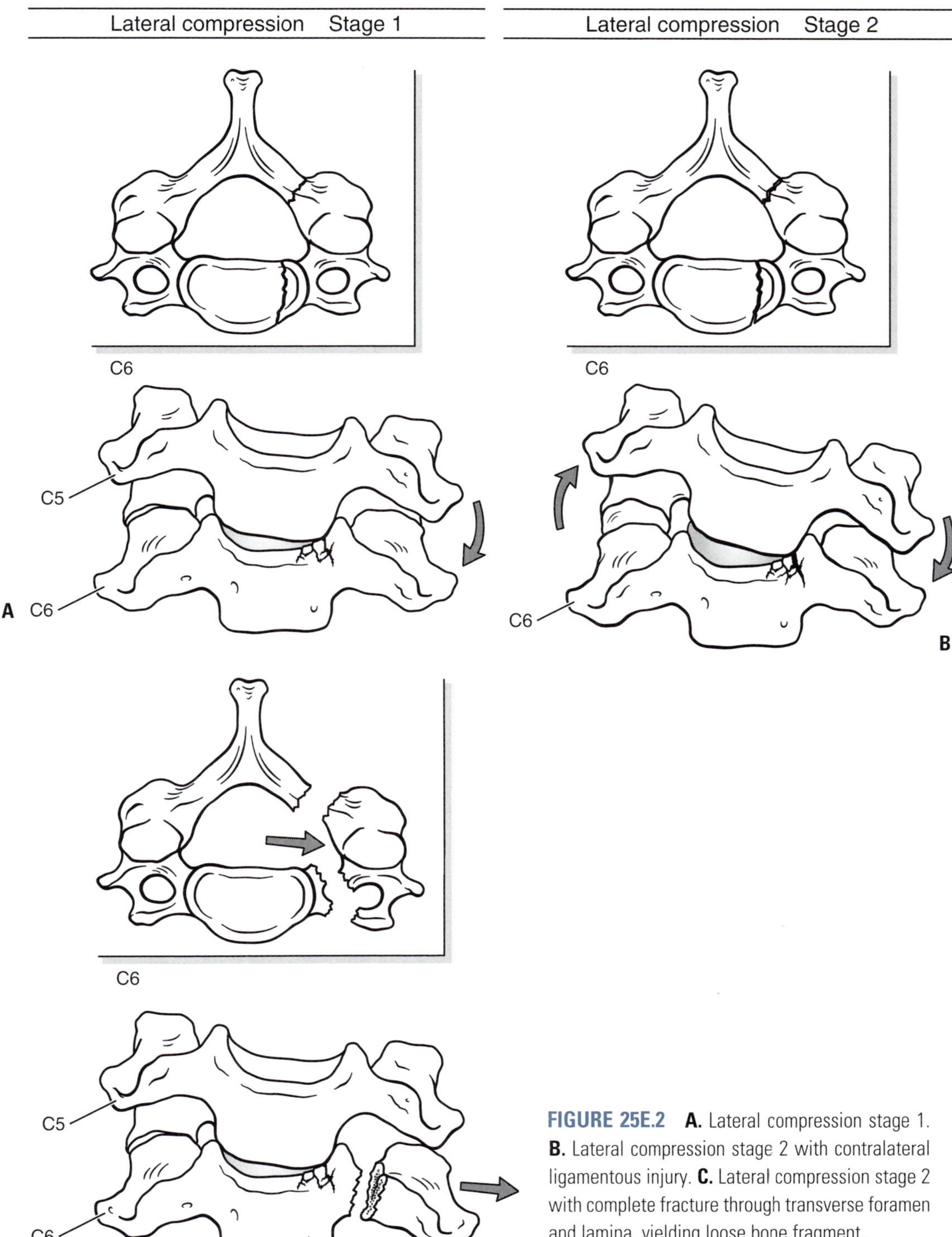

FIGURE 25E.2 **A.** Lateral compression stage 1. **B.** Lateral compression stage 2 with contralateral ligamentous injury. **C.** Lateral compression stage 2 with complete fracture through transverse foramen and lamina, yielding loose bone fragment.

set of cervical, thoracic, and lumbar radiographs should be obtained at a minimum. CT is required if an injury to the spine is detected.

Initially these patients should be immobilized. This should follow the protocol of cervical spine immobilization with a cervical collar or halo vest, bed rest, and possibly a Rotarest bed with log-roll precautions. This should be continued until a better understanding of the fracture is obtained. In addition to the general neurologic evaluation, careful evaluation should be performed for isolated cervical nerve root injuries.

DEFINITIVE TREATMENT

Most of these injuries are stable injuries without neurologic compromise. Thus, the vast majority are treated nonoperatively. However, to develop a treatment plan for this injury pattern, a sense of the stability of the fracture must be determined. Most of the lateral flexion stage 1 fractures would appear to be stable. In the absence of a neurologic injury, it would be expected that the osseous structures and soft tissues should heal in 6 to 12 weeks. If, as expected, this injury appears stable, immobilization for 6 to 12 weeks should suffice. Immobilization in either a halo vest or rigid cervical orthosis should be adequate. No study could be found in the literature comparing or suggesting an advantage of one type of immobilization over the other for this injury pattern.

If, on evaluation, cervical root involvement or other neurologic injury is found, treatment may be directed by the presenting neurology rather than the stability of this injury pattern. This would require assessing the neurologic injury and developing a plan to restore normal function. In the case of nerve root compression, this may be by direct posterior decompression (foraminotomy) and fusion. Additionally, anterior indirect decompression by way of an anterior cervical discectomy and fusion with a plate may also be appropriate. Again, each individual fracture must be scrutinized for the most appropriate treatment plan.

Patients with a lateral flexion stage 2 injury pattern have a more unstable injury. As is the case in patients with a lateral flexion stage 2 injury, a sense for the stability of the fracture must be developed by evaluating both the osseous and ligamentous injuries. Although the osseous injuries will often heal primarily, the contralateral facet separation or dislocation is concerning. This type of injury is associated with a fair amount of soft tissue disruption, and a posterior fusion is the treatment of choice. The displaced lateral mass fracture is also of concern. There is a high probability for early instability in these fractures, and again early surgical intervention is warranted. It is important in displaced lateral mass fractures to be aware that two motion segments are involved. This free lateral mass will lead to instability of the vertebrae above and below the level of the fracture. Therefore, a displaced lateral mass of the sixth cervical vertebra will require a fusion from the fifth cervical vertebra to the seventh cervical vertebra posteriorly. The surgical approach (anterior or posterior) depends on surgeon preference and the individual characteristics of each fracture. Anterior surgical intervention may be required if there is associated anterior spinal cord compression. Root injuries may be addressed either through a foraminotomy or facetectomy and fusion, or anteriorly through an indirect decompression of the foramen with distraction between the two adjacent vertebral bodies. Instrumentation techniques useful with this injury include anterior cervical plates and lateral mass screws and wiring techniques.[6] Because of the rarity of this injury pattern, there are no predefined treatment algorithms, and each fracture again must be evaluated on an individual basis.

PROGNOSIS

Overall, the prognosis for lateral flexion injuries is good. As noted previously, there is a relatively low rate of neurologic injury. No long-term study of this fracture subset can be found in the literature. This is likely because of the overall low incidence of this injury pattern.

COMPLICATIONS

Although neurologic compromise has been shown to be relatively rare in lateral flexion injuries, there are case reports in the literature. In patients treated nonoperatively, there is always the risk for malunion and nonunion. This may be associated with chronic neck pain or neurologic injury. The overall complication rate is low, and most go on to heal without a problem. The operative complications are similar to those seen in all posterior and anterior cervical fusion surgeries. These include, but are not limited to, neurologic compromise, nonunion, and loss of reduction. Again, with the overall low incidence of this fracture subset, clinical evidence and follow-up data are scarce.

REFERENCES

1. Allen B, Ferguson R. A mechanistic classification of closed, indirect fractures and dislocations of the lower cervical spine. *Spine* 1982;7:1–27.
2. Roaf R. Lateral flexion injuries of the cervical spine. *J Bone Joint Surg Br* 1963;45:36–38.
3. Dai L. Disc degeneration and cervical instability: correlation of magnetic resonance imaging with radiography. *Spine* 1998;23:1734–1738.
4. Lee C, Woodring JH. Sagittally oriented fractures of the lateral masses of the cervical vertebrae. *Trauma Injury Infect Crit Care* 1991;31:1638–1643.
5. Hovis D, Limbird T. An evaluation of cervical orthoses in limiting hyperextension and lateral flexion in football. *Med Sci Sports Exerc* 1994;26:872–876.
6. Roy-Cammille R, Mazel G, Salliant G. Les fractures-separation du massif articulatire. In: Roy-Cammile R, ed. *Rachis Cervical Inferiur: Sixiemes Journees D'Orthopedie de la Pitie.* Paris: Masson, 1988:94–103.

CHAPTER 25F

Subaxial Injuries: Pillar (Pedicle and Lateral Mass) Fractures

Kuniyoshi Abumi, Yoshihisa Kotani, Manabu Ito, and Alexander R. Vaccaro

INTRODUCTION

With the recent progression of medical imaging technologies, an increasing number of pillar fractures in the cervical spine are clinically detected in the cervical spine. These often require a conservative treatment; however, surgical treatment is indicated when there is a neurologic disturbance or definite segmental spinal instability at the injured segment. The purpose of this chapter is to discuss the pathological condition, diagnosis, classification, and treatment of pillar fracture of the cervical spine.

MECHANISM OF INJURY

Pillar fractures in the cervical spine, which include fractures of the lateral mass, articular process, and pedicle, were generally accepted as being produced by hyperextension or hyperextension combined with a rotational injury mechanism, involving mostly unilateral structures of the cervical vertebra.[1–3] According to Allen's classification, most pillar injuries are classified into compressive-extension injuries or lateral flexion injuries.[4,5] In lateral flexion injuries, lateral mass fractures are often comminuted and associated with asymmetric vertebral body fractures. Purely symmetric hyperextension mechanisms may occasionally produce a traumatic spondylolysis of the posterior elements.

CLASSIFICATION

Allen's mechanistic classification describes in detail the proposed mechanisms of traumatic subaxial cervical spine injuries; however, it is often difficult to envision a particular fracture type with this classification system. In this chapter a classification of pillar fractures of the cervical spine is presented.[5] The classification divides pillar fractures into the following four subtypes: (a) separation, (b) comminution, (c) split, and (d) traumatic spondylolysis (Fig. 25F.1). In addition, isolated superior and inferior articular process fractures may also occur, often produced by asymmetric cervical hyperextension mechanisms.

SEPARATION FRACTURE

In a separation type of injury, a fracture line passes through one pedicle perpendicular to the axis of the pedicle and another fracture line passes vertically through the ipsilateral lamina (Fig. 25F.2).

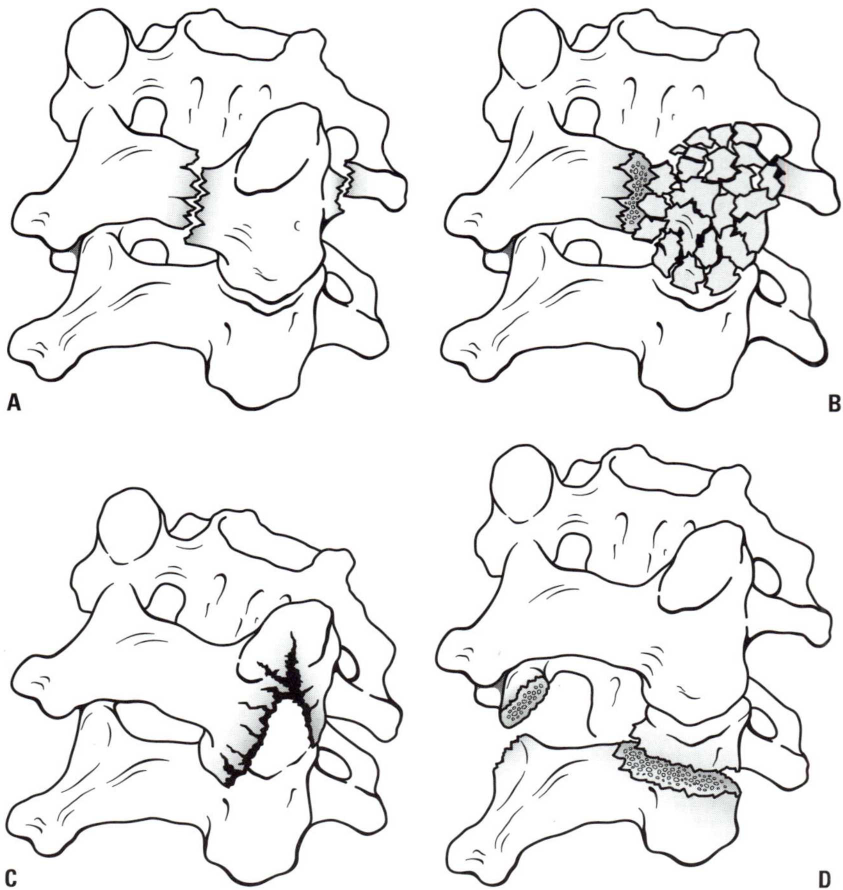

FIGURE 25F.1. Subtypes of lateral mass fractures. **A.** Separation fracture. **B.** Comminution type. **C.** Split type. **D.** Traumatic spondylolysis. There are bilateral horizontal fracture lines at the pars interarticularis, leading to a separation between anterior and posterior spinal elements. (Kotani K, Abumi K, Ito M, et al. Cervical spine injuries associated with lateral mass and facet joint fracture: new classification and surgical treatment with pedicle screw fixation. *Eur Spine J* 2005;14:69–77.)

This, in essence, isolates an articular mass and separates it from the rest of the cervical vertebra. A fracture of this type minimizes the stabilizing capacity of both the cephalad and caudad facet joints because of the location of the fracture lines.[6,7] Levine et al.[8] reported a high incidence of anterior vertebral translation at the fractured level (79%) and the cephalad-adjacent vertebra (21%) in 24 cases of lateral mass fracture separations.

COMMINUTION FRACTURE

The comminution type of fracture consists of multiple fracture lines in the lateral mass, with significant fragmentation frequently accompanying a lateral wedge deformity in the coronal plane (Fig. 25F.3). Both the superior and inferior articular processes are also compromised, and, therefore, the stabilizing capacity of both adjacent facet joints to the abrupted vertebra is reduced to some extent.

SPLIT FRACTURE

The split type of fracture has a vertical fracture line in the coronal plane through a unilateral lateral mass extending up through the inferior articular process, creating an anterior-posterior separation of the articular pillar. This fracture subtype is similar to the fracture type previously reported by Sim[9]

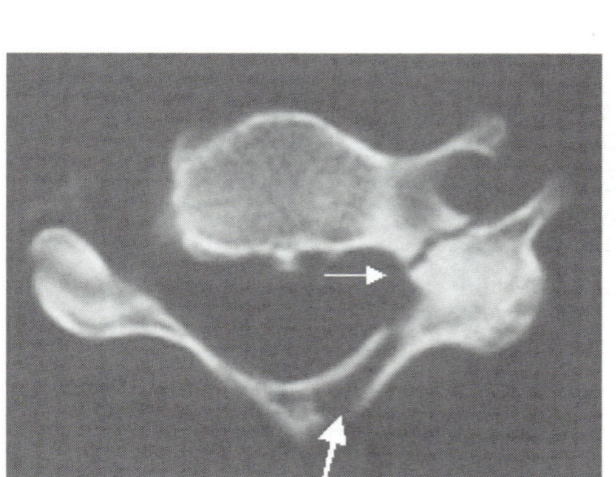
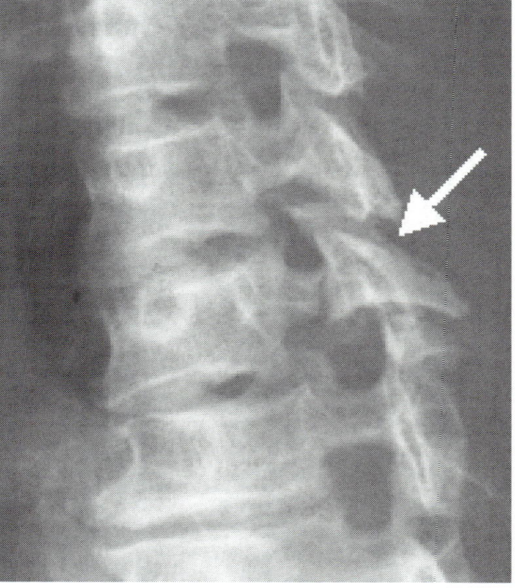

FIGURE 25F.2. Separation fracture. **A.** Separation fracture is defined as two fracture lines of unilateral lamina and pedicle, thereby isolating and separating the unilateral entire articular mass. **B.** The nerve root in the neural foramen is compressed by leaned articular process by horizontalization of the floating lateral mass.

and Yetkin et al.[10]; however, this injury type was never recognized as a subtype of a lateral mass fracture. Sim[9] reported five cases of this type of injury and noted that segmental stability was likely to be adequate with nonsurgical intervention. This injury type usually presents with some degree of anterior translation, axial rotational deformity, and local lateral wedging in the coronal plane. Some authors have recommended surgical intervention in this fracture subtype because of the potential for recognized persistent neck pain (Fig. 25F.4).

TRAUMATIC SPONDYLOLYSIS

A traumatic spondylolysis of the subaxial cervical spine involves a bilateral horizontal fracture through the pars interarticularis, or lateral mass, that may lead to a separation (listhesis) between the anterior

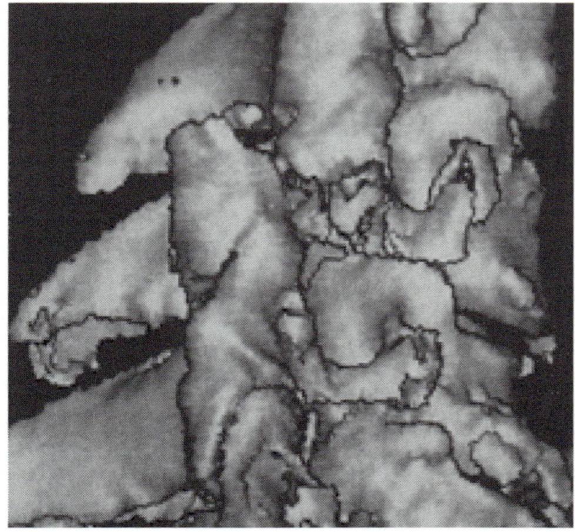
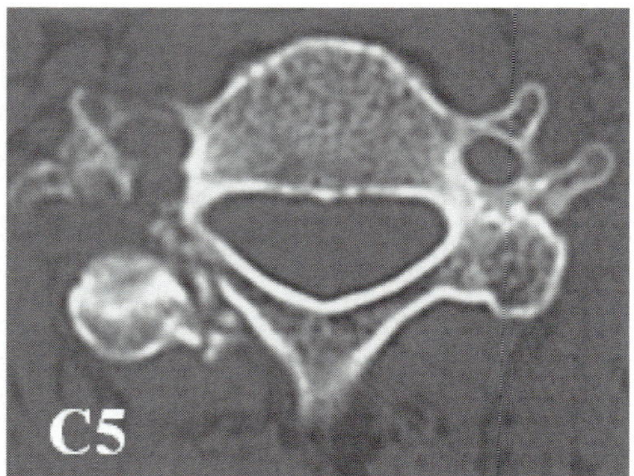

FIGURE 25F.3. Comminution fracture. The comminution type of fracture consists of multiple fracture lines in the lateral mass with significant fragmentations.

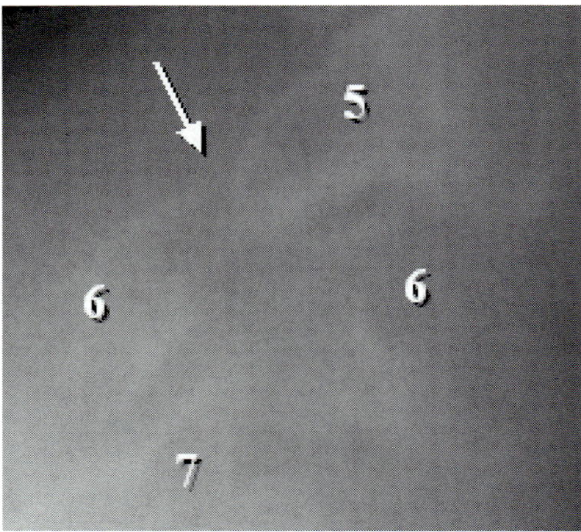

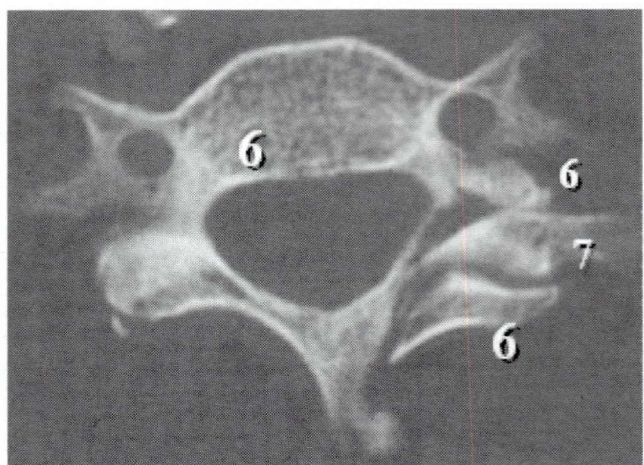

FIGURE 25F.4. Split fracture. There is vertical fracture line on a coronal plane in the unilateral lateral mass, creating an anterior-posterior separation with the invagination of superior articular process of caudal adjacent vertebra.

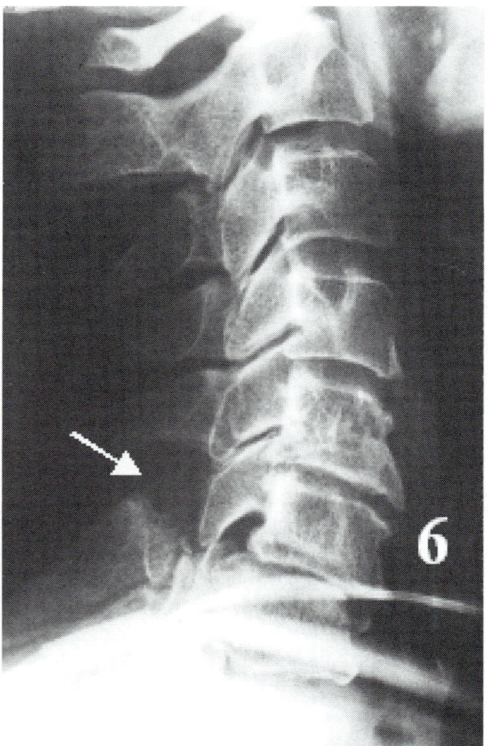

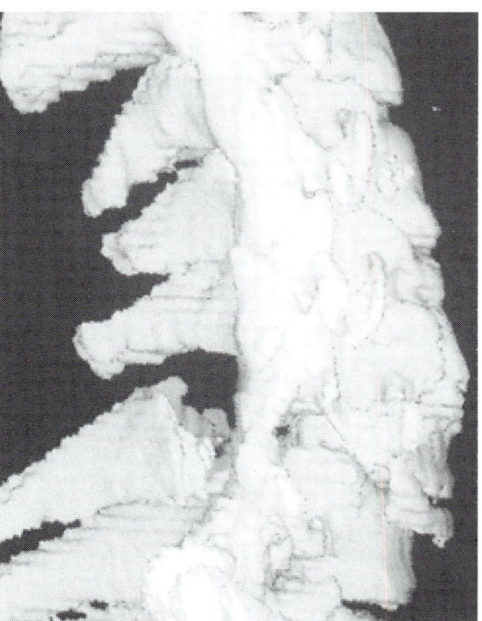

FIGURE 25F.5. Traumatic spondylolysis. Bilateral horizontal fracture lines appear at the pars interarticularis, leading to a separation between anterior and posterior spinal elements. The anterior portion of injured vertebra is displaced with partial vertebral body width.

and posterior spinal elements. This injury subtype may also involve bilateral superior and inferior articular process fractures or a combination of both fractures at consecutive vertebrae (Fig. 25F.5). This fracture type is classified as a compressive-extension injury by the Allen classification system. The vertebral body of the injured vertebra level may slip anteriorly in more severe injuries (traumatic spondylolisthesis).

ISOLATED ARTICULAR PROCESS FRACTURES

A linear fracture through a unilateral articular process represents this fracture subtype. There may or may not be an associated anterorotary displacement of the vertebral body (Fig. 25F.6). This type of injury has been classified as a stage 1 compressive-extension injury in Allen's classification. There may be a single nerve root lesion with this injury type resulting from superior articular process displacement into the neural foramen.

STABILITY OF PILLAR FRACTURE

Injuries of the true lateral mass often present with a higher incidence of sagittal plane deformity than that seen with isolated articular process fractures. Levine et al.[8] reported a high incidence of anterior vertebral translation in 24 cases of lateral mass fracture separation. As noted previously, anterior translation of the fractured vertebra was observed in 79% of patients along with a 21% incidence of sagittal plane deformity in cephalad-adjacent vertebra. These data were similar to the findings of Kotani et al.[5] The split and comminution fracture subtypes have a significantly higher rate of spinal malalignment compared to the separation fracture subtype.[5] This may be a reflection of the higher energy transfer seen in the split and comminution fracture subtypes.

According to the study by Kotani et al.,[5] 76% of cases had injury to the anterior longitudinal ligament (ALL) and disc, 35% to the posterior longitudinal ligament (PLL), and 12% to the supraspinous ligament (SSL) and interspinous ligament (ISL) on MRI at the injury level. Halliday et al.[11] reported that 50% of cases had injury to the ALL, 29% to the PLL, and 75% to the ISL in 24 cases of lateral mass and facet fractures. It is not unusual to note the higher frequency of ALL and

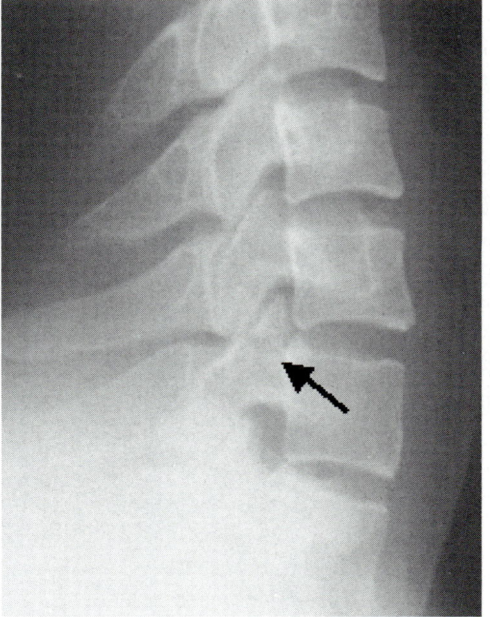

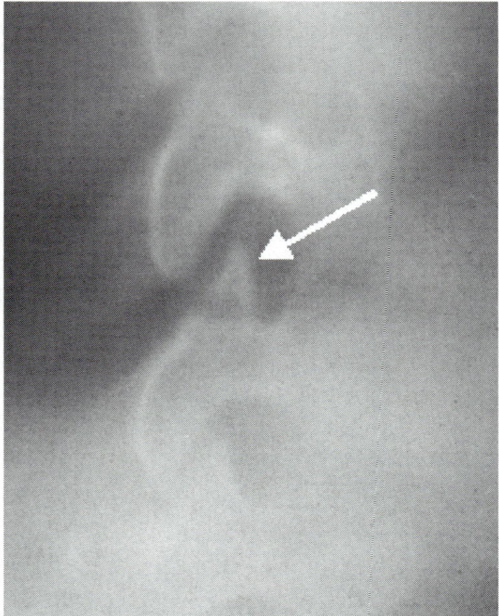

FIGURE 25F.6. Isolated articular process fractures. A linear fracture through the ipsilateral superior or inferior articular process represents this type of fracture.

disc injuries in the setting of a compressive-extension mechanism, common to these injury subtypes, than injuries to the SSL or ISL. Stability to two motion segments is often compromised in separation or comminution fracture subtypes. Injury to the intervertebral disc is often limited to one level with pillar injuries. Understanding the level of compromise to the motion segment is extremely important because it has significant implications on the extent of fusion that may be necessary. This makes the use of MRI extremely valuable when assessing disc integrity. In the setting of a traumatic spondylolysis or listhesis, instability is confined to the caudad motion segment with concomitant injury to the intervertebral disc. With regard to articular process fractures, instability is limited to the motion segment of the particular articular process. For example, a superior articular process injury may result in instability to the cephalad motion segment, whereas an inferior articular process fracture may lead to instability of the caudal vertebral body.

TREATMENT

INITIAL TREATMENT

Initial treatment of pillar fracture is often guided by associated injuries such as the presence or absence of a neurologic deficit and associated spinal injuries. Spinal stability is often not severely compromised in most types of pillar fractures except in advanced-grade spondylolisthesis. Initial spinal immobilization is often adequately conferred with a cervical orthosis (e.g., Philadelphia collar, SOMI orthosis, Minerva jacket, etc.) in those without a neurologic deficit or severe radicular pain. Surgical intervention is often selected in cases with associated neurologic compromise or a significant translational or kyphotic deformity. In these situations, immobilization via skeletal traction or halo-vest immobilization is often recommended until surgical intervention.

DEFINITIVE TREATMENT

Separation Fracture

If a patient has no neurologic deficit, nonsurgical treatment using a cervical orthosis for 6 to 10 weeks is often recommended. The bony fractures and floating lateral mass can be expected to heal with minimal translational deformity. Delayed instability or nerve root injury may occur in the setting of intervertebral disc injury, especially during orthosis immobilization. This delayed complication may be managed surgically at any point during treatment before fracture healing. Surgical stabilization anteriorly consisting of a single-level fusion involving the caudal motion segment or the level above and below the injury level with a posterior approach may be necessary with unstable injuries or in the presence of a neurologic deficit. The posterior approach ensures more optimal nerve root decompression when a nerve root injury is identified on direct visualization of the nerve root. Various fixation methods may be used posteriorly, such as spinous process wiring or unilateral or bilateral lateral mass, facet, or pedicle screw fixation[12,13] (Fig. 25F.7). A single screw osteosynthesis may be attempted to reduce the injured level vertebral body to the involved pedicle.[6] However, residual anterior translation of the repaired vertebra may still persist, especially if there is injury to the caudad intervertebral disc.[15] Therefore, this method of treatment is recommended only in separation-type injuries with a minimum of disc damage demonstrated on MRI.

Comminution Fracture

Nonsurgical treatment using a cervical orthosis for 6 to 10 weeks is recommended for this fracture type in the absence of a neurologic deficit. Surgical intervention should be considered for the comminuted fracture type in the presence of a neurologic deficit. In this setting, a posterior approach is often adequate to ensure nerve root decompression. Both the superior and inferior articular processes are often compromised in severely comminuted fractures, which require a two-motion segment stabilization procedure. If minimal comminution is present or if there is only minimal injury to the cranial or caudal facet joint, a single-level fixation procedure can often be selected. Nerve

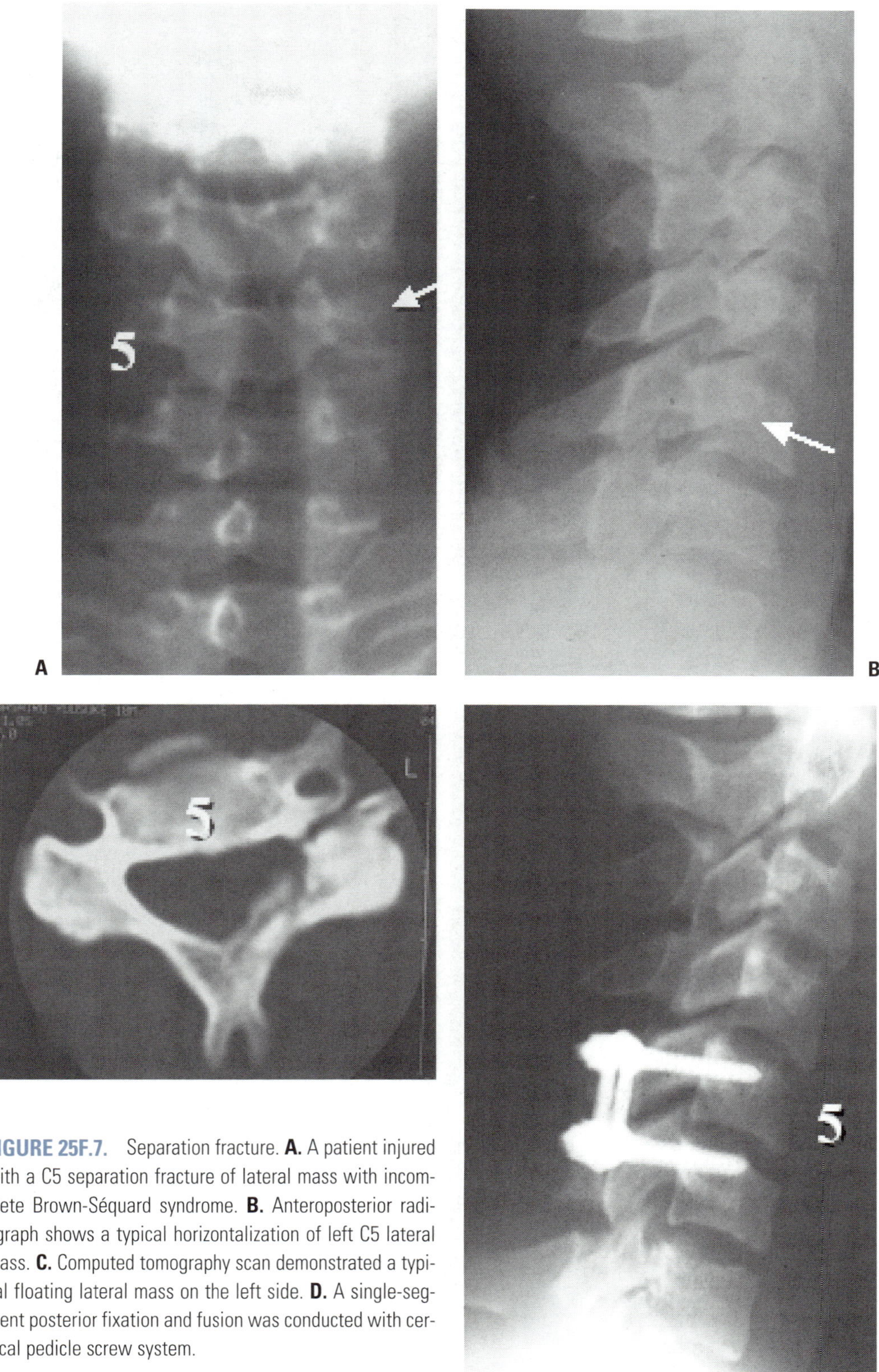

FIGURE 25F.7. Separation fracture. **A.** A patient injured with a C5 separation fracture of lateral mass with incomplete Brown-Séquard syndrome. **B.** Anteroposterior radiograph shows a typical horizontalization of left C5 lateral mass. **C.** Computed tomography scan demonstrated a typical floating lateral mass on the left side. **D.** A single-segment posterior fixation and fusion was conducted with cervical pedicle screw system.

A,B

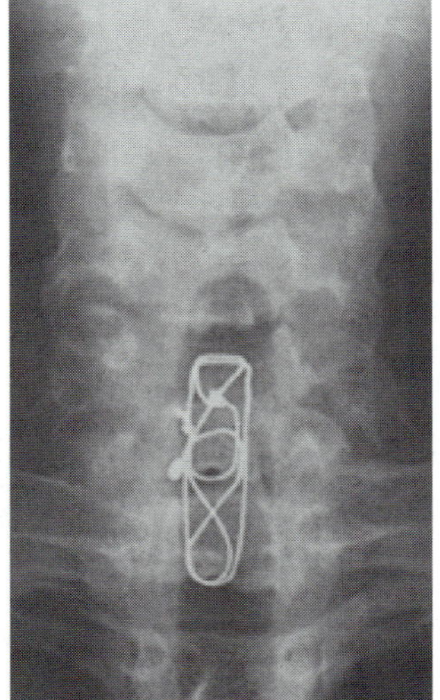

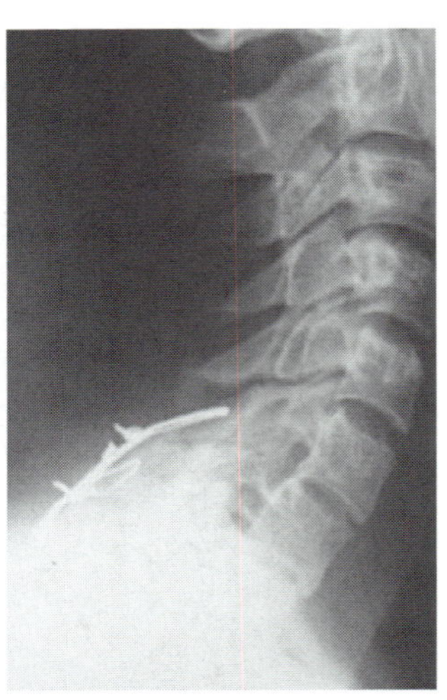

C

FIGURE 25F.8. Comminution type fracture. A patient had a comminution-type C7 lateral mass fracture with a C7 nerve root lesion. A two-level posterior fixation and fusion was conducted, with spinous process wiring.

decompression can be performed via a posterior foraminotomy with or without a laminotomy, considering the degree of nerve root compression. Spinous process wiring or a combination of spinous process wiring, lateral mass, facet screw, and pedicle screw fixation may be employed (Fig. 25F.8). Lateral mass and pedicle screw fixation is unsuitable at the level of a comminuted lateral mass, and therefore, screw fixation would be required above and below the injury level.

Split Fracture

Split fractures may be managed nonoperatively in the absence of significant vertebral translation. In the setting of vertebral translation, surgical stabilization is recommended, with the number of immobilized motion segments contingent on the anatomic structures disrupted. Spinous process wiring, lateral mass screw fixation, or pedicle screw fixation may all be employed as surgical anchors with this injury type (Fig. 25F.9).

Traumatic Spondylolysis

Traumatic subaxial cervical spondylolysis without anterior vertebral displacement may be treated adequately by nonsurgical methods in the absence of a neurologic deficit. In the setting of a listhesis, surgical intervention is often recommended because of the presumed injury to the posterior bony elements and intervertebral disc. This injury subtype may be stabilized via an anterior approach stabilizing the caudal vertebral motion segment. Because of the degree of instability present with this injury (listhesis), adjunctive halo immobilization should be considered when using an anterior stand-alone surgical procedure. Often an adjunctive posterior stabilizing procedure is recommended with displaced injuries. This requires, in the majority of cases, extension to the cephalad motion segment to obtain adequate stability. If pedicle screw fixation is chosen for surgical stabilization, because of this method of fixation's greater pull-out strength, a stand-alone posterior stabilization procedure often is sufficient with displaced injuries (Fig. 25F.10).[15,16]

Isolated Articular Process Fractures

Isolated articular process injuries can be managed adequately nonoperatively with a cervical orthosis for 6 to 10 weeks. Surgical intervention is considered an option in the setting of a nerve root injury.

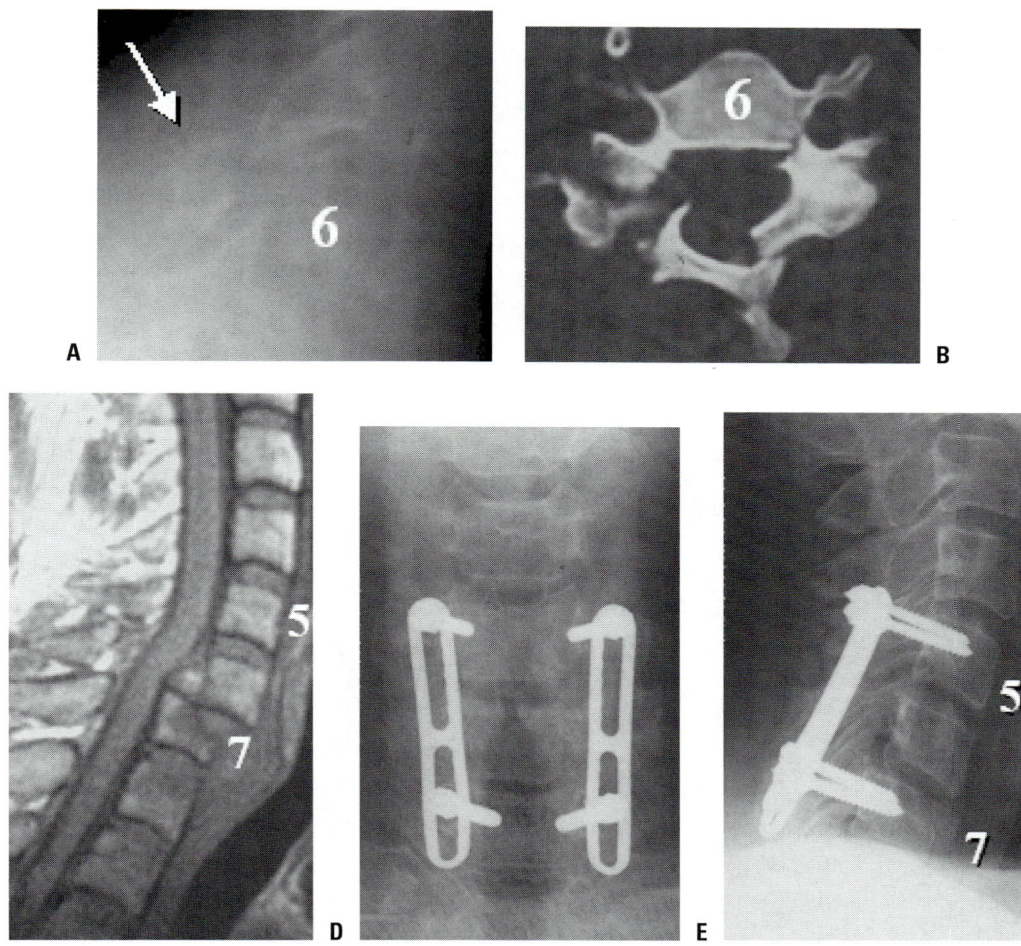

FIGURE 25F.9. Split-type fracture. **A,B.** A patient with split-type lateral mass fracture of C6 sustained an incomplete spinal cord lesion. Lateral laminogram and computed tomography image demonstrate splitting of C6 lateral mass by invagination of the superior articular process of C7. **C.** Magnetic resonance image showing anterior slipping of C6, destruction of the cephalad portion of C7 vertebral body, and spinal cord compression. **D,E.** Two-level posterior fixation and fusion was performed with a cervical pedicle screw system.

Isolated inferior articular process fractures often are not associated with a nerve root deficit. This may occur with these injuries in the setting of a traumatic disc herniation or narrowed spinal canal. Isolated superior articular process fractures may be associated with a nerve root lesion caused by a ventrally migrated articular process fragment. Surgical decompression via a posterior foraminotomy with removal of the fractured articular process is recommended with this injury subtype. Simple spinous process wiring, and lateral mass, facet, or pedicle screw fixation may all be used as stabilizing anchors.

PROGNOSIS

Patterns of neurologic deficits associated with pillar fracture are mostly nerve root lesions or, infrequently, an incomplete spinal cord lesion. Neurologic prognosis is often satisfactory after cervical stabilization following fracture healing or surgical intervention.

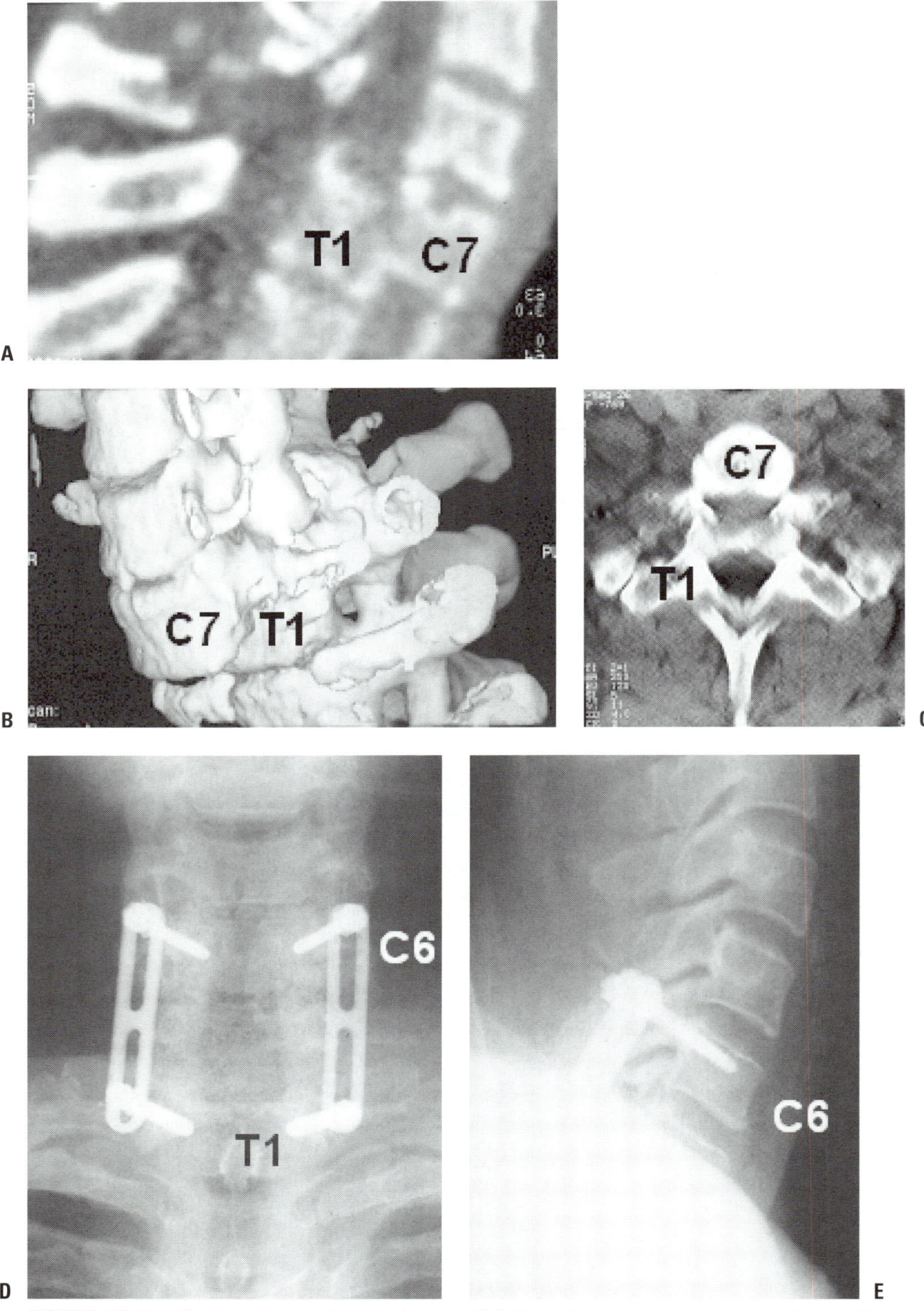

FIGURE 25F.10. High-grade traumatic spondylolysis. **A,B,C.** The patient sustained a complete spinal cord lesion in a traffic collision. Reconstructive computed tomography (CT) scans demonstrate anterior displacement of C7 vertebral body with bilateral pedicles and cephalad portion of the lateral masses with full vertebral body width displacement. **D,E.** Application of distraction force between screws inserted into the bilateral pedicle of C6 and T1 provided sufficient reduction of C7 on T1. *(continued)*

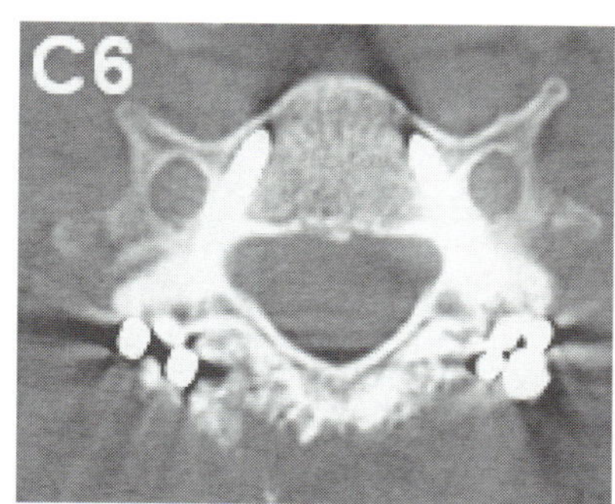

F

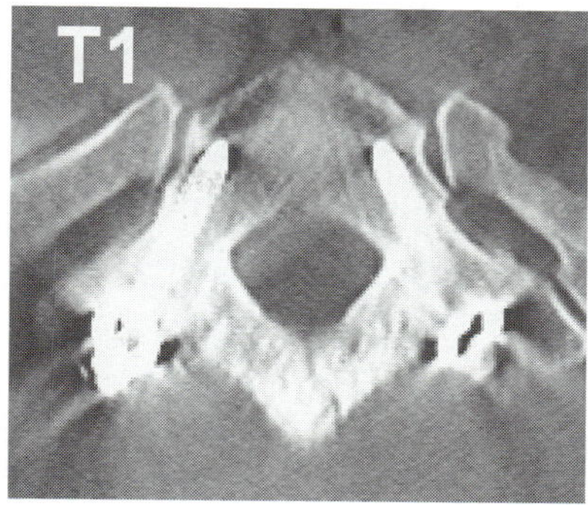

G

FIGURE 25F.10. *(continued)* **F,G.** CT scans demonstrate proper screw location and trajectory. (Courtesy of Dr. H Taneichi, Department of Orthopaedics, Dokkyo University, Tochigi, Japan.)

REFERENCES

1. Harris JH, Mirvis SE. *Radiology of Acute Cervical Spine Trauma.* 3rd ed. Baltimore: William & Wilkins, 1996: 320–339.
2. Whitley JE, Forsyth HF. The classification of cervical spine injuries. *AJR Am J Roentgenol* 1960;83:633–644.
3. Woodring JH, Lee C. Limitations of cervical radiography in the evaluation of acute cervical trauma. *J Trauma* 1993;34:32–39.
4. Allen B Jr, Ferguson RL, Lehmann TR. A mechanistic classification of closed, indirect fractures and dislocations of the lower cervical spine. *Spine* 1982;7:1–27.
5. Kotani K, Abumi K, Ito M, et al. Cervical spine injuries associated with lateral mass and facet joint fracture: new classification and surgical treatment with pedicle screw fixation. *Eur Spine J* 2005;14:69–77.
6. Jeanneret B, Gebhard JS, Magerl F. Transpedicular screw fixation of articular mass fracture-separation: results of an anatomical study and operative technique. *J Spinal Disord* 1994;7:222–229.
7. Judet R, Roy-Camille R, Zerah JC. Fracture du rachis cervical, fracture separation du massif articulaire. *Rev Chir Orthop* 1970;56:155–164.
8. Levine AM, Mazel C, Roy-Camille R. Management of fracture separations of the articular mass using posterior cervical plating. *Spine* 1992;17:S447–S454.
9. Sim E. Vertical facet splitting: a special variant of rotatory dislocations of the cervical spine. *J Neurosurg* 1995;82:239–243.
10. Yetkin Z, Osborn AG, Giles D. Uncovertebral and facet joint dislocations in cervical articular pillar fractures: CT evaluation. *AJNR Am J Neuroradiol* 1985;6:633–637.
11. Halliday AL, Henderson BR, Hart BL, et al. The management of unilateral lateral mass/facet fractures of the subaxial cervical spine: the use of magnetic resonance imaging to predict instability. *Spine* 1997;22:2614–1621.
12. Abumi K, Ito H, Taneichi H. Transpedicular screw fixations for traumatic lesions of the middle and lower cervical spine: description of the techniques and preliminary report. *J Spinal Disord* 1994;7:19–28.
13. Abumi K, Ito M, Kotani Y. Cervical pedicle screw fixation. In: Cervical Spine Research Society, eds. *The Cervical Spine Surgery Atlas.* 2nd ed. Philadelphia: Lippincott Williams Wilkins, 2004.
14. Kotani Y, Cunningham BW, Abumi K, et al. Biomechanical analysis of cervical stabilization systems: an assessment of transpediclar screw fixation in the cervical spine. *Spine* 1994;19:2529–2539.
15. Jones EL, Heller JG, Silcox DH, et al. Cervical pedicle screws versus lateral mass screws: anatomic feasibility and biomechanical comparison. *Spine* 1997;22:977–982.
16. Smith GR, Beckly DE, Abel MS. Articular mass fracture: a neglected cause of post-traumatic neck pain? *Clin Radiol* 1976;27:335–340.

CHAPTER 26

Cervicothoracic Junction

Rod J. Oskouian Jr., Sumon Bhattacharjee, Alexander R. Vaccaro, and Christopher I. Shaffrey

INTRODUCTION

The true incidence of fractures involving the cervicothoracic spine is not clearly known but has been reported to be approximately 9%. With the advent of fast spiral computerized tomography (CT) scanners and the routine use of magnetic resonance imaging (MRI) in the setting of trauma, there has been an increasing frequency in the diagnosis of these injuries.[1–3] These injuries are sometimes missed or overlooked on the initial lateral radiograph because it may not adequately visualize the cervicothoracic junction, especially in a patient with a depressed level of consciousness or other distracting injuries[1,4–6] (Fig. 26.1). Trauma centers with defined trauma protocols using spiral CT technology of the head and cervical spine including the cervicothoracic junction have contributed toward rapid recognition of these injuries (Fig. 26.2).

RADIOLOGIC EVALUATION

Clear radiographic evaluation of the cervicothoracic junction is often a challenge, especially in patients with wide and short necks. Adequate visualization of this area is technically difficult with plain radiographs. Although cervical spine fractures are relatively uncommon, occurring in 1% to 5% of blunt trauma patients, the devastating consequences of a missed fracture requires a high index of suspicion. Current clinical criteria exist to assist clinicians in selecting awake patients who are at low risk for cervical spine injury and are therefore suitable for cervical spine clearance via only clinical examination and history.[6,7] The imaging study of choice when there is a high suspicion for injury must be sensitive, cost-effective, widely available, easily performed, and anatomically complete. For those patients who are at high risk or in whom the physical examination is unreliable, current guidelines recommend a three-view series of plain cervical spine radiographs, including an open-mouth odontoid view, an anteroposterior view, and a cross-table lateral view. Technical adequacy is essential to the reliability of these radiographs and is usually the limiting factor. Current guidelines further recommend using CT to study the occiput-C2 region in patients who undergo head CT examinations and supplemental cervical spine CT for other areas poorly visualized or in which fracture is suspected on plain radiographs.[4,8]

In at least 26% of all trauma patients, the C7-T1 disc space is not adequately visualized on the three-view plain radiograph series. This evaluation is particularly difficult in obtunded patients who are intubated. With the advent of rapid sequence CT scanners at most North American trauma centers, detailed imaging evaluation of the entire spinal axis is easily obtainable. CT imaging is superior in detecting osseous injury to the spinal column. Spiral CT with multiplanar reformatting capability has improved the detection of occult injuries, especially at spinal junctions. Multiple studies have confirmed that plain radiographs are unreliable in the unconscious patient.

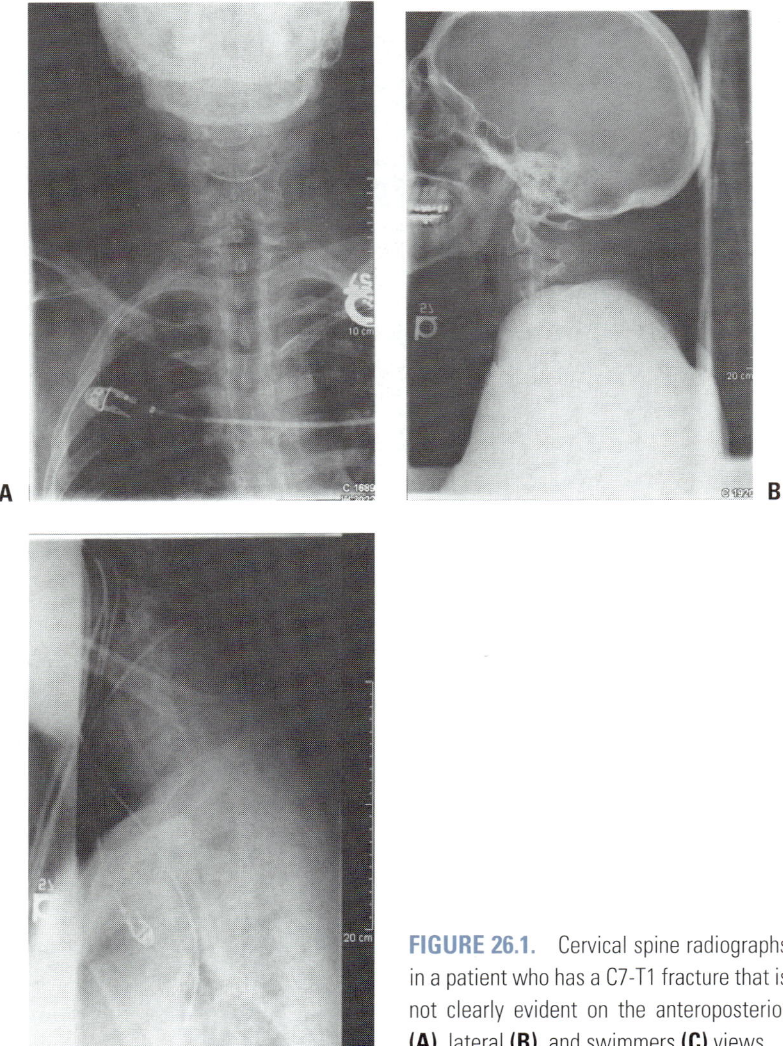

FIGURE 26.1. Cervical spine radiographs in a patient who has a C7-T1 fracture that is not clearly evident on the anteroposterior **(A)**, lateral **(B)**, and swimmers **(C)** views.

MECHANISM OF INJURY

The cervicothoracic region is predominantly exposed to flexion and compressive forces. The location and type of cervical spine injury that may occur in this region is intimately associated with the surrounding anatomy. The cervical spine is mobile and lordotic and abruptly transitions to the kyphotic and rigid thoracic spine. The rigidity of the upper thoracic spine is the result of its articulation with the ribs and sternum. Recent CT kinematics studies demonstrate that the cervicothoracic junction is twice as stiff as the remainder of the cervical spine. However, the angular motions in this region are comparable to those of the subaxial cervical area[9] (Fig. 26.3).

CLASSIFICATION

The cervicothoracic region is described as including the vertebral segments of C7 through T1 or as low as T4. The patterns of injury frequently seen at this junction include rotatory subluxations of C7 on T1, fracture-dislocations, unilateral and bilateral facet dislocations, and burst fractures.

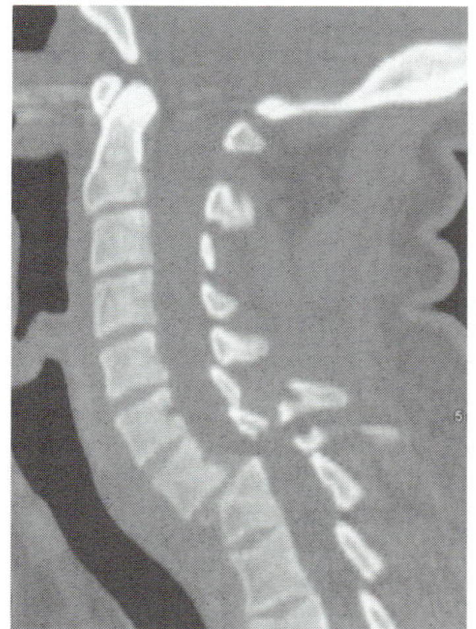
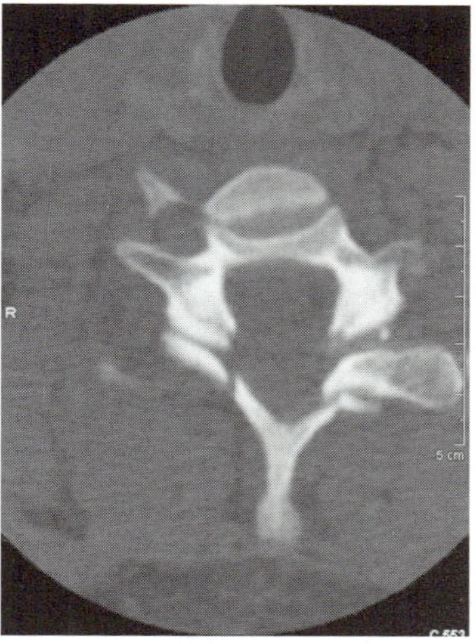

FIGURE 26.2. Computed tomography in the patient in Figure 26.1 demonstrating **(A)** C7-T1 dislocation and other osseous injuries and gross malalignment of the cervical spine with **(B)** bilateral jumped facets at the cervicothoracic junction with severe compromise of the central canal. Note posteriorly displaced fractures of the lamina, facets, and spinous processes and teardrop fractures.

Fractures involving T1 through T4 are rare. The Allen and Ferguson mechanistic classification of the subaxial spine is often applied in injuries involving the cervicothoracic junction.[10] This classification system is based on six major classes that are further divided into subclassifications.[11]

Anterior wedge compression fractures are caused by axial loading of the spine in flexion. These injuries can often be treated conservatively; however there is a risk for developing a progressive kyphotic deformity if vertebral fracture angulation is greater than 11 degrees or if there is a greater than 25% loss of vertebral body height. Cervical burst fractures are caused by a substantial axial compressive load. This injury morphology is often associated with incomplete and complete spinal cord injuries (SCIs) as a result of extrusion of bony fragments into the spinal canal. The treatment of cervical burst fractures is based primarily on the neurologic status of the patient. Patients with a neurologic deficit are often treated surgically with an anterior approach to decompress the spinal

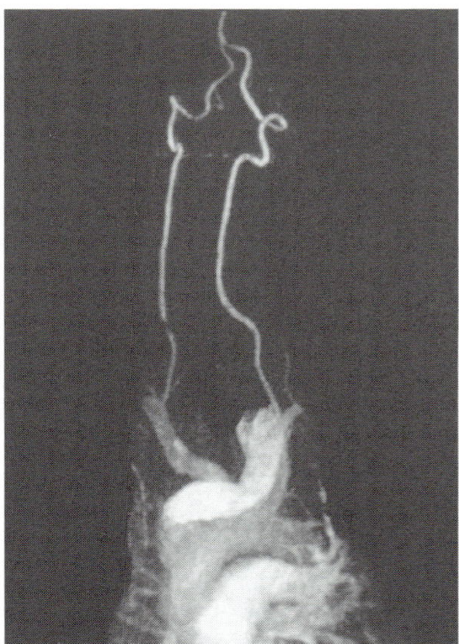

FIGURE 26.3. Magnetic resonance angiography in a patient with cervicothoracic subluxation who developed a right vertebral artery dissection following the injury.

canal through a cervical corpectomy and fusion with a structural graft, as well as internal fixation with an anterior cervical plate. The design of anterior plating systems has improved a great deal over the last decade, and stand-alone anterior internal fixation devices often can be used unless there is substantial posterior column injury, in which case an anteroposterior approach is desirable.

Facet injuries are one of the most common injuries seen in patients with cervical spine trauma. Unilateral facet fractures can involve either the inferior or superior facet and are often caused by rotational forces with the neck in a slightly flexed position. Superior facet fractures are more common than inferior facet fractures, and disruption of the facet capsule inherently implies some translational forces with disruption of the interspinous ligament and possibly the disc space. The treatment of unilateral facet injuries depends on the degree of instability caused by the fracture as well as cervical spine alignment. A nondisplaced fracture that involves only the facet joint can often be treated with a cervical orthosis. Facet fractures with significant angulation and translation are best treated with reduction and fusion over the injured levels. The surgical options include a stand-alone anterior or posterior fusion procedure or a combined approach if there is a significant three-column injury. Bilateral facet fractures are caused by shear and translational forces. These fractures are often associated with severe discal disruption and SCI.

Unilateral and bilateral facet subluxations or dislocations are flexion-distraction injuries that may result in disruption of the posterior longitudinal ligament (bilateral facet dislocation), facet capsule, or disc space (unilateral and bilateral facet dislocation). These injuries are almost universally treated surgically in the presence of objective ligamentous disruption.[4,12]

TREATMENT

INITIAL TREATMENT

The early identification and recognition of any associated spinal injury is crucial in the management of a patient with a cervicothoracic spine injury. The incidence of complete SCI in the setting of a spinal injury at this level of the spine is extremely high. The principles of initial intervention involve early closed reduction of the spinal deformity and establishing spinal alignment. Relocation of a cervicothoracic junction dislocation routinely requires a greater traction force than midcervical dislocation, and weights up to 120 lb have frequently been used to successfully achieve a closed reduction. Chapman et al.[13] recommend applying traction weight of up to 60% of the patient's body weight to achieve reduction. The authors of this series did not notice any adverse outcome from such traction weight. If closed reduction is unsuccessful, operative reduction is recommended on a timely basis in the setting of a neurologic deficit.

OPERATIVE SELECTIVE CRITERIA

The selection criteria for surgical intervention for trauma involving the cervicothoracic junction are not well defined. There is no level I or level II medical evidence that delineates surgical indications in the management of trauma to this junction. Individual retrospective series have suggested treatment recommendations for specific fracture patterns only.

The basic tenets of spinal trauma care are applicable to this level of the spine, that is, early spinal alignment in the setting of a neurologic deficit and the restoration of spinal stability.[14–18]

CT imaging is crucial in determining the bony architecture and biomechanical characteristics of a fracture. MRI is extremely valuable in assessing injury to the spinal cord, surrounding soft tissues, and intervertebral disc. Three-column injuries often require surgical stabilization because of the potential for progressive cervical kyphosis at this level of the spine. The prevention of progressive kyphosis is paramount, especially in the setting of a neurologic deficit. Recent animal studies have demonstrated that progressive kyphosis of the cervical spine results in demyelination of nerve fibers and anterior horn cell loss as a result of chronic compression. Therefore, prevention of deformity progression is an important goal of treatment that is often not well maintained with any form of external immobilization at the cervicothoracic junction. Unfortunately, it is not clear as to the extent of kyphosis in the acute setting that requires early correction and stabilization.

If nonoperative treatment is chosen carefully, follow-up is necessary to assess for fracture displacement or progression of deformity.

In the setting of a complete SCI, the goal of treatment is early mobilization and the prevention of progressive kyphosis and posttraumatic syrinx formation.

OPERATIVE TREATMENT

Stabilization of the cervicothoracic junction can be difficult, and a variety of techniques and approaches have been described for this level of the spine. Cervicothoracic fixation of the unstable spine is challenging because of the change of cervical lordosis to thoracic kyphosis. One of the technical challenges has been that instrumentation designed for the cervical spine is significantly smaller and less strong than instrumentation designed for the thoracolumbar spine. Differences in the entry point location for C6 lateral mass, C7 pedicle and lateral mass, and T1 pedicle screws and the potential for implant crowding in this location, indicates that compromises such as skipping the C7 screws may be needed to successfully use the existing instrumentation systems. One strategy is to bridge separate cervical and thoracic implants at the cervicothoracic junction with potentially bulky connectors. A second option is to extend a cervical lateral mass plate down into the thoracic spine and place screws out laterally into the thoracic transverse processes on the thoracic pedicles. Neither approach is totally satisfactory in terms of the strength needed at this level to restore native biomechanical stability. The development of dual-diameter or tapered rods has somewhat obviated this problem. This approach enables the surgeon to use appropriate-sized and placed spinal anchors and to connect these implants with a longitudinal connector of the appropriate strength.[13–16,19–21] Posterior spinal implants have proved to provide adequate stability to this junction in the absence of marked anterior column instability. Rhee et al[22] biomechanically compared the stiffness of several posterior fixation strategies at the cervicothoracic junction. They found that a C7 and T1 pedicle screw implant strategy was stronger than using a lateral mass screw at C7. Additionally, extending fixation to C6 further stiffened the construct in compression. Wiring augmentation did not provide any further increase in rigidity.

The problem with anterior plating at this junction is the difficulty in affixing screws in the upper thoracic spine because of visualization problems and the fact that the upper thoracic spine moves away from the surgical field and surgeon as a result of upper thoracic kyphosis.

SCREW PLACEMENT AT THE CERVICAL LEVEL

In the cervical spine, screws may be placed posteriorly either in the lateral masses or the pedicles. Various authors have described different methods of lateral mass fixation. Biomechanically, the utility of lateral mass screw fixation has been tested in animal and human cadaver models.[23] The literature is sparse on clinical studies that specifically refer to the use of posterior screw fixation across the cervicothoracic junction.[22] Biomechanical studies have shown that cervical pedicle screw fixation provides the most rigid form of internal fixation in unstable cervical spine injuries.

The specific risks of cervical pedicle screw versus lateral mass screw must be considered. Cadaveric morphometric analyses have shown that the cervical nerve roots from C3 to C8 lie between the posterior midpoints of the lateral masses.[24] From C3 to C5, the vertebral artery is normally situated medially to the posterior midpoint of the lateral mass, whereas it is located anterior to the midpoint of the lateral mass at the C6 level. The foramen transversarium, the conduit for the vertebral vein and artery, which routinely enter the foramen transversarium at C7 and C6, respectively, are at risk in cervical lateral mass screws directed anteromedially or anteriorly starting at the midpoint of the cervical lateral mass.[25] The Magerl technique is a safe and effective method for placing posterior cervical lateral mass screws. The starting point for screw insertion is 1 to 2 mm medial and caudal to the center of the lateral mass, with the drill direction aimed 25 degrees lateral and 40 degrees cephalad. The trajectory is intended to orient the screw parallel to the facet joint. Screws are usually placed in a bicortical fashion to improve screw purchase.[24]

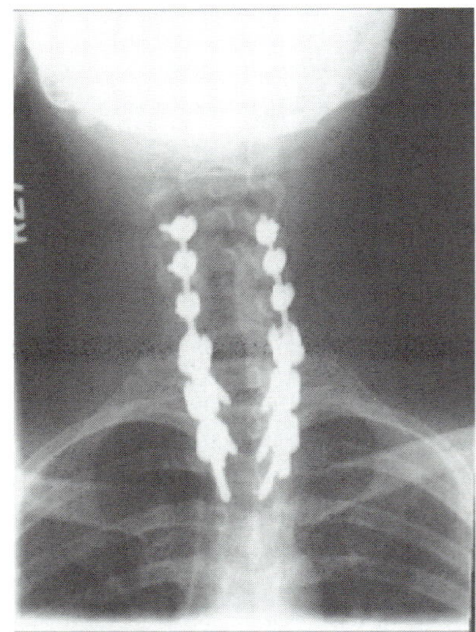

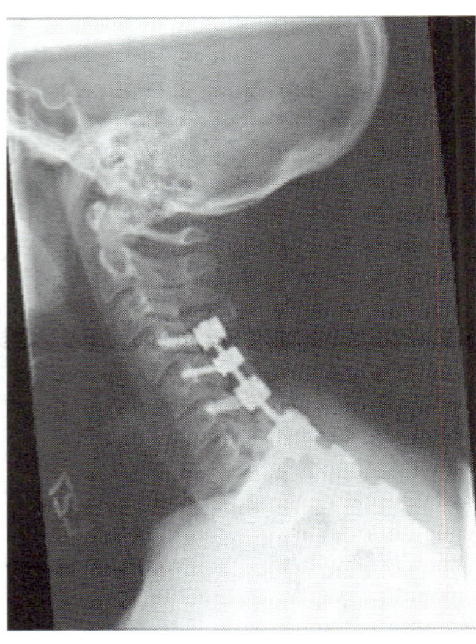

A B

FIGURE 26.4. A,B. Postoperative anteroposterior and lateral plain radiographs in a patient who had a C7-T1 subluxation and complete spinal cord injury with fractures of the posterior elements extending down to T2. After 110 lb of traction failed to reduce the subluxation, the patient was taken emergently to the operating room where a C4-T4 posterior segmental fusion was performed.

C7 SCREW PLACEMENT

Morphometric analysis of the C7 pedicle has demonstrated that the mediolateral and superoinferior outer pedicle diameters average 6.9 and 7.5 mm, respectively. The average mediolateral inner diameter is approximately 5.2 mm. The overall length of the pedicle averages 9.1 mm and the medial angulation or trajectory of the pedicle in relationship to the vertebral body is approximately 34 degrees. These dimensions routinely allow the safe placement of pedicle screws at this level of the spine if pedicle screw fixation is chosen.[26] During screw insertion the shoulder unfortunately often obstructs a clear intraoperative lateral radiographic image of the C7 pedicle, body, and facet joint. If a pedicle screw is to be used at C7, T1, or T2, precise knowledge of the entry points, pedicle diameters, and medial angulation for screw insertion based on preoperative image analysis is imperative. We recommend a pedicle entry point for the C7 pedicle 1 mm inferior to the midportion of the C6-C7 facet joint, with drill angulation 25 to 30 degrees medially and perpendicular to the posterior arch (Fig. 26.4).

UPPER THORACIC SPINE SCREW PLACEMENT

In the thoracic spine, screws are placed in the pedicles because the transverse processes are considerably weaker and the pedicles are much larger. As is often the case in cervicothoracic trauma, there may be lamina or facet fractures, making pedicle screw fixation the optimal spinal anchor at this level. From a morphometric perspective, the T1 and T2 pedicles are larger than those of T4 through T7. Pedicle width decreases proceeding caudally from T1 to T5 from an average of 7.8 to 4.4 mm. For T1 and T2 pedicle screw fixation, the projection point of the pedicle axis is slightly lateral to the midfacet joint and superior to the midline of the transverse process in the transverse plane (see Fig. 26.4).

CONCLUSION

The evaluation and treatment of injuries of the cervicothoracic junction require extra vigilance to improve injury surveillance. Biomechanically, the treating physician should become familiar with the unique anatomic constraints of this junction and the requirements necessary to treat these injuries successfully nonoperatively and surgically. Contemporary spinal implants have allowed successful reconstruction of this region of the spine and have virtually obviated the need for prolonged halo vest application during the recovery period.

REFERENCES

1. Bach CM, Steingruber IE, Peer S, et al. Radiographic evaluation of cervical spine trauma: plain radiography and conventional tomography versus computed tomography. *Arch Orthop Trauma Surg* 2001;121:385–387.
2. Takhtani D, Melhem ER. MR imaging in cervical spine trauma. *Clin Sports Med* 2002;21:49–75, vi.
3. Takhtani D, Melhem ER. MR imaging in cervical spine trauma. *Magn Reson Imaging Clin North Am* 2000;8: 615–634.
4. Gale SC, Gracias VH, Reilly PM, et al. The inefficiency of plain radiography to evaluate the cervical spine after blunt trauma. *J Trauma* 2005;59:1121–1125.
5. Kaiser JA, Holland BA. Imaging of the cervical spine. *Spine* 1998;23:2701–2712.
6. Keats TE, Dalinka MK, Alazraki N, et al. Cervical spine trauma: American College of Radiology appropriateness criteria. *Radiology* 2000;215(suppl):243–246.
7. Goergen SK, Fong C, Dalziel K, et al. Development of an evidence-based guideline for imaging in cervical spine trauma. *Australas Radiol* 2003;47:240–246.
8. Sanchez B, Waxman K, Jones T, et al. Cervical spine clearance in blunt trauma: evaluation of a computed tomography-based protocol. *J Trauma* 2005;59:179–183.
9. Simon S, Davis M, Odhner D, et al. CT imaging techniques for describing motions of the cervicothoracic junction and cervical spine during flexion, extension, and cervical traction. *Spine* 2006;31:44–50.
10. Allen BL Jr, Ferguson RL, Lehmann TR, et al. A mechanistic classification of closed, indirect fractures and dislocations of the lower cervical spine. *Spine* 1982;7:1–27.
11. Budorick TE, Anderson PA, Rivara FP, et al. Flexion-distraction fracture of the cervical spine: a case report. *J Bone Joint Surg Am* 1991;73:1097–1100.
12. Schenarts PJ, Diaz J, Kaiser C, et al. Prospective comparison of admission computed tomographic scan and plain films of the upper cervical spine in trauma patients with altered mental status. *J Trauma* 2001;51:663–668.
13. Chapman JR, Anderson PA, Pepin C, et al. Posterior instrumentation of the unstable cervicothoracic spine. *J Neurosurg* 1996;84:552–558.
14. Anderson PA, Bohlman HH. Anterior decompression and arthrodesis of the cervical spine: long-term motor improvement. II: Improvement in complete traumatic quadriplegia. *J Bone Joint Surg Am* 1992;74:683–692.
15. Bohlman HH, Anderson PA. Anterior decompression and arthrodesis of the cervical spine: long-term motor improvement. I: Improvement in incomplete traumatic quadriparesis. *J Bone Joint Surg Am* 1002;74:671–682.
16. Brodke DS, Anderson PA, Newell DW, et al. Comparison of anterior and posterior approaches in cervical spinal cord injuries. *J Spinal Disord Tech* 2003;16:229–235.
17. Cotler HB. The treatment of cervical spine trauma: a century of progress. *Orthopedics* 1002;15:279–283.
18. Do KY, Lim TH, Won YJ, et al. A biomechanical comparison of modern anterior and posterior plate fixation of the cervical spine. *Spine* 2001;26:15–21.
19. Anderson PA, Henley MB, Grady MS, et al. Posterior cervical arthrodesis with AO reconstruction plates and bone graft. *Spine* 1991;16:S72–S79.
20. Lowery GL, McDonough RF. The significance of hardware failure in anterior cervical plate fixation: patients with 2- to 7-year follow-up. *Spine* 1998;23:181–186.
21. McNamara MJ, Devito DP, Spengler DM. Circumferential fusion for the management of acute cervical spine trauma. *J Spinal Disord* 1991;4:467–471.
22. Rhee JM, Kraiwattanapong C, Hutton WC. A comparison of pedicle and lateral mass screw construct stiffnesses at the cervicothoracic junction: a biomechanical study. *Spine* 2005;30:E636–E640.
23. Xu R, Ebraheim NA, Klausner T, et al. Modified Magerl technique of lateral mass screw placement in the lower cervical spine: an anatomic study. *J Spinal Disord* 1998;11:237–240.
24. Xu R, Haman SP, Ebraheim NA, et al. The anatomic relation of lateral mass screws to the spinal nerves: a comparison of the Magerl, Anderson, and An techniques. *Spine* 1999;24:2057–2061.
25. Xu R, Kang A, Ebraheim NA, et al. Anatomic relation between the cervical pedicle and the adjacent neural structures. *Spine* 1999;24:451–454.
26. Xu R, Ebraheim NA, Yeasting R, et al. Anatomy of C7 lateral mass and projection of pedicle axis on its posterior aspect. *J Spinal Disord* 1995;8:116–120.

SECTION VIII

Posttraumatic Cervical Deformities

CHAPTER 27

Management of Posttraumatic Cervical Kyphosis

Alpesh A. Patel, Derek J. Donegan, and Todd J. Albert

INTRODUCTION

The potential development of deformity is a recognized complication of cervical spine trauma. Progressive deformity may be seen in the setting of an unrecognized or underappreciated injury. Additionally, deformity may be due to iatrogenic injury during operative treatment. Unfortunately, a thorough discussion of cervical deformity is not well represented in the current literature related to the treatment of sagittal plane deformities.

The combination of deformity, cervical instability, and potential neurologic compromise makes the correction of posttraumatic cervical imbalance difficult. This chapter will address the biomechanics, clinical evaluation, and treatment options for posttraumatic cervical imbalance.

BIOMECHANICS

A discussion of normal cervical alignment and anatomy is important in understanding the development of cervical kyphosis. Normal cervical lordosis measures an average of 14.4 degrees but has been shown to range from 10 to 30 degrees, with a large degree of variability.[1,2] A loss of normal lordosis may be seen in association with both acute and chronic pain.[3] However, kyphosis of the cervical spine, especially when focal, should be considered abnormal.

The normal weight-bearing axis of the cervical spine typically falls behind C2-C7, thereby accentuating lordotic alignment and minimizing the demands on the posterior cervical musculature.[4,5] Normal load transmission, as shown in a cadaveric experiment by Pal and Sherk,[6] occurs primarily through the posterior elements (64%) compared with the anterior elements (36%).

The development of cervical kyphosis can be attributed to mechanical failure of the posterior or anterior anatomic structures. This instability may be directly related to traumatic or iatrogenic disruption of normal stabilizing structures. Incompetence of the posterior elements can cause significant instability of the cervical spine.[7,8] The facet joint is the most significant stabilizer of the posterior elements; the spinous processes and interspinous ligaments act in a secondary, yet still important, role.

The importance of facet joint integrity to cervical spine stability is well recognized in the clinical literature. Nowinski et al.[9] reported that, when combined with laminectomy, facetectomy of as little as 25% can result in kyphosis. Fager[10,11] and Epstein[12] also stressed the importance of maintaining facet integrity during cervical laminectomy; Epstein[12] warned against resecting more than one quarter to one third of the facet. In a clinical review of patients treated for spondylotic myelopathy, Herkowitz[13] reported a 25% incidence of kyphosis in patients with bilateral facetectomy.

These clinical findings have been supported by animal and cadaveric studies. In a primate study, Munechika[14] showed that unilateral facet resection significantly increased the risk for developing a kyphotic deformity. In an examination of human specimens, Zdeblick et al.[8] showed that more than 50% facet capsule release caused significant instability. Additionally, in a similar anatomic study, Zdeblick et al.[8] showed that more than 50% facetectomy caused a statistically significant loss of stability in flexion and torsion.[1] Studies by Cusick et al.[15] and White and Panjabi[16] further support the relationship between progressive facet resection and cervical instability.

Integrity of the spinous process and interspinous ligament is also important in the maintenance of normal cervical alignment. Disruption of these structures has been shown to increase tensile forces across the facet joints.[17] The development of tensile forces at the facet joints can lead to injury or can accentuate the deformity across an injured joint.

Instability produced by injury to the posterior elements will, either acutely or progressively, lead to an anterior shift of the weight-bearing axis with a coupled shift of load transmission to the vertebral bodies and disks. The status of the anterior column, therefore, is also a critical factor in the development of kyphosis. Cervical extensors can temporarily counter small changes in sagittal alignment as a result of posterior disruptions when the anterior column remains intact. Ultimately, progressive kyphosis will develop as pain and muscle fatigue which will limit the ability of the extensors to maintain alignment.[18,19] Failure of the anterior column, through vertebral fracture or intervertebral disc disruption, eliminates the ability of the cervical extensors to maintain balance and results in acute deformity.

As the spine assumes a kyphotic position, tensile forces posteriorly and compressive forces anteriorly increase. A vicious cycle then ensues as these forces cause further kyphotic deformity across a mechanically incompetent spine.

CLINICAL EVALUATION

Patient presentation can vary. In common with sagittal plane deformities of the thoracic and lumbar spine, typical symptoms can include pain, neurologic dysfunction, and cosmetic deformity. Because of the critical importance of head position in daily life, some of the functional problems that occur are unique to the cervical spine.

Pain location can be focal or diffuse. Focal pain can be related to nonunion of fractured posterior or anterior elements. Additionally, the large forces acting at the apex of the deformity may result in painful degenerative changes in the facet and uncovertebral joints.

A more diffuse, axial pain may be due to paraspinal muscle fatigue and dysfunction associated with the anatomic deformity. Facet overload at compensatory adjacent levels may also account for diffuse pain symptoms. Occipital headaches can be attributed to excessive compensatory occipitocervical extension as the patient attempts to maintain normal head position. The exact cause of both focal and diffuse pain, however, may be difficult to define.

Neurologic dysfunction can develop with a progressive cervical deformity. Development of symptoms may be quick after injury or may be delayed by many years.[20] Symptoms may be radicular because of foraminal stenosis and neural stretch that can occur with kyphosis and secondary degenerative changes. Of greater concern is the development of cervical myelopathy. The degree of neurologic dysfunction and the rate of progression should be determined from the patient's history. Symptoms may be subtle or overt. Loss of manual dexterity, loss of gait and balance, loss of bowel or bladder control, or loss of sexual function may all be more obvious presenting symptoms. More subtle complaints should be taken just as seriously. Additionally, physical examination should include a diligent search for evidence of spinal cord dysfunction: pathologic reflexes (hyperreflexia, Hoffman sign, inverted radial reflex), difficulty with posture and balance (Romberg sign, gait analysis), motor weakness, and poor motor coordination (disdiadochokinesia).

Cosmetic deformity may also be a presenting complaint. Unique to the cervical spine, severe functional disability may accompany cosmetic, most notably severe sagittal plane, deformities. This is a reflection of the importance of head position to such basic functions as vision, speech, and the ability

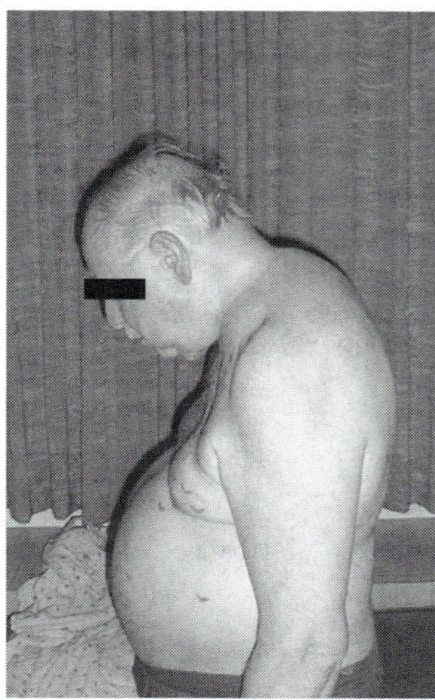

FIGURE 27.1. A patient with posttraumatic "chin-on-chest" deformity.

to eat, drink, and breathe. The progressive change in forward gaze angle overpowers the ability of the eyes to compensate. Severe "chin-on-chest" deformity may further impair the ability to open and close the jaw, in addition to swallowing dysfunction. The loss of these basic abilities can have a profound impact on nearly all daily activities from hygiene and nourishment to hand-eye coordination and work. Additionally, these individuals lose the ability to be self-sufficient because they can no longer travel or communicate independently. The psychological impact of severe chin-on-chest deformity can be quite significant (Fig. 27.1).

Coronal plane and rotational deformities can also result in an aesthetically unappealing head position. Functional disability is typically limited. Freedom of jaw motion and the ability of the cerebellum and extraocular muscles to accommodate for rotatory changes in gaze angle account for this (Fig. 27.2).

RADIOLOGIC EVALUATION

Diagnostic evaluation begins with plain radiographs. Anteroposterior (AP), lateral, and flexion-extension films must allow for clear visualization of the end and neutral vertebrae. Small localized areas of kyphosis can be differentiated from more global kyphosis. Flexion-extension radiographs will aid in

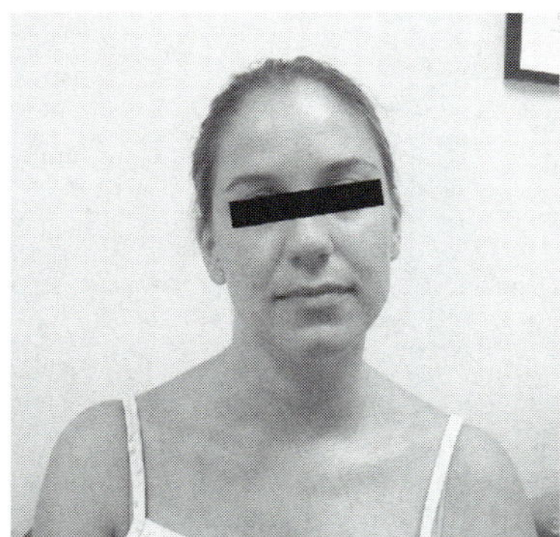

FIGURE 27.2. A patient with a posttraumatic coronal plane deformity. The functional consequences of this deformity are less severe than the "chin-on-chest" deformity shown in Figure 27.1.

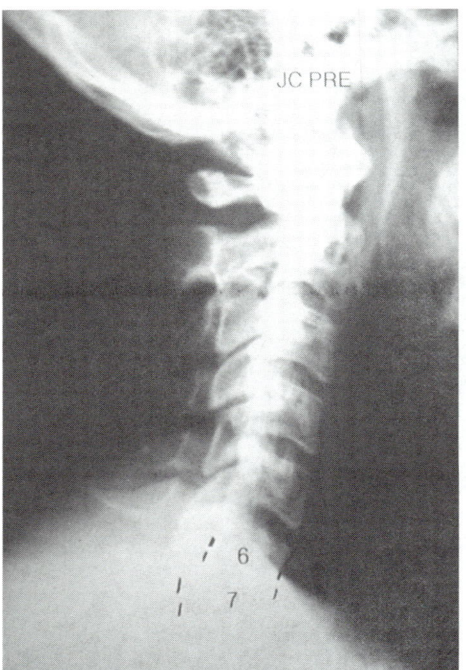

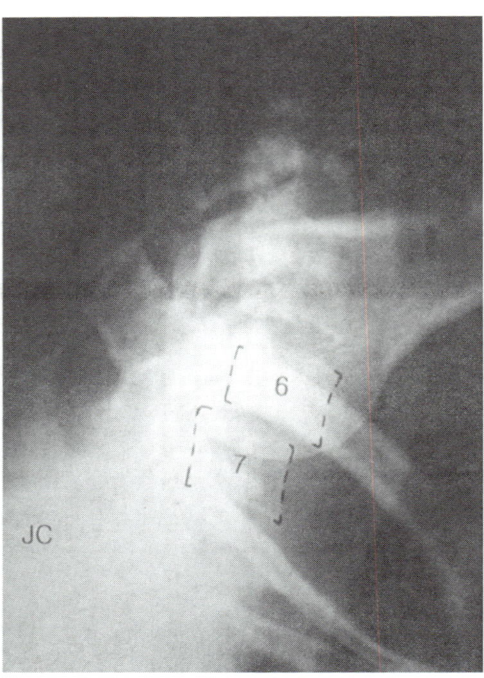

FIGURE 27.3. Radiographs showing anterior displacement of C6 with respect to C7.

differentiating fixed and flexible deformities. Additionally, fixed curves with or without flexion ankylosis can be differentiated. Lastly, standing AP and lateral 36-inch cassette radiographs can assess concurrent thoracolumbar deformity that may contribute to the patient's global deformity (Figs. 27.3 and 27.4).

Magnetic resonance imaging (MRI) plays a critical role in assessing the cervical spine. Spinal cord compression can be identified and localized. Additional cord changes that can account for neurologic changes such as myelomalacia, cord atrophy, syrinx formation, or tethered cord can be

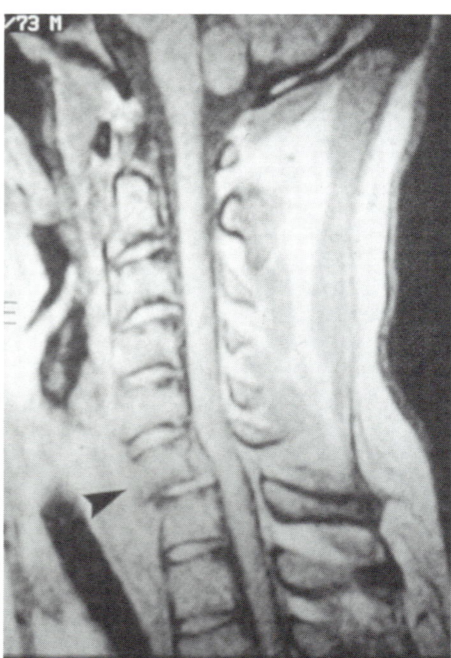

FIGURE 27.4. Lateral MRI showing anterior vertebral displacement, or posttraumatic cervical kyphosis.

visualized. The status of the intervertebral discs can also be assessed and may influence end fusion levels. Magnetic resonance angiography (MRA) can define the vertebral artery system. The absence of vertebral artery patency can influence operative treatment or mandate preoperative intervention. Additionally, the patient can be maximally educated on perioperative risk.

Computed tomography (CT) aids in the visualization of bony anatomy, especially when otherwise limited by plain radiographs. Thin-cut (1 to 3 mm) axial images, when combined with sagittal and coronal reconstructions, allow for an improved understanding of the fracture pattern and posttraumatic anatomic changes. The location of the vertebral arteries, status of the facet joints, and anatomy of the cervical pedicles can be identified. Additionally, CT can demonstrate the presence of bony ankylosis or fracture nonunion. The use of CT with contrast myelography improves visualization of spinal cord and nerve roots that may otherwise be difficult to assess, especially in patients with prior surgical treatment.

CLASSIFICATION

There are no reported classification schemes for posttraumatic cervical deformity. The deformity is best described by defining (a) the initial traumatic injury, (b) the current anatomy, and (c) the neurologic status of the patient.

Knowledge of the initial fracture pattern aids in understanding the degree of cervical instability. Vertebral body fractures may necessitate anterior corpectomy, whereas injuries involving the disc space may be treated with interbody releases and grafting. Additionally, rotational deformity associated with facet or lateral mass injuries may be better defined. The details of prior operative treatment should also be ascertained to define sources of iatrogenic instability (e.g., laminectomy) that may mandate circumferential fusion.[21]

The current anatomy of the deformity is best described by defining the location, flexibility, and principal plane of the deformity, as well as any functional limitations resulting from the deformity. The end and neutral vertebrae of the deformity should be clearly defined. The degenerative status of the intervertebral discs should also be noted. Lastly, the degree of spinal canal and neural foraminal compression is defined.

The neurologic status of the patient is of critical importance. Severe cord compression and myelopathic symptoms may necessitate a decompressive procedure antecedent to correction of deformity.

SURGICAL TREATMENT AND OUTCOMES

The goals of operative treatment are correction of deformity, relief of neural compression, and stable reconstruction of the spine.

The principals of surgical correction of thoracolumbar kyphosis are applicable to the cervical spine. Anterior column lengthening combined with posterior column shortening will address the kyphotic malalignment. Additional decompressive procedures may be required to relieve or prevent spinal cord compression. Unique to the cervical spine, surgical planning must also address functional disabilities and rotational deformities. Difficulty with jaw opening will generally be addressed with kyphosis correction. Restoration of gaze angle requires specific attention. Rotational deformities are more common in the neck and challenging to correct at a later stage.

Surgical technique will depend on the specific pathologic condition. Flexible deformities can be corrected by traction or postural correction with fusion in the corrected position. Most cases of posttraumatic deformity will, however, involve a fixed deformity. The presence of a fixed deformity can significantly change the surgical management. A deformity that is fixed but not globally ankylosed in flexion can be treated with anterior release and multilevel anterior interbody fusion or corpectomies.

The decision between multilevel discectomy and corpectomy is, on the surface, a difficult one. Multiple anterior interbody grafts restore more lordosis to the cervical spine than long, straight structural grafts. However, the increased rate of pseudarthrosis in multilevel anterior discectomy is well documented. Additionally, both procedures have potentially high complication rates. The decision between discectomy and corpectomy should therefore be guided primarily by the location of neurologic compression. If significant compression is present posterior to the vertebral body, as with ossified posterior longitudinal ligament, corpectomy is indicated. If neurologic compression is localized to the disc level or if neurologic compromise is caused by draping of the spinal cord across the area of kyphosis, multiple discectomies are preferred.

Whether multilevel anterior interbody fusion or corpectomy is selected, the surgical reconstruction should be augmented with posterior instrumented arthrodesis.[22–24] Anterior release in the setting of posterior instability, either iatrogenic of traumatic, produces circumferential instability and increases the incidence of complications in anterior-only reconstruction. Emery et al.[22] reviewed 16 patients who underwent three-level anterior interbody discectomy and fusion with iliac crest autograft. At an average of 37 months follow-up, 7 of 16 (44%) patients displayed symptomatic pseudarthroses. Riew et al.[24] found that anterior-only reconstruction, after cervical corpectomy in the setting of prior laminectomy, was associated with an unacceptable high rate of complications. Of 18 patients, 11 within an average of 2.7 years of follow-up, had complications, with 9 of 11 having graft-related complications, which included extrusion or collapse of the graft, pseudarthrosis, and progressive kyphosis. Zdeblick and Bohlman,[25] in a review of anterior corpectomy and structural grafting, found the highest risk for graft extrusion to be among those patients with prior cervical laminectomy.

The benefit of anterior instrumentation to a large anterior-only reconstruction remains controversial. Anterior plating has been shown by some to improve outcomes in postlaminectomy patients undergoing cervical corpectomy.[26] A critical look at this study, however, reveals that no clear fusion criteria were stated and that the prevalence of graft subsidence was not reported. Furthermore, others have reported significant complications such as graft and plate displacement with long anterior-only instrumented arthrodesis.[27] The use of multilevel discectomy or corpectomy and discectomy with segmental instrumentation has shown improved mechanical properties compared with long corpectomy and end-point fixation.[28] However, Boelesta et al.,[29] in a review of 15 patients who underwent multilevel, segmental anterior instrumented fusion, found pseudarthrosis in 8 of 15 patients. The role of dynamic anterior instrumentation remains unclear. The use of dynamic anterior instrumentation has been shown to increase compressive loads in cadaveric specimens after three level discectomy.[30] There is, however, no clear evidence to support an improved clinical outcome.

Circumferential fusion, by comparison, has shown good results. McAfee et al.[31] reported results on 100 patients, including tumor, trauma, and postlaminectomy patients, undergoing combined anterior and posterior arthrodesis. Although the results of the traumatic and postlaminectomy patients were not reported separately, only 2 of 100 patients developed pseudarthrosis. McAfee and Bohlman[32] described 24 patients with fixed cervical kyphosis, resulting from either tumor or trauma, and neurologic injury or cervical instability who underwent a single-stage circumferential arthrodesis with anterior decompression and posterior stabilization. They reported successful fusion in all patients and improved neurologic findings in 22 of 24 patients, including patients who were treated more than 10 months after initial injury. The remaining patients, both quadriplegics, showed no deterioration (Fig. 27.5).

The addition of posterior instrumentation has also shown superior mechanical properties compared with anterior-only reconstructions, with or without a plate.[23] The improved mechanical properties of circumferential instrumentation can maximize stability of the reconstructed spine and thereby decrease the risk for graft-related complications. The addition of posterior instrumented fusion is therefore strongly indicated for multilevel anterior arthrodesis in the setting of posttraumatic deformity.

A fixed deformity with ankylosis in flexion, although uncommon among patients with posttraumatic deformity, requires special attention. These patients typically present with severe deformity and functional disabilities. The severe degree of kyphosis cannot be corrected with anterior releases, anterior corpectomy, or anterior interbody fusion alone. The severity of the deformity requires a posterior extension osteotomy to correct sagittal alignment.

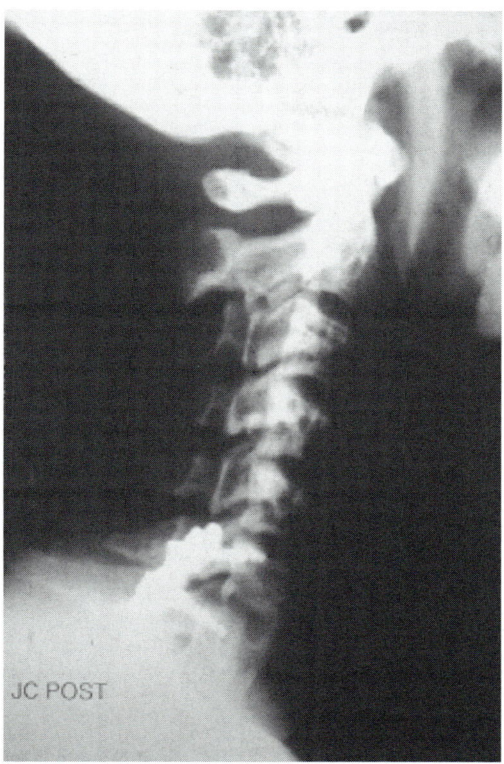

FIGURE 27.5. Instrumented fusion to correct posttraumatic cervical kyphosis (anterior decompression and posterior stabilization).

The use of cervicothoracic osteotomy has been most widely described in the setting of ankylosing spondylitis. Although differences exist, knowledge of this procedure can be applied to severe cases of posttraumatic deformity. One of the earliest descriptions of posterior cervical osteotomy was by Mason et al.[33] They stressed the importance of performing the osteotomy at the cervicothoracic junction, below the entrance of the vertebral arteries in the C6 transverse foramina. The osteotomy is intended to hinge at the posterior longitudinal ligament, with resultant posterior column shortening and anterior column lengthening.

The use of this technique has shown good results. Belanger et al.[34] reported 26 patients with an average 4.5-year follow-up after extension osteotomy for chin-on-chest deformity. Posterior osteotomy was performed under local anesthesia with the patient awake in a halo orthosis, as described by Urist.[35] The procedure was augmented with wired instrumentation in 19 patients and with anterior osteoclasis in all patients. Patients were maintained in halo jacket immobilization. Postoperative sagittal alignment improved by an average of 38 degrees. At final follow-up, an average of 2.6 degrees of correction was lost; greater than 5 degrees loss of correction was noted with nonunion of osteotomy or with new trauma. Of 10 patients with preoperative myelopathy, 9 showed functional improvements. Of 24 patients with preoperative neck pain, 21 showed mild to no neck pain postoperatively.

Simmons[36] reported 11 patients treated with extension osteotomy under local anesthetic. No internal fixation was used and halo jacket immobilization was used postoperatively. Although no objective data were given, he reported improved head position, gaze, and functional capacity in all patients. He reported one nonunion that ultimately required an anterior fusion.

McMaster[37] reviewed 15 patients treated with extension osteotomy at the cervicothoracic junction for severe flexion deformity. The procedure was performed under general anesthesia with the patient in the prone position; three patients had posterior Luque wire augmentation. McMaster reported that closure of the osteotomy resulted in fracture through the anterior column, thereby obviating the need

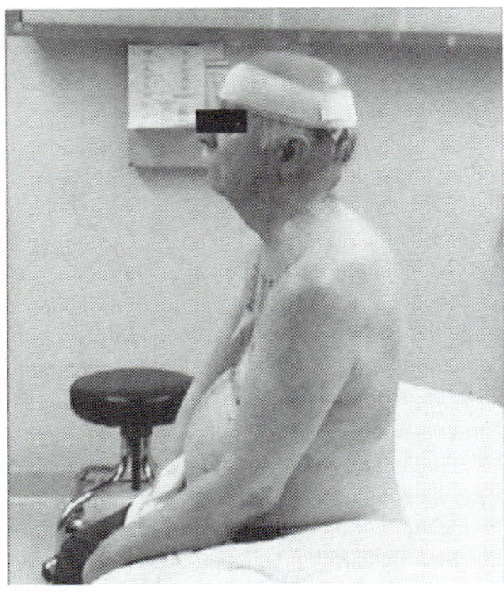

FIGURE 27.6. Corrected chin-brow to vertical angle <10 degrees (see Fig. 27.1 for preoperative condition).

for anterior osteotomy. Patients were immobilized in a halo jacket orthosis postoperatively. The mean preoperative cervical kyphosis of 23 degrees was corrected to a mean of 31 degress of lordosis, for an overall mean correction of 54 degrees. Nonunion was observed in two patients and felt to be associated with translation at the osteotomy during closure.

In a more recent review, the role of instrumented posterior fusion was further addressed. Langeloo et al.[38] reviewed 16 patients with C7 osteotomy treated with posterior instrumented fusion. Eleven patients were treated with halo immobilization in the seated position with local anesthetic; five patients were treated prone under a general anesthetic. The authors state that the prone position allows for instrumented fusion toward T4-T6. The improved rigidity of the internal construct obviated the need for halo jacket immobilization postoperatively. All patients obtained fusion without translation.

In addition to correction of sagittal alignment, operative treatment must also address associated functional limitations of jaw movement, swallowing, and vision. Improvement in head position obtained with kyphosis correction will readily improve jaw opening. Although transient dysphagia has been reported, the restoration of a more normal head position will also improve pharyngoesophageal function.[34,37] Belanger et al.[34] reported improved swallowing function, horizontal gaze, and visual field in all patients by final follow-up examination. McMaster[37] and Simmons[36] described visual field improvements in all patients after extension osteotomy. Simmons[36] described a secondary procedure of halo adjustment, performed postoperatively with the patient under a general anesthetic, to perfect head positioning according to the patient's preference.

More recently, in discussing sagittal correction, it has become evident that angular correction of kyphosis does not necessarily correlate with correction of horizontal gaze.[39] Although no standardized methods exist for determining a gaze angle to the horizon, Suk et al.[40] described a chin-brow angle measured from clinical pictures to objectively define head position: the angle between the vertical and a tangential line from the chin and brow. In a review of 34 patients, chin-brow angle improved from a mean of 35.5 degrees to 1.8 degrees. Patients reported good satisfaction with their results. Langeloo et al.[38] reported a mean postoperative chin-brow to vertical angle of 5 degrees (range 0 to 15); they reported no unsatisfied patients. We strive for a postoperative chin-brow to vertical angle of 5 to 10 degrees. This angle allows for ease in reading, walking up or down stairs, and other daily activities that require a subtle downward gaze (Fig. 27.6).

COMPLICATIONS

Complications specific to the treatment of posttraumatic cervical deformity can be related to the graft or instrumentation, overcorrection or undercorrection of the kyphosis correction, or neurologic deterioration. As discussed previously, long anterior reconstructions should be augmented with posterior instrumented fusion to decrease the risk for nonunion and minimize graft and plate complications.

Malalignment of the cervical spine after surgical reconstruction can result in significant functional problems. Although jaw opening and swallowing function may improve, visual field may remain limited if the gaze angle is not adequately addressed. When done under local anesthetic, the patient can be questioned as to optimal head positioning.[34–36] The majority of surgical cases for posttraumatic cervical deformity, however, are performed under a general anesthetic. The use of a general anesthetic requires the surgeon to determine optimal head positioning.

Undercorrection has been attributed to tightness of the anterior cervical musculature, surgeon and patient concerns regarding overcorrection, or loss of operative correction.[36] Overcorrection of the sagittal alignment will result in difficulty looking ahead, looking down, and ambulating down stairs. Suk et al.[40] reported significant difficulty in going down stairs in patients with overcorrection. Sengupta et al.[41] described a technique of cervicothoracic flexion osteotomy to correct to a neutral gaze angle; they suggested that the use of clear drapes intraoperatively may improve surgeon assessment of optimal head positioning. Combined with a sitting position, this does decrease the chance for overcorrection or undercorrection.

Neurologic complications, although rare, are the most devastating complications associated with treating cervical deformity. The location of the deformity places the spinal cord at risk. Additionally, chronic injury to the cord, resulting from progressive stretch and a potentially compromised blood supply, further place the patient at risk for cord injury perioperatively. Cervical cord injury has, therefore, been described across the spectrum of operative treatment options.

Assessment of neurologic status is critical in determining safety of operative treatment. Intraoperative neurologic exam can be performed in the awake patient. Simmons[36] reported no neurologic complications within his group of patients with cervicothoracic osteotomy treated under local anesthetic. Belanger et al.[34] reported permanent quadriplegia in 1 of 16 normal preoperative patients. Any neurologic symptoms expressed by the patient intraoperatively can allow for immediate surgical correction. Yet, despite its purported benefits, cord injury has been seen in surgery in the awake patient.

The immediate neurologic feedback of the awake patient is lost when the procedure is performed with the patient under a general anesthetic. McMaster[37] reported one patient who developed complete quadriplegia 1 week after surgery. The use of intraoperative neural monitoring is thought to allow early detection of neurologic injury in an anesthetized patient. Wenger et al.[42] report a temporary spinal artery syndrome during correction of posttraumatic cervical kyphosis. Despite normal somatosensory evoked potential monitoring intraoperatively, the patient awoke with tetraplegia. The patient showed neurologic recovery with months, and by 3-year follow-up showed no deficits. The addition of transcranial motor evoked potentials has been shown to improve detection of cord injury in the cervical spine.[43] Langeloo et al.[38] reported nine neurologic events during intraoperative motor evoked potential monitoring. Eight of nine resolved either spontaneously or after surgical correction. One patient showed no resolution and awoke with an incomplete cord injury. The use of transcranial motor evoked potentials intraoperatively may diminish the risk of cervical cord injury during corrective surgery. We use motor evoked potentials, somatosensory evoked potentials, and free-run electromyelographic monitoring to help offset the risk for neurologic injury.

In addition to cervical cord injury, attention also must be directed toward the cervical nerve roots. Traction injury after curve correction may occur, most commonly at the C5 root. Compressive injury to the C8 nerve root has been described after closure of the extension osteotomy; deficits have been reported to be both transient and permanent.[34,37] Wide decompression of bilateral nerve roots at the site of osteotomy is therefore recommended.

CONCLUSION

Treatment of posttraumatic cervical kyphosis requires a thorough understanding of the pathologic condition. In addition to radiographic analysis, neurologic compromise and function limitations associated with the deformity must be clearly defined.

Surgical correction will require combined anterior and posterior arthrodesis of the spine with instrumentation to improve union rates and decrease graft complications. Severe fixed deformities require a posterior closing osteotomy.

Cosmetic and functional outcomes can be excellent with restoration of normal jaw opening, swallowing function, and vision. Significant complications are associated with operative treatment, with devastating neurologic injury as a potential adverse outcome. Patients should be educated very clearly about this risk. Additionally, when a primary indication for surgery is neck pain in addition to deformity, the resolution of pain is less predictable. This is due to lack of understanding of the source of pain and the potential multiple causes of neck pain.

REFERENCES

1. Zdeblick, TA, Zou D, Warden KE, et al. Cervical instability after foraminotomy: a biomechanical in vitro analysis. *J Bone Joint Surg Am* 1992;74:22–27.
2. Loder RT. Profiles of the cervical, thoracic, and lumbosacral spine in children and adolescents with lumbosacral spondylolisthesis. *J Spinal Disord* 2001;14:465–471.
3. Harrison DD, Harrison DE, Janik TJ, et al. Modeling of the sagittal cervical spine as a method to discriminate hypolordosis: results of elliptical and circular modeling in 72 asymptomatic subjects, 52 acute neck pain subjects, and 70 chronic neck pain subjects. *Spine* 2004;29:2485–2492.
4. Panjabi MM, White AA, Johnson RM. Cervical spine biomechanics as a function of transection of components. *J Biomechan* 1975;8:327–336.
5. Panjabi MM, Summer DJ, Pelker RR, et al. Three-dimensional load-displacement curves due to forces on the cervical spine. *J Orthop Res* 1986;4:151–152.
6. Pal GP, Sherk HH. The vertical stability of the cervical spine. *Spine* 1988;13:447–449.
7. Raynor RB, Moskovich T, Zidel P, et al. Alterations in primary and coupled neck motions after facetectomy. *Neurogsurgery* 1987;21:681–686.
8. Zdeblick TA, Abitbol J-J, Kunz DN, et al. Cervical stability after sequential capsule resection. *Spine* 1993;18: 2005–2008.
9. Nowinski, GP, Visarious H, Nolte P, et al. A biomechanical comparison of cervical laminaplasty and cervical laminectomy with progressive facetectomy. *Spine* 1993;18:1995–2004.
10. Fager CA. Results of adequate posterior decompression in relief of spondylotic cervical myelopathy. *J Neurosurg* 1973;8:684–692.
11. Fager CA. Management of cervical lesions and spondylosis by posterior approaches. *Clin Neurosurg* 1977;24: 488–507.
12. Epstein JA. The surgical management of cervical spinal stenosis, spondylosis, and myeloradiculopathy by means of the posterior approach. *Spine* 1988;13:864–869.
13. Herkowitz HN. A comparison of anterior cervical fusion, cervical laminectomy, and cervical laminoplasty for the surgical management of multiple level spondylitic myelopathy. *Spine* 1988;13:774–780.
14. Munechika Y. Influence of laminectomy on the stability of the spine: an experimental study with special reference to the extent of laminectomy and the resection of the intervertebral joint. *J Japan Orthop Assoc* 1973;47:111–125.
15. Cusick JF, Yoganandan N, Pintar F, et al. Biomechanics of cervical spine facetectomy and fixation techniques. *Spine* 1988;13:808–812.
16. White AA, Panjabi MM. Biomechanic considerations in the surgical management of cervical spondylotic myelopathy. *Spine* 1988;13:856–860.
17. Saito T, Yamamuro T, Shikata J, et al. Analysis and prevention of spinal column deformity following cervical laminectomy. I: Pathogenetic analysis of postlaminectomy deformities. *Spine* 1991;19:494–502.
18. Nolan JP, Sherk HH. Biomechanical evaluation of extensor musculature of the cervical spine. *Spine* 1988;13:9–11.
19. Albert T, Vacarro A. Postlaminectomy kyphosis. *Spine* 1998;23:2738–2745.
20. Kalbhenn T, Mittlmeier T, Woiciechowsky C. Late neurological deterioration 30 years following conservative treatment of a lower cervical spine fracture: a case report. *Zentralbl Neurochir* 2002;63:77–80.
21. Riew KD, Hilibrand AS, Palumbo MA, et al. Anterior cervical corpectomy in patients previously managed with a laminectomy: short-term complications. *J Bone Joint Surg Am* 1999;81:950–957.
22. Emery SE, Fisher JR, Bohlman HH. Three-level anterior cervical discectomy and fusion: radiographic and clinical results. *Spine* 1997;22:2622–2624.
23. Kirkpatrick JS, Levy JA, Carillo J, et al. Reconstruction after multilevel corpectomy in the cervical spine: a sagittal plane biomechanical study. *Spine* 1999;24:1186–1190.
24. Riew KD, Hilibrand AS, Palumbo MA, et al. Anterior cervical corpectomy in patients previously managed with a laminectomy: short-term complications. *J Bone Joint Surg Am* 1999;81:950–957.

25. Zdeblick TA, Bohlman HH. Myelopathy, cervical kyphosis, and treatment by anterior corpectomy and strut grafting. *J Bone Joint Surg Am* 1989;71:170–182.
26. Herman JM, Sonntag VKH. Cervical corpectomy and plate fixation for postlaminectomy kyphosis. *J Neurosurg* 1994;80:963–970.
27. Vaccaro AR, Falatyn SP, Scuderi GJ, et al. Early failure of long segment anterior cervical plate fixation. *J Spinal Disord* 1998;11:410–415.
28. Singh K, Vaccaro AR, Kim J, et al. Enhancement of stability following anterior cervical corpectomy: a biomechanical study. *Spine* 2004;29:845–849.
29. Bolesta MJ, Rechtine GR, Chrin AM. Three- and four-level anterior cervical discectomy and fusion with plate fixation: a prospective study. *Spine* 2000;25(16):2040–2044.
30. Truumees E, Demetropoulos CK, Yang KH, et al. Effects of a cervical compression plate on graft forces in an anterior cervical discectomy model. *Spine* 2003;28:1097–1102.
31. McAfee PC, Bohlman HH, Ducker TB, et al. One-stage anterior cervical decompression and posterior stabilization: a study of one hundred patients with a minimum of two years of follow-up. *J Bone and Joint Surg Am* 1995;77:1791–1800.
32. McAfee PC, Bohlman HH. One-stage anterior cervical decompression and posterior stabilization with circumferential arthrodesis: a study of twenty-four patients who had a traumatic or a neoplastic lesion. *J Bone Joint Surg Am* 1989;71:78–88.
33. Mason C, Cozen L, Adelstein L. Surgical correction of flexion deformity of the cervical spine. *Calif Med* 1953;79:244–246.
34. Belanger TA, Milam RA 4th, Roh JS, et al. Cervicothoracic extension osteotomy for chin-on-chest deformity in ankylosing spondylitis. *J Bone Joint Surg* 2005;87:1732–738.
35. Urist MR. Osteotomy of the cervical spine; report of a case of ankylosing rheumatoid spondylitis. *J Bone Joint Surg Am* 1958;40:833–843.
36. Simmons EH. The surgical correction of flexion deformity of the cervical spine in ankylosing spondylitis. *Clin Orthop Relat Res* 1972;86:132–143.
37. McMaster MJ. Osteotomy of the cervical spine in ankylosing spondylitis. *J Bone Joint Surg Br* 1997;79:197–203.
38. Langeloo DD, Journee HL, Pavlov PW, et al. Cervical osteotomy in ankylosing spondylitis: evaluation of new developments. *Eur Spine J* 2006;15:493:500.
39. von Royen BJ, Slot GM. Closing-wedge posterior osteotomy for ankylosing spondylitis. *J Bone Joint Surg Br* 1995;77:117–121
40. Suk KS, Kim KT, Lee SH, et al. Significance of chin-brow vertical angle in correction of kyphotic deformity of ankylosing spondylitis patients. *Spine* 2003;28:2001–2005.
41. Sengupta DK, Khazim R, Grevitt MP, et al. Flexion osteotomy of the cervical spine: a new technique for correction of iatrogenic extension deformity in ankylosing spondylitis. *Spine* 2001;26:1068–1072.
42. Wenger M, Braun M, Markwalder T. Post-traumatic cervical kyphosis with surgical correction complicated by temporary anterior spinal artery syndrome. *J Clin Neurosci* 2005;12:193–196.
43. Hillbrand AS, Schwartz DM, Sethuraman V, et al. Comparison of transcranial electric motor and somatosensory evoked potential monitoring during cervical spine surgery. *J Bone Joint Surg Am* 2004;86:1248–1253.

SECTION IX

Fractures in Metabolic Bone Disease

CHAPTER 28

Ankylosing Spondylitis

Aditya Pandey, Alexander R. Vaccaro, and James S. Harrop

INTRODUCTION

Spondyloarthropathies represent a group of inflammatory disorders that are clinically manifested as inflammatory changes to the axial spinal skeleton and peripheral joints. Such disorders include: ankylosing spondylitis, reactive arthritis, psoriatic arthritis, enteropathic arthritis, and juvenile arthritis. This chapter discusses ankylosing spondylitis (Bechterew's disease) in the context of traumatic injuries to the cervical spine.[1] Ankylosing spondylitis is an uncommon entity, with a prevalence in the general population of approximately 1.4%.[2] Approximately 1% of all cervical spinal disorders seen by spine surgeons are related to ankylosing spondylitis.[3]

Ankylosing spondylitis was originally described in Russia as a disease in which inflammation leads to ossification of the joints and ligaments.[4] These inflammatory changes typically begin in the sacroiliac joints, where sclerosis and fusion can be illustrated on plain radiographs. With progression of the disease process, the axial spinal column is also involved. There is ossification of the longitudinal ligaments and subsequent disc space calcification, thus creating immobility of the spinal segments. This process advances to multiple spinal segments, creating long rigid lever arms that are extremely brittle biomechanically (Fig. 28.1).[2] Thus, when the patient is subjected to external forces, there is a tendency for the spinal column to fracture and translate, resulting in injury to the neural elements. A similar pattern of injury occurs in patients with ankylosed spines from spondylosis, surgery, or diffuse idiopathic skeletal hyperostosis (DISH).

Ankylosing spondylitis tends to be a disease process affecting young male individuals, although fractures are seen in older age groups. The male to female ratio is reported to vary from 4:1 to 10:1, and the majority of cases present clinically in the fourth decade of life with axial skeletal pain.[4] Ankylosing spondylitis uniformly involves the sacroiliac joints, but in male patients tends to also involve the thoracolumbar spine (Fig. 28.2) and in female patients the cervical spine. Symptoms tend to reflect the distribution of inflammatory changes. The sacroiliac joints and the lumbar spine are first to be affected; thus, patients commonly present with back and hip pain. Along with other constitutional symptoms, most patients will describe morning stiffness that progressively improves with activity. Nonsteroidal anti-inflammatory drugs (NSAIDs) are typically beneficial for pain control in this patient population.

DIAGNOSIS

The diagnosis of ankylosing spondylitis is defined by clinical symptoms in the setting of appropriate radiologic criteria. Biopsy of an affected joint is not required, but if performed would illustrate findings of inflammatory changes: synovial hyperplasia, edema, and lymphocytic infiltrate. These

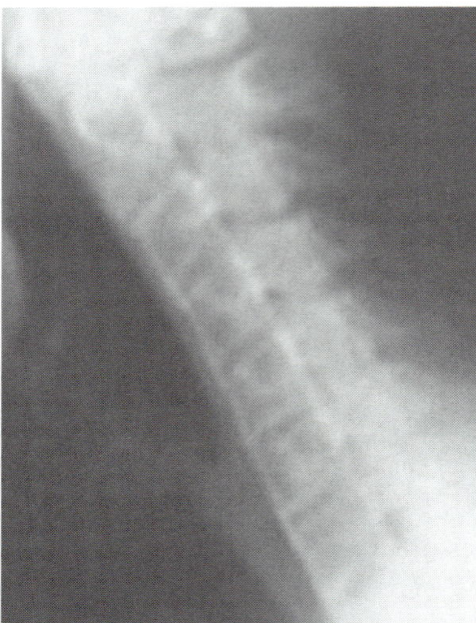

FIGURE 28.1. Lateral radiograph of the cervical spine demonstrating ankylosis of the cervical spine.

histologic changes then further progress to fibrous destruction of the joint and subsequent ankylosis. The demographic characteristics of patients with ankylosing spondylitis were well described by Vosse et al.[2]: mean age at time of diagnosis was 32 years of age and mean age at the time of first symptomatic fracture was 50 years.

Genetic markers over the last several decades have been a further diagnostic instrument in defining the ankylosing spondylitis patient population. Of all men with ankylosing spondylitis, 81% are positive for HLA-B27.[2] Specifically, the HLA-B27 haplotype has been isolated in 90% of individuals meeting the clinical diagnosis of ankylosing spondylitis, but is seen in less than 7% of individuals not affected by the disease.[2,5] Although the HLA-B27 marker appears to be a strong predictor of the ankylosing spondylitis phenotype, unfortunately the molecular product of the HLA-B27 haplotype has yet to be defined in the pathogenesis of ankylosing spondylitis.

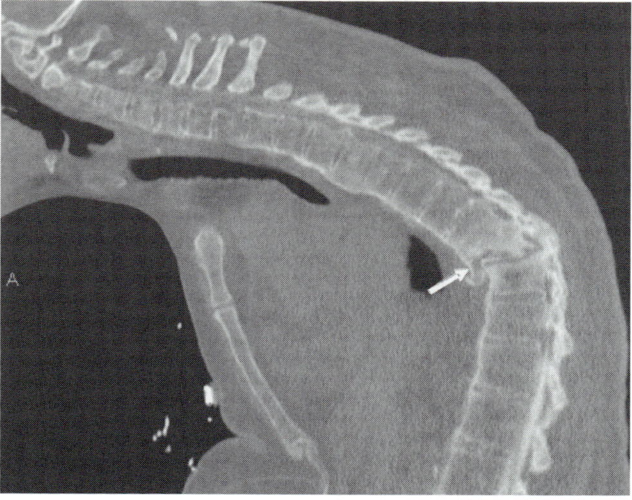

FIGURE 28.2. Lateral radiograph of the cervical and thoracic spine in a patient with ankylosing spondylitis.

PROGRESSION OF DISEASE AND SYMPTOMS

As ankylosing spondylitis advances, ossification of the ligaments and disc spaces occurs, creating loss of mobile spinal motion segments. The spine radiographically appears as a solid ossified column and has been referred to as a bamboo spine because of this appearance (Fig. 28.3). The resulting non-mobile spine loses its ability to dissipate or accommodate external traumatic forces. Stresses are not absorbed by the dysfunctional discs or calcified ligamentous structures, and thus fractures are common even with minimal trauma. This is further complicated by the long lever arms of the ossified spine, where small movements of the fractured spine will result in translational forces and shear injury to the spinal cord and neural elements.[5] Thus, a flexion injury frequently leads to tensile failure of the posterior elements, resulting in a shear-type fracture involving the posterior and anterior elements. Such a fracture is similar to the seat belt injury described in the lumbar spine.

Ankylosis of the spine, combined with the poor bone stock and alteration in spinal biomechanics, creates the environment for low-energy forces to produce devastating spinal column fractures. In the report by Vosse et al.,[2] in 56% of patients with ankylosing spondylitis, traumatic spinal fractures were created through low- to medium-energy forces.[2] These authors further stated that the low-energy spinal fractures in this population were typically more complicated and severe than higher energy traumas. This was due to a combination of an ankylosed spine and significant osteoporosis. Thus, in an individual with ankylosing spondylitis and osteoporosis the spinal column's ability to absorb external forces and retain tensile strength is lost, leading to complex spinal fractures with minimal trauma such as a fall from a standing position. Furthermore, the preexisting kyphotic posture causes loss of balance, making falls more likely. Kyphosis also protrudes the head forward, potentially subjecting it to direct facial trauma and creating hyperextension forces and extension cervical fractures.

Fractures in this population can be difficult to diagnose because they tend to be hairline fractures through the ossified disc space and posterior facets. Plain images typically are nondiagnostic because of the osteoporotic nature of the bone and the architectural changes usually associated with ankylosing spondylitis. Therefore, any patient with ankylosing spondylitis who presents with spinal axial pain after a traumatic injury should be suspected of having a spinal fracture, and additional advanced imaging modalities should be employed.[6] This is particularly true for the cervical spine, where any injury can have a catastrophic effect if left untreated. Cooper et al.[7] noted a relative risk of

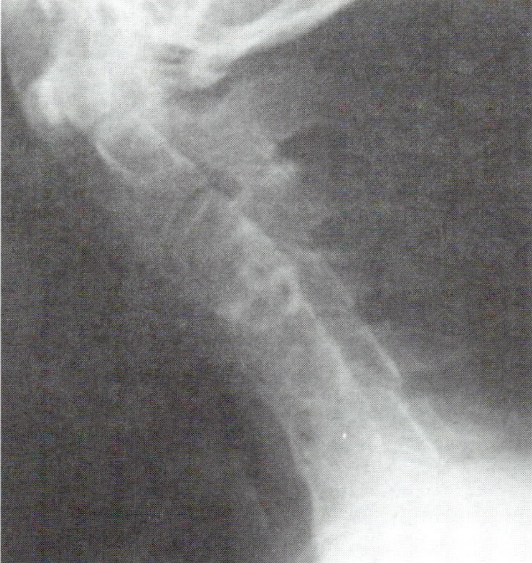

FIGURE 28.3. Lateral radiograph of the cervical spine demonstrating ankylosis of the cervical spine.

7.6 (95% CI, 4.3 to 12.6) in developing a spinal fracture in the setting of ankylosing spondylitis following trauma.

Although there is agreement that all cervical fractures in patients with ankylosing spondylitis are potentially unstable, patients may clinically present anywhere along a spectrum of minor neck discomfort to a severe neurologic deficit from spinal cord injury. In the series by Vosse et al.,[2] 47% of patients with ankylosing spondylitis with spinal fractures at presentation had neurologic deficits ranging from sensory disturbance to paralysis.[2]

In patients whose initial acute cervical fractures are not diagnosed, there is the possibility of developing a chronic nonhealed cervical fracture or a cervicothoracic kyphotic deformity. This progressive kyphosis may result in the development of a chin-on-chest deformity in which the patient is unable to open the mouth or view the horizon because the line of sight is altered. This chin-on-chest deformity is thought to develop from minor flexion injuries to the cervical spine that may not be obvious to the patient initially. Extreme kyphotic deformities at the cervicothoracic junction can clinically be devastating for the patient. The angulation of the neck and head prevents the patient from looking upward or forward. In addition, patients with ankylosing spondylitis typically develop swallowing difficulty because of mandibular dysfunction. This, associated with cervical kyphosis, may result in angulation of the trachea or esophagus, leading to further dysphagia and odynophagia.[3]

TYPES OF FRACTURES

Arthropathies are a progressive disease process, and patients with ankylosing spondylitis who are clinically symptomatic for more than 20 years tend to have an increased incidence of cervical ankylosis.[8] With ankylosis of the cervical spine, even minor trauma can lead to devastating cervical fracture. Descriptions of minor trauma have included falling out of bed, falling out of a chair, driving over speed bumps, simple falls, and chiropractic maneuvers.[9] Patients with ankylosing spondylitis may present with a fracture without specific knowledge of any traumatic or antecedent event. The amount of manipulation required to induce a fracture of these fragile ankylosed spines is minimal; in fact, there are case examples of patients with ankylosing spondylitis developing cervical fractures during emergent intubation.[9]

Spinal fractures are approximately 3 to 3.5 times more common in the ankylosing spondylitis population than the general population.[10,11] Hunter and Dubo[12,13] noted that the majority of spinal fractures in the ankylosing spondylitis population occur in the cervical spine, specifically at the cervicothoracic junction. The long, rigid lever arm of the immobile cervical spine, osteoporosis, and kyphotic posture that transitions into the rigid thoracic spine all predispose the patient with ankylosing spondylitis to a higher incidence of cervical fractures. In the general population, the highest incidence of cervical fractures (33%) occurs between the occiput and C2 because of the transition of external forces from the mobile cranium to the mobile cervical spine.[14] However, in the ankylosing spondylitis patient population, as a result of the spontaneous arthrodesis and immobility between the occiput and C2, fractures at this level are infrequent, occurring with an incidence of 17%.[1] In most ankylosing spondylitis cervical trauma series, fractures of the cervical spine occur more frequently between C5 and C7 (Fig. 28.4).[9] Unrecognized noncontiguous fractures (such as at the thoracolumbar junction) are not uncommon in patients with traumatic cervical spine injuries.

Chronic fractures in the ankylosing spondylitis population are referred to as spondylodiscitis, which is a misnomer, because it describes the erosive and sclerotic appearance of a nonhealed fracture seen on plain radiographs. This term is a historic reference describing the radiographic characteristics seen in discitis and osteomyelitis and shared by the radiographic appearance of a chronically nonhealed fracture in the setting of ankylosing spondylitis. This entity in ankylosing spondylitis is in no way related to an infectious process. Instead, it is due to a combination of inflammation and excessive loads on discs that have not yet fused. These lesions are fractures that progress to a pseudarthrosis as a result of the long lever arms creating constant motion at these sites.[3] Patients present because of pain at the injury site or the development of a neurologic deficit.

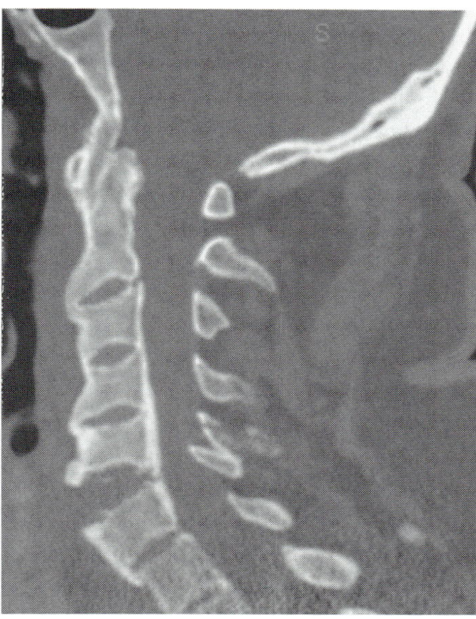

FIGURE 28.4. Acute fracture involving the C5 and C6 vertebral bodies in a patient with ankylosing spondylitis.

RADIOLOGIC FINDINGS

All patients with ankylosing spondylitis who present with spinal axial symptoms should undergo a thorough physical examination and a detailed radiologic evaluation to exclude the possibility of an occult fracture. The patient's radiographic evaluation should consist of initial plain radiographs of the involved segment of spine. In a suspected cervical fracture, the plain radiographs should be assessed for evidence of prevertebral soft tissue swelling as an indicator of traumatic injury. Unfortunately, in the ankylosing spondylitis population, these plain radiographs can be difficult to assess because of the presence of calcified ligaments and disc spaces, as well as the limited resolution of osteoporotic bone. Cervical fractures in patients with ankylosing spondylitis typically involve the cervicothoracic junction, the C5-T1 segment. Because of the patient's body habitus and poor bone quality, it is often difficult to visualize the bony anatomy at these levels. Koivikko et al.[1] illustrated this point in their series of 18 patients with progressive ankylosing spondylitis. Only 8% of the patients had lateral radiographs that clearly visualized the cervicothoracic junction. Plain radiographs in this series had a sensitivity of 48%, which was reduced to 33% when the fracture line was transverse. In another retrospective analysis, 9 of 11 traumatic ankylosing spondylitis patients were diagnosed with cervical traumatic fractures using plain radiographs; however, all 11 patients were diagnosed with a cervical fracture using more sophisticated imaging modalities such as computed tomography (CT) and magnetic resonance imaging (MRI).[11]

CT provides detailed imaging of the anatomy of a cervical fracture, including the bony architecture and status of the spinal canal. In addition, sagittal and coronal reformatted images can be reconstructed to better understand overall spinal alignment. The emergence of multidetector CT has further aided in the detection of occult cervical spinal injuries in this patient population.[6] If a spinal fracture is present, consideration should be given to obtaining thoracic and lumbar CT with reformatting, because many patients will have unsuspected noncontiguous fractures. MRI provides detailed imaging of the cervical spinal cord and its relationship to the bony spinal fracture. It allows for an understanding of nonosseous compression of the cervical spinal cord by either a disc herniation or epidural hematoma (Fig. 28.5). Although MRI is a valuable imaging modality, it is not always feasible in the ankylosing spondylitis population. In the series by Koivikko et al.,[1] only 61% of

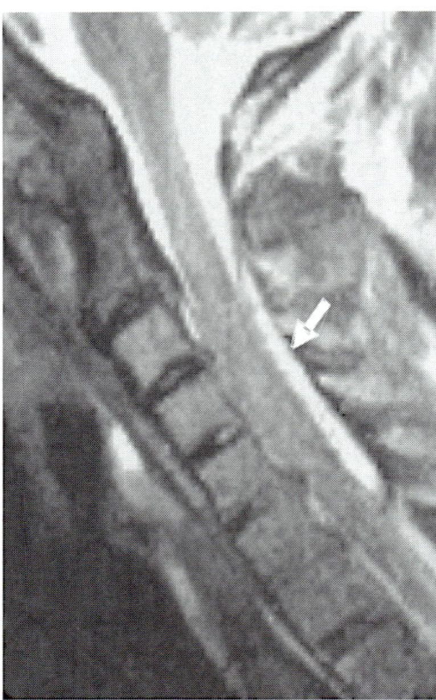

FIGURE 28.5. Magnetic resonance imaging of the cervical spine showing an acute spinal epidural hematoma located dorsally.

patients were able to undergo MRI evaluation. Some precluding factors included longer time for evaluation, MRI-incompatible equipment (traction devices, anesthesia equipment, pacemakers), and kyphotic deformities leading to inability to lie flat.

Nonetheless, MRI can provide detailed visualization of the neural elements that may influence surgical approach for an unstable injury.

TREATMENT AND OUTCOME

Poor bone quality and the long lever arm of fused bone above and below a fracture make any spinal fracture in the setting of ankylosing spondylitis an unstable lesion with a high potential for neurologic injury.[15,16] Rowed[17] illustrated the susceptibility of patients with ankylosing spondylitis to developing a symptomatic spinal cord injury (SCI) following trauma. In their series of 21 patients with cervical fractures, 16 (76%) developed a spinal cord injury. In the same series, a similar group of trauma patients without ankylosing spondylitis had only an 18% incidence of SCI.[15] Bohlman et al.[15] noted a 66% incidence of SCI following a fracture in the setting of ankylosing spondylitis. Other series of patients with ankylosing spondylitis have reported an incidence of SCI between 50% and 73% in the setting of a cervical fracture.

The neurologic injury is caused by the primary injury mechanism or is delayed as a result of instability, deformity, or epidural hematoma. The incidence of traumatic spinal epidural hematoma (SEH) in patients with ankylosing spondylitis is reported to range from 10% to 50% following trauma.[18] These epidural hematomas usually form as the result of fracturing of calcified posterior epidural arterial vessels following trauma. Some authors have postulated that venous oozing from disrupted trabeculae may also be the cause of the increased incidence of epidural hematomas in this patient group.[17]

Patients with ankylosing spondylitis may sustain asymptomatic cervical spinal fractures following trivial trauma and thus may not seek medical attention. These patients typically sustain flexion compression injuries that can lead to an incompetence of the anterior column and development of a kyphotic deformity. Grisola et al.[19] described six patients with fractures in the setting of ankylosing spondylitis, five of whom were asymptomatic by history. Surin[20] noted that flexion compression injuries in the cervical spine tend to go unnoticed because they are usually not associated with neurologic deficits. These injuries, however, may present in a delayed manner when the patient develops a kyphotic deformity leading to a chin-on-chest deformity, the loss of horizontal sight, mandibular dysfunction, or symptoms resulting from kinking of the esophagus or trachea.

Treatment options for cervical fractures in the setting of ankylosing spondylitis include both nonoperative management and surgical stabilization. Conservative measures or nonoperative strategies include cervical spine immobilization through the use of collars, cervical traction, and halo vest orthosis. There is increased risk for neurologic injury in the ankylosing spondylitis population over the general population with the use of cervical traction following fracture. This is a result of the long lever arms of fused vertebrae surrounding the fracture site that predispose to a large transmission of forces at the injury site potentially leading to neurologic injury.

The indications for surgical intervention in the patient with ankylosing spondylitis include progressive kyphotic deformities, neurologic deficits, and unstable fractures. However, the majority of injuries are best treated with surgical stabilization.

Rowed[17] reported on 11 patients with a traumatic injury in the setting of ankylosing spondylitis treated conservatively. Three patients had a complete neurologic injury, and eight had an incomplete neurologic injury. All patients were treated with halo vest immobilization. At follow-up, seven patients (64%) eventually went on to a productive lifestyle and return to work, one patient suffered neurologic deterioration, two patients died, and one remained hospitalized. The incomplete neurologic injuries were not described in detail; thus no conclusion could be made regarding neurologic improvement. However, four patients did develop recurrent dislocations and one patient developed a new-onset neurologic deficit. Because of the unstable nature of cervical fractures in the ankylosing spondylitis population, most clinical series recommend against pure axial distraction forces through traction. Initial nonoperative treatment often involves gentle traction reduction of the deformity followed by halo vest application.

The majority of traumatic cervical fractures in the ankylosing spondylitis population involve a certain degree of translation displacement. The options for surgical stabilization in this setting include (a) an initial anterior decompression with fusion, followed by a posterior stabilization procedure, or (b) an initial posterior decompression, reduction, and stabilization procedure, followed (if necessary) by an anterior decompression and fusion. Fox et al.[21] reported on the successful use of posterior spinous process wiring and bone grafting followed by external immobilization for 3 to 6 months in this patient population following a cervical spine fracture. Taggard and Traynelis[22] reported on the use of lateral mass screw fixation as a method of rigid internal fixation, followed by cervical collar immobilization, thereby avoiding the discomfort and morbidity of the halo vest. The posterior fixation strategy included lateral mass plating two levels above and below the level of fracture, supplemented with a rib autograft fixated to the lamina and spinous process. When the C7, T1, or T2 levels were included in the fusion mass, pedicle screw instrumentation was used. All patients who underwent posterior cervical instrumentation maintained or improved their neurologic status, and no patient experienced neurologic deterioration. At follow-up, all patients demonstrated evidence of stable bony fusion on dynamic plain imaging.

Although the authors mentioned earlier have had great success with lateral mass fixation, it is important to realize the anatomic complexity of identifying posterior landmarks in the patient with ankylosing spondylitis. Because of the natural ossification of the posterior lateral masses and facet joints, there is often a paucity of anatomic landmarks to assist in hardware placement. Thus, familiarity with such anatomy is essential in performing posterior fixation in the ankylosing spondylitis patient population. Taggard and Traynelis[22] recommended that 13-mm screws be used to decrease the risk for nerve root injury. In addition, in the lower cervical spine, pedicle screw instrumentation was recommended to further improve the stability of the construct. Because all joints are already fused, longer multilevel constructs can be used to increase strength of fixation.

Often, because of circumferential instability, a combined surgical approach may be necessary or recommended. Posterior instrumented fusions are often successful over the long term in the absence of kyphotic deformity.[22] Unfortunately, a posterior-only instrumentation construct may not be able to overcome the gravitational forces and biomechanical disadvantages of a kyphotic deformity. In this setting, consideration of spinal realignment is necessary at the site of the fracture or supplemental anterior column support is needed at the anterior fracture gap for further fracture site stabilization and support.[10]

Typically, a posterior stabilization procedure involves multilevel fixation (three levels above and below the cervical fracture site) to obtain adequate purchase above and below the fracture level. The length of the construct will not result in loss of spinal motion because the patient's cervical spine is already autofused. If a significant anterior column gap is present after posterior instrumentation, often it is subsequently grafted with or without plate fixation. The decision to proceed with a decompression is based on the presence of a symptomatic disc herniation or epidural hematoma as delineated by MRI. If there is no cord compression, the goal of surgery is to stabilize the fracture.

Although patients with ankylosing spondylitis who sustain fractures have an increased mortality risk, very rarely does the fracture actually contribute directly to this. Hollin et al.[23] describe a 45% acute mortality rate in patients with ankylosing spondylitis with vertebral body fractures. Similarly, Rowed[17] found that patients with ankylosing spondylitis with cervical fractures had a twofold increase in mortality rate (30% to 35%) compared to controls (17%). In the majority of these cases, patient mortality was directly attributed to respiratory failure. In fact, Radford et al.[24] attributed only 3 of 146 deaths in a series of 836 patients with ankylosing spondylitis to vertebral column fracture.

The functional outcome after cervical fractures in the ankylosing spondylitis population has also been described. Broom and Raycroft reported that approximately 20% of their patients achieved independence, and Hunter and Murray reported good outcomes with functional recovery in 43% to 45% of their patients.[8] Further studies are needed to accurately assess the effects of early surgical stabilization and mobilization on functional improvement and long-term morbidity and mortality.

CONCLUSION

Spinal fractures in patients with ankylosing spondylitis are highly unstable, and complications such as displacement, neurologic deterioration, epidural hematoma, and death are common. Delays in diagnosis stem from difficultly in imaging and often only subtle manifestations of fracture. Any patient with ankylosing spondylitis with a history of trauma and new pain should be critically evaluated with radiologic imaging, including CT or MRI. Initial treatment for cervical fractures should be immobilization, although standard traction techniques may be dangerous. Definitive treatment can be by orthosis such as a halo vest, although the authors recommend internal stabilization, usually with a posterior technique.

REFERENCES

1. Koivikko MP, Kiuru MJ, Koskinen SK. Multidetector computed tomography of cervical spine fractures in ankylosing spondylitis. *Acta Radiol* 2004;45:751–759.
2. Vosse D, Feldtkeller E, Erlendsson J, et al. Clinical vertebral fractures in patients with ankylosing spondylitis. *J Rheumatol* 2004;31:1981–1985.
3. Szpalski M, Gunzburg R. What are the advances for surgical therapy of inflammatory diseases of the spine? *Best Pract Res Clin Rheumatol* 2002;16:141–154.
4. Schmidek HH, Roberts DW. *Operative Neurosurgical Techniques: Indications, Methods, and Results.* New York: Saunders; 2000, 1822–1830.
5. Graham B, Van Peteghem PK. Fractures of the spine in ankylosing spondylitis. Diagnosis, treatment, and complications. *Spine* 1989;14:803–807.
6. Harrop JS, Sharan A, Anderson G, et al. Failure of standard imaging to detect a cervical fracture in a patient with ankylosing spondylitis. *Spine* 2005;30:E417–E419.
7. Cooper C, Carbone L, Michet CJ, et al. Fracture risk in patients with ankylosing spondylitis: a population based study. *J Rheumatol* 1994;21:1877–1882.

8. Murray GC, Persellin RH. Cervical fracture complicating ankylosing spondylitis: a report of eight cases and review of the literature. *Am J Med* 1981;70:1033–1041.
9. Salathe M, Johr M. Unsuspected cervical fractures: a common problem in ankylosing spondylitis. *Anesthesiology* 1989;70:869–870.
10. El Masry MA, Badawy WS, Chan D. Combined anterior and posterior stabilization for treating an unstable cervical spine fracture in a patient with long standing ankylosing spondylitis. *Injury* 2004;35:1064–1067.
11. Nakstad PH, Server A, Josefsen R. Traumatic cervical injuries in ankylosing spondylitis. *Acta Radiol* 2004;45: 222–226.
12. Hunter T, Dubo H. Spinal fractures complicating ankylosing spondylitis. *Ann Intern Med* 1978;88:546–549.
13. Hunter T, Dubo HI. Spinal fractures complicating ankylosing spondylitis: a long-term follow-up study. *Arthritis Rheum* 1983;26:751–759.
14. Goldberg W, Mueller C, Panacek E, et al. Distribution and patterns of blunt traumatic cervical spine injury. *Ann Emerg Med* 2001;38:17–21.
15. Bohlman HH. Acute fractures and dislocations of the cervical spine: an analysis of three hundred hospitalized patients and review of the literature. *J Bone Joint Surg Am* 1979;61:1119–1142.
16. Detwiler KN, Loftus CM, Godersky JC, et al. Management of cervical spine injuries in patients with ankylosing spondylitis. *J Neurosurg* 1990;72:210–215.
17. Rowed DW. Management of cervical spinal cord injury in ankylosing spondylitis: the intervertebral disc as a cause of cord compression. *J Neurosurg* 1992;77:241–246.
18. Jacobs WB, Fehlings MG. Ankylosing spondylitis and spinal cord injury: origin, incidence, management, and avoidance. *Neurosurg Focus* 2008;24(1):E12.
19. Grisola A, Bell RL, Peltier LF. Fractures and dislocations of the spine complicating ankylosing spondylitis: a report of six cases. *Clin Orthop Relat Res* 2004;422:129–134.
20. Surin VV. Fractures of the cervical spine in patients with ankylosing spondylitis. *Acta Orthop Scand* 1980;51:79–84.
21. Fox MW, Onofrio BM, Kilgore JE. Neurological complications of ankylosing spondylitis. *J Neurosurg* 1993;78: 871–878.
22. Taggard DA, Traynelis VC. Management of cervical spinal fractures in ankylosing spondylitis with posterior fixation. *Spine* 2000;25:2035–2039.
23. Hollin SA, Gross SW, Levin P. Fractures of the cervical spine in patients with rheumatoid spondylitis. *Am Surg* 1965;31:532–536.
24. Radford EP, Doll R, Smith PG. Mortality among patients with ankylosing spondylitis not given X-ray therapy. *N Engl J Med* 1977;297:572–576.

SUGGESTED READINGS

Belanger TA, Milam RA 4th, Roh JS, et al. Cervicothoracic extension osteotomy for chin-on-chest deformity in ankylosing spondylitis. *J Bone Joint Surg Am* 2005;87:1732–1738.

Coleman JA. Cervical spine fracture in the ankylosing spondylitis patient. *J Am Coll Surg* 2005;201:318.

Exner G, Botel U, Kluger P, et al. Treatment of fracture and complication of cervical spine with ankylosing spondylitis. *Spinal Cord* 1998;36:377–379.

Frymoyer JW, Weisel SW. *The Adult and Pediatric*. Philadelphia: Lippincott Williams & Wilkins, 2004:484.

Good AE. Nontraumatic fracture of the thoracic spine in ankylosing spondylitis. *Arthritis Rheum* 1967;10:467–469.

Hansen ST Jr, Taylor TK, Honet JC, et al. Fracture-dislocations of the ankylosed thoracic spine in rheumatoid spondylitis, ankylosing spondylitis, Marie-Strumpell disease. *J Trauma* 1967;7:827–837.

Harding JR, McCall IW, Park WM, et al. Fracture of the cervical spine in ankylosing spondylitis. *Br J Radiol* 1985;58:3–7.

Ho EK, Chan FL, Leong JC. Post surgical recurrent stress fracture in the spine affected by ankylosing spondylitis. *Clin Orthop Relat Res* 1989;247:87–89.

Osgood C, Martin LG, Ackerman E. Fracture-dislocation of the cervical spine with ankylosing spondylitis. Report of two cases. *J Neurosurg* 1973;39:764–769.

Peh WC, Ho EK. Fracture of the odontoid peg in ankylosing spondylitis: case report. *J Trauma* 1995;38:361–363.

Podolsky SM, Hoffman JR, Pietrafesa CA. Neurologic complications following immobilization of cervical spine fracture in a patient with ankylosing spondylitis. *Ann Emerg Med* 1983;12:578–580.

Tait TJ, Barlow G, Iveson JM. Cervical spine fracture in ankylosing spondylitis: a case of 'autofracture.' *Br J Rheumatol* 1998;37:467–468.

Ueno Y, Nishimura A, Ogawa Y, et al. [Fracture of the cervical spine caused by blow in patient with ankylosing spondylitis: a report of an autopsy case.] *Nippon Hoigaku Zasshi* 1992;46:321–326.

Woodruff FP, Dewing SB. Fracture of the cervical spine in patients with ankylosing spondylitis. *Radiology* 1963;80:17–21.

Zimmermann-Gorska I, Koperska M. [Fracture of cervical spine in ankylosing spondylitis]. *Reumatologia* 1973;11:67–69.

CHAPTER 29

Diffuse Idiopathic Skeletal Hyperostosis

Kirkham B. Wood and Alexander R. Vaccaro

INTRODUCTION

Diffuse idiopathic skeletal hyperostosis (DISH) is a disorder of the spine often mistaken for ankylosing spondylitis, first coined by Resnick et al.[1,2] It is a bone-forming disorder most often seen in the thoracic and lumbar regions but also found in the more cephalad cervical spine.[1–3] Unlike ankylosing spondylitis, however, it is not a true arthropathy, which has not only skeletal inflammation but also frequently peripheral joint and extraarticular pathology. DISH is a simple bone-forming process seen predominantly in male individuals and principally limited to the axial skeleton, although in most instances, there is association with some mild degenerative intervertebral disc pathology. In the cervical spine it is considered part of the spectrum of conditions involving ossification of the vertebral ligaments, such as ossification of the posterior longitudinal ligament (OPLL).

Radiographically, DISH is typified by ossification of the spinal ligaments and immediate surrounding soft tissues. Its appearance is classically described as a "flowing" or "candle wax" pattern along at least four vertebral bodies. Large osteophytes—syndesmophytes—are trabecular bone that extend from the vertebral margins and the anulus fibrosus caused by repeated episodes of inflammation and repair that connect with similar processes caudally and cranially. Articular cartilage, the intervertebral disc, and synovial joint surfaces, including the apophyseal and sacroiliac joints, are spared erosive changes.

DISH is not rare, being reported in up to 12% of the elderly population.[1,2] Extensive ossification of the cervical spine can result in some loss of motion, although not as dramatic as in ankylosing spondylitis. It has been reported that these conditions may coexist in up to 20% of affected individuals.[3] The thickness of appositional bony growth can range from a few millimeters to as thick as 20 mm. Patients with extensive DISH of the cervical spine may complain of dysphagia most commonly, but also dyspnea or stridor.[2,4]

The primary goals of treatment are to try to maintain a reasonable range of motion and reduce discomfort. Physical therapy should be consulted to maintain muscle strength, condition, and flexibility. There is no established medical treatment for DISH, beyond that of anti-inflammatory nonsteroidal medications. Patients should be counseled on the expectations over time. Psychosocial issues can often be an overlooked burden in conditions such as DISH.

Although somewhat less common than ankylosing spondylitis, the cervical spine involved with DISH may be quite susceptible to trauma, with fracture patterns mimicking those of the appendicular skeleton. Because of the brittle nature of the relatively osteopenic segmentally ankylosed bone,

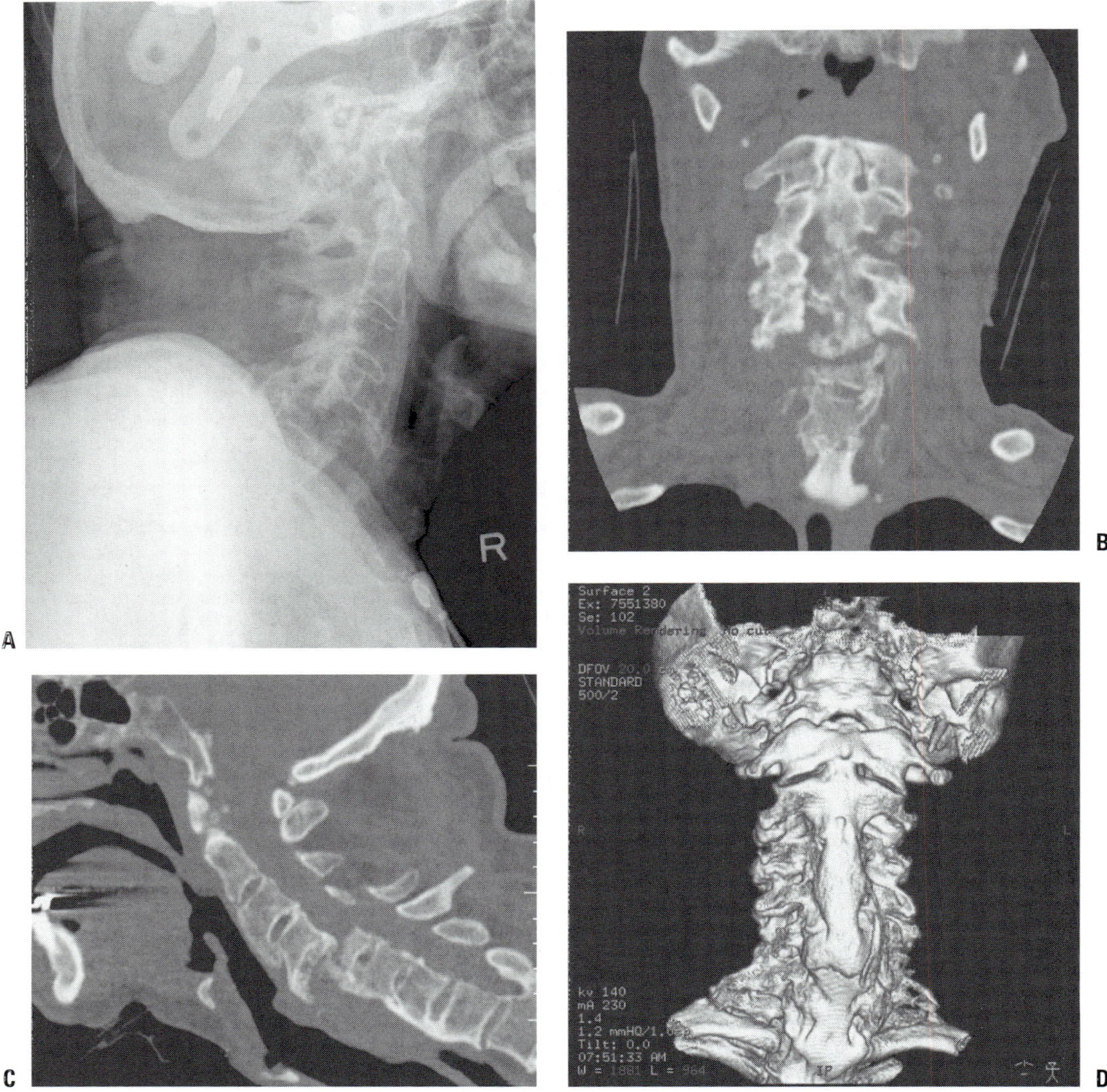

FIGURE 29.1. A 77-year-old man with fracture dislocation through C4-C5 suffered after a fall down stairs resulting in complete paraplegia. **A.** Lateral radiograph. Coronal **(B)** and sagittal **(C)** computed tomography showing complete anteroposterior translation. **D.** Three-dimensional reconstruction of the fractured spine illustrating the multisegmental involvement. The patient died 9 days postoperatively.

minor trauma acts with a long lever arm and can result in significant fractures (Fig. 29.1).[5] The circumferential ossification often results in disruption of both the anterior weight-bearing column as well as the posterior osteoligamentous complex. Computed and conventional tomography enable the diagnosis in most instances. Magnetic resonance imaging (MRI) is especially useful in describing ligamentous disruption and discal disruption and assessing the spinal canal for hematoma or bony fragments.

Following a cervical spine fracture subluxation, there is often a transverse shift of the fractured segment and resultant myelopathy.[5] Of 14 cervical fractures reported by Hendrix et al.[5] from

Northwestern University's Trauma Center, 12 had either complete or incomplete paraplegia. Patients with shorter ankylosed segments had relatively less severe spinal cord injuries.

Because the affected population is typically older and the causative mechanism of injury is frequently a fall, a distractive hyperextension-type injury with complete disruption of the anterior longitudinal ligament is a resultant common injury pattern. Even in a subtle extension-distraction injury, MRI will often demonstrate intradiscal and/or intravertebral fluid–like collections localized to the injury level.[6]

Distractive extension injuries through the disc are often unstable and frequently require surgical stabilization. The resultant fracture configuration is reminiscent of a long bone fracture because of the long juxtaposed fused segments, and as a result, the instrumentation scheme is preferably one of multiple points of fixation proximal and distal to the injury site (Fig. 29.2). In less severe injuries without marked displacement, an anterior tension band reconstruction with an interbody spacer and anterior cervical plate is often sufficient. In the setting of displacement or concomitant symptomatic multilevel stenosis, a posterior approach with or without a decompressive procedure is often preferred. As in ankylosing spondylitis, attention should be given to the potential for a postfracture epidural hematoma and resultant compromised neurologic function.

The overall mortality following a cervical spine fracture in the setting of DISH can be significant, aided in part because of the elevated age of those involved, associated medical comorbidities, and the degree of neurologic pathology. In literature reports, there was an overall perifracture mortality rate of 10% to 25%.[5,7] It is suggested, thus, that all elderly patients with DISH-like pathologic findings and a history of either trivial trauma or any new complaints of neck pain be examined carefully for the presence of an occult injury, because the mortality rates increase sharply for patients with impaired neurologic function that may develop insidiously with gradual fracture displacement.

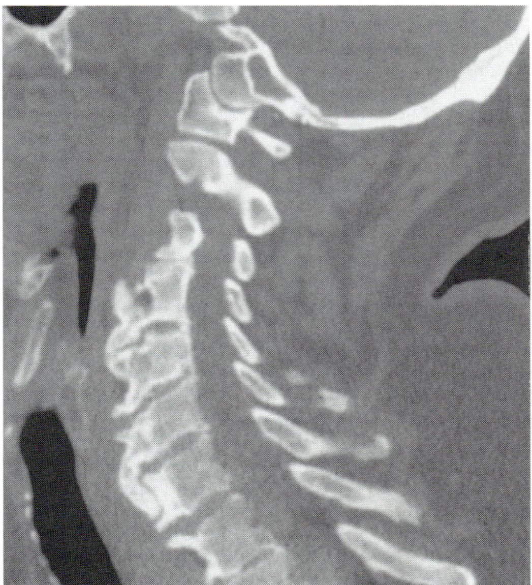

A

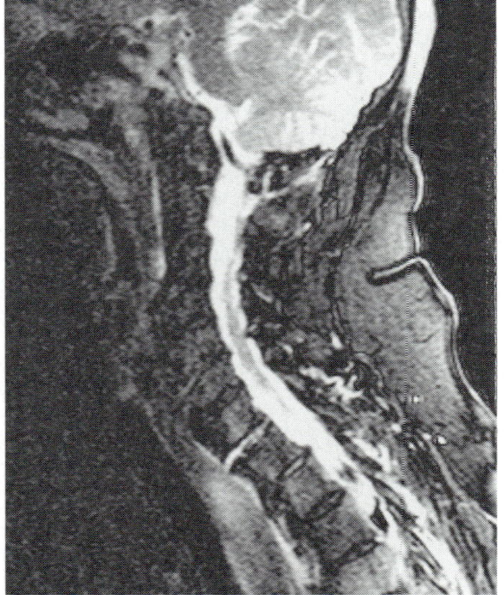

B

FIGURE 29.2. After a relatively minor fall, this 75-year-old man presented with a two-column extension-distraction injury through C6-C7 **(A)**. **B.** Magnetic resonance imaging confirms pathologic findings in both the anterior weight-bearing column (note the intervertebral fluid collection) and the posterior osteoligamentous complex. *(continued)*

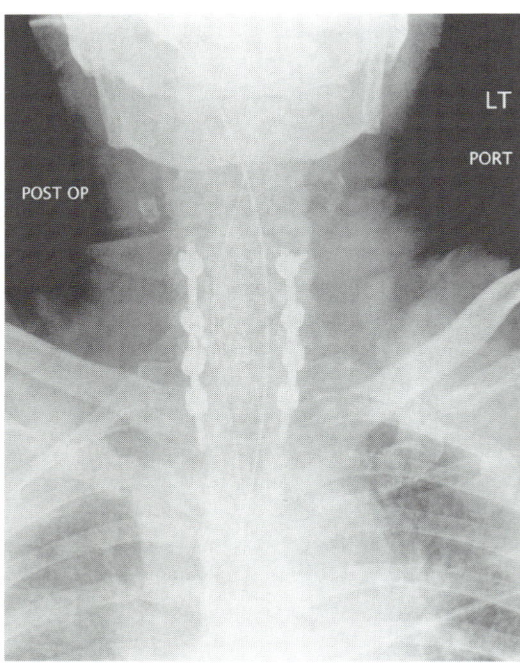

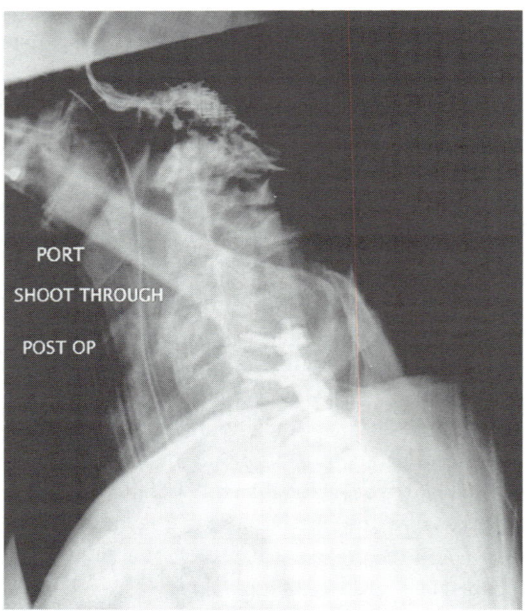

C D

FIGURE 29.2. *(continued)* Anteroposterior **(C)** and lateral **(D)** radiography illustrating multisegmental posterior fixation and fusion.

REFERENCES

1. Resnick D, Shaul SR, Wiesner K, et al. Diffuse idiopathic skeletal hyperostosis (DISH): Forestier's disease with extraspinal manifestations. *Radiology* 1975;115:513–524.
2. Resnick D, Shapiro RF, Wiesner KB, et al. Diffuse idiopathic skeletal hyperostosis (DISH). *Semin Arthritis Rheum* 1978;7:153–187.
3. Shaikh SA, Clauw DJ. Inflammatory diseases A: Diagnosis and management. In: Fymoyer JW, Weisel SW, eds. *The Adult and Pediatric Spine.* 3rd ed. Philadelphia: Lippincott Williams & Wilkins, 2004:147.
4. Mader R. Clinical manifestations of diffuse idiopathic skeletal hyperostosis of the cervical spine. *Semin Arthritis Rheum* 2002;32:130–135.
5. Hendrix RW, Melany M, Miller F, et al. Fracture of the spine in patients with ankylosis due to diffuse skeletal hyperostosis: clinical and imaging findings. *Am J Roentgenol* 1994;162:899–904.
6. Le Hir PX, Sautet A, Le Gars L, et al. Hyperextension vertebral body fractures in diffuse idiopathic skeletal hyperostosis: a cause of intravertebral fluidlike collections on MR imaging. *Am J Roentgenol* 1999;173: 1679–1683.
7. Meyer PR. Diffuse idiopathic skeletal hyperostosis in the cervical spine. *Clin Orthop Relat Res* 1999;359:49–57.

CHAPTER 30

Rheumatoid Arthritis

Jim A. Youssef, Stacey L. Forsythe, Nicole Glover, and Andrew J. Paterson

INTRODUCTION

Rheumatoid arthritis (RA) affects more than 2 million people in the United States. The prevalence of RA is approximately 1% to 2% of the world's adult population.[1] A systematic autoimmune disease, RA is characterized by chronic, symmetric, and erosive synovitis of peripheral joints. Progression to later stages is characterized by destructive synovitis leading to ligamentous laxity and bony erosions, which may also result in instability and subluxation in the cervical spine. RA is the most common inflammatory disorder to affect the cervical spine. It can significantly alter cervical spine biomechanics.[2] Depending on the diagnostic criteria applied, 25% to 80% of patients diagnosed with RA have cervical spine involvement.[3] Because of the degenerative effects of the disease, physicians treating patients with RA, especially in the context of cervical trauma, must be cognizant of compromised bone quality and healing capabilities. Given the high prevalence of cervical spine involvement in RA, it is essential that surgeons develop effective treatment protocols for cervical spine trauma in this challenging group of patients. This chapter will briefly discuss the pathophysiology of RA and provide a summary of clinical aspects of diagnosis and treatment of patients with preexisting cervical RA who present with comorbid cervical spine trauma.

PATHOPHYSIOLOGY

The rheumatoid synovium consists of two distinct cell populations, type A cells, which are morphologically similar to macrophages, and type B cells, which are similar to fibroblasts.[4] Type A cells are equipped for phagocytosis, whereas type B cells are mainly equipped for protein synthesis. In the early stages of erosive synovitis, a cascade of events occurs leading to a hyperplastic, multilayered synovium. The cells in this layer are metabolically active and produce collagenase, interleukins, and cytokines.[5] Histologic evaluation of tissue taken during surgical resection of the dens and retrodental soft tissues demonstrates a unique vascular synoviocyte layer on a subsynovial core and, unlike early active rheumatoid synovium, formation of hyperplastic synovium (type I). These specimens did not show significant lymphocyte infiltration. In the majority of the specimens harvested during surgical excision, an end-stage or chronic, inactive synovium was seen (type II). Patients with mild, stable myelopathy with complaints of radiculopathy within the C2 distribution caused by increasing hypermobility of the atlantoaxial joint presented as type I. Patients with type II were older, with more advanced neurologic and mechanical deterioration of the osseoligamentous structures at the craniocervical junction.[6] Erosive changes in the synovium (panus) affect not only joint surfaces but also the other soft tissue structures such as ligaments, tendons, and capsules.

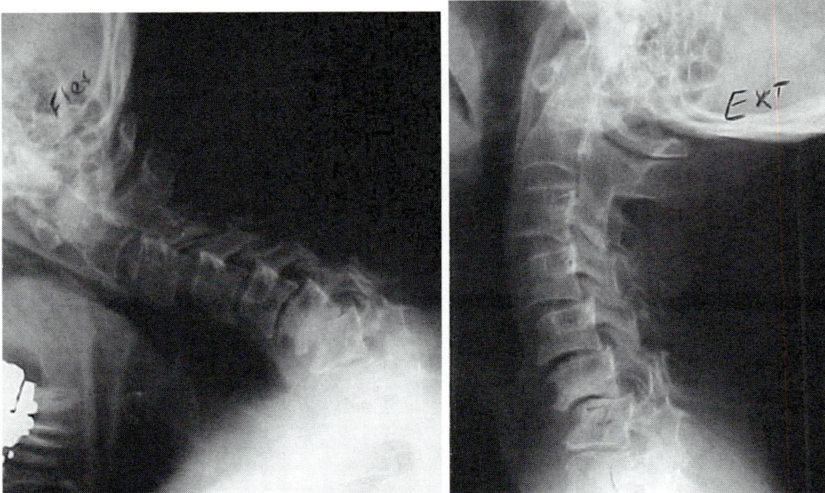

FIGURE 30.1. A 49-year-old woman with preexisting rheumatoid arthritis after sustaining a motor vehicle collision with neck pain and radiculopathy. Lateral flexion and extension cervical radiographs demonstrate classic "staircase" appearance with new fracture-subluxation of C6-C7.

PATHOMECHANICS

Early stages of RA begin as erosive synovitis involving multiple joints.[7] The upper cervical spine is particularly vulnerable to the effects of RA because of the presence of unique synovium-lined joints not seen elsewhere in the spine.[8] Because the craniocervical junction (C0, C1, C2) depends on ligamentous structures for stability, early instability in this region is due to the soft tissue destruction caused by this erosive synovitis of the cruciform-alar ligamentous complex. This leads to degenerative changes imposed on the occipitocervical junction.[9] The most common deformities include atlantoaxial subluxations, and advanced disease leads to superior migration of the odontoid and basilar invagination.[2] In the subaxial spine (C3-C7), the inflammatory process affects the uncovertebral joints and ligamentous structures, resulting in subaxial instability. The hallmark "staircase" radiographic appearance of the subaxial spine is due to progressive subluxation as a result of instability initiated by ligamentous damage and degenerative changes occurring during the inflammatory phase of the disease process[10] (Fig. 30.1). Later, in more advanced stages, progressive disc space collapse can lead to subaxial ankylosis.[11] Panus formation and subsequent subaxial spinal cord compression may occur, leading to myelopathy in addition to neck pain.[12]

IMAGING AND TREATMENT ALGORITHMS

Patients with RA may present with few symptoms related to their neck after trauma. The goal during patient evaluation is to differentiate new trauma from preexisting deformity. In the presence of neck pain, plain radiographs are the basis for evaluation. Radiographic instability usually develops within the first decade of diagnosis. Clinically, 40% to 80% of patients with RA have neck pain, and subluxation is appreciated on 43% to 86% of radiographic images. However, neurologic deficit resulting from spinal stenosis is reported in only 7% to 34% of patients with RA.[8,13–15]

Magnetic resonance imaging (MRI) scans should be obtained for any patient presenting with neurologic deficit and in patients with evidence of basilar invagination noted on plain radiographs (Fig. 30.2). Distinguishing trauma from preexisting deformity may be difficult. MRI short tau inversion recovery (STIR) images, in particular, are very sensitive not only for bony and soft tissue

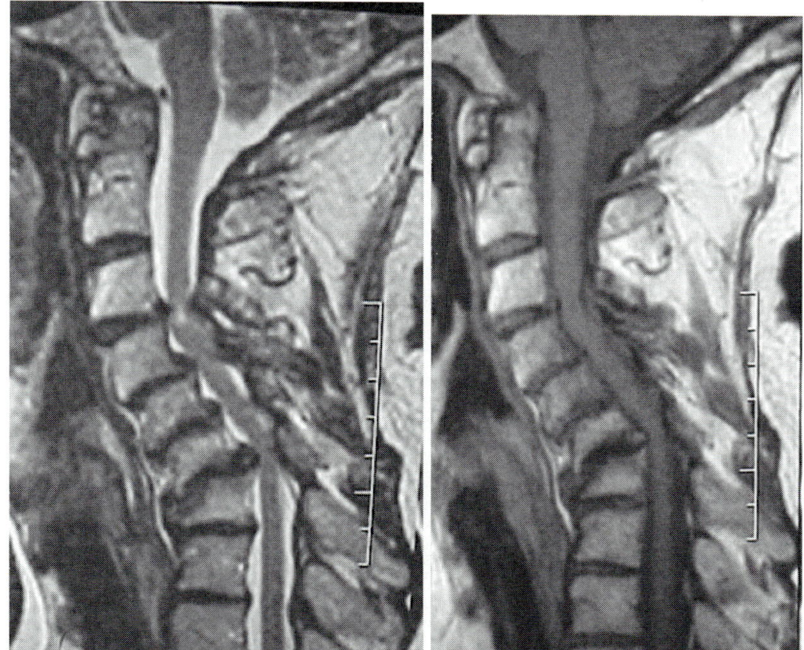

FIGURE 30.2. MRI demonstrates underlying myelomalacia at C2-C3, focal kyphosis, and severe spinal stenosis at the level of the injury.

edema associated with trauma but also for degenerative changes. MRI is also sensitive for spinal cord compression. Numerous measurements can be made to determine disease progression, including the anterior atlantodens interval (AADI) and posterior atlantodens interval (PADI). The McGregor Line, Ranawat Index, Redlund-Johnell measurements, and Clark Station are all used to assess cranial settling.[15] Treatment algorithms differ in the patient with active RA disease that may have a neurologic component, such patients with RA involving the cervical spine. Evaluating the RA patient with cervical trauma is similar to a standard cervical trauma evaluation; however, in patients with RA, trauma can exacerbate degenerative changes and dynamic instability of the cervical spine. Increased pain can be the result of an aggravation of a preexisting injury or due to new trauma. Patients carrying an advanced diagnosis of RA are more susceptible to spinal cord compression and abnormal spinal cord signal seen on MRI resulting from preexisting spinal deformity. Treatment algorithms differ in patients with RA with preexisting spinal deformity, instability, or neurologic deficit and in those with normal radiographs and active disease. The following section will delineate treatment protocols in these two groups of patients.

PATIENTS WITH RHEUMATOID ARTHRITIS WITHOUT PREEXISTING RADIOGRAPHIC FINDINGS

Unimpaired patients with cervical trauma who are alert and have normal mental status still require systematic evaluation protocols. A thorough patient history evaluation should note the presence of an RA diagnosis. All patients who present with cervical trauma should be examined for distracting injuries, including radiographic imaging in the presence of injury. In the absence of distracting injury, the patient's neurologic status should be assessed. If no signs of neurologic impairment are present, neck pain should be assessed with high clinical acuity. The presence of neck pain to palpation should lead the clinician to obtain the appropriate imaging studies, including anteroposterior and lateral plain radiographs, computed tomography (CT), and MRI.

The following flowcharts summarize treatment protocols specific for cervical trauma patients with RA.[13]

RA patients without pre-existing radiographic abnormalities and comorbid cervical trauma:

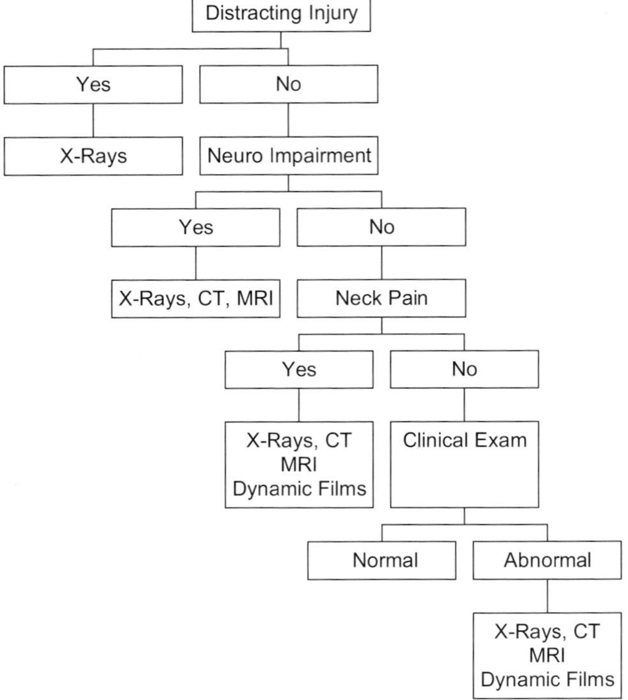

RA patients with classic radiographic deformities and comorbid cervical trauma:

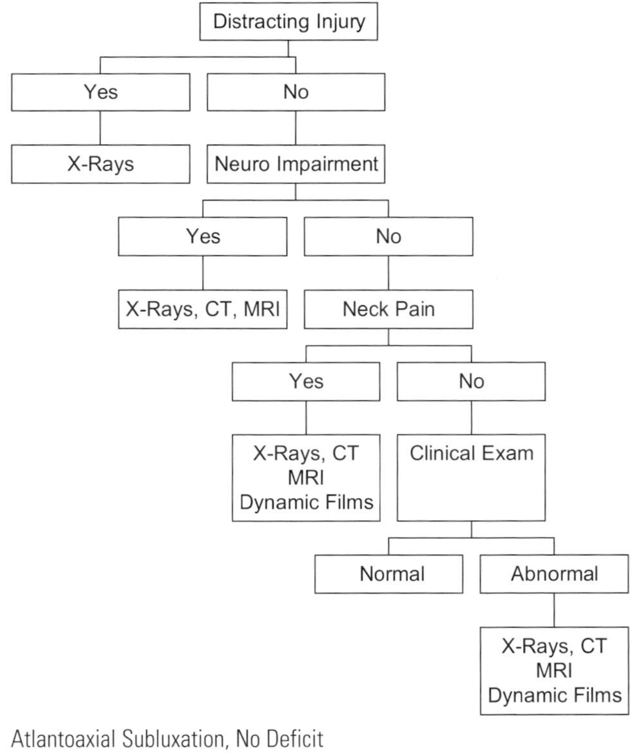

Atlantoaxial Subluxation, No Deficit

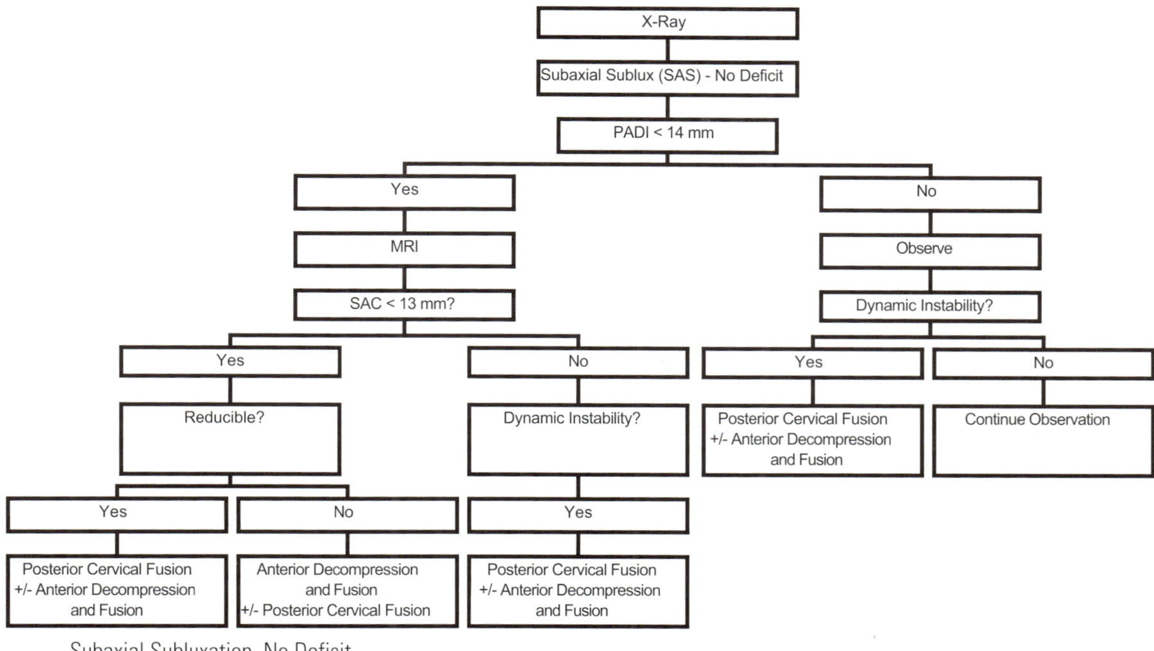

Subaxial Subluxation, No Deficit

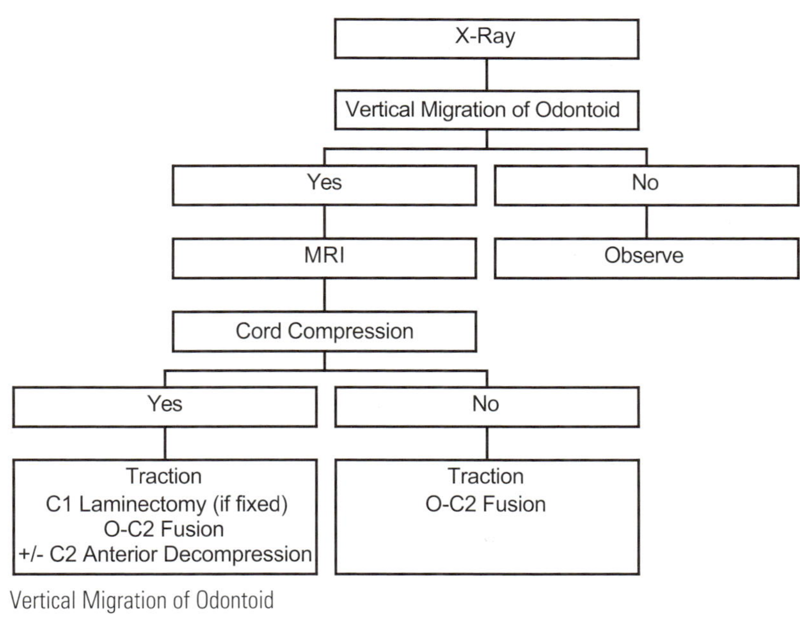

Vertical Migration of Odontoid

CLINICAL EVALUATION AND TREATMENT

Neck pain at the craniocervical junction and occipital headaches are the most common symptoms in patients with RA.[13] Patients may also present with myelopathic features, including weakness, loss of endurance, gait disturbance, loss of dexterity, and paresthesias of their hands. When a patient with RA presents in a clinical setting, a detailed history is required, including the date of RA diagnosis, current medication management (well controlled vs. poorly controlled), effectiveness of current medical treatment, surgical history, preexiting symptoms including neck and back pain, and review of any previous imaging studies to assess preexisting deformity.

The evaluation of patients with RA with comorbid cervical trauma should adhere to the aforementioned principles of medical assessment while further investigating the presence of traumatic injury. Imaging studies should include static and dynamic plain radiographs when possible, especially in the upright position. Appropriate CT and MRI studies are imperative in making an accurate diagnosis of cervical trauma in these challenging patients. Treatment of specific cervical spine injury patterns should adhere to standard cervical trauma protocols. Nonoperative treatment may include cervical orthosis immobilization or halo vest treatment. However, surgical intervention may be necessary in treating certain fracture patterns.

Effective surgical treatment in patients with RA who have comorbid trauma frequently requires anterior and posterior fixation. Bone quality is especially poor in patients with RA. Anterior instrumentation alone is at high risk for failure. The posterior elements of the spine are more dense and therefore potentially provide better fixation points for the rigid instrumentation.[17] As the previous algorithms demonstrate, treatment for cervical trauma patients and cervical trauma patients with RA is similar; however, special precautions must be taken when the patient has active RA, particularly when there is preexisting spinal deformity, instability, or neurologic deficit.

Consideration of a patient's medical condition, bone quality, underlying preexisting deformity, and stenosis can make the surgical treatment of cervical spine trauma more challenging in patients with RA. Whether anterior or posterior procedures are intended, the treating physician should make every attempt to restore sagittal alignment to near anatomic parameters (Fig. 30.3). Presurgical halo traction may be necessary to help achieve such goals. The realignment is necessary to maximize the ability of the vertebral column to load share with the newly introduced instrumentation. In addition

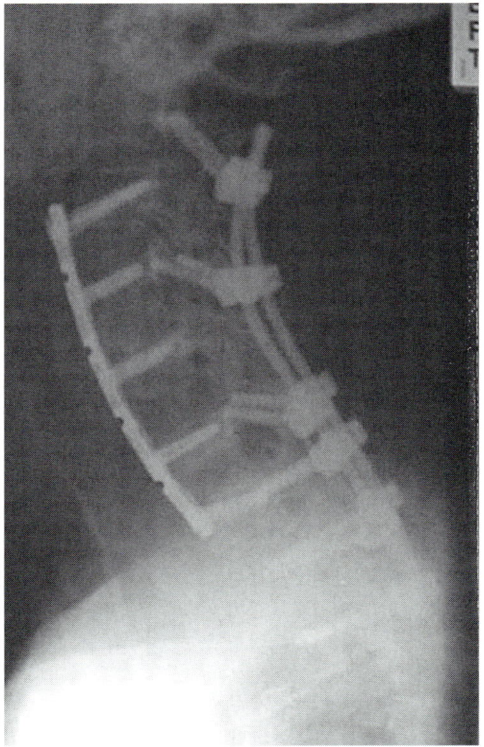

FIGURE 30.3. Postoperative lateral radiograph demonstrate restoration of sagittal alignment and anterior-posterior arthrodesis.

to autologous iliac crest bone graft, adjunctive bone graft extenders may be necessary because patients with RA may have underlying osteoporosis and poor bone quality. Prolonged postoperative immobilization may also be required to achieve a solid arthrodesis.

After a patient with cervical trauma has undergone effective triage and treatment, several considerations should be taken into account when assisting with their recovery. Patients dealing with active RA and cervical trauma face unique obstacles. Complications are not uncommon; however, complications seem to decrease if surgical intervention occurs before the onset of myelopathy. Without severe compression of the cord and the presence of solid arthrodesis, patients experience good pain relief and better neurologic recovery. However, nonunion rates have been noted to be as high as 20% to 30% when fusion is attempted. The presence of adjacent segment disease is also common following surgery in the setting of RA.[18] Furthermore, the treating physician should take into account the difficulties that can arise during rehabilitation. Many patients with advanced RA will face challenges during physical therapy as a result of physical weakness and limb deformity.

CONCLUSION

RA is a pervasive chronic disease with devastating physical and economic consequences. The primary goal in management of patients with RA who sustain cervical trauma is to prevent progressive deformity or irreversible neurologic deficit. In the treatment of cervical spine trauma, it is imperative that treating physicians are cognizant of the effects of RA on the cervical spine. Treatment protocols for cervical spine trauma are similar for patients with and without RA; however, the physician must be vigilant in treatment of the patient with RA to avoid increasing the risk for development of more serious problems, including permanent neurologic deficit and even death.

REFERENCES

1. Linos AA, Worthington JW, O'Fallen WM, et al. The epidemiology of rheumatoid arthritis in Rochester Minnesota: a study of incidence, prevalence and mortality. *Am J Epidemiol* 1980;111:87–98.
2. Reiter MF, Boden S. Inflammatory disorders of the cervical spine. *Spine* 1998;23:2755–66.
3. Rajangamk K, Thomas IM. Frequency of cervical spine involvement in rheumatoid arthritis. *J Indian Med Assoc* 1995;93:138–139.
4. Rooney M, Condell D, Quinlan W, et al. Analysis of the histologic variation of synovitis in rheumatoid arthritis. *Arthritis Rheum* 1988;31:956–963.
5. Soden M, Rooney M, Whalen A, et al. Immunohistological analysis of the synovial membrane: search for the clinical course in rheumatoid arthritis. *Ann Rheum Dis* 1991;5673:673–676.
6. Crockard HA. Spine update: surgical management of cervical rheumatoid problems. *Spine* 1995;20:2584–2590 [abstract].
7. Nguyen HV, Ludwig S, Silber J, et al. Rheumatoid arthritis of the cervical spine. *Spine J* 1994;20:329–334.
8. Morizono Y, Sakou T, Kawaida H. Upper cervical involvement in rheumatoid arthritis. *Spine* 1987;12:721–725 [abstract].
9. Yonezawa T, Tsuji H, Matsui H, et al. Subluxation lesions in rheumatoid arthritis: radiographic factors suggestive of lower cervical myelopathy. *Spine* 1995;20:208–215.
10. Redlund-Johnell I, Pettersson H. Subaxial antero-posterior dislocation of the cervical spine in rheumatoid arthritis. *Scand J Rheumatol* 1985;14(4):355–363.
11. Olerud C, Larsson BE, Rodriguez M. Subaxial cervical spine subluxation in rheumatoid arthritis: a retrospective analysis of 16 operated patients after 1–5 years. *Acta Orthop Scand* 1997;68(2):109–115.
12. Boden SD, Clark CR. Rheumatoid arthritis of the cervical spine. In: The Cervical Spine Research Society Education Committee, ed. *The Cervical Spine*, 3rd ed. Philadelphia: Lippincott-Raven; 1998.
13. Boden SD, Dodge LD, Bohlman HH, et al. Rheumatoid arthritis of the cervical spine. *J Bone Joint Surg Am* 1993;75:1282–1297.
14. Boden S. Rheumatoid arthritis of the cervical spine. *Spine* 1994;1920:2275–2280.
15. Monsey RD. Rheumatoid arthritis of the cervical spine. *J Am Acad Orthop Surg* 1997;5(5):240–248.
16. O'Brein MF, Sutterlin III CE. Occipitocervical biomechanics: clinical and biomechanical implications for posterior occipitocervical stabilization and fusion. *Spine* 1996;135:25–31.
17. Moskovich R, Crockhard HA, Shott S, et al. Occipitalocervical stabilization for myelopathy in patients with rheumatoid arthritis. *J Bone Joint Surg Am* 2000;82:349–365.

CHAPTER 31

Osteoporosis

F. Cumhur Öner

INTRODUCTION

Osteoporosis is a progressive systemic disease characterized by loss of bone mass, diminishing bone density, and progressive loss of normal bone architecture. The resulting reduced mechanical strength of bone leads to an increased risk for bone fracturing under even minor stress, particularly in the spine, distal radius, and hip. Osteoporosis is also called the silent epidemic and is estimated to affect 75 million people in the United States, Europe, and Japan, including one in three postmenopausal women, the majority of elderly people, and a substantial number of men. The increasing number of elderly people all around the world makes osteoporosis-related disorders of the skeleton one of the major challenges of the health care systems. In the European Union, it is estimated that the number of people over age 65 will rise from 8.9 million women and 4.5 million men in 1995 to 26.4 million women and 17.4 million men by 2050. Also, the number of patients using medications causing osteoporosis such as corticosteroids, cytostatics, and antiviral agents is constantly growing. Worldwide, the lifetime risk for osteoporotic fractures in women is about 40%, whereas in men it is only 13%; however, according to recent studies, European men are catching up. Osteoporosis is a silent, asymptomatic disease and is usually not detected until fractures occur. Osteoporotic fractures are commonly associated with considerable morbidity, mortality, and cost. The most common localizations for osteoporotic fractures are vertebrae, wrist, and hip. Although the hip fracture rate increases exponentially with age, vertebral fractures are the most common type of osteoporotic fractures, occur earlier in the natural history of the disease, and are one of the important clinical manifestations of osteoporosis. The consequences of vertebral fractures include back pain and disability, physical deformity (e.g., kyphosis, abdominal protrusion, and loss of height), diminished quality of life, and increasing rates of hospitalization, long-term care, and other kinds of resource utilization.

The anterior column of the spine, consisting of the vertebral bodies and discs, is responsible for absorbing compressive forces. The vertebral bodies consist of predominantly cancellous bone within a relatively thin cortical shell. The relative amount of cancellous bone is the highest in the vertebral bodies of the thoracic and lumbar spine. Posterior elements, such as the pedicles, laminae, and lateral processes, contain a higher proportion of cortical bone and are mechanically stronger (Fig. 31.1). The mechanical strength of cancellous bone is more dependent on the microarchitecture, which is first affected by osteoporosis. Cortical bone is affected only late in the osteoporosis process. It is thus no wonder that the incidence of osteoporotic fractures is highest in the regions with a high proportion of cancellous bone, such as distal radius, femoral head, and vertebral bodies.

In the spine, osteoporotic fractures occur most frequently at two sites: the midthoracic region (T5-T8) and the thoracolumbar junction (T11-L1). These are the most biomechanically compromised regions of the vertebral column where compression forces on the anterior column are maximal and the proportion of the cancellous bone is highest. Thoracic kyphosis is most pronounced at

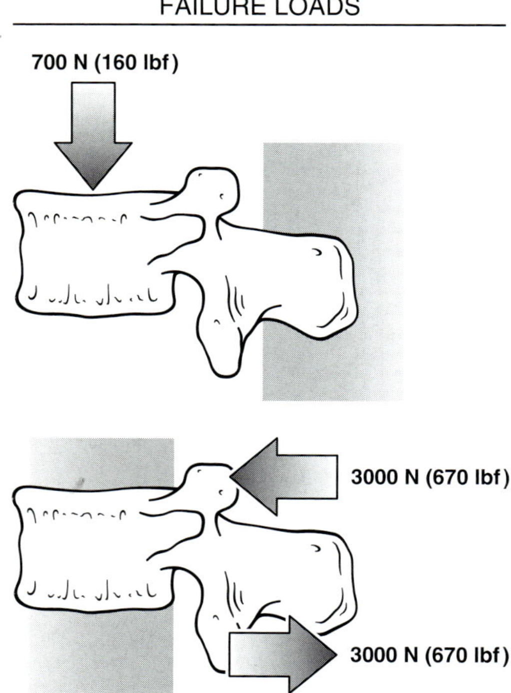

FIGURE 31.1. Failure loads of the anterior column and the posterior elements differ significantly. (Adapted from White AA, Panjabi MM. *Clinical Biomechanics of Spine.* Philadelphia: Lippincott, 1978, 31.)

the midthoracic region, around T5-T8, so that loading is accentuated in flexion. The thoracolumbar junction consists of an articulation between the relatively rigid thoracic spine (bolstered by the thoracic cage) and the freely mobile lumbar segment, again maximizing compressive stresses. In the lordotic regions the compression forces on the anterior column are relatively weaker, and a greater portion of these forces is transmitted through the stronger posterior elements. Also in the lordotic regions, the arthrosis of the facet joints is more pronounced. Arthrosis leads to thickening of the subchondral bone causing an increase in bone mineral density. Just like in the hips, where arthrotic joints do not usually suffer osteoporotic fractures, facet arthrosis in the lumbar and cervical regions in the spine confers a protective effect against an osteoporotic fracture. The cervical spine, with its lordotic posture, relatively high proportion of cortical bone because of the presence of the lateral masses, and high incidence of facet arthrosis in combination with the relatively low loads in this spinal area, is less affected by osteoporosis. The compression-type osteoporotic fractures of the anterior column, commonly seen in the thoracic and thoracolumbar spine, are indeed very rare in the cervical spine (Fig. 31.2). However, there are two regions of the cervical spine that are exceptions to this general rule: the atlantoaxial complex and the cervicothoracic junction.

The central part of the body of C1 is fused to C2, forming the odontoid process, and the rest of the disc space is transformed into a horizontal joint, allowing the unique ability of the atlantoaxial joint complex to show the most extreme rotation of the whole spine. There is no true facet joint between C1 and C2. This anatomic configuration makes the proportion of cancellous bone exceptionally high in C2 and leaves this segment vulnerable without the protection of a true facet joint. Arthrosis of the horizontal C1-C2 joints increases further the translational stress on the odontoid. Because of these reasons, odontoid fractures, which make up no more than 10% of cervical fractures, are the most common cervical fracture in patients older than 70 years. Usually these fractures are a result of a minor injury in the elderly and are often highly comminuted and may be accompanied by C1 fractures (Fig. 31.3). Elderly people with osteoporosis usually develop a hyperkyphosis of the thoracic spine, with a compensated hyperlordosis of the cervical spine.

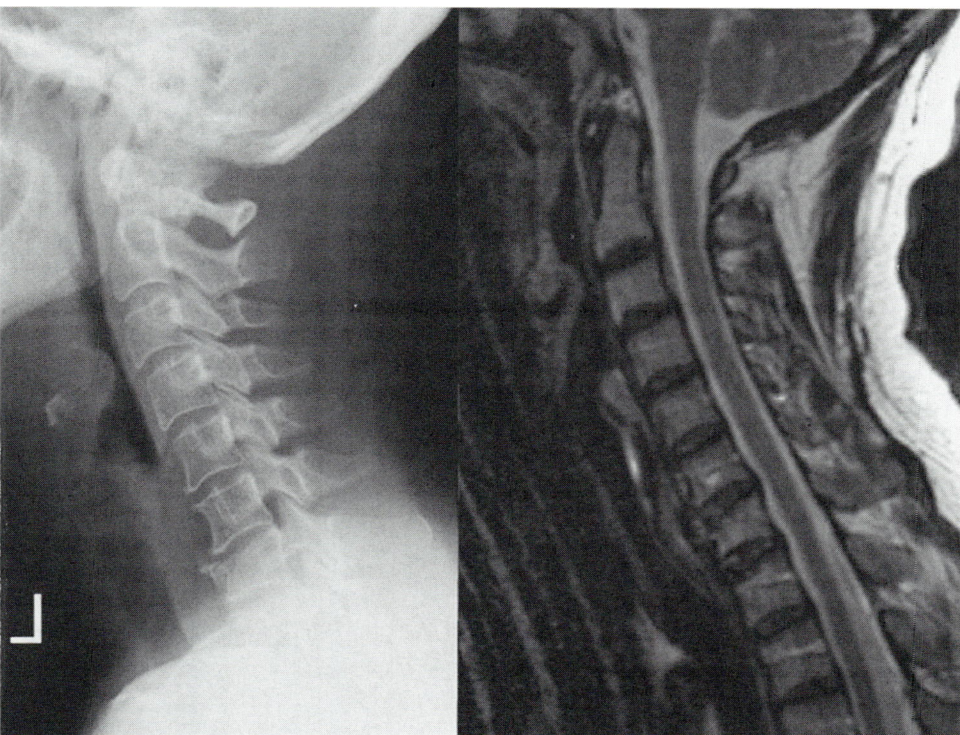

FIGURE 31.2. Compression-type vertebral body fracture, the most common pattern in thoracic and thoracolumbar spine, is rarely seen in the cervical spine. This 58-year-old woman fell in her bathroom and suffered compression fractures of C7 and T1. Further analysis revealed serious osteoporosis requiring medical treatment.

Although this hyperlordosis may protect the cervical spine against compression fractures, it also predisposes the atlantoaxial complex to hyperextension injuries with minor falls. Although there are no reliable studies, the general impression is that there is a steep increase in the incidence of this type of injury in the elderly. Neurologic involvement is uncommon, probably because of a high likelihood of acute fatality resulting from such an injury. Treatment of these injuries should follow the general principles of odontoid fracture management. However, some factors may

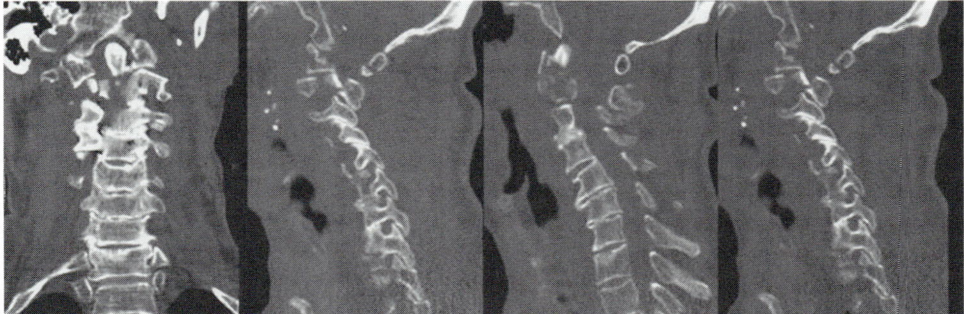

FIGURE 31.3. A "typical" high cervical fracture in the elderly osteoporotic spine. This 82-year-old woman was admitted after a fall down stairs. Note the serious comminution of the C1-C2 complex and the stiff, arthrotic subaxial spine typical of this age group. She tolerated halo vest treatment well, and the fractures healed without residual instability.

complicate the treatment in the elderly. The rate of nonunion of odontoid fractures is higher in the elderly probably because of the stiffness of the rest of the cervical spine. Halo vest treatment may not be tolerated well by these patients, especially if they have concomitant pulmonary problems because of their thoracic deformity. Operative treatment options are problematic too. Anterior odontoid screw fixation may not be possible because of the thoracic deformity and cervical stiffness. Careful preoperative planning including assessment of computed tomography (CT) reconstructions or magnetic resonance imaging (MRI) of the cervical and thoracic spine is mandatory to assess whether screw fixation is possible. There is no salvage anteriorly if one realizes during surgery that the dens is not accessible for screw fixation because of anatomic constraints. Also, screw fixation of the osteoporotic odontoid may not be strong enough. Posterior C1-C2 fusion is usually feasible in the elderly, but the functional limitations of this procedure in an already stiff neck should be considered. The elderly with osteoporotic C1-C2 fractures may best be treated with a collar and "benign neglect" because the alternatives may result in prohibitive neck stiffness. In patients with serious comorbidities, permanent collar use in cases of abnormal C1-C2 motion is a defendable option.

Another region where osteoporotic fractures can seriously affect cervical function is the cervicothoracic junction. Even low-energy traumas can cause serious deformity in the upper thoracic junction leading to a drop-head in the elderly. Because of the difficulties of imaging this area, especially in osteoporotic spine, many fractures may be missed (Fig. 31.4). In combination with pretrauma hyperkyphosis of the thoracic spine, these fractures tend to lead to progressive kyphosis. In the elderly patient with any suspicion for a fracture in this region, even after seemingly minor injuries, CT or MRI of this region should be obtained.

Last but not least, one should never forget that osteoporosis and old age do not protect people against trauma. The combination of high-energy trauma and osteoporosis is rapidly increasing because many elderly people enjoy active lives participating in all kinds of social and sportive activities. Considering that an average European woman can enjoy at least 31 active and healthy years after her menopause, we can expect more patients with osteoporosis of varying degrees getting

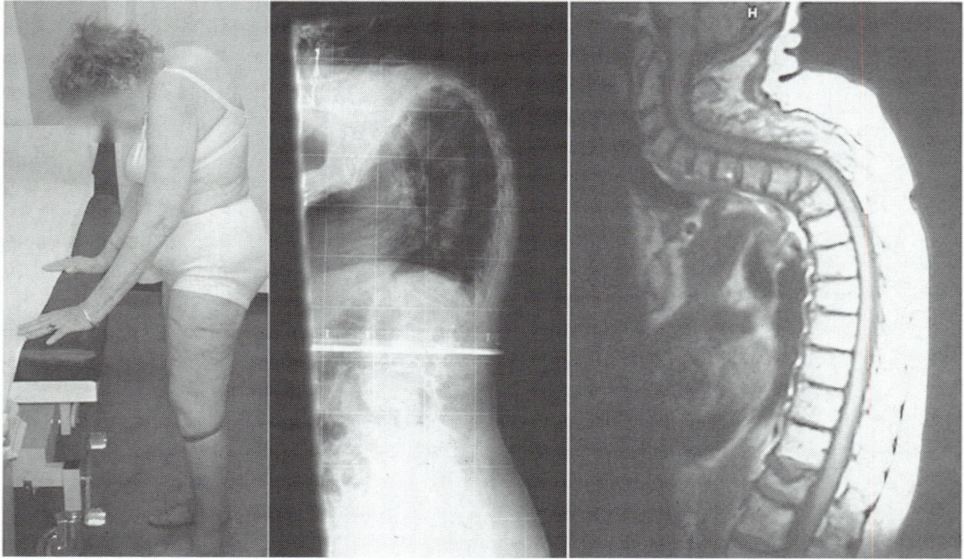

FIGURE 31.4. Unrecognized fractures of the cervicothoracic junction may cause serious deformity. This 78-year-old woman fell with her bicycle. The high thoracic fractures were not recognized at the emergency department. She developed progressive kyphosis and respiratory insufficiency. Although the deformity was corrected successfully with pedicle subtraction osteotomy, she died 9 months after surgery because of respiratory insufficiency.

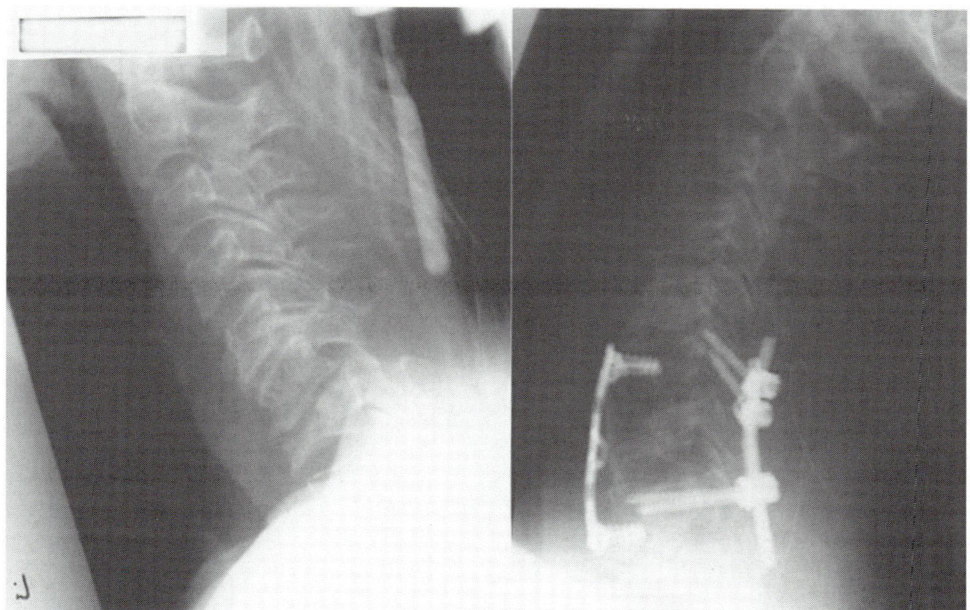

FIGURE 31.5. Traumatic fractures may behave unpredictably in the osteoporotic spine. A flexion-compression injury of C7 in this 70-year-old woman after an accident driving her car was treated conservatively with a collar but progressed to serious kyphosis requiring anterior and posterior surgery. Note the pullout of the distal screws of the anterior plate.

involved in accidents leading to spinal fractures (Fig. 31.5). In fact, there has been a steady increase in the average age of spinal injury victims in North America and Europe during the last three decades. That means that we should be prepared to see all kinds of cervical fractures in these osteoporotic spines. The challenges are numerous. Surgical treatment of these injuries is more difficult, and multiple-level fixations and anteroposterior constructs may need to be used to achieve the same mechanical stability. Considerable increase in complication rates of both surgical and conservative treatment regimens should be anticipated.

We should also not forget the responsibility of orthopaedic surgeons and neurosurgeons in the treatment of osteoporosis. Osteoporosis is a systemic disease that can be successfully treated. However, it is usually the trauma and spinal surgeons who are first confronted with the symptoms of this disorder, which is taking on epidemic proportions. In some North European countries, new programs are being initiated in cooperation with trauma and emergency medicine departments to screen for osteoporosis all patients over the age of 50 years with any fracture. Trauma and spinal surgeons all around the world should be encouraged to take an active role in these kinds of programs.

SUGGESTED READINGS

Blauth M, Lange UF, Knop C, et al. Spinal fractures in the elderly and their treatment. *Orthopäde* 2000;29:302–317.

Glassman SD, Alegre GM. Adult spinal deformity in the osteoporotic spine: options and pitfalls. *Instr Course Lect* 2003;52:579–588.

Haczynski J, Jakimiuk A. Vertebral fractures: a hidden problem of osteoporosis. *Med Sci Monit* 2001;7:1108–1117.

Lakshmanan P, Jones A, Howes J, et al. CT evaluation of the pattern of odontoid fractures in the elderly: relationship to upper cervical spine osteoarthritis. *Eur Spine J* 2005;14:78–83.

Nagashima H, Morio Y, Hasegawa K, et al. Teshima R. Odontoid fractures complicated by fractures of the posterior arch of the atlas in the elderly over 85 years with severe thoracic kyphosis secondary to osteoporosis. *Injury* 2001;32:501–504.

Vieweg U, Schultheiss R. A review of halo vest treatment of upper cervical spine injuries. *Arch Orthop Trauma Surg* 2001;121:50–55.

SECTION X

Pediatric Cervical Spine

CHAPTER 32

Cervical Spine Injuries in Children: Attention to Radiographic Differences and Stability Compared to the Adult Patient

Steve Chang, Pankaj A. Gore, and Nicholas Theodore

INTRODUCTION

Cervical spine trauma accounts for approximately 1.5% of pediatric trauma admissions.[1] The medical, psychological, and societal costs of severe pediatric cervical spine trauma can be vastly disproportionate to this small percentage.[2–5] An understanding of the unique anatomic, radiographic, and biomechanical characteristics of the pediatric cervical spine is essential to the appropriate care of these challenging patients.

EPIDEMIOLOGY

Most pediatric cervical spine injuries are a result of blunt trauma.[1] In large series, males outnumber females 1.5 to 1.9:1.[1,6–8] Motor vehicle–related accidents, which account for 48% to 61% of all injuries, are the most common mechanism of injury in children both older and younger than 8 years of age.[1,6,7] Of these, injuries to occupants (31% to 42%) predominate over those to pedestrians (11% to 16%) and bicycle riders (5% to 6%).[1,6–8]

Falls account for 18% to 30% of cervical spine injuries in the younger age group (<8 years) and 11% in the older age group (>8 years).[1,6] Sports injuries are more prevalent in the older group (20% to 38%) and uncommon in the younger group (3%). Nonaccidental trauma and penetrating injuries are also found in small numbers of very young children and adolescents, respectively.[7,9]

The largest reported series of pediatric cervical spine injury patients (n = 1098) was gleaned from a 10-year interval of the National Pediatric Trauma Registry and probably represents the best epidemiologic data from this patient population.[1] Of these patients, 83% had bony cervical spine injuries. Fractures were more common in all age groups, although dislocations were more prevalent in younger children than older children. Upper cervical spine injuries (C1-C4) were almost twice as common as lower cervical injuries (C5-C7). Seven percent of the patients had both an upper and lower cervical spine injury. Spinal cord injury (SCI) occurred in 35% of the pediatric cervical spine injuries. About half of these demonstrated no radiographic evidence of bony injury. Of the SCIs, 75% were incomplete and 25% were complete.[1]

EMBRYOLOGY AND DEVELOPMENT

An understanding of the developmental anatomy of the pediatric cervical spine facilitates the interpretation of its imaging and the conceptualization of its biomechanical properties. The vertebral bodies undergo chondrification around the fifth or sixth week of gestation.[10] By the fourth month, ossification centers have appeared in all of the vertebral bodies. Ossification continues through adolescence. Most vertebrae originate from four primary ossification centers: one in each hemi-arch and two within the centrum. The body of each vertebra develops from the fusion of the dorsal and ventral ossification centers within the centrum, an event that occurs by the twenty-fourth week of gestation.[11]

THE ATLAS

Ossification of the anterior arch of the atlas begins in 33% of children by 3 months and in 81% of children by 1 year (Fig. 32.1).[12] Complete ossification of the posterior arch occurs by 3 years of age. The synchondroses between the body and the posterior elements fuse by 7 years of age.[13]

THE AXIS

The axis is unique in that there are two additional ossification centers that fuse in the midline to form the odontoid process by the seventh gestational month. The body of C2 fuses to the odontoid between 3 and 6 years of age. The fusion line often is visible until the age of 11 years and is visible throughout life in a third of the population (Fig. 32.2).[13] The secondary ossification center at the apex of the odontoid appears between 6 and 8 years of age and fuses with the dens around 12 years of age.[14] Failure of fusion at this location results in ossiculum terminale, a condition that is usually benign but has been associated with atlantoaxial instability.[15]

The C2 posterior arches fuse in the midline by 2 to 3 years and fuse with the body by 3 to 6 years. The inferior epiphyseal ring is a secondary ossification center that appears at the inferior endplate of C2 at puberty and fuses with the body by 25 years of age.

THE SUBAXIAL CERVICAL SPINE

The development of the subaxial cervical spine is highly conserved between C3 and C7. Ossification of the centrum is present by the fifth gestational month. The arches fuse in the midline by the second to third year and fuse to the body between the third and the sixth year. Secondary ossification centers develop at the anterior transverse processes, spinous process apices, and superior and inferior epiphyseal rings. The anterior transverse process fuses with the vertebrae by the sixth year. The latter three centers fuse by the twenty-fifth year (Fig. 32.3).[13]

IMAGING CHARACTERISTICS OF THE PEDIATRIC CERVICAL SPINE

Incomplete ossification and physiologic hypermobility of the pediatric cervical spine contribute to imaging findings that can be confused with pathologic conditions. Lateral and anteroposterior (AP) radiographs of the cervical spine are frequently used as a primary screening study. Imaging findings within the realm of normal variants in children include prevertebral soft tissue thickening, increased atlantodens interval (ADI), overriding C1 anterior arch on the dens, pseudospread of the C1 lateral masses on C2, pseudosubluxation of C2 on C3 and of C3 on C4, any radiolucent synchondrosis, wedging of subaxial cervical vertebral bodies, and the absence of cervical lordosis.

Prevertebral soft tissue swelling in adults can indicate adjacent cervical spine injury. In children, a thickened prevertebral shadow on plain radiographs can result from expiration, especially if a child is crying.[11] If repeat radiographs during inspiration are infeasible, computed tomography (CT) of the region is indicated.

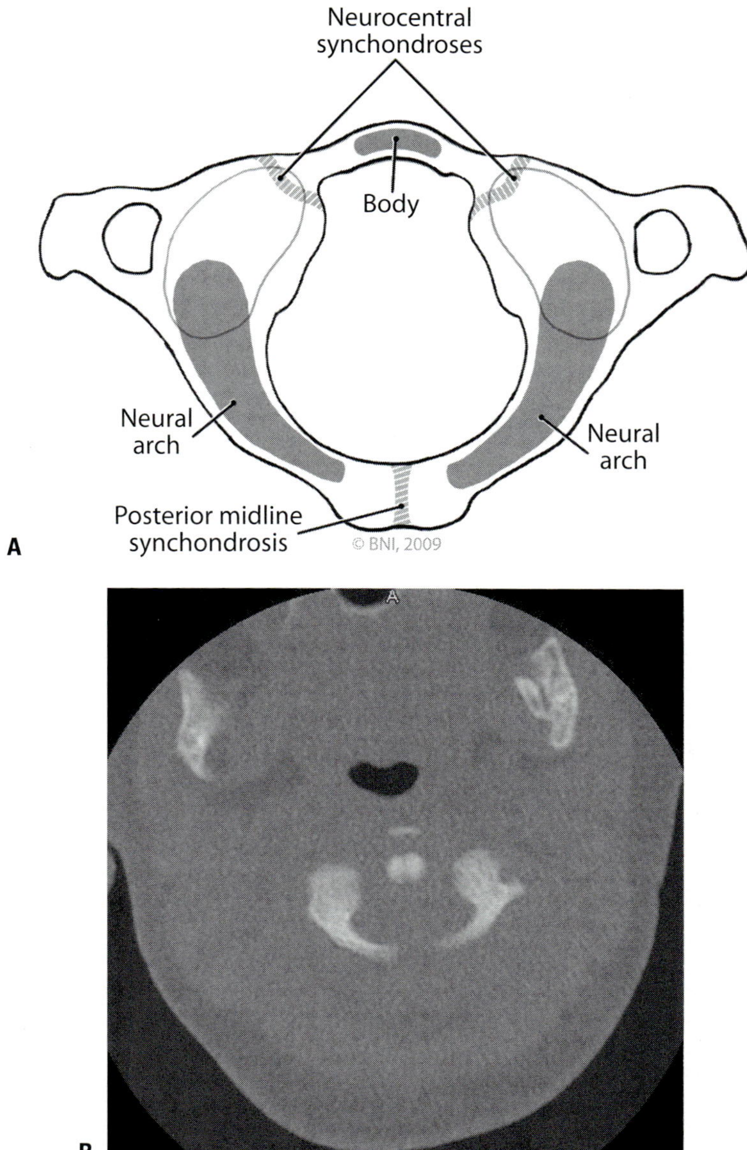

FIGURE 32.1. **A.** Illustration showing the ossification centers and synchondroses of the atlas. The neural arch ossification centers form during the seventh fetal week, and the ossification center within the body of C1 becomes visible during the first year of life. The posterior midline synchondrosis fuses at about the third year of life. The neurocentral synchondroses about the atlas body fuse around the age of 7 years. **B.** Correlative axial computed tomography scan from a 24-week-old child. (With permission from Barrow Neurological Institute.)

In the adult population the normal ADI is less than 3 mm. On plain radiographs of the pediatric cervical spine, this distance should be less than 5 mm.[16] However, some authors report a more stringent 4 mm.[12,17] The exaggeration in ADI potentially reflects incomplete ossification of the dens and laxity of the transverse ligament. Overriding of the anterior arch of C1 on the dens during extension also can be mistaken for atlantoaxial instability. This finding is normal in 20% of children younger than 8 years.[18]

C1 lateral mass displacement more than 6.9 mm on open-mouth views is the classic radiographic indicator of transverse ligament disruption in adults,[19] although magnetic resonance imaging (MRI)

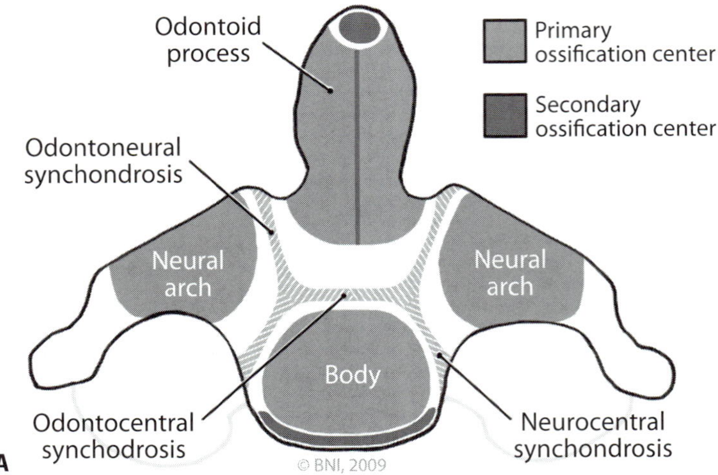

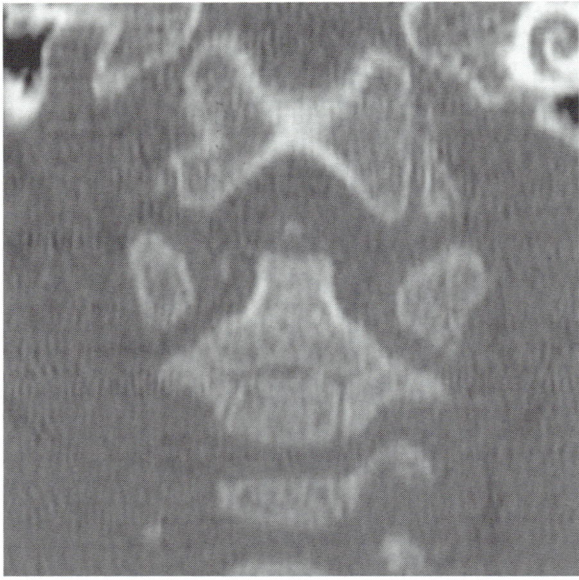

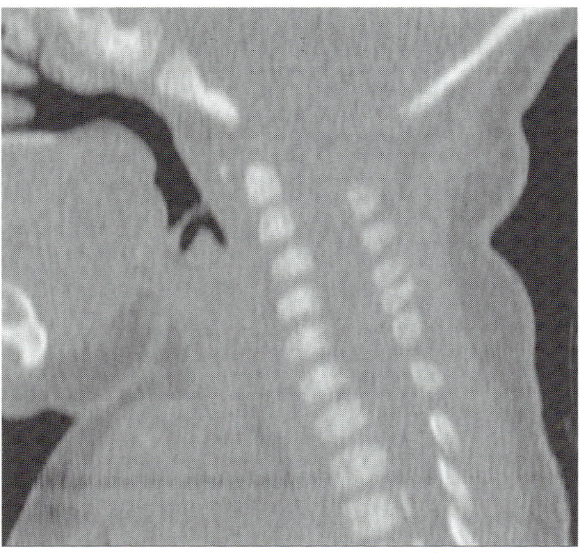

FIGURE 32.2. **A.** Illustration showing the ossification centers and synchondroses of the axis. Two ossification centers fuse in the midline to form the odontoid process by the seventh gestational month. The body of C2 fuses to the odontoid between 3 and 6 years of age. The neurocentral synchondroses about the body also fuse between 3 and 6 years of age. The secondary ossification center at the apex of the odontoid appears between 6 and 8 years of age and fuses with the dens around 12 years of age. **B.** Correlative coronal computed tomography (CT) scan from a 6-month-old child shows the synchondrosis between the odontoid and body of C2, the neurocentral synchondroses, and an early apical ossification center for the odontoid. **C.** Correlative sagittal CT from a 24-week-old child shows the synchondrosis between the odontoid and body of C2. Note the absence of an apical ossification center. (With permission from Barrow Neurological Institute.)

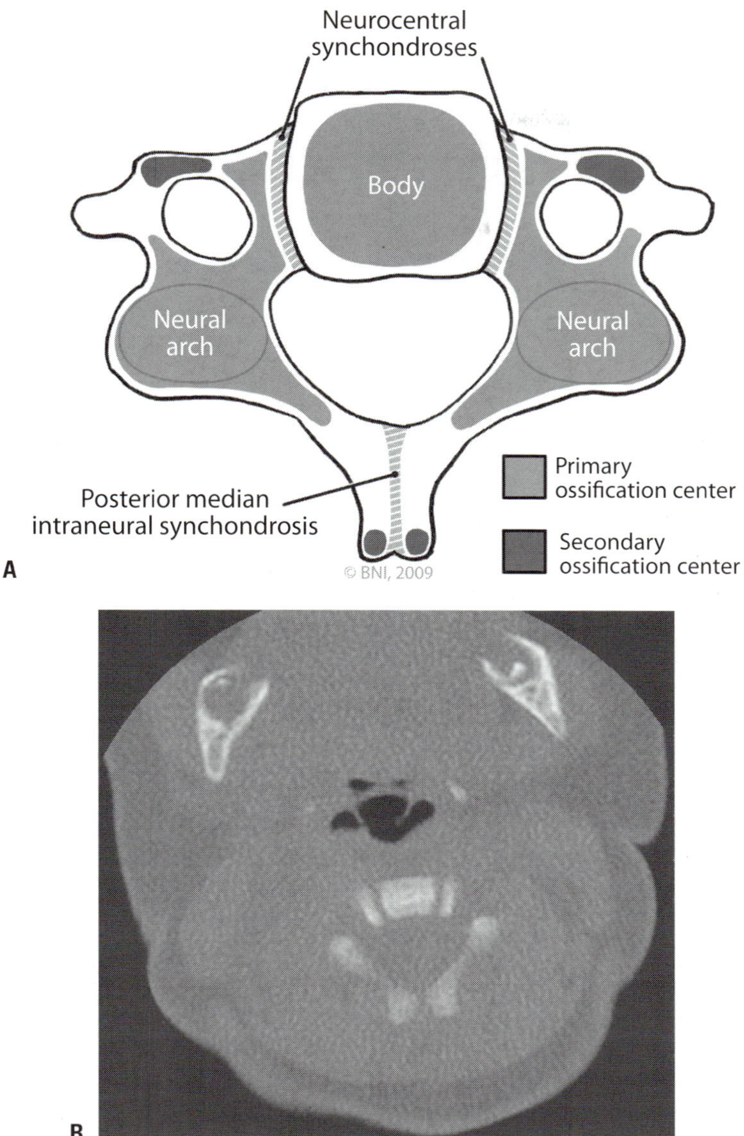

FIGURE 32.3. A. Illustration showing the ossification centers and synchondroses of a subaxial vertebrae. The development of the subaxial cervical spine is highly conserved from C3 through C7. Ossification of the centrum is present by the fifth gestational month. The arches fuse in the midline by the second to third year of age. The neurocentral synchondroses fuse between the third and the sixth year of age. **B.** Correlative sagittal computed tomography scan from a 24-week-old child. Discontinuity within bilateral neural arches is due to plane of section. (With permission from Barrow Neurologic Institute.)

has demonstrated the low sensitivity of this technique.[20] As much as 6 mm of C1 lateral mass displacement is common in children younger than 4 years and may be present until the age of 7 years.[21,22]

Pseudosubluxation of C2 on C3 is present in 22% to 24% of normal pediatric static cervical spine radiographs.[18,23,24] Although this finding diminishes with increasing age, it has been noted in children as old as 14 years (Fig. 32.4).[23] On dynamic films, as many as 46% of normal children under 8 years of age have 3 mm of motion of C2 on C3. On lateral radiographs, 14% of children

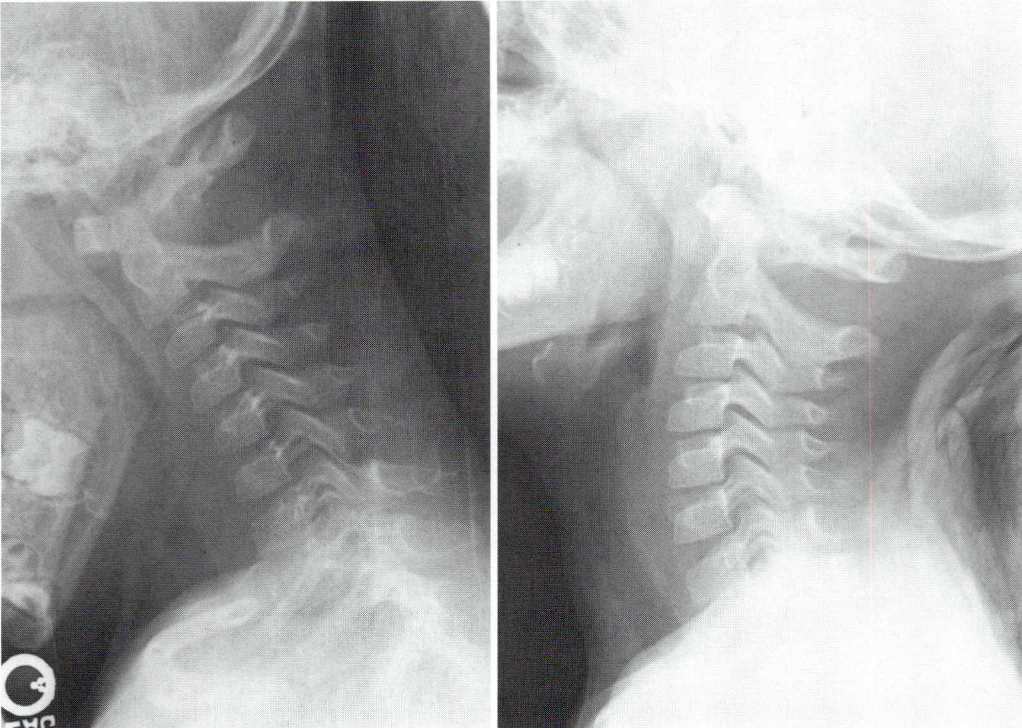

FIGURE 32.4. Normal flexion-extension views from a 12-year-old boy. Note the persistent mild anterior wedging of C3. (With permission from Barrow Neurological Institute.)

have pseudosubluxation of C3 on C4.[18] Pseudosubluxation does not correlate with intubation status, injury severity score, or gender.[23,24] Full reduction of displacement on extension suggests pseudosubluxation rather than true instability.[11]

Swischuk[25] proposed a method to differentiate pseudosubluxation of C2 on C3 from instability caused by a hangman fracture. A line is drawn from the anterior cortex of the posterior arch of C1 to the anterior cortex of the posterior arch of C3. This line typically travels less than 1 mm anterior to the posterior arch of C2. If this distance is more than 2 mm, a disconnection of the anteriorly displaced C2 body from the C2 posterior elements is suggested. Pang and Sun[26] proposed that more than 4.5 mm of horizontal displacement at C2-C3 or C3-C4 should be considered unstable in children younger than 8 years. In children older than 8 years, more than 3.5 mm of horizontal displacement at any cervical level reflects instability.[27]

On both CT and plain radiographs, synchondroses can be mistaken for fracture lines. Conversely, fractures through synchondroses can be misinterpreted as within the realm of normal. The dens–C2 body synchondrosis is well corticated and lies below the level of the superior facets of C2, but it can be mistaken for a type II dens fracture. Fractures through the dens–C2 body synchondrosis may be missed in pediatric patients.[28] This is the most common injury involving the odontoid process in children younger than 7 years.[29–31] Similarly, the C1 synchondroses can be misinterpreted as fractures or abnormally separated.[32] Epiphyseal growth plates of vertebral bodies can be mistaken for fractures. They also may be the sites of shearing injuries. A working knowledge of the location and evolution of synchondroses is essential to the accurate interpretation of pediatric spine imaging.

In newborns, cervical vertebral bodies have an ovoid appearance, with the vertebral interspaces equivalent to the height of the vertebral bodies. With increasing age the vertebral bodies assume a more rectangular shape. A wedge appearance of the anterior aspect of the vertebral body is a common intermediate stage. In particular, mild C3 wedging can persist until 12 years of age.[33]

Loss of cervical lordosis, which can indicate injury in adults, is a normal finding in 14% of children.[18]

BIOMECHANICAL PROPERTIES OF THE DEVELOPING CERVICAL SPINE

Compared to the extensive literature on the biomechanics of the adult cervical spine, biomechanical studies of the pediatric cervical spine are rare. It is generally accepted that the pediatric cervical spine demonstrates an age-dependent hypermobility resulting from underdeveloped bony anatomy, ligaments, and musculature. Furthermore, forces applied to a proportionally larger head enable a larger moment arm to act on the underdeveloped spine.

In the 0- to 8-year-old group, large series have demonstrated a tendency toward involvement of the occipitoatlantoaxial complex[1,6–9] and pure ligamentous injuries rather than fractures. The craniocervical junction is vulnerable in young children for the following reasons:

1. The occipital condyles are smaller.
2. The articulation with the lateral masses of C1 is more planar than cuplike, and it is biased toward the axial plane.[27,34]
3. The relatively large head size coupled with the upper cervical hypermobility places the fulcrum of flexion in the craniocervical region.[13,27]
4. The odontoid synchondrosis is susceptible to translational forces.

In children older than 8 years, injury patterns approach an adult distribution. With increasing age, the fulcrum moves caudally until it reaches the adult position at C5-C7.[27] In older children, cervical spine injuries below the craniovertebral junction tend to be osseous, although pure ligamentous injuries still occur. Subaxial hypermobility arises for the following reasons:

1. The facet joints are biased toward the axial plane.[35]
2. The anterior wedging of vertebral bodies permits added flexion.
3. The disc-annulus complex allows greater longitudinal expansion and distraction.[27,36]
4. In children younger than 10 years, undeveloped uncinate processes permit greater susceptibility to lateral and rotational forces.[27]
5. The joint capsules and ligaments are more elastic.[7,13]

EARLY EVALUATION AND MANAGEMENT

PREHOSPITAL IMMOBILIZATION

Establishment of an airway, adequate ventilation, and cardiovascular support are cardinal principles in the management of any trauma patient. Apnea, cardiorespiratory arrest, or severe hypotension can result from injury to the high cervical spinal cord.[37] Immediate in-the-field spinal immobilization of any patient with a suspicious mechanism of injury or with a neurologic disability is essential to prevent repetitive spinal cord or spinal column injury.

As in adults, the goal of immobilization is to retain the pediatric cervical spine in neutral position. In children younger than 8 years who are immobilized on a spine board, the relatively large head compared to the shoulder girdle and torso places the cervical spine into flexion regardless of the presence of a collar.[38] In one series, more than 20% of children 8 years and older immobilized on a backboard demonstrated more than 10 degrees of cervical flexion (C2-C6 Cobb angle).[39] Herzenberg et al.[40] recommended the use of an occipital recess or thoracic elevation to eliminate the backboard-induced flexion. Nypaver and Treloar[41] determined that children younger than 8 years require a mean of 2.5 cm of thoracic elevation with respect to the occiput to achieve neutral position.

In a trauma setting, infants and young children are often uncooperative and restless. Immobilization with a rigid collar alone may allow more than 15 degrees of flexion and extension.[42] A rigid collar combined with supplemental devices that partially enclose the head (e.g., Kendrick Extrication Device) and tape provide the best prehospital immobilization of the pediatric cervical spine.[42] Cervical collars can lead to supraphysiologic distraction and neurologic injury in the presence of occipitoatlantal dislocation.[43] Sandbags and tape should be used in this situation instead.

CLINICAL CLEARANCE OF THE CERVICAL SPINE

Clinical clearance of the cervical spine can be undertaken in a subset of pediatric trauma patients. Laham et al.[44] established criteria for clinical clearance of the cervical spine in a retrospective series of 268 head-injured pediatric patients. Patients with isolated head injuries who were able to communicate and who had no neck pain or neurologic deficits were classified as low risk (n = 135). High-risk patients (n = 133) were those younger than 2 years, those incapable of verbal communication, and those with neck pain. All patients underwent cervical spine radiographs. No injuries were found in the low-risk group, and 10 injuries were found in the high-risk group. Laham et al.[44] concluded that cervical spine radiographs are unnecessary in pediatric patients who fulfill the low-risk criteria.

Viccellio et al.[45] reported 3065 pediatric patients in a multicenter prospective trial that assessed the utility of cervical spine imaging. Six hundred and three patients met five low-risk criteria, which were defined as each of the following: (a) the absence of midline cervical tenderness, (b) evidence of intoxication, (c) altered level of alertness or intubation, (d) focal neurologic deficits, and (e) painful distracting injury. All patients underwent at least three-view cervical spine imaging. No patient who met all five low-risk criteria had a cervical spine injury.

At our institution, we use the five low-risk criteria studied by Viccellio et al.[45] in combination with a sixth criterion, which requires the ability for appropriate verbal communication before the cervical spine can be cleared.

IMAGING

All children who do not meet the above low-risk criteria should undergo at least AP and lateral cervical spine radiography with swimmers views as necessary. Swischuk et al.[46] have questioned the utility of open-mouth views in children under 5 years of age. In a series of 51 pediatric patients with cervical spine injuries, Buhs et al.[47] concluded that open-mouth views provided no additional information beyond that found on AP and lateral views in children younger than 9 years. Instead, the authors recommended eliminating the open-mouth view and obtaining a CT scan in this patient population.[47]

The use of CT as a primary tool for cervical spine imaging is controversial. Management guidelines from the American Association of Neurological Surgeons/Congress of Neurological Surgeons[24] suggest that "CT of the cervical spine should be used judiciously to define bony anatomy at specific levels but is not recommended as a means to clear the entire cervical spine in children." In adults a growing body of literature indicates the significantly higher sensitivity of CT compared to radiography for the evaluation of cervical spine injuries, especially in obtunded or intubated patients.[48–51] Similar studies in the pediatric population are lacking. CT-based protocols have replaced plain films in adults who cannot be cleared clinically.[52]

Slack and Clancy[53] have advocated CT imaging in obtunded pediatric patients. Although the cervical spine in young children is often easily visualized on plain radiographs,[24] missed fractures on plain films alone have led to neurologic injury in this population.[54] Given the potentially devastating clinical consequences of a missed pediatric cervical spine injury, we recommend CT imaging in all patients who do not satisfy the low-risk criteria discussed in the previous section. Furthermore, CT imaging can prove useful in preoperative planning.

MRI is far superior to CT in delineating nonosseous anatomy. Flynn et al.[55] examined the use of MRI in the evaluation of pediatric cervical spine injury. By institutional protocol, MRI was obtained if at least one of four criteria was met: (a) an obtunded or nonverbal child with a suspicious mechanism of injury, (b) equivocal plain films, (c) neurologic symptoms without radiographic findings, or (d) an inability to clear the cervical spine based on clinical or radiographic evidence within 3 days of injury. MRI altered the diagnosis based on plain radiography in 34% of cases. Frank et al.[56] reported that the use of MRI is associated with more rapid cervical spine clearance and shorter stays in the intensive care unit in obtunded and intubated pediatric trauma patients. Of 52 pediatric trauma patients with normal plain radiographs and CT scans of the cervical spine, 31% demonstrated changes on MRI.[57] These findings ranged from soft tissue or ligamentous signal changes to a bulging disc. The MRI findings influenced surgical planning in four patients. MRI is useful in the evaluation of SCI without radiographic abnormality (SCIWORA),[58] although findings may appear normal in the pediatric population with this injury.[59]

The authors use MRI when a neurologic deficit is present and to assess the extent of ligamentous involvement, particularly with craniovertebral junction injuries. We have a low threshold for obtaining MRIs of the cervical spine in obtunded young children with mechanisms of injury that are high risk for injury to the craniovertebral junction. However, MRI is a static test and does not necessarily predict cervical spine instability.[60] The extent of injury demonstrated on MRI can be used to guide management (Fig. 32.5).[57] Special attention should be directed at the craniocervical junction because injuries in this location are more common in children. T2 or fat suppression sequences such as short tau inversion recovery (STIR) are more sensitive in identifying ligamentous injuries.

Flexion-extension films enable the determination of dynamic instability. Several authors have questioned their use in the face of adequate normal static films. Dwek and Chung[61] reported a series of 247 pediatric trauma patients. No child with normal neutral radiographs demonstrated instability on flexion-extension views. Ralston et al.[62] similarly reported 129 pediatric trauma patients and concluded that flexion-extension radiography was unlikely to be abnormal when isolated loss of lordosis or no acute abnormality was evident on AP and lateral cervical spine radiographs. Woods et al.[63] concluded that flexion-extension films were not useful in the setting of normal static cervical spine films.

METHYLPREDNISOLONE

There are few data on the use of methylprednisolone specific to pediatric patients. The Second National Acute Spinal Cord Injury Study included 13- to 19-year-old patients, but this demographic group composed only 15% of the overall study population. Methylprednisolone is used at the discretion of the treating physician.

PATTERNS OF PEDIATRIC CERVICAL SPINE INJURY

OCCIPITOATLANTAL AND ATLANTOAXIAL DISLOCATION

When distraction injuries are considered, the occipitoatlantoaxial complex can be regarded as one unit. The O-C1 and C1-C2 joint capsules and the atlantooccipital and atlantoaxial membrane do not contribute significantly to the vertical stability of the craniocervical junction.[16,64] The tectorial ligament, alar ligaments, and surrounding musculature appear to have the biggest roles in stabilizing this segment.[65–68]

Although occipitoatlantal and atlantoaxial dislocation injuries are uncommon, they are often seen in young children involved in high-speed motor vehicle collisions, auto-versus-pedestrian accidents, or in airbag-related injuries.[69] Associated neurologic deficits are partial or absent. Complete neurologic injury at this level usually results in rapid death. In this patient population, traction and a cervical collar can lead to overdistraction and worsening neurologic injury and should be avoided.[43]

Diagnosis of occipitoatlantoaxial dislocation (OAAD) in children requires a high index of suspicion, especially in victims of auto-versus-pedestrian accidents and motor vehicle collisions with or without ejection. Reconstructed coronal and sagittal CT images can demonstrate unilateral or bilateral joint widening at O-C1 or C1-C2. At C2, widening of the retropharyngeal space beyond 7 mm is a subtle sign of high cervical injury. MRI can define abnormalities of joints, ligaments, and soft tissues at O-C1 and C1-C2. Sun et al.[70] emphasized the integrity of the tectorial membrane on MRI as a critical factor in determining both occipitoatlantal and atlantoaxial stability against vertical distraction. Definitive treatment of occipitoatlantoaxial instability requires surgical fusion, although cases of children treated nonoperatively have been reported.

A wide range of sensitivities has been reported for the techniques used to diagnose OAD, [71–74] and none of these criteria are fail proof. Available methods include Power's ratio, X-line method, condylar gap method, basion-dens interval (BDI), and basion-axial interval (BAI) (Fig. 32.6). The BDI and BAI measurements are also known as Harris lines. We most commonly use the BDI, BAI, and Power's ratio.

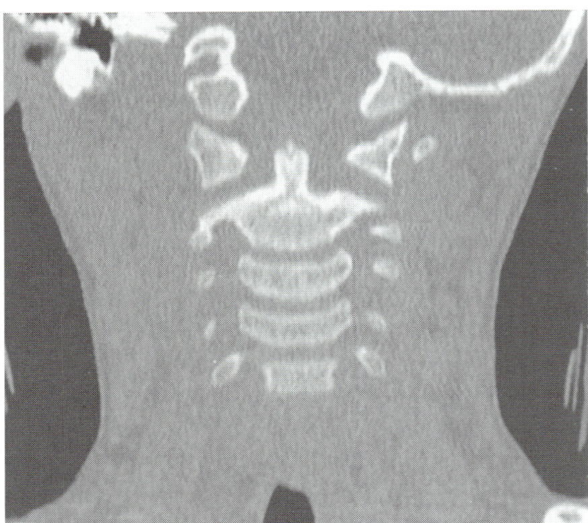

A

FIGURE 32.5. A. Coronal computed tomography scan from a 4-year-old girl who was an unrestrained passenger in a motor vehicle collision showing widening of the bilateral atlantoaxial joints. **B** Sagittal magnetic resonance imaging (MRI) short tau inversion recovery (STIR) images show signal changes within the bilateral atlantoaxial joints and within the right occipitoatlantal joint. MRI confirmed that the transverse ligament was intact (not shown). *(continued)*

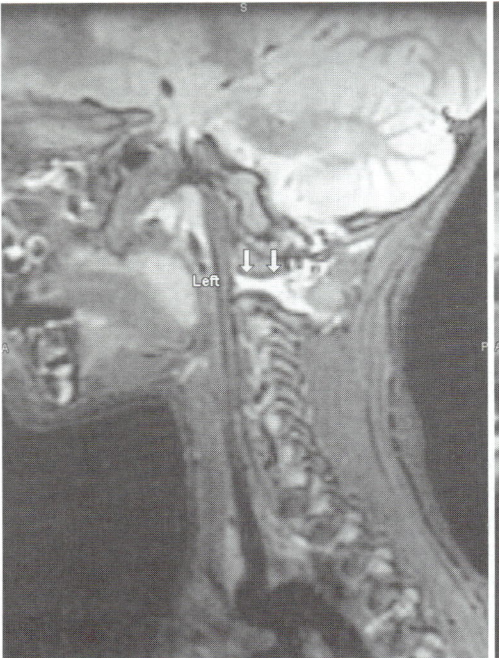

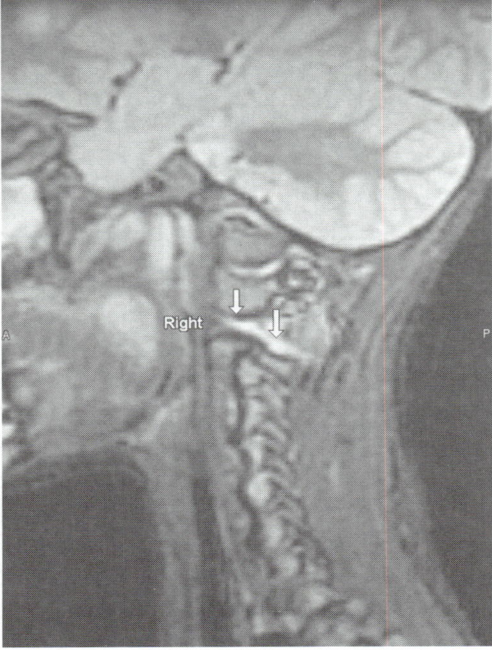

B

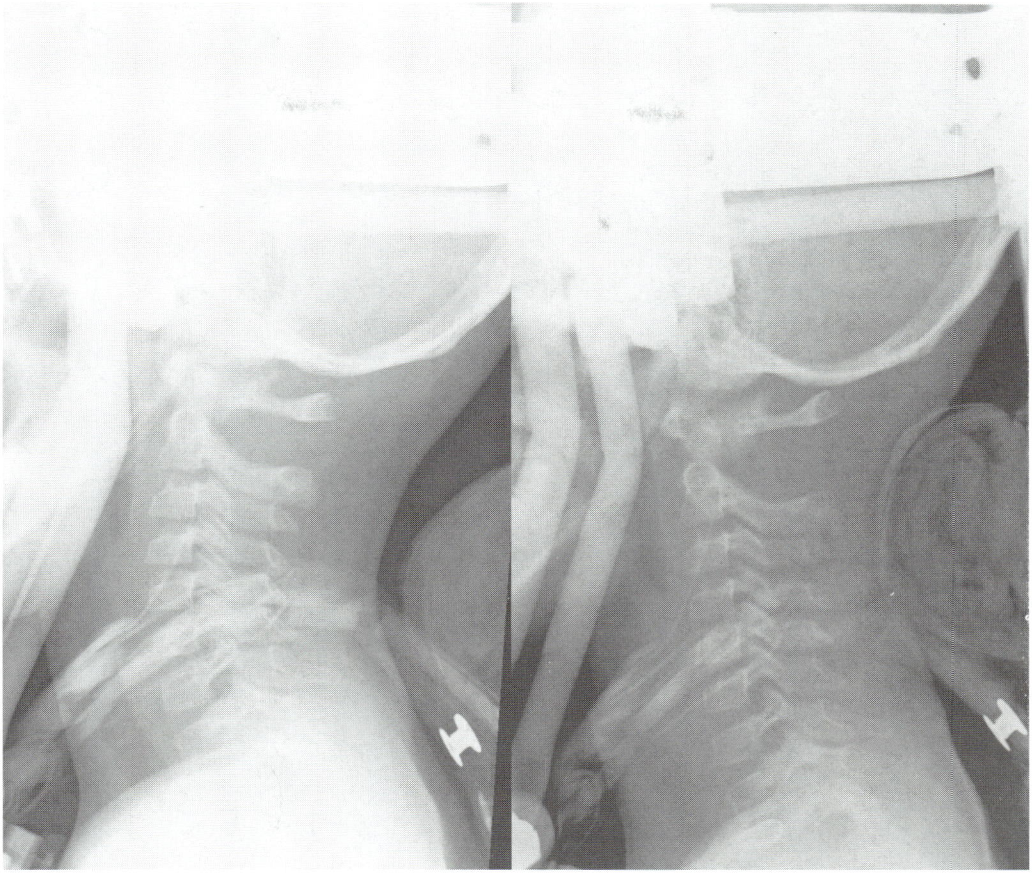

C

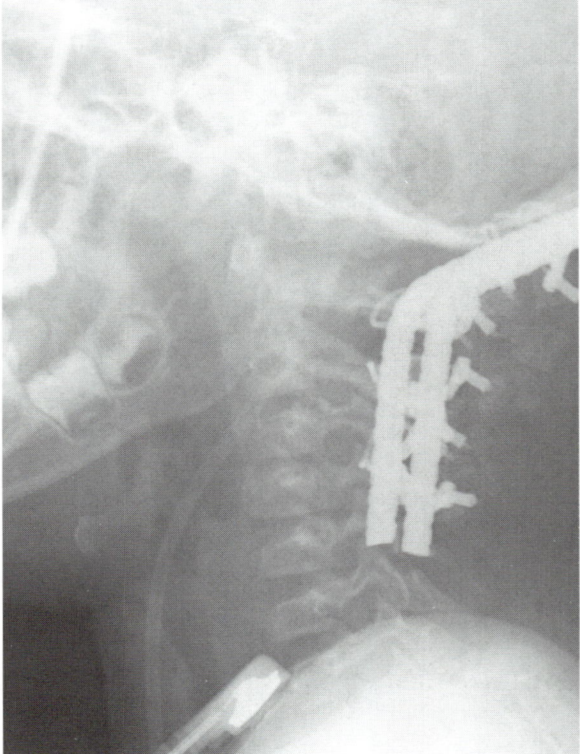

D

FIGURE 32.5. *(continued)* **C.** Halo immobilization was unsuccessful as evidenced by persistent vertical translocation at C1-C2 between upright *(left)* and supine *(right)* films. **D.** Surgical stabilization was achieved with occiput-to-C4 titanium rod fixation and autograft fusion. (With permission from Barrow Neurological Institute.)

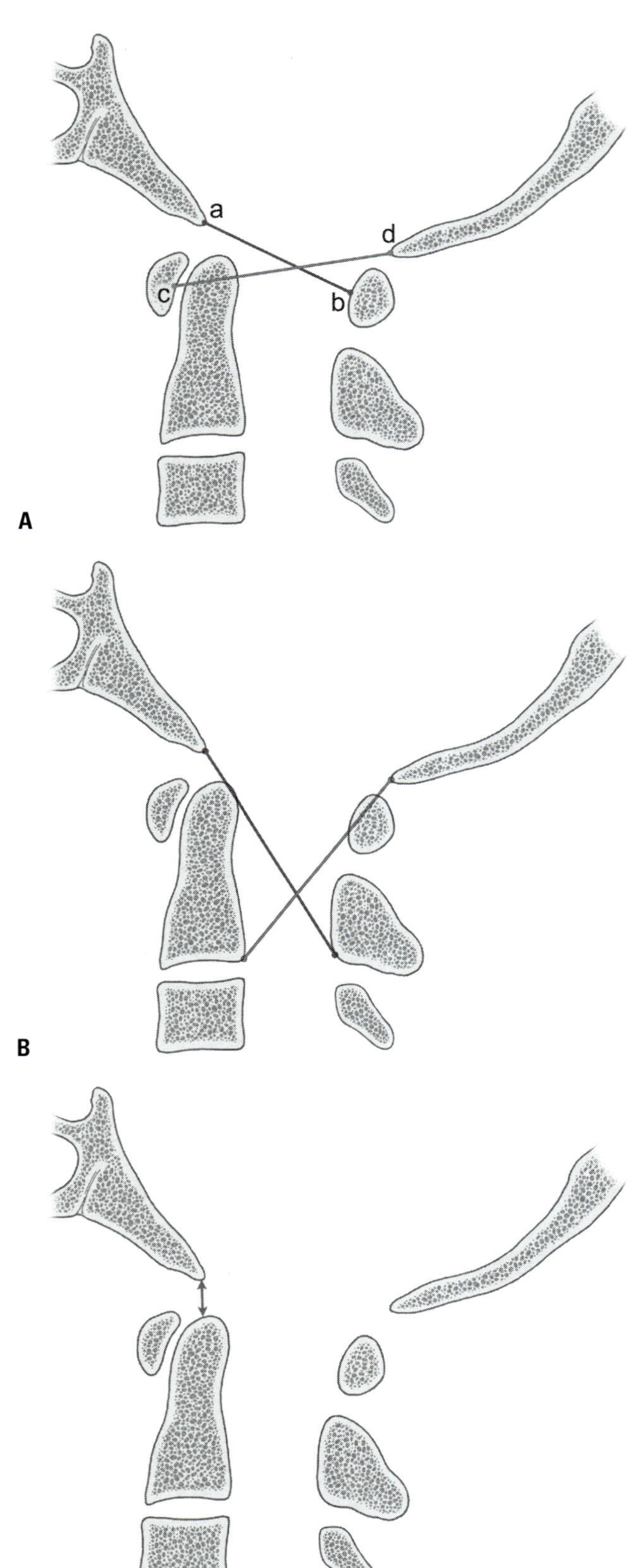

FIGURE 32.6. Traditional lateral cervical radiographic techniques for diagnosis of OAAD: **A.** Power's ratio is the ratio of the basion-posterior atlas arch to the opisthion-anterior arch (*ab/cd*) and is abnormal at values greater than 1.[91] **B.** The X-line method is considered abnormal if the line from the basion to the axis spinolaminar junction does not intersect C2 and if a line from the opisthion to the posterior inferior corner of the body of the axis does not intersect C1.[63] **C.** The basion-dens interval (BDI) is abnormal in the presence of a displacement between the basion and the dens of >10 mm in adults or >12 mm in pediatric patients.[134] *(continued)*

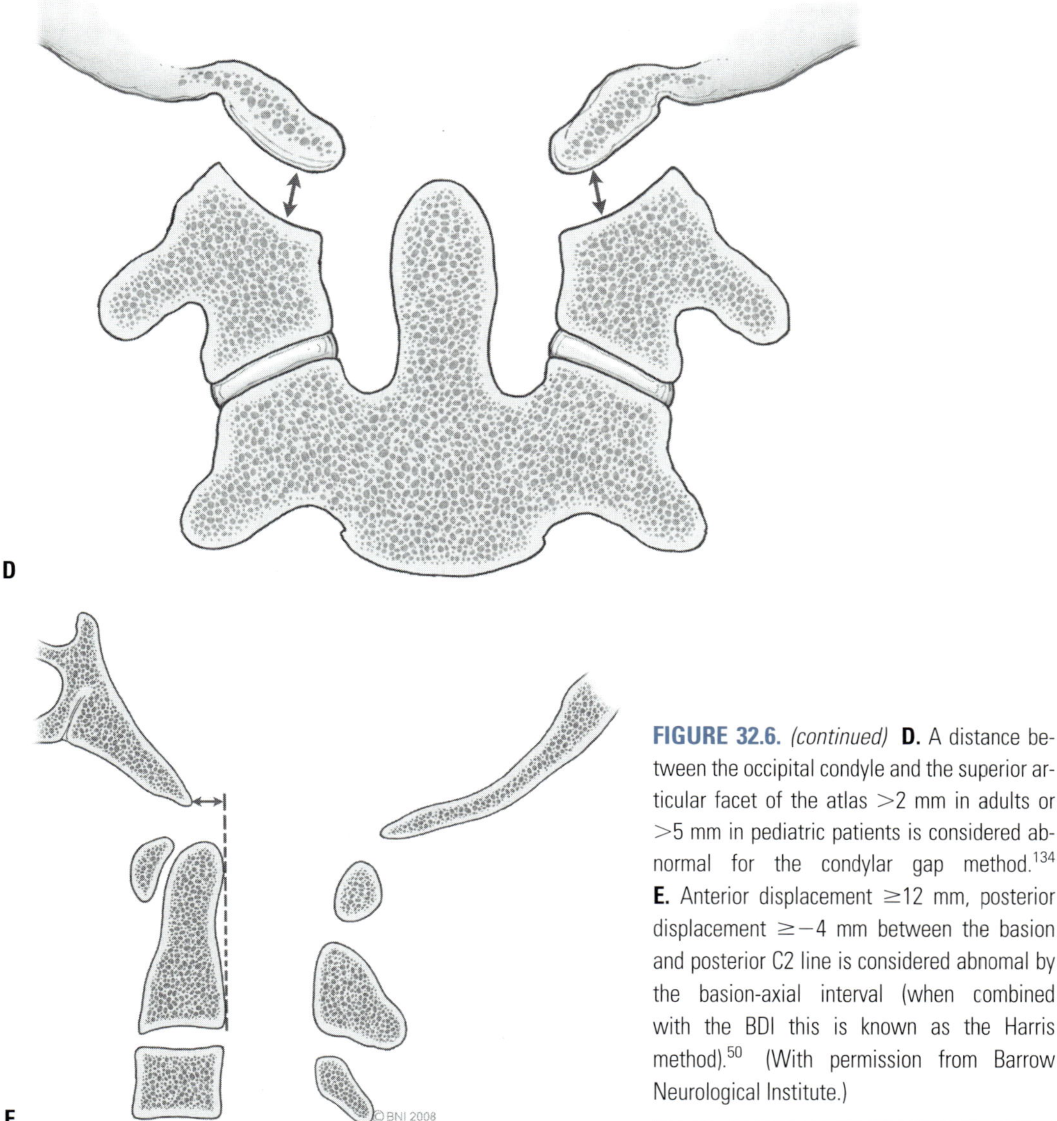

FIGURE 32.6. *(continued)* **D.** A distance between the occipital condyle and the superior articular facet of the atlas >2 mm in adults or >5 mm in pediatric patients is considered abnormal for the condylar gap method.[134] **E.** Anterior displacement ≥12 mm, posterior displacement ≥−4 mm between the basion and posterior C2 line is considered abnomal by the basion-axial interval (when combined with the BDI this is known as the Harris method).[50] (With permission from Barrow Neurological Institute.)

A universal theme underlying the difficulties in diagnosing OAD using plain lateral cervical radiographs is the ability to visualize the anatomic landmarks required for application of these methods. Diagnostic tests rely on bony landmarks that are remote from the injured occipitoatlantal joint. During patient positioning, these landmarks could inadvertently align and conceal actual disruption of the joint. With respect to the initial cross-table lateral radiograph of the cervical spine, landmarks may be indistinct and magnification error may invalidate several of the indices commonly used for diagnosis. Poor visualization of the relevant anatomic structures on lateral cervical radiographs may lead to missed injuries. Congenital anomalies of C1, C2, and at the foramen magnum and immature or delayed ossification of the odontoid segments also preclude use of many radiologic criteria.

Based on class III evidence, *The Guidelines for the Management of Acute Cervical Spine and Spinal Cord Injuries*[46] recommends applying the BAI-BDI (Harris method) to a plain lateral cervical radiograph. In the event of a nondiagnostic film in the presence of clinical suspicion or swelling of vertebral soft tissue, CT or MRI is recommended. Additional diagnostic clues include the following: enlargement of the predental space; neurological abnormalities, including lower cranial nerve paresis (particularly cranial nerves VI, X, and XII); monoparesis, hemiparesis, and quadriparesis; respiratory dysfunction including apnea; complete high cervical cord motor deficits in the setting of normal plain spinal x-rays; subarachnoid hemorrhage at the craniovertebral junction on CT scans; ligamentous abnormalities of the tectorial, alar, and transverse ligaments; and short tau inversion recovery (STIR) changes of the posterior interspinous ligament of the occipitoatlantal joint capsule on MRI.[75,76]

Since these guidelines were published, the number of publications documenting the use of CT as the diagnostic imaging of choice in patients suspected of having OAD has increased.[71,76–78] Dedicated studies using CT to diagnose OAD have supported the use of the BDI (with 10 mm as the cutoff)[71] and the occipital condyle-C1 interval (CCI) (>4 mm is abnormal) as the diagnostic tests of choice.[76]

Pang et al.[78] described normative data for the occipitoatlantal joint in 89 children, in whom the normal occipitoatlantal joint was tightly apposed with a mean CCI of 1.28 mm. There was considerable left-right symmetry, and the CCI was stable from ages 0–18 years. On high-resolution CT scans in all individual joint measurements, the normal CCI was less than 2 mm. No single measurement among all 1424 data points was greater than 2.5 mm. Similar to the lateral mass interval as a diagnostic standard for atlanto-axial distraction injuries,[79] the CCI is the only test that directly measures the integrity of the actual joint injured in OAD. Furthermore, a widened CCI cannot be concealed by positioning after injury.

Pang et al.[76] subsequently applied the CCI method to 16 patients with OAD and found pathologic widening ranging from 5 to 34 mm. The CCI criterion was positive in all of their 16 patients with OAD with a diagnostic sensitivity of 100%. The authors have advocated treatment of patients with pathological widening greater than the upper normal limit of CCI of 4 mm. Given the variability in ossification and fusion at the craniocervical junction, this method is especially applicable to the pediatric population.

Harris et al.[72] found the BDI diagnostically unreliable in children under the age of 13 years. However, the BAI was reproducible and normally did not exceed 12 mm. In fact, the CCI may become the diagnostic criterion of choice even in adults as the normative data reported did not show a statistical change from birth to 18 years. Current studies are underway to determine the diagnostic sensitivity and specificity of the CCI method in adults.

ATLANTOAXIAL ROTATORY FIXATION

Atlantoaxial rotatory fixation (AARF) is an alteration of the normal rotational relationship between the atlas and axis. This condition ranges from significant limitation of motion to absolute fixation. Trauma, upper respiratory infections, and head and neck surgery are the main causes for this disorder.

Fielding and Hawkins[80] established a four-tier classification system (Fig. 32.7). Type I AARF is defined by an intact transverse ligament. Types II and III injuries are defined by the disruption of the transverse ligament alone and by disruption of the transverse and alar ligaments, respectively. These injuries are associated with a progressively widened ADI corresponding to increased displacement of the atlas on C2. Type IV AARF is defined as a posterior rotatory displacement of the atlas on C2. This injury is very rare and can occur only in the setting of a hypoplastic odontoid process. Types II, III, and IV AARF are easily defined on CT and MRI and usually require surgical stabilization of the atlantoaxial complex.

Type I AARF is most difficult to diagnose because the pathologic C1-C2 fixation can appear within the range of physiologically normal on static imaging.[81] In this largely pediatric disorder, patients have painful torticollis in the "cock-robin" position with the head turned to one side and the neck laterally flexed in the opposite direction. Ligamentous laxity and shallow C1-C2 lateral mass articulations predispose children to initial overrotation and subluxation.[82] Spasms of cervical

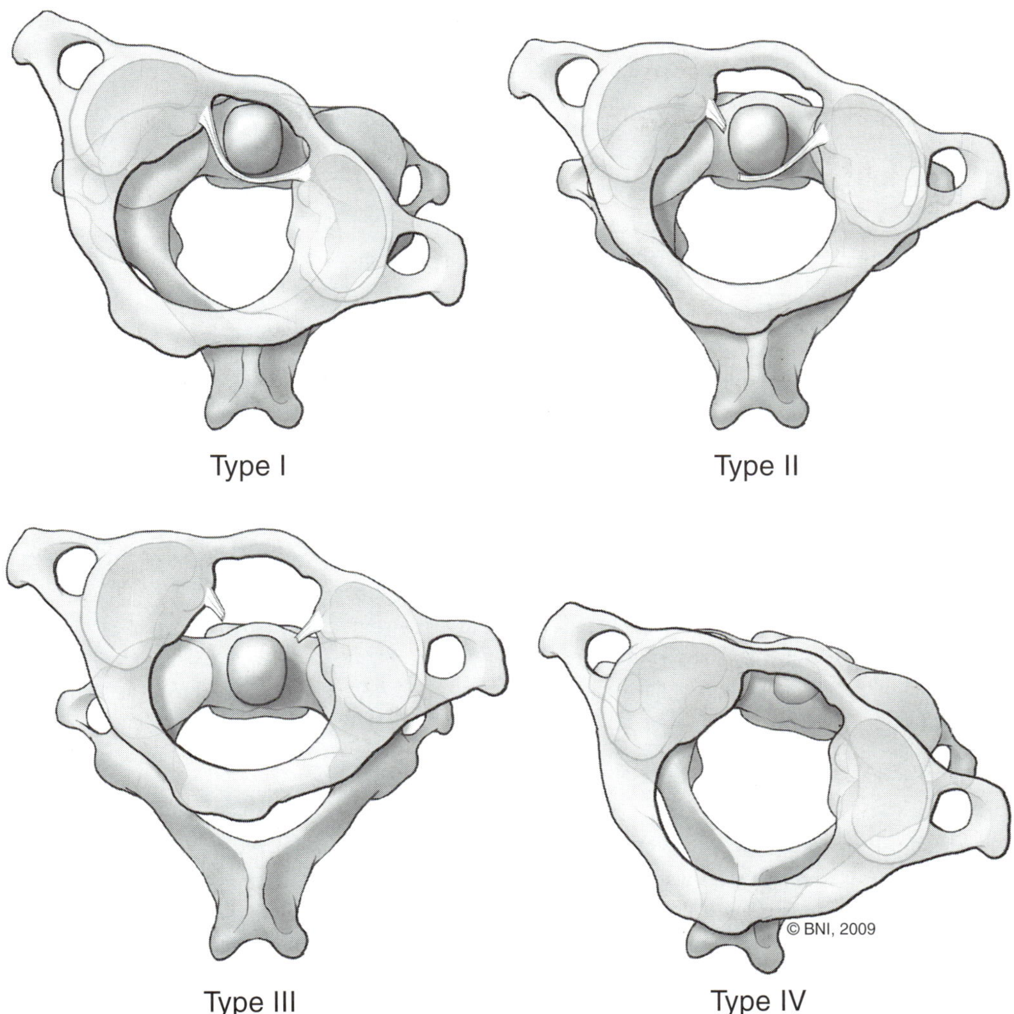

FIGURE 32.7. Fielding and Hawkins classification scheme for atlantoaxial rotatory fixation (AARF). Type I AARF is defined by an intact transverse ligament. Types II and III injuries are defined by the disruption of the transverse ligament alone and by disruption of the transverse and alar ligaments, respectively. These injuries are associated with a progressively widened atlantodens interval. Type IV AARF is a posterior rotatory displacement of the atlas on C2, in the setting of odontoid hypoplasia. (With permission from Barrow Neurological Institute.)

musculature, synovial inflammation, or mechanical obstruction of the C1-C2 articular surfaces have all been implicated in maintenance of the deformity.[82]

Traditionally, dynamic CT is used to evaluate AARF.[83] In this protocol, fine-cut CT imaging is used to image the atlantoaxial span in the presenting position and at the limits of rotation in either direction, as dictated by the patient's discomfort. Limitation or absence of motion is used to diagnose AARF, but the reliability of this technique has been questioned.[16,84]

Pang and Li[81] refined the conceptualization of Fielding and Hawkins type I AARF from that of a locked angle of rotation of C1 on C2 to that of a "pathological stickiness" between C1 and C2 that leads to abnormal motion on rotation. In normal individuals, axial rotation of the head results in three discrete phases of C1 motion on C2 (Fig. 32.8).[81] From 0 degrees (defined by the head

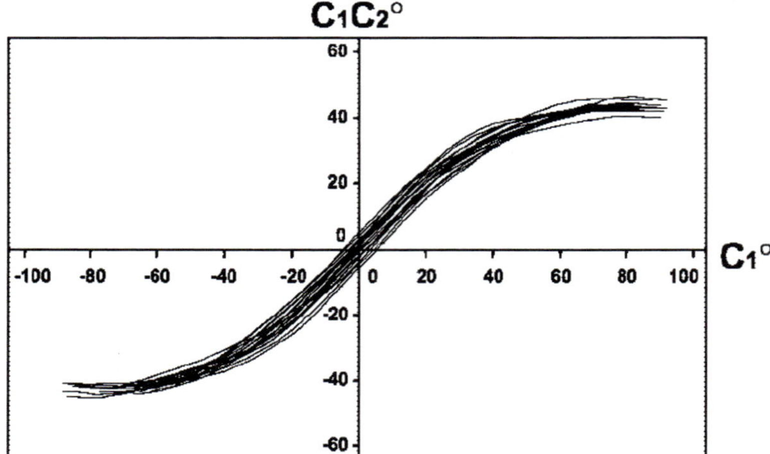

FIGURE 32.8. Superimposed C1-C2 motion curves from 18 normal patients. X axis denotes head position and, therefore, C1 position relative to body. Y axis denotes rotational angle between C1 and C2. From 0 degrees (defined by the head facing straight forward) to 23 degrees head rotation, C1 rotates independently of an immobile C2. From 23 to 65 degrees, C2 rotates with C1, albeit more slowly. At 65 degrees head rotation, a fixed angle (43 degrees) of C1-C2 rotational separation is reached. Further head rotation from 65 to 90 degrees is characterized by lock-step motion of C1 with C2 and results wholly from subaxial rotational mobility. (From Pang D, Li V. Atlantoaxial rotatory fixation. I: Biomechanics of normal rotation at the atlantoaxial joint in children. *Neurosurgery* 2004;55:620. With permission from Lippincott Williams & Wilkins.)

facing straight forward) to 23 degrees of head rotation, C1 rotates independently while C2 remains immobile. From 23 to 65 degrees, C2 rotates with C1, albeit more slowly. At 65 degrees of head rotation, the angle of C1-C2 rotational separation reaches a maximum of 43 degrees. Further head rotation from 65 to 90 degrees is characterized by lock-step motion of C1 with C2 and is entirely provided by subaxial rotational mobility.

Based on an analysis of 40 pediatric patients presenting with torticollis, Pang and Li[85] refined the dynamic CT protocol and classified Fielding and Hawkins type I AARF into three subtypes corresponding to decreasing amounts of "pathological stickiness." Atlantoaxial scans are obtained in the presenting position, with the nose pointing directly forward and with the head turned to the contralateral side as much as the patient can tolerate. The C1-C2 rotational angle is assessed at each position. In subtype I AARF there is no motion between C1 and C2. In subtype II AARF the C1-C2 rotational angle will decrease but never approach zero despite maximal contralateral neck rotation. In subtype III AARF the C1-C2 rotational angle will reduce to zero but only with rotation of the head greater than 20 degrees past midline to the contralateral side. A fourth group of patients demonstrated indeterminate pathology between subtype III AARF and normal.

Delays in treatment of AARF lead to worsening C1-C2 adherence. Severity and chronicity of AARF are both independently associated with more difficult and longer treatment, a greater chance of recurrence, higher rates of irreducibility, greater need for surgical stabilization, and higher rates of complete C1-C2 motion segment loss.[86] Patients with chronic subtype I AARF should undergo halo-ring traction followed by halo vest immobilization for 3 months. Patients with chronic subtype II should undergo halter or halo traction followed by halo vest immobilization for 3 months. Patients with subtype III AARF should undergo halter traction followed by immobilization in a cervicothoracic orthosis for 3 months. First recurrences in the orthosis are treated with repeat traction and immobilization. During or after halo vest immobilization, irreducible deformity or recurrence is treated with surgical fusion of C1-C2.

ODONTOID INJURIES

In children younger than 7 years, odontoid injuries are typically avulsions of the synchondrosis between the body of C2 and the dens (Fig. 32.9).[29–31,87] Falls and high-speed motor vehicle collisions, especially with children secured in forward-facing car seats, have been implicated in this injury pattern.[88] Many patients with odontoid synchondrosis are neurologically intact because a high cervical SCI is otherwise fatal. Lateral radiographs often show an anteriorly displaced odontoid peg.[89] Reconstructed CT images may show widening of the synchondrosis.

Epiphyseal injuries appear to have a high likelihood of healing with closed reduction and immobilization. Several authors have used halo or plaster-cast immobilization as first-line treatment, with most patients achieving stable fusions.[87–89] This management strategy preserves the motion segment and avoids surgery in this very young population. C1-C2 fusion may be necessary when nonoperative treatment fails.

SUBAXIAL LIGAMENTOUS INJURIES

Injuries to the subaxial cervical spine have been reported in children under 8 years of age but are generally rare.[7,81] As the pediatric spine matures toward adultlike biomechanics, subaxial injuries become more common, with an increasing proportion of bony rather than ligamentous injuries.

The severity of subaxial soft tissue and ligamentous injuries varies. Mild forms may present with neck pain but no abnormality on CT or dynamic plain films of the cervical spine. More severe injuries may be associated with widening of facet joints, widening or collapse of the disc space, and separation of the spinous process. MRI STIR sequences delineate ligamentous, soft tissue, joint capsule, and epiphyseal endplate injury but may not correlate well with cervical stability.[60] White and Panjabi[90] suggested that more than 11 degrees of angulation and/or 3.5 mm of subluxation between adjacent vertebrae implies significant ligamentous injury with the likelihood of instability. Based on unpublished data from Pang and Brockmeyer, it is suggested that more than 7 degrees of kyphotic angulation between adjacent vertebral bodies in the pediatric spine implies unstable ligamentous injury.[91] This poor tolerance for angulation reflects the increased recoil forces within the intact pediatric cervical spine.

Soft tissue and ligamentous injury without radiographic abnormality on CT or dynamic radiographs is managed with analgesics and a soft collar, as necessary. If neck pain limits sufficient excursion on dynamic films, the patient is placed in a hard cervical collar and reevaluated with dynamic films after a 2-week interval.

Patients with more substantial soft tissue and ligamentous injury with evidence of widened facet joints, disc spaces, or spinous processes must be evaluated carefully. Pennecot et al.[92] reported that 8 of 11 patients with such injuries who were initially managed with reduction and a collar required surgical fusion for instability. MRI may help delineate the extent of injury and influence management. If nonoperative management is undertaken, we recommend hard-collar immobilization and meticulous long-term follow-up with dynamic radiographs to evaluate for late instability. Any neurologic deficits resulting from spinal column instability should be treated with operative stabilization.

Unilateral or bilateral facet dislocation is a relatively common injury pattern of the adolescent pediatric cervical spine. It is caused by a flexion-distraction mechanism and complete disruption of facet capsules. In a patient with bilateral jumped facets and motor-complete SCI, we use emergent manual reduction followed by immediate MRI to evaluate for an epidural hematoma or herniated disc. Although the literature supports the lack of need for a prereduction MRI if the patient is alert and cooperative, we first obtain an MRI to evaluate for a herniated disc or hematoma within the spinal canal in a neurologically intact patient with jumped facet(s). In the absence of such a lesion, the patient is placed in tongs or halo traction for closed reduction of the deformity. In patients with motor-incomplete SCI and jumped facet(s), we immediately obtain an MRI to evaluate for disc material or hematoma within the spinal canal. In their absence, manual or weighted traction can be used to reduce the deformity, based on the severity of motor injury. In all cases, anterior and/or posterior surgical stabilization at the level of injury is necessary. Surgery can be undertaken on an

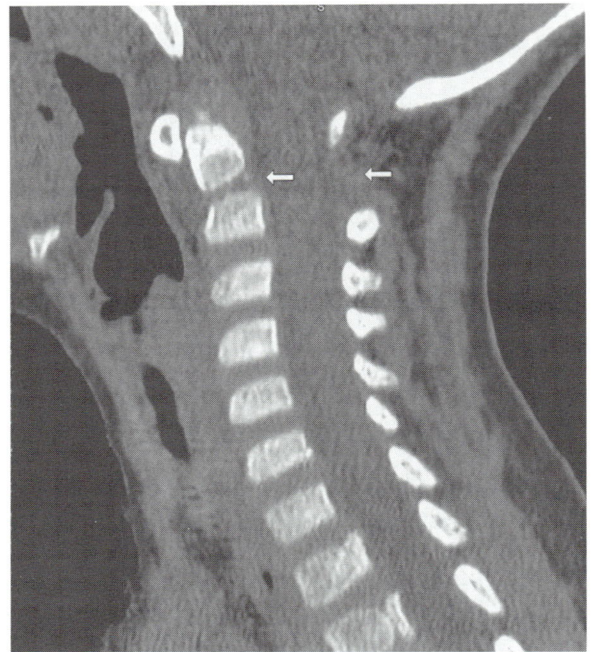

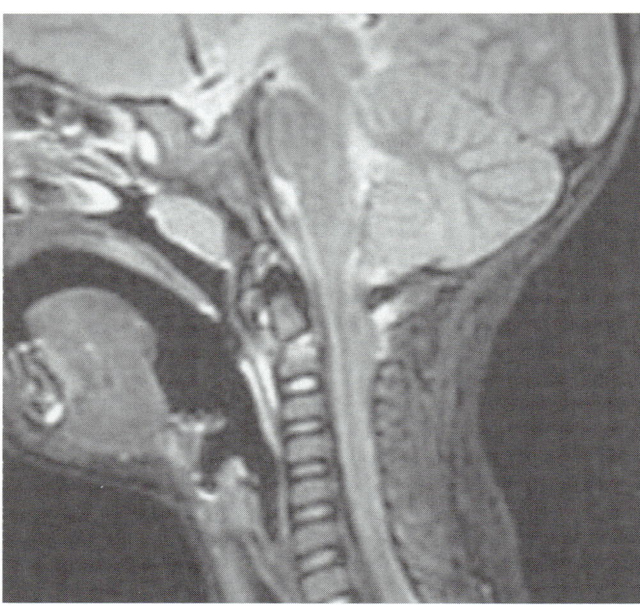

FIGURE 32.9. **A.** Sagittal CT scan of a 3-year-old boy who was a restrained passenger in a motor vehicle collision shows disruption of the synchondrosis between the odontoid process and body of C2. Note the widening of the posterior elements of C1 and C2. **B.** Sagittal MRI short tau inversion recovery confirms fracture across the odontoid synchondrosis and posterior ligamentous injury at C1-C2.

emergent basis to treat compressive pathology within the spinal canal, although the optimal timing of surgical intervention is unclear.

SPINAL CORD INJURY WITHOUT RADIOLOGIC ABNORMALITY

SCIWORA was described by Pang and Wilberger[93] in 1982. The incidence of SCIWORA in pediatric patients with SCI has been estimated at between 5% and 67%.[94] A meta-analysis conducted by Pang[94] places this number at about 35%. In younger patients, falls and auto-versus-pedestrian accidents are a common cause of SCIWORA. In adolescents, sports injuries and motor vehicle collisions are more common. In neonates, hyperflexion and hyperextension resulting from child abuse can lead to devastating SCIWORA.

The pathophysiologic basis for SCIWORA is the hypermobility of the pediatric cervical spine. When subjected to traumatic hyperflexion, hyperextension, or distraction, the spine recoils to its physiologic state while the spinal cord, with little tolerance for deformation, sustains varying amounts of injury.[94,95] Spinal cord ischemia from vertebral artery injury has also been proposed as an underlying mechanism.[49] Patients present with a spectrum of neurologic manifestations ranging from mild transient sensory symptoms to quadriplegia. Children younger than 8 years are much more likely to have more rostral and severe SCIWORA than older children.[49,96] In 8- to 16-year-olds, SCIWORA tends to occur at lower levels and to be less severe than in younger children.[49,96,97]

Fundamental to the definition of SCIWORA is the absence of abnormality on static and dynamic flexion-extension films, CT imaging, and CT myelography. Also excluded are injuries from penetrating trauma, obstetric complications, and electrical shock. MRI enables superior characterization of both the spinal cord and surrounding nonosseous support structures.

Pang[94] reported the high prognostic utility of MRI in 50 patients with SCIWORA. At presentation, MRI findings within the spinal cord were divided into major hemorrhage, minor hemorrhage, edema, and no-abnormality categories. Patients with major hemorrhage on MRI presented as Frankel grades B and C (severe deficits) and remained at this level of impairment long term. Patients with minor spinal cord hemorrhage also presented as Frankel grades B and C, but 40% improved to grade D at 6 months. Of patients with edema only, 44% presented as Frankel grade B and C and 56% presented as grade D (minor deficits). At 6 months, 75% percent of patients who had presented with edema only were Frankel grade D and 25% were grade E (normal). There were no MRI findings in 23 patients with clinical SCIWORA. These patients universally made a complete recovery.

MRI is useful in characterizing nonneural injury to the cervical ligamentous and soft tissues in SCIWORA. Injuries to the anterior and posterior longitudinal ligaments, epiphyseal growth plate, facet joints, tectorial membrane, and disc spaces have been documented on MRI.[94] Pang[94] proposed the concept of "occult" instability of the spine in patients with SCIWORA, even in the setting of normal dynamic films with sufficient excursion. In occult instability, the ligamentous and soft tissue structures are injured but not destroyed. They are able to withstand moderate physiologic forces but are vulnerable to significant stress. The literature provides scant direct evidence for this concept,[96] but occult instability is proposed as a possible cause of the delayed neurologic deterioration that has been reported in patients with SCIWORA.[94,97,98] Occult instability has also been implicated in recurrent SCIWORA.[99] In this entity, a minor trauma after an initial SCIWORA episode causes recurrent symptoms. Ostensibly, the injured spinal cord is more vulnerable to recurrent injury and the weakened nonneural structures may facilitate the recurrence.

In the clinical setting of SCIWORA, MRI can be completely normal.[58,59] Pang[94] reported that MRI was positive in 64% of pediatric patients with SCIWORA with persistent motor deficits lasting more than 24 hours, in 27% of patients with deficits lasting fewer than 24 hours, and in 6% of patients with only sensory symptoms. He advocates repeating MRI 6 to 9 days after injury because edema may take 3 to 4 hours to develop after the initial insult, and small foci of hemorrhage within the spinal cord may not manifest until converted to methemoglobin.[99]

Cervical immobilization of patients with SCIWORA is controversial. If dynamic films sufficiently demonstrate stability of the cervical spine, the role of cervical immobilization is unclear.[100] Pang and Pollack[95] advocated 12 weeks of immobilization in a Guilford brace to allow ligamentous injuries to heal and to prevent recurrent SCIWORA. Bosch et al.[101] reported that rigid braces, including the Guilford, Aspen, Miami J, and Minerva cast, did not prevent recurrent SCIWORA. They questioned the theory of occult instability as a causative factor. In the setting of only extraneural MRI findings, neurologic recovery, and no neck pain, the authors recommend hard-collar immobilization for 2 weeks followed by dynamic films. With neural findings on MRI, 12 weeks of immobilization followed by dynamic films is appropriate.

CERVICAL CORD NEURAPRAXIA

Cervical cord neurapraxia, also known as spinal cord concussion or a stinger, likely represents a mild form of SCIWORA that occurs in athletes playing contact sports. Sensory and motor symptoms involving both arms, both legs, or all four extremities can occur.[102] The symptoms usually last 10 to 15 minutes but can persist as long as 48 hours.[103] In adult athletes, cervical cord neurapraxia is often related to cervical stenosis. The relative risk for an athlete sustaining cervical cord neurapraxia a second time increases exponentially compared to the risk for sustaining cervical cord neurapraxia the first time.[104] Boockvar et al.[105] reported 13 children, aged 7 to 15 years, with cervical cord neurapraxia with no evidence of spinal stenosis. In this population, cervical cord neurapraxia was attributed to cervical hypermobility. Most patients were managed with 2 weeks of cervical immobilization in a hard cervical collar followed by dynamic films. At a mean follow-up of 15 months after injury, all children had returned to sports without restriction, with no recurrence of cervical cord neurapraxia or neck pain.

NEONATAL INJURIES

The incidence of birth-related SCIs is approximately 1 in 60,000.[106] The upper cervical spine is the most susceptible to injury[107] and is associated with cephalic presentation and the use of forceps.[107,108] Infants present with flaccidity and absence of spontaneous motion. Injured infants who do not make respiratory efforts during the first day of life tend to remain ventilator dependent.[24,106] Spinal immobilization with a thermoplastic molded device spanning from the occiput to the thorax has been used in the management of this difficult problem.[24]

OS ODONTOIDEUM

Os odontoideum is a well-corticated odontoid process that lacks continuity with the body of C2. Both traumatic and congenital causes of os odontoideum have been documented.[109,110] Two anatomic subsets of os odontoideum exist: orthotopic and dystopic. An orthotopic os moves with C1, whereas a dystopic os is fixed to the basion. Patients can present with occipitocervical pain, myelopathy, or vertebrobasilar ischemia.[111] The natural history of os odontoideum has not been adequately defined, leading to significant controversy about its appropriate management.

The initial diagnosis can be easily made with lateral radiography. Multiple authors have reported that the degree of C1-C2 instability on flexion-extension films does not correlate with the presence of myelopathy.[112–114] However, these authors also reported that a sagittal diameter of the spinal canal of 13 mm or less on plain radiographs is strongly associated with myelopathy.[112,114]

Spierings and Braakman[112] reported nonoperative management of 16 patients with os odontoideum without myelopathy. At a median follow-up of 7 years, no patient had suffered neurologic deterioration. As an option, the Guidelines for the Management of Acute Cervical Spine and Spinal Cord Injuries suggest that patients without neurologic deficits, but with instability at C1-C2 on flexion-extension studies, can be managed without operative intervention.[111] Given the potential for neurologic injury in children with os odontoideum resulting from minor trauma,[115] Brockmeyer[91] believes that the risks of untreated os odontoideum outweigh the risks of C1-C2 fusion.

OPERATIVE AND NONOPERATIVE MANAGEMENT CONSIDERATIONS

Many pediatric cervical spine injuries can be treated with halo or hard-collar immobilization.[97,116] Indications for surgical intervention include an unstable injury, irreducible fracture or dislocation, progressive neurologic deficit from compression, and progressive deformity.[7,107,108] Within the last decade, the percentage of pediatric patients with cervical spine trauma managed surgically has increased as a result of advances in fixation systems and techniques.[6,117] Surgical stabilization of the spine, combined with early mobilization of pediatric patients with SCI, likely reduces the risk for deep venous thrombosis, decubitus ulcers, and respiratory infections.[117,118]

Historically, pediatric cervical spinal fusion was limited to posterior bone and wire techniques followed by halo or cervicothoracic immobilization. These techniques have a higher rate of failed fusion than contemporary rigid fixation techniques.[117,119,120] However, the smaller anatomy and greater proportion of cartilage in the young pediatric spine demand great accuracy in the placement of any screw. Additional concerns in pediatric spine fusion are the development of adjacent level disease and the "crankshaft" phenomenon characterized by continued growth of bone at fixated levels, resulting in a deformity.

OCCIPITOCERVICAL SURGICAL STABILIZATION

Occipitocervical fusion with threaded contoured rods and wiring has proved effective in stabilizing the adult craniocervical junction.[121] Schultz et al.[122] advocated this technique in children older than 12 months, suggesting that the rigidity afforded by this method may eliminate the need for a halo. We have used this technique in children as young as 11 months with success.[123] Several authors also have used C1-C2 transarticular screws or C2 pedicle screws coupled with rigid loops and plate or rod constructs in pediatric patients with excellent success.[91,118,124] We have also used keel screws coupled with C1 lateral mass screws and C2 pars screws for occipitoatlantoaxial stabilization in young pediatric patients (Fig. 32.10).

ATLANTOAXIAL SURGICAL STABILIZATION

Traditionally, atlantoaxial fusion in the pediatric population was accomplished by posterior wiring using Sonntag and Gallie-type constructs.[125,126] Gluf and Brockmeyer[118] reported 67 pediatric patients who underwent C1-C2 transarticular screw fixation. Of these 67 patients, 65 developed successful fusion without application of a halo. Two unilateral vertebral artery injuries occurred without permanent neurologic deficit. One hardware failure occurred, attributed to a novel fixation device, and four infections developed. The authors successfully placed transarticular screws in 13 patients younger than 4 years old, the youngest being 18 months old. Brockmeyer[91] emphasized the importance of obtaining preoperative multiplanar reconstructions of thin-cut CT scans to determine the appropriate screw size, its entry point, and its trajectory. In a series of more than 50 patients who underwent C1-C2 transarticular fixation, growth was arrested at the fused atlantoaxial level and no craniovertebral deformities developed.

SUBAXIAL SURGICAL STABILIZATION

Increasingly, anterior and posterior subaxial instrumentation and techniques are used for pediatric applications. To date there has been little rigorous examination of the use of these techniques in children. Short stature and low-profile anterior plating systems have been placed in children as young as 3 years old.[91] Small vertebral bodies and cartilaginous endplates provide little margin for error when placing anterior screws in young children.[91] Shacked et al.[127] successfully used the anterior cervical approach for autograft arthrodesis of cervical segments in six pediatric trauma patients. No instrumentation was placed, but the patients underwent postoperative rigid immobilization in a halo or Minerva cast. Posterior instrumentation is also limited by the constraints of small anatomy.

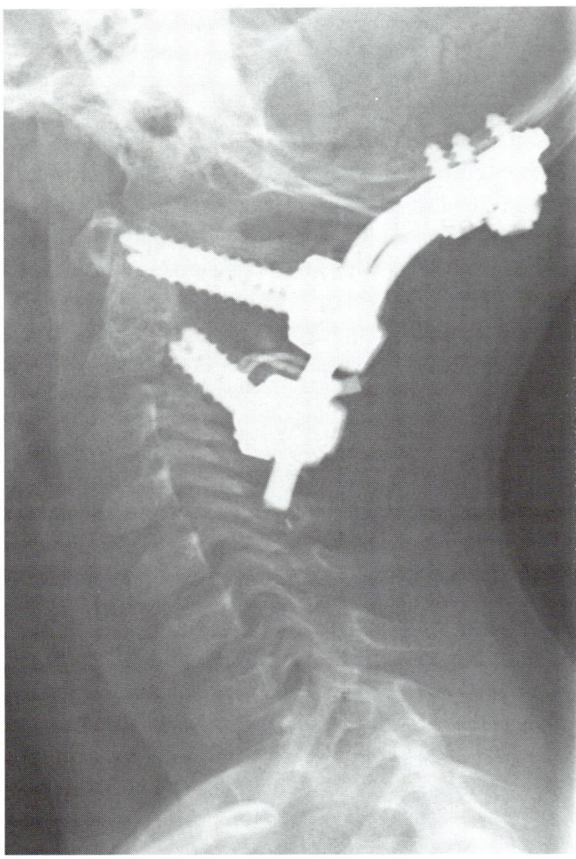

FIGURE 32.10. Postoperative lateral radiograph of a 3-year-old girl with both occipitoatlantal and atlantoaxial dislocation fixated via an occipital keel screw, C1 lateral mass screws, and C2 pars screws.

Brockmeyer[91] reported that pedicle or lateral mass screws can be placed in children as young as 4 years old. In very young patients, posterior bone and wiring techniques followed by immobilization may still represent the best treatment option.

BONE GRAFTS

Autograft has been shown to be superior to allograft for use in posterior cervical fusion constructs.[128,129] Much of this work predates the current era of rigid internal fixation. Composite bone grafts, consisting of demineralized bone matrix and aspirated bone marrow, may reduce morbidity and still maintain the rates of fusion associated with iliac crest autograft.[130] Options for autograft harvest in pediatric patients include the iliac crest, rib, and split- and full-thickness calvarial grafts. In young children, iliac crest harvest may not provide sufficient bone. Both iliac crest and rib harvest can cause severe postoperative pain, the latter potentially resulting in postoperative splinting. Chadduck and Boop[131] advocated rostral extension of the posterior midline cervical incision and harvest of parietal bone. The lambdoid suture may not be ossified and should not be incorporated in the graft.

TRACTION AND IMMOBILIZATION DEVICES

The use of traction in young children has not been well studied.[24] The thin calvarium in this population increases the risk for skull penetration with pin placement. Low body weight decreases resistance to traction, and lax ligaments and underdeveloped musculature increase the risk for overdistraction. Biparietal sets of burr holes with 22-gauge wire have been used to achieve skull purchase in infants.[132] For slightly older children, the use of a halo ring with 8 to 10 pins may be appropriate. Weight should be administered judiciously with frequent neurologic examinations and radiographic imaging.

Halo immobilization has been reported in children as young as 7 months, with 10 pins placed to finger-tightness only.[133] Children aged 16 and 24 months were also immobilized successfully in halos with 2 ft-lb of torque applied at each of 10 pins.[133] Minor complications such as pin-site infections are common.[134] Mandabach et al.[87] reported successful fusion of 8 of 10 odontoid epiphyseal fractures managed in a halo. This group recommends 1 ft-lb of torque per year of age until 5 ft-lb is reached. The thermoplastic Minerva body jacket is an alternative to halo immobilization in the very young. This device permits 2.1 degrees of flexion-extension compared to 1.3 degrees with a halo vest.[87] No pins are used and no artifact is created on MRI and CT scan.

CONCLUSION

Appropriate management of cervical spine trauma in children requires an understanding of the unique anatomic, biomechanic, radiographic, and pathophysiologic characteristics of pediatric patients. Almost all literature on this subject is Class III standard. There are many areas for further study, including the use of steroids in pediatric SCI, optimization of neck clearance in head-injured pediatric patients, and the appropriate management of SCIWORA. The relative rarity of pediatric cervical spine injuries demands multicenter involvement for well-designed studies.

REFERENCES

1. Patel JC, Tepas JJ III, Mollitt DL, et al. Pediatric cervical spine injuries: defining the disease. *J Pediatr Surg* 2001;36:373–376.
2. Taniguchi MH, Schlosser GA. Adolescent spinal cord injury: considerations for post-acute management. *Adolesc Med* 1994;5:327–344.
3. Vogel LC, Krajci KA, Anderson CJ. Adults with pediatric-onset spinal cord injury: part 1: prevalence of medical complications. *J Spinal Cord Med* 2002;25:106–116.
4. Vogel LC, Krajci KA, Anderson CJ. Adults with pediatric-onset spinal cord injury: part 2: musculoskeletal and neurological complications. *J Spinal Cord Med* 2002;25:117-123.
5. Vogel LC, Krajci KA, Anderson CJ. Adults with pediatric-onset spinal cord injuries: part 3: impact of medical complications. *J Spinal Cord Med* 2002;25:297–305.
6. Eleraky MA, Theodore N, Adams M, et al. Pediatric cervical spine injuries: report of 102 cases and review of the literature. *J Neurosurg* 2000;92:12–17.
7. Brown RL, Brunn MA, Garcia VF. Cervical spine injuries in children: a review of 103 patients treated consecutively at a level 1 pediatric trauma center. *J Pediatr Surg* 2001;36:1107–1114.
8. Kokoska ER, Keller MS, Rallo MC, et al. Characteristics of pediatric cervical spine injuries. *J Pediatr Surg* 2001;36:100–105.
9. Cirak B, Ziegfeld S, Knight VM, et al. Spinal injuries in children. *J Pediatr Surg* 2004;39:607–612.
10. Bullough PG, Boachie-Adjei O. *Atlas of Spinal Diseases*. New York: Lippincott; 1988.
11. Grabb PA, Hadley MN. Spinal column trauma in children. In Albright AL, Pollack IF, Adelson PD (Eds). *Principles and Practice of Pediatric Neurosurgery*. New York: Thieme; 1999, 935–953.
12. Wang JC, Nuccion SL, Feighan JE, et al. Growth and development of the pediatric cervical spine documented radiographically. *J Bone Surg Am* 2001;83-A:1212–1218.
13. Fesmire FM, Luten RC. The pediatric cervical spine: developmental anatomy and clinical aspects. *J Emerg Med* 1989;7:133–142.
14. Ogden JA. Radiology of postnatal skeletal development. XII. The second cervical vertebra. *Skeletal Radiol* 1984;12:169–177.
15. Liang CL, Lui CC, Lu K, et al. Atlantoaxial stability in ossiculum terminale. Case report. *J Neurosurg* 2001;95:119–121.
16. White AA, Panjabi MM. *Clinical Biomechanics of the Spine*. Philadelphia: JB Lippincott; 1990.
17. Locke GR, Gardner JI, Van Epps EF. Atlas-dens interval (ADI) in children: a survey based on 200 normal cervical spines. *Am J Roentgenol Radium Ther Nucl Med* 1966;97:135–140.
18. Cattell HS, Filtzer DL. Pseudosubluxation and other normal variations in the cervical spine in children. A study of one hundred and sixty children. *J Bone Joint Surg Am* 1965;47:1295–1309.

19. Spence KF Jr, Decker S, Sell KW. Bursting atlantal fracture associated with rupture of the transverse ligament. *J Bone Joint Surg Am* 1970;52:543–549.
20. Dickman CA, Greene KA, Sonntag VK. Injuries involving the transverse atlantal ligament: classification and treatment guidelines based upon experience with 39 injuries. *Neurosurgery* 1996;38:44–50.
21. Suss RA, Zimmerman RD, Leeds NE. Pseudospread of the atlas: false sign of Jefferson fracture in young children. *AJR Am J Roentgenol* 1983;140:1079–1082.
22. Lustrin ES, Karakas SP, Ortiz AO, et al. Pediatric cervical spine: normal anatomy, variants, and trauma. *Radiographics* 2003;23:539–560.
23. Shaw M, Burnett H, Wilson A, et al. Pseudosubluxation of C2 on C3 in polytraumatized children—prevalence and significance. *Clin Radiol* 54:377-380, 1999.
24. Management of pediatric cervical spine and spinal cord injuries. *Neurosurgery* 2002;50:S85–S99.
25. Swischuk LE. Anterior displacement of C2 in children: physiologic or pathologic. *Radiology* 1977;122:759–763.
26. Pang D, Sun PP. Pediatric vertebral column and spinal cord injuries. In Winn HR (Ed). *Neurological Surgery.* Philadelphia: WB Saunders; 2004, 3515–3557.
27. Ware ML, Gupta N, Sun PP, et al. Clinical biomechanics of the pediatric craniocervical junction and the subaxial spine. In Brockmeyer DL (Ed). *Advanced Pediatric Craniocervical Surgery.* New York: Thieme; 2006, 27–42.
28. Sherburn EW, Day RA, Kaufman BA, et al. Subdental synchondrosis fracture in children: the value of 3-dimensional computerized tomography. *Pediatr Neurosurg* 1996;25:256–259.
29. Schippers N, Konings P, Hassler W, et al. Typical and atypical fractures of the odontoid process in young children. Report of two cases and a review of the literature. *Acta Neurochir (Wien)* 1996;138:524–530.
30. Blauth M, Schmidt U, Otte D, et al. Fractures of the odontoid process in small children: biomechanical analysis and report of three cases. *Eur Spine J* 1996;5:63–70.
31. Connolly B, Emery D, Armstrong D. The odontoid synchondrotic slip: an injury unique to young children. *Pediatr Radiol* 1995;25(Suppl 1):S129–S133.
32. Judd DB, Liem LK, Petermann G. Pediatric atlas fracture: a case of fracture through a synchondrosis and review of the literature. *Neurosurgery* 2000;46:991–994.
33. Swischuk LE, Swischuk PN, John SD. Wedging of C-3 in infants and children: usually a normal finding and not a fracture. *Radiology* 1993;188:523–526.
34. Englander O. Nontraumatic occipito-atlanto-axial dislocation: a contribution to the radiology of the atlas. *Br J Radiology* 1942;15:341–345.
35. Townsend EH Jr, Rowe ML. Mobility of the upper cervical spine in health and disease. *Pediatrics* 1952;10:567–574.
36. Kalfas I, Wilberger J, Goldberg A, et al. Magnetic resonance imaging in acute spinal cord trauma. *Neurosurgery* 1988;23:295–299.
37. Bohn D, Armstrong D, Becker L, et al. Cervical spine injuries in children. *J Trauma* 1990;30:463–469.
38. Treloar DJ, Nypaver M. Angulation of the pediatric cervical spine with and without cervical collar. *Pediatr Emerg Care* 1997;13:5–8.
39. Curran C, Dietrich AM, Bowman MJ, et al. Pediatric cervical-spine immobilization: achieving neutral position? *J Trauma* 1995;39:729–732.
40. Herzenberg JE, Hensinger RN, Dedrick DK, et al. Emergency transport and positioning of young children who have an injury of the cervical spine. The standard backboard may be hazardous. *J Bone Joint Surg Am* 1989;71:15–22.
41. Nypaver M, Treloar D. Neutral cervical spine positioning in children. *Ann Emerg Med* 1994;23:208–211.
42. Huerta C, Griffith R, Joyce SM. Cervical spine stabilization in pediatric patients: evaluation of current techniques. *Ann Emerg Med* 1987;16:1121–1126.
43. Dickman CA, Papadopoulos SM, Sonntag VK, et al. Traumatic occipitoatlantal dislocations. *J Spinal Disord* 1993;6:300–313.
44. Laham JL, Cotcamp DH, Gibbons PA, et al. Isolated head injuries versus multiple trauma in pediatric patients: do the same indications for cervical spine evaluation apply? *Pediatr Neurosurg* 1994;21:221–226.
45. Viccellio P, Simon H, Pressman BD, et al. A prospective multicenter study of cervical spine injury in children. *Pediatrics* 2001;108:E20.
46. Swischuk LE, John SD, Hendrick EP. Is the open-mouth odontoid view necessary in children under 5 years? *Pediatr Radiol* 2000;30:186–189.
47. Buhs C, Cullen M, Klein M, et al. The pediatric trauma C-spine: is the 'odontoid' view necessary? *J Pediatr Surg* 2000;35:994–997.
48. Griffen MM, Frykberg ER, Kerwin AJ, et al. Radiographic clearance of blunt cervical spine injury: plain radiograph or computed tomography scan? *J Trauma* 2003;55:222–226.
49. Widder S, Doig C, Burrowes P, et al. Prospective evaluation of computed tomographic scanning for the spinal clearance of obtunded trauma patients: preliminary results. *J Trauma* 2004;56:1179–1184.
50. Brohi K, Healy M, Fotheringham T, et al. Helical computed tomographic scanning for the evaluation of the cervical spine in the unconscious, intubated trauma patient. *J Trauma* 2005;58:897–901.

51. Schenarts PJ, Diaz J, Kaiser C, et al. Prospective comparison of admission computed tomographic scan and plain films of the upper cervical spine in trauma patients with altered mental status. *J Trauma* 2001;51:663–668.
52. Sanchez B, Waxman K, Jones T, et al. Cervical spine clearance in blunt trauma: evaluation of a computed tomography-based protocol. *J Trauma* 2005;59:179–183.
53. Slack SE, Clancy MJ: Clearing the cervical spine of paediatric trauma patients. *Emerg Med J* 2004;21:189–193.
54. Avellino AM, Mann FA, Grady MS, et al. The misdiagnosis of acute cervical spine injuries and fractures in infants and children: the 12-year experience of a level I pediatric and adult trauma center. *Childs Nerv Syst* 2005;21:122–127.
55. Flynn JM, Closkey RF, Mahboubi S, et al. Role of magnetic resonance imaging in the assessment of pediatric cervical spine injuries. *J Pediatr Orthop* 2002;22:573–577.
56. Frank JB, Lim CK, Flynn JM, et al. The efficacy of magnetic resonance imaging in pediatric cervical spine clearance. *Spine* 2002;27:1176–1179.
57. Keiper MD, Zimmerman RA, Bilaniuk LT. MRI in the assessment of the supportive soft tissues of the cervical spine in acute trauma in children. *Neuroradiology* 1998;40:359–363.
58. Grabb PA, Pang D. Magnetic resonance imaging in the evaluation of spinal cord injury without radiographic abnormality in children. *Neurosurgery* 1994;35:406–414.
59. Dare AO, Dias MS, Li V. Magnetic resonance imaging correlation in pediatric spinal cord injury without radiographic abnormality. *J Neurosurg* 2002;97:33–39.
60. Horn EM, Lekovic GP, Feiz-Erfan I, et al. Cervical magnetic resonance imaging abnormalities not predictive of cervical spine instability in traumatically injured patients. Invited submission from the Joint Section Meeting on Disorders of the Spine and Peripheral Nerves, March 2004. *J Neurosurg Spine* 2004;1:39–42.
61. Dwek JR, Chung CB. Radiography of cervical spine injury in children: are flexion-extension radiographs useful for acute trauma? *AJR Am J Roentgenol* 2000;174:1617–1619.
62. Ralston ME, Chung K, Barnes PD, et al. Role of flexion-extension radiographs in blunt pediatric cervical spine injury. *Acad Emerg Med* 2001;8:237–245.
63. Woods WA, Brady WJ, Pollock G, et al. Flexion-extension cervical spine radiography in pediatric blunt trauma. *Emerg Radiol* 1998;5:381–384.
64. Crisco JJ III, Oda T, Panjabi MM, et al. Transections of the C1-C2 joint capsular ligaments in the cadaveric spine. *Spine* 1991;16:S474–S479.
65. Werne S. Studies in spontaneous atlas dislocation. *Acta Orthop Scand Suppl* 1957;23:1–150.
66. Harris MB, Duval MJ, Davis JA Jr, et al. Anatomical and roentgenographic features of atlantooccipital instability. *J Spinal Disord* 1993;6:5–10.
67. Dvorak J, Schneider E, Saldinger P, et al. Biomechanics of the craniocervical region: the alar and transverse ligaments. *J Orthop Res* 1988;6:452–461.
68. Panjabi M, Dvorak J, Crisco J III, et al. Flexion, extension, and lateral bending of the upper cervical spine in response to alar ligament transections. *J Spinal Disord* 1991;4:157–167.
69. Marshall KW, Koch BL, Egelhoff JC. Air bag-related deaths and serious injuries in children: injury patterns and imaging findings. *AJNR Am J Neuroradiol* 1998;19:1599–1607.
70. Sun PP, Poffenbarger GJ, Durham S, et al. Spectrum of occipitoatlantoaxial injury in young children. *J Neurosurg* 2000;93:28–39.
71. Dziurzynski K, Anderson PA, Bean DB, et al. A blinded assessment of radiographic criteria for atlanto-occipital dislocation. *Spine* 2005;30:1427–1432.
72. Harris JH Jr, Carson GC, Wagner LK. Radiologic diagnosis of traumatic occipitovertebral dissociation: 1. Normal occipitovertebral relationships on lateral radiographs of supine subjects. *AJR Am J Roentgenol* 1994;162:881–886.
73. Harris JH Jr, Carson GC, Wagner LK, et al. Radiologic diagnosis of traumatic occipitovertebral dissociation: 2. Comparison of three methods of detecting occipitovertebral relationships on lateral radiographs of supine subjects. *AJR Am J Roentgenol* 1994;162:887–892.
74. Lee C, Woodring JH, Goldstein SJ, et al. Evaluation of traumatic atlantooccipital dislocations. *AJNR Am J Neuroradiol* 1987;8:19–26.
75. Diagnosis and management of traumatic atlanto-occipital dislocation injuries. *Neurosurgery* 2002;50: S105–S113.
76. Pang D, Nemzek WR, Zovickian J. Atlanto-occipital dislocation—part 2: The clinical use of (occipital) condyle-C1 interval, comparison with other diagnostic methods, and the manifestation, management, and outcome of atlanto-occipital dislocation in children. *Neurosurgery* 2007;61:995–1015.
77. Horn EM, Feiz-Erfan I, Lekovic GP, et al. Survivors of occipitoatlantal dislocation injuries: imaging and clinical correlates. *J Neurosurg Spine* 2007;6:113–120.
78. Pang D, Nemzek WR, Zovickian J. Atlanto-occipital dislocation: part 1—normal occipital condyle-C1 interval in 89 children. *Neurosurgery* 2007;61:514–521.
79. Gonzalez LF, Fiorella D, Crawford NR, et al. Vertical atlantoaxial distraction injuries: radiological criteria and clinical implications. *J Neurosurg Spine* 2004;1:273–280.

80. Fielding JW, Hawkins RJ. Atlanto-axial rotatory fixation. (Fixed rotatory subluxation of the atlanto-axial joint.) *J Bone Joint Surg Am* 1977;59:37–44.
81. Pang D, Li V. Atlantoaxial rotatory fixation: part 1—biomechanics of normal rotation at the atlantoaxial joint in children. *Neurosurgery* 2004;55:614–625.
82. Subach BR, McLaughlin MR, Albright AL, et al. Current management of pediatric atlantoaxial rotatory subluxation. *Spine* 1998;23:2174–2179.
83. Rinaldi I, Mullins WJ Jr, Delaney WF, et al. Computerized tomographic demonstration of rotational atlanto-axial fixation. Case report. *J Neurosurg* 1979;50:115–119.
84. Alanay A, Hicazi A, Acaroglu E, et al. Reliability and necessity of dynamic computerized tomography in diagnosis of atlantoaxial rotatory subluxation. *J Pediatr Orthop* 2002;22:763–765.
85. Pang D, Li V. Atlantoaxial rotatory fixation: part 2—new diagnostic paradigm and a new classification based on motion analysis using computed tomographic imaging. *Neurosurgery* 2005;57:941–953.
86. Pang D, Li V. Atlantoaxial rotatory fixation: part 3—a prospective study of the clinical manifestation, diagnosis, management, and outcome of children with alantoaxial rotatory fixation. *Neurosurgery* 2005;57:954–972.
87. Mandabach M, Ruge JR, Hahn YS, et al. Pediatric axis fractures: early halo immobilization, management and outcome. *Pediatr Neurosurg* 1993;19:225–232.
88. Odent T, Langlais J, Glorion C, et al. Fractures of the odontoid process: a report of 15 cases in children younger than 6 years. *J Pediatr Orthop* 1999;19:51–54.
89. Sherk HH, Nicholson JT, Chung SM. Fractures of the odontoid process in young children. *J Bone Joint Surg Am* 1978;60:921–924.
90. White AA III, Panjabi MM. The basic kinematics of the human spine. A review of past and current knowledge. *Spine* 1978;3:12–20.
91. Brockmeyer DL. Advanced atlantoaxial surgery in children. In Brockmeyer DL (Ed). *Advanced Pediatric Craniocervical Surgery.* New York: Thieme; 2006, 75–92.
92. Pennecot GF, Leonard P, Peyrot Des GS, et al. Traumatic ligamentous instability of the cervical spine in children. *J Pediatr Orthop* 1984;4:339–345.
93. Pang D, Wilberger JE Jr. Spinal cord injury without radiographic abnormalities in children. *J Neurosurg* 1982;57:114–129.
94. Pang D. Spinal cord injury without radiographic abnormality in children, 2 decades later. *Neurosurgery* 2004;55:1325–1342.
95. Pang D, Pollack IF. Spinal cord injury without radiographic abnormality in children—the SCIWORA syndrome. *J Trauma* 1989;29:654–664.
96. Dickman CA, Zabramski JM, Hadley MN, et al. Pediatric spinal cord injury without radiographic abnormalities: report of 26 cases and review of the literature. *J Spinal Disord* 1991;4:296–305.
97. Osenbach RK, Menezes AH. Spinal cord injury without radiographic abnormality in children. *Pediatr Neurosci* 1989;15:168–174.
98. Hamilton MG, Myles ST. Pediatric spinal injury: review of 174 hospital admissions. *J Neurosurg* 1992;77:700–704.
99. Pollack IF, Pang D, Sclabassi R. Recurrent spinal cord injury without radiographic abnormalities in children. *J Neurosurg* 1988;69:177–182.
100. Spinal cord injury without radiographic abnormality. *Neurosurgery* 2002;50:S100–S104.
101. Bosch PP, Vogt MT, Ward WT. Pediatric spinal cord injury without radiographic abnormality (SCIWORA): the absence of occult instability and lack of indication for bracing. *Spine* 2002;27:2788–2800.
102. Torg JS, Corcoran TA, Thibault LE, et al. Cervical cord neurapraxia: classification, pathomechanics, morbidity, and management guidelines. *J Neurosurg* 1997;87:843–850.
103. Torg JS, Pavlov H, Genuario SE, et al. Neurapraxia of the cervical spinal cord with transient quadriplegia. *J Bone Joint Surg Am* 1986;68:1354–1370.
104. Castro FP Jr. Stingers, cervical cord neurapraxia, and stenosis. *Clin Sports Med* 2003;22:483–492.
105. Boockvar JA, Durham SR, Sun PP. Cervical spinal stenosis and sports-related cervical cord neurapraxia in children. *Spine* 2001;26:2709–2712.
106. Vogel LC. Unique management needs of pediatric spinal cord injury patients: etiology and pathophysiology. *J Spinal Cord Med* 1997;20:10–13.
107. MacKinnon JA, Perlman M, Kirpalani H, et al. Spinal cord injury at birth: diagnostic and prognostic data in twenty-two patients. *J Pediatr* 1993;122:431–437.
108. Menticoglou SM, Perlman M, Manning FA. High cervical spinal cord injury in neonates delivered with forceps: report of 15 cases. *Obstet Gynecol* 1995;86:589–594.
109. Verska JM, Anderson PA. Os odontoideum. A case report of one identical twin. *Spine* 1997;22:706–709.
110. Currarino G. Segmentation defect in the midodontoid process and its possible relationship to the congenital type of os odontoideum. *Pediatr Radiol* 2002;32:34–40.
111. Os odontoideum. *Neurosurgery* 2002;50:S148–S155.

112. Spierings EL, Braakman R. The management of os odontoideum. Analysis of 37 cases. *J Bone Joint Surg Br* 1982;64:422–428.
113. Watanabe M, Toyama Y, Fujimura Y. Atlantoaxial instability in os odontoideum with myelopathy. *Spine* 1996; 21:1435–1439.
114. Shirasaki N, Okada K, Oka S, et al. Os odontoideum with posterior atlantoaxial instability. *Spine* 1991;16: 706–715.
115. Choit RL, Jamieson DH, Reilly CW. Os odontoideum: a significant radiographic finding. *Pediatr Radiol* 2005;35:803–807.
116. Hadley MN, Zabramski JM, Browner CM, et al. Pediatric spinal trauma. Review of 122 cases of spinal cord and vertebral column injuries. *J Neurosurg* 1988;68:18–24.
117. Brockmeyer D, Apfelbaum R, Tippets R, et al. Pediatric cervical spine instrumentation using screw fixation. *Pediatr Neurosurg* 1995;22:147–157.
118. Gluf WM, Brockmeyer DL. Atlantoaxial transarticular screw fixation: a review of surgical indications, fusion rate, complications, and lessons learned in 67 pediatric patients. *J Neurosurg Spine* 2005;2:164–169.
119. Rockswold GL, Bergman TA, Ford SE. Halo immobilization and surgical fusion: relative indications and effectiveness in the treatment of 140 cervical spine injuries. *J Trauma* 1990;30:893–898.
120. Smith MD, Phillips WA, Hensinger RN. Fusion of the upper cervical spine in children and adolescents. An analysis of 17 patients. *Spine* 1991;16:695–701.
121. Apostolides PJ, Dickman CA, Golfinos JG, et al. Threaded Steinmann pin fusion of the craniovertebral junction. *Spine* 1996;21:1630–1637.
122. Schultz KD Jr, Petronio J, Haid RW, et al. Pediatric occipitocervical arthrodesis. A review of current options and early evaluation of rigid internal fixation techniques. *Pediatr Neurosurg* 2000;33:169–181.
123. Rekate HL, Theodore N, Sonntag VK, et al. Pediatric spine and spinal cord trauma. State of the art for the third millennium. *Childs Nerv Syst* 1999;15:743–750.
124. Pait TG, Al Mefty O, Boop FA, et al. Inside-outside technique for posterior occipitocervical spine instrumentation and stabilization: preliminary results. *J Neurosurg* 1999;90:1–7.
125. Dickman CA, Sonntag VK, Papadopoulos SM, et al. The interspinous method of posterior atlantoaxial arthrodesis. *J Neurosurg* 1991;74:190–198.
126. Parisini P, Di Silvestre M, Greggi T, et al. C1-C2 posterior fusion in growing patients: long-term follow-up. *Spine* 2003;28:566–572.
127. Shacked I, Ram Z, Hadani M. The anterior cervical approach for traumatic injuries to the cervical spine in children. *Clin Orthop Relat Res* 1993;292:144–150.
128. Koop SE, Winter RB, Lonstein JE. The surgical treatment of instability of the upper part of the cervical spine in children and adolescents. *J Bone Joint Surg Am* 1984;66:403–411.
129. Stabler CL, Eismont FJ, Brown MD, et al. Failure of posterior cervical fusions using cadaveric bone graft in children. *J Bone Joint Surg Am* 1985;67:371–375.
130. Price CT, Connolly JF, Carantzas AC, et al. Comparison of bone grafts for posterior spinal fusion in adolescent idiopathic scoliosis. *Spine* 2003;28:793–798.
131. Chadduck WM, Boop FA. Use of full-thickness calvarial bone grafts for cervical spinal fusions in pediatric patients. *Pediatr Neurosurg* 1994;20:107–112.
132. Gaufin LM, Goodman SJ. Cervical spine injuries in infants. Problems in management. *J Neurosurg* 1975;42:179–184.
133. Mubarak SJ, Camp JF, Vuletich W, et al. Halo application in the infant. *J Pediatr Orthop* 1989;9:612–614.
134. Dormans JP, Criscitiello AA, Drummond DS, et al. Complications in children managed with immobilization in a halo vest. *J Bone Joint Surg Am* 1995;77:1370–1373.

SECTION XI

Complication Awareness and Management

CHAPTER 33

Management of Posttraumatic Cerebrospinal Fluid Leakage

John Heller and Jason E. Lowenstein

INTRODUCTION

Dural tears are a well-recognized consequence of spinal trauma. Although tears associated with thoracolumbar fractures and dislocations are well documented in the literature, little has been written regarding these issues in the cervical spine. The purpose of this chapter is to discuss the evaluation and management of dural tears associated with either blunt or penetrating cervical spine trauma.

Blunt spinal trauma can result in a spectrum of injuries, ranging from simple muscular strains to comminuted fracture-dislocations with significant displacement and neurologic injury. A dural defect may be an associated injury and present an additional challenge to successful treatment. Persistent cerebrospinal fluid (CSF) leakage may result in several long-term sequelae, including psuedomeningocele, arachnoiditis, subarachnoid-cutaneous fistula, meningitis, and further neurologic dysfunction.[1,2]

Penetrating trauma to the cervical region may also be a source of dural injury. The possibility might be reasonably considered in the face of gunshot wounds or stabbings that have involved the cervical spine, particularly in the presence of a neurologic deficit. More so than with blunt trauma, it seems reasonable to presume the presence of a dural laceration when a stab wound has caused a spinal cord injury. Similarly, bullets may be presumed to have disrupted the meninges under various circumstances. This would be a virtual certainty if a bullet has traversed the spinal canal. Imaging studies that suggest such a path of the projectile, or those demonstrating bullet fragments or shards of bone within the spinal canal, are obvious evidence of dural disruption. What to do or whether to do anything for these patients must be factored into their treatment recommendations. Thankfully, in the case of penetrating trauma to the cervical spine, surgical treatment is not often required and these presumed defects seal themselves.

In the case of blunt trauma to the thoracolumbar spine, there is a body of evidence that dural tears are generally correlated with higher energy injuries and coupled with neurologic deficits. Cammisa et al.[3] retrospectively reviewed 60 patients with thoracic or lumbar burst fractures and found that there was a significant association between dural laceration and neurologic compromise, with 100% of patients with a neurologic deficit having a dural tear. Pickett and Blumenkopf[4] also reported on their experience with treatment of thoracolumbar fractures. They found a significant association between a severe neurologic deficit and the presence of a dural laceration. They commented that dural tears were commonly found in patients who required operative intervention in their spinal fracture. Aydinli et al.[5] reviewed their experience with lumbar trauma and associated dural injury. They evaluated 45 patients with greenstick laminar fractures and found that although the majority of dural ruptures were found in patients with neurologic compromise, three neurologically intact patients were found to have dural tears at the time of surgery. Therefore, in the setting of thoracolumbar trauma, the presence of a neurologic deficit implies the possibility of a dural rupture or laceration. This is particularly likely in the presence of marked disruption of the vertebral column, especially splaying of laminar fracture fragments. In the absence of a body of literature devoted to the cervical spine, experience and logic suggest that these lessons must be reasonably translated to the cervical spine. The consulting surgeon must keep this in mind when planning treatment, be it open or closed.

The presence of a dural tear may be difficult, if not impossible, to determine by clinical examination or radiographic studies. Classically, the symptoms of CSF leaks include postural headaches, nausea, vomiting, dizziness, photophobia, tinnitus, and vertigo.[6] These symptoms are presumed to be due to changes in intrathecal pressure and resultant strain on the supporting structures of the central nervous system.[7] However, in the setting of cervical spinal trauma, sorting out such symptoms may be difficult, if not impossible. First, concomitant injury to the head and neck may mask such symptoms. Most of these classic symptoms are position dependent, and the fact that patients with cervical spine injuries are kept supine and immobilized if not in traction will further cloud the ability to recognize any CSF leak symptoms. To further confuse the issue, these symptoms may be absent, even in the presence of a dural tear. Therefore, although these symptoms could theoretically alert the physician to a possible dural injury, it is more likely that information regarding the victim's neurologic status and the kinetic force of the cervical injury (e.g., high-energy motor vehicle collision versus a low-energy fall) combined with appropriate imaging studies may help suggest the presence of a tear.

Imaging modalities may offer some information regarding possible dural injury. Pickett and Blumenkopf[4] retrospectively reviewed the computed tomography (CT) scans and intraoperative data concerning 25 patients with thoracolumbar burst fractures. They found that although there was no relationship between the degree of canal compromise and risk for dural injury, there was a significant relationship between fracture of the posterior elements and dural tears. It is likely that injury to the dura occurs at the time of force impact, at which time there may frequently be disruption of the posterior elements. Posterior surgical exploration often reveals either a vertical split of the dura, as if split by tensile forces at impact, or tearing or shredding of the nerve root sleeve. Less commonly there is a puncture of the dura from a displaced fracture fragment. Finally, there may be evidence of CSF leakage as a result of a tear that is not within the field of exposure, that is, an anterior tear when opening the canal from a posterior approach or vice versa. Alternatively, one could theorize that the dura may become entrapped in a widening laminar fracture at the moment of displacement, which then results in laceration as the fracture site recoils to a closed position, as implied by Pickett and Blumenkopf.[4] However, it seems more likely that the same bursting mechanism that creates the posterior element fractures ruptures the dura as the fracture happens, thus rendering the neural elements vulnerable to entrapment.

Dural laceration caused by anterior bone fragments retropulsed into the canal has been described as well. Carl et al.[8] retrospectively reviewed 60 patients with thoracolumbar burst fractures treated with anterior approaches. They observed that 10% of their patients had traumatic dural tears when explored surgically. The degree of canal compromise measured by CT scan ranged from 50% to 95% and was not reported to be correlated with dural tear incidence. However, in each case, asymmetry of the fracture fragments and sharp fragment edges were found, which they believed to be the cause of the lacerations. Fortunately, anterior dural tears associated with burst fractures are rather uncommon, despite the degree of fracture displacement.

These reports offer observations and concepts that may be useful in the evaluation and treatment of cervical spine fractures. The presence of marked posterior element disruption, certainly when associated with a neurologic injury, should alert the treating physician that an underlying dural injury may be coupled with the cervical spine fracture. And although severity of canal compromise may not be correlated with the presence of a dural laceration, the surgeon preparing to operate on such injuries must be cognizant of the relationship between displaced bone fragments and the possibility of dural defects. Whereas not all retropulsed fragments cause ventral tears, scans that reveal asymmetric and sharp fragments within the canal may be associated with some probability of dural injury. Perhaps even more probable is the likelihood of dural lacerations in the presence of sharp posterior element fragments displaced into the dorsal aspect of the canal. Under such circumstances the authors have encountered not only dural lacerations but shredded or amputated nerve root sleeves with CSF leaks.

The management of a traumatic dural defect in the cervical spine is largely determined by the severity of the injury and the need for operative treatment of the spinal injury. Stable cervical spine fractures that can otherwise be treated nonoperatively that are found to have concomitant dural tears diagnosed either by physical examination or imaging studies may benefit from closed treatment of the CSF leak. Carlson et al.[9] studied the effect of position on CSF pressure using a canine model. Measuring subarachnoid pressure at C3 and L4, they found that as body inclination increased from 0 to 90 degrees, cervical CSF pressure significantly decreased (from 10.0 to 7.1 cm H_2O). Conversely, lumbar CSF pressure increased significantly with inclination (from 8.8 to 18.4). Lumbar durotomy was performed to simulate lumbar subarachnoid drainage. This provided for an additional 23% decrease in cervical CSF pressure at 90 degrees, with a combined 46% decrease in pressure from baseline (from 10.0 to 5.4).[9] Whereas lumbar dural tears are associated with increased hydrostatic pressure at the bottom of the water column and persistent leakage of CSF, cervical tears that occur at the top of the column are subjected to decreased pressure at the point of rupture when the head is elevated. As a result, small cervical tears may have greater potential to heal closed than those occurring within the lumbar spine.[7] Simply positioning the patient with the head of the bed elevated may reduce the intradural pressure and contribute to healing of the tear.

Dural healing is a complex process, beginning with acute inflammation and proceeding though fibroblastic bridging and remodeling of the dural defect. Cain et al.[10] observed the histopathologic events associated with dural repair in the canine model. Primary dural healing was found to be slow, with fibrous bridging of the durotomy detected on postoperative day 6, and closure of the defect occurring on postoperative day 10. Internal sealing of the durotomy was found to occur though adherence of the pia and arachnoid meninges to the tear, which was found to be present by postoperative day 2. In 59 of 63 durotomies occurring at the spinal cord level, meningeal adhesions to the dural defect were found. In contrast, 9 of 23 durotomies at the cauda equina had similar adhesions. Pressurization testing at postoperative days 2 and 4 revealed significant increase in bursting pressure in durotomies performed at the spinal cord level when compared to the cauda equina level. This was attributed to the increased meningeal "plugging" effect at the cord level,[10] which might explain the lower likelihood of clinically apparent CSF leaks in cervical trauma, as well as the paucity of literature on the topic.

A lumbar subarachnoid drain may be inserted to decrease the hydrostatic pressure at the point of CSF leakage. Lumbar drains provide a path of lesser resistance by allowing for shunting of CSF away from the tear, providing an improved opportunity for meningeal healing. An intradural catheter is placed percutaneously under sterile conditions. CSF is then drained at a continuous rate (approximately 10 mL/hr), matching the CSF production of the choroid plexus. The major risk associated with in-dwelling CSF drains is meningitis. Most often the patient is administered prophylactic antibiotics during the period of drain use. The antibiotics selected should have reliable blood–brain barrier penetration. Symptoms or signs suggestive of meningitis should be regularly sought and taken seriously if present. They are a call to immediate action. A CSF sample should be sent for emergent analysis, including cell count, differential, Gram stain, culture, and glucose and protein levels. Consideration might be given to adjusting the antibiotic coverage pending the results of the evaluation. Eismont et al.[11] recommended removal of the catheter in the face of a significant rise in CSF white blood cell count. Though not completely benign, the advantage of CSF diversion with a lumbar drain is that it may allow for the avoidance of a general anesthetic and an open surgical repair of the dura, when surgery is not otherwise indicated by the cervical injury, such as for a persistent CSF leak with penetrating trauma.

When a cervical spine injury requires operative intervention, accessible dural injuries warrant repair. Direct dural approximation and primary suture repair is the strategy of first choice. Various techniques can be employed, but most commonly a nonabsorbable suture (from 5-0 to 8-0) is recommended. A simple running or locked running suture technique is most often employed. Other circumstances may call for an interrupted suture technique.[11] The suturing technique will need to be tailored to the size, shape, and location of the tear(s). Alternatively, dural staples may be used. Although quick and easy to place, they require removal once the tear has healed.[7] Thus, we do not favor this option.

In the lumbar spine, the cauda equina elements are often herniated through the dural defects, especially when the canal is first opened and the fracture fragments are still displaced. The neural elements must be reduced inside the thecal sac before closure, which typically follows satisfactory fracture fragment reduction or removal. This is often achieved with a small patty placement over the involved roots at the margin of the tear, with closure over the patty and its distal migration as the repair continues. Patty migration continues simultaneously with the repair until it can safely be removed without reherniation of the cauda equina. Cervical spine defects are less often associated with nerve root evagination because of the direct lateral root take-off and decreased root excursion at this level of the spine. As a result, root herniation is less often a problem, but certain laterally placed durotomies may be associated with this issue, and techniques of closure as in the lumbar repair may be used. Ideally a tension-free repair is obtained to allow for optimal healing while preventing iatrogenic stenosis at the level of the repair. Once completed, the repair can be tested using a Valsalva maneuver. Once the surgical site is meticulously dried, the anesthesiologist can provide a Valsalva of approximately 30 to 40 mm Hg. The repair is carefully checked for any sign of CSF leakage. Persistent leakage suggests further suturing or other adjunctive measures may be necessary, whereas a clean and dry field indicates an acceptable dural repair.

Suture repairs are commonly supplemented with a fibrin adhesive sealant, also known as fibrin glue. This glue was originally made from a mixture of cryoprecipitate and thrombin solution.[11] Once coagulated, the clot acts as a tissue sealant, impeding extravasation of CSF at the site of the tear. Cain et al.[1] performed a study to compare both cadaveric and in vitro rabbit dural repair using suture, fibrin glue, or a combination of the two. They found that fibrin glue supplementation of a running locked stitch resulted in a significantly increased failure pressure of 90.5 mm Hg compared to a running locked stitch alone, which failed at 13.6 mm Hg, and the combined glue and suture was superior to glue alone, which failed at 80.0 mm Hg. Cain et al.[1] also investigated the use of cyanoacrylate, or Krazy Glue, a polymer that provided for superior failure pressures (up to 290 mm Hg combined with suture repair), but because of its neurotoxic effects, it is not recommended for clinical use. Fibrin adhesive sealant allows for an immediate seal over a dural defect. It results in a minimal inflammatory host response, and reabsorbs during the healing phase. The major risk associated with its use is possible viral transmission associated with its use of an allograft cryoprecipitate, although to date, no cases have been reported.[7] It greatly improves the initial failure pressure compared to suture alone and may provide for superior clinical healing rate. Campbell et al.[12] evaluated the sealing properties of three commercially available fibrin adhesives, DuraSeal, CoSeal, and HemaSeel fibrin sealant. Preparation time, mechanical strength, water uptake, and burst pressure strength were tested. Evaluation was performed immediately after preparation, and at 1, 2, and 3 days after soaking in 37° phosphate buffered saline to simulate a physiologic environment. DuraSeal was found to have the fastest preparation time (1.0 minute) and averaged 5 times stronger than CoSeal and 3 times stronger than HemaSeel comparing energy to failure in a physiologic environment at 1, 2, and 3 days. CoSeal showed the greatest water uptake, with a 558% gain in weight at 3 days, compared to 98% increased for DuraSeal and 3% for HemaSeel. Theoretically, this water uptake could lead to a compression of adjacent neural tissue and potentially result in neurologic compromise, especially in the less forgiving cervical spine, and care should be taken to apply only the amount required to cover the tear.[12]

Patch grafts may be used in the case of an irreparable dural tear. Although durotomies are generally amenable to primary closure, high-energy tears with associated "shredding" of the dura may be unsuitable for direct suture repair. In these cases, when a tension-free closure with suture alone is not possible, patch grafts may be sewn into the defect to achieve closure. As well, some dural tears are located in difficult to reach locations, such as along the far lateral sac, and grafting may provide an option for dural repair. Several graft options are available, including autogenous tissues, allograft, and synthetic material. All grafts are placed over the durotomy and are then secured in place using either interrupted or running suture techniques. Muscle, fat, and fascia can all be obtained from the local surgical site or harvested from a distant site to provide closure of a dural defect. In the anterior cervical spine, Riew and Khanna[7] described the use of local platysma muscle with its overlying fascia as an option for patch grafting. Mayfield and Kurokawa[13] described the use of an intentional midline durotomy to allow for a fat graft to be placed in the case of a difficult to reach, far lateral tear. Once the intentional opening is made, a fat graft is directed into the dural tear, from inside-out, to plug the defect, and then is sutured into place.

Several synthetic graft materials are available for dural repair. Keller et al.[14] compared the use of two synthetic materials, Mersilene polyester fiber mesh and silicone-coated Dacron, with autologous fat graft for dural closure using a dog model. Using histologic examination, they found that both the Mersilene and autologous fat grafts provided excellent substrates for dural repair, whereas the Dacron grafts became encapsulated in soft tissue, resulting in worse healing and frequent compression of the underlying spinal cord.

Narotam et al.[15] described their use of collagen matrix graft (Duragen) in the repair of dural tears. They retrospectively reviewed 110 patients over an 8-year period who underwent dural repair using only collagen matrix grafting for dural repair. In 80% of patients, collagen matrix was the sole method of duraplasty, whereas 20% had additional suture placement. Graft failure with persistent leakage was found in 3 patients (2.7%), 4 patients developed psuedomeningoceles (3.6%), and wound infections were seen in 2 patients (1 superficial and 1 deep). The authors described the sole use of collagen matrix as a novel approach to duraplasty that may avoid the need for suture repair.[15] Synthetic grafts obviate the minimal risk for donor site morbidity, yet they introduce a foreign body and possibly increase the risk for infection. Synthetics also add significant cost. As a result, it is the author's opinion that autogenous grafts be used whenever possible.

A difficult treatment decision is presented when a clinically significant dural tear is found in association with a cervical spine injury that can be managed conservatively. Certain dural tears, possibly as a result of a sharp retropulsed vertebral body fragment, may be of a critical size that would render conservative management ineffective. It is difficult to measure these tears using clinical information and imaging studies and even more difficult to identify which tear may be amenable to conservative management versus surgical repair. It is the author's recommendation that in the face of a stable fracture that should otherwise be treated conservatively, a trial of nonoperative management of the traumatic durotomy should be attempted, including positioning changes, as well as a percutaneous lumbar drain. If these measures are inadequate to provide for dural closure, formal repair can then be pursued, in association with internal fixation for fracture stabilization.

A second difficult scenario is presented when a dural tear is identified at a site distant from the planned operative field. De Gelb et al.[16] described a case in which a patient with a C4-C5 dislocation was first treated with an anterior stabilization procedure, followed by posterior fusion. Although no evidence of a CSF leak was noticed during the anterior procedure, the posterior approach revealed an irreparable tear from C4 to C7, requiring allograft dural patch and fibrin glue supplementation, along with a lumbar drain. In retrospect, they postulated that avoidance of the posterior procedure and treatment with isolated anterior fusion and halo placement might have been a superior treatment method, allowing the tear to seal primarily. In the case of a severe dural injury, if a durotomy can be identified in advance, avoidance of the tear during a stabilization procedure coupled with a lumbar drain to shunt flow away from the laceration site may be beneficial and allow for improved healing potential. Although compromise of fracture stability is unacceptable, if adequate fixation can be achieved surgically, with or without the use of a halo or orthosis, avoidance of the tear and use of a shunt may be the best treatment option when confronted with an irreparable dural laceration. This notion is bolstered by the observed plugging effect of leaks at the spinal cord level described earlier by Cain et al.[10]

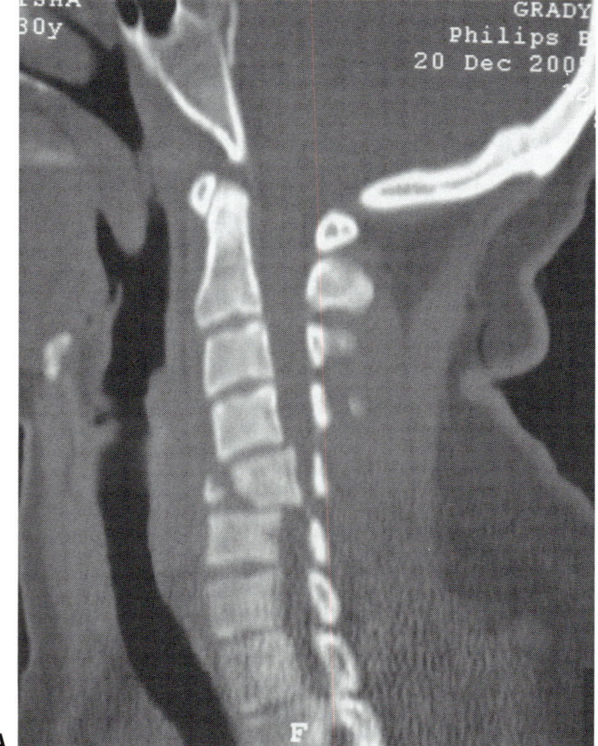

A

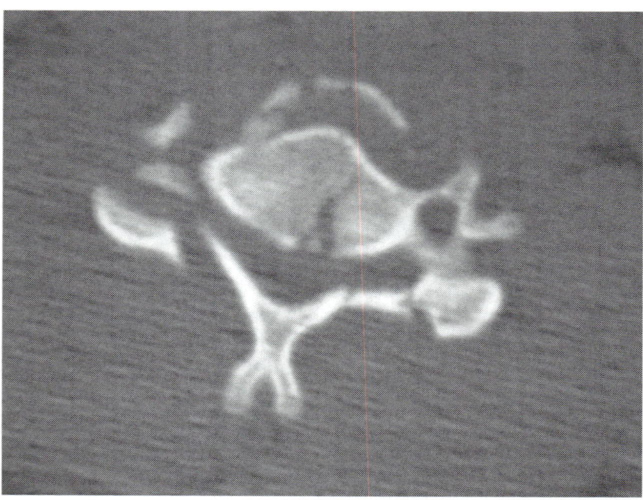

B

FIGURE 33.1. Sagittal reformation **(A)** and axial computed tomography scan **(B)** in a patient who sustained C5 complete quadriplegia because of a C5-C6 fracture-subluxation. At the time of her initial anterior procedure, a cerebrospinal fluid leak was appreciated as a result of an inaccessible dural tear. It was presumed that the leak was either secondary to puncture from the spike of laminar bone from the displaced laminar fracture or possibly a nerve root sleeve injury. No additional treatment was deemed necessary. The leak presumably sealed perioperatively, because there were no symptoms or signs associated with persistent leakage.

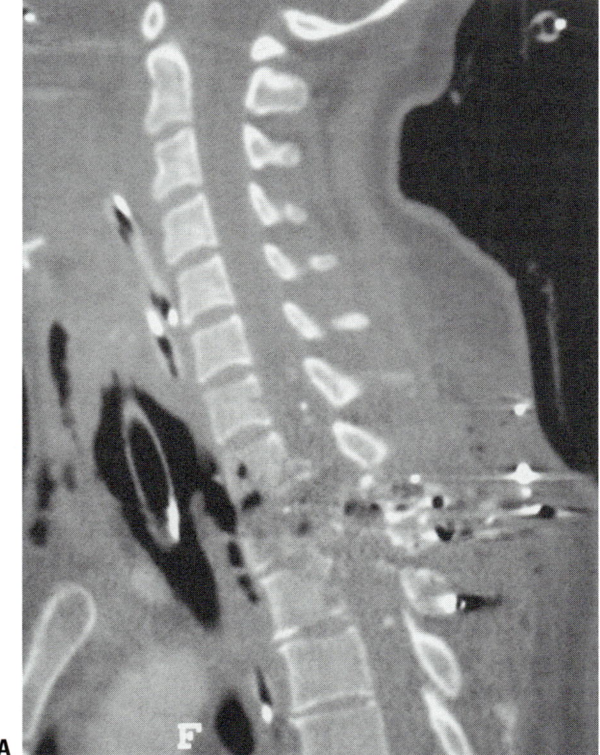

A

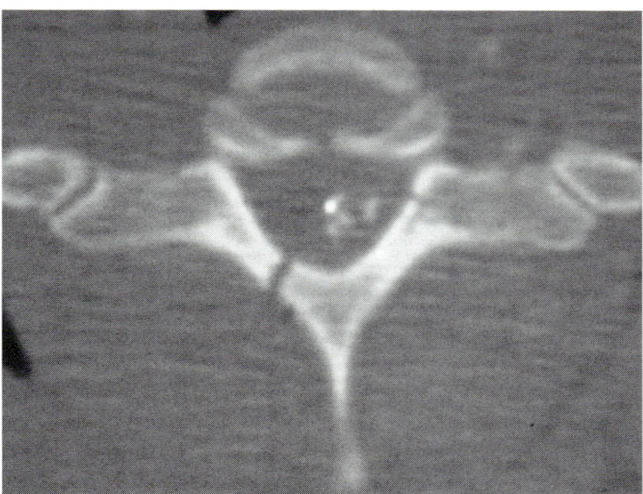

B

FIGURE 33.2. A sagittal **(A)** and axial **(B)** computed tomography scan in a patient who sustained a complete spinal cord injury from a gunshot wound to the cervical spine. Note that dural injury and cerebrospinal fluid (CSF) leakage are a virtual certainty in such instances, but treatment directed toward the CSF leak is rarely ever indicated.

CONCLUSION

Dural tears associated with cervical trauma provide an additional treatment challenge. Although repair of an incidental durotomy during elective surgery has been shown to have little evidence of increased effect on long-term outcomes,[17] the situation is less clear in the instance of CSF leaks associated with cervical trauma. In the case of blunt cervical trauma, extrapolation from observations in thoracolumbar trauma and anecdotal experience suggest that the likelihood of dural tears increases in proportion to the magnitude of the applied force and cervical column displacement at the instant of injury, which in turn will dictate the need for open treatment. When encountered, every reasonable effort should be made to repair or patch accessible defects. If persistent CSF leaks are anticipated, whether due to inadequate repair, lack of surgical access to the defects, or some combination thereof, CSF diversion via a lumbar cisternal drain should be seriously considered. Diversionary drains may also be effective in managing CSF leaks associated with penetrating trauma that would not otherwise require spinal surgery, or to avoid repeat surgery in the event of CSF leaks presenting postoperatively. Whatever steps are required, every effort should be made to prevent or eliminate cutaneous fistulae that might result in the potentially profound consequences of bacterial meningitis.

REFERENCES

1. Cain JE Jr, Dryer RF, Barton BR. Evaluation of dural closure techniques: suture methods, fibrin adhesive sealant, and cyanoacrylate polymer. *Spine* 1988;13:720–725.
2. Stambough JL, Templin CR, Collins J. Subarachnoid drainage of an established or chronic pseudomeningocele. *J Spinal Disord* 2000;13:39–41.
3. Cammisa FP Jr, Eismont FJ, Green BA. Dural laceration occurring with burst fractures and associated laminar fractures. *J Bone Joint Surg Am* 1989;71:1044–1052.
4. Pickett J, Blumenkopf B. Dural lacerations and thoracolumbar fractures. *J Spinal Disord* 1989;2:99–103.
5. Aydinli U, Karaeminogullari O, Ozerdemoglu RA, et al. Dural tears in lumbar burst fractures with greenstick lamina fractures. *Spine* 2001;26:E410–E415.
6. Clark CR, ed. *The Cervical Spine.* 4th ed. Philadelphia: Lippincott Williams & Wilkins, 2005.
7. Riew KD, Khanna N. Treatment of cerebrospinal fluid leaks. In: Vaccaro AR, Zeidman SM, eds. *Principles and Practice of Spine Surgery.* Philadelphia: Mosby, 2003:735–743.
8. Carl AL, Matsumoto M, Whalen JT. Anterior dural laceration caused by thoracolumbar and lumbar burst fractures. *J Spinal Disord* 2000;13:399–403.
9. Carlson GD, Oliff HS, Gorden C, et al. Cerebral spinal fluid pressure: effects of body position and lumbar subarachnoid drainage in a canine model. *Spine* 2003;28:119–122.
10. Cain JE Jr, Lauerman WC, Rosenthal HG, et al. The histomorphologic sequence of dural repair: observations in the canine model. *Spine* 1991;16(suppl 8):S319–S323.
11. Eismont FJ, Wiesel SW, Rothman RH. Treatment of dural tears associated with spinal surgery. *J Bone Joint Surg Am* 1981;63:1132–1136.
12. Campbell PK, Bennett SL, Driscoll A, et al. Evaluation of absorbable surgical sealants: in vitro testing. Available at: http://www.confluentsurgical.com/pdf/ds/6070_DuraSeal_Invitro_WP13=25.pdf. Accessed May 1, 2009.
13. Mayfield FH, Kurokawa K. Watertight closure of spinal dura mater. Technical note. *J Neurosurg* 1975;43:639–640.
14. Keller JT, Ongkiko CM Jr, Saunders MC, et al. Repair of spinal dural defects: an experimental study. *J Neurosurg* 1984;60:1022–1028.
15. Narotam PK, José S, Nathoo N, et al. Collagen matrix (DuraGen) in dural repair: analysis of a new modified technique. *Spine* 2004;29:2861–2867, discussion 2868–2869.
16. De Gelb D, Lenke L, Pond J. Dural tear associated with a flexion distraction subluxation to the cervical spine without neurologic injury. *Acta Orthop Belg* 1998;64:224–228.
17. Wang JC, Bohlman HH, Riew KD. Dural tears secondary to operations on the lumbar spine: management and results after a two-year-minimum follow-up of eighty-eight patients. *J Bone Joint Surg Am* 1998;80:1728–1732.

CHAPTER 34

Neurologic Deterioration in the Nonoperated Patient

Michael Nikolakis and Marcel Dvorak

INTRODUCTION

Neurologic deterioration, whether it occurs after a spinal cord injury (SCI) or following an initially neurologically intact cervical spinal column injury, is one of the most devastating complications of cervical spine trauma. The typical pattern is one of ascending myelopathy rostral to the last normal neurologic level, although motor and/or sensory loss in more caudal spinal segments is possible, particularly in incomplete SCI.[1–5] This feared complication occurs in 1.8% to 10.4% of patients admitted to the hospital with cervical spine trauma and is associated with a mortality rate of 25% to 42%.[1–13] The morbidity related to this neurologic deterioration can range from a reversible loss of function at a single spinal segment to permanent high cervical paralysis with permanent dependence on a respirator. It is hoped that increased vigilance, reliable and regular standardized neurologic assessments, early identification of high-risk patients, and improved immobilization and stabilization techniques from the point of injury through acute care will reduce the incidence of neurologic deterioration. This chapter will identify factors to reduce the incidence of this complication, while acknowledging that only some of these instances are preventable.

The various causes of neurologic deterioration can be categorized broadly according to the time at which the problems typically present after the acute injury. Early deterioration, occurring within the first 24 hours after injury, may be related to spontaneous fluctuation or evolution of the secondary SCI or may be associated with iatrogenic intervention. Subacute deterioration, which occurs between 24 hours and 20 days after injury, is most commonly the result of ascending myelopathy, hematoma, or soft tissue cord compression. Associated carotid or vertebral arterial injury will also present in the subacute window. Late deterioration, occurring after 20 days postinjury, may be due to progressive instability (most often kyphosis) or syringomyelia.

EARLY DETERIORATION FOLLOWING CERVICAL SPINE INJURY

Early deterioration following cervical spine trauma can be defined as deterioration in motor and/or sensory function occurring within the first 24 hours after the injury and can be broadly classified into deterioration occurring before the definitive diagnosis of SCI; spontaneous fluctuation in neurologic function; and intervention-related deterioration.

NEUROLOGIC DETERIORATION OCCURRING BEFORE DEFINITIVE SPINAL DIAGNOSIS

Tremendous advances have been made in the care of injured patients at the point of injury. Highly trained emergency health personnel apply cervical spine precautions before extraction of patients from vehicles and before moving those injured from other mechanisms (sport, falls, work related). In the authors' experience, we continue to see instances in which bystanders will move an injured individual in a way that likely contributes to neurologic injury or worsening of an existing deficit. Often, inebriation with alcohol or drugs affects the judgment of both the injured and nearby bystanders. Because no objective examinations are available in these environments, few conclusions can be drawn other than to state that in some cases lack of appropriate protocols at the scene of the injury may contribute to neurologic injury and deterioration.

Of even more concern are the cases in which the diagnosis of cervical injury is delayed because of altered levels of consciousness, most frequently as a result of head injury but also influenced by alcohol and drug use. There have been reports describing the failure to maintain cervical spine precautions in the obtunded patient resulting in neurologic deterioration.[14] In some cases this may result in a catastrophic permanent deterioration (Fig. 34.1). Either failure to appropriately clear the cervical spine in the obtunded patient or misreading of radiographic studies can lead to progressive subluxation, dislocation, deformity, and neurologic injury or deterioration of an existing deficit.

EARLY SPONTANEOUS DETERIORATION OF NEUROLOGIC FUNCTION

Marshall et al.[1] and others[4,5] have reported neurologic deterioration occurring within the first 24 hours after injury. Because of the presence of spinal shock, which can last up to 48 hours, the initial neurologic evaluation, particularly in the patient with incomplete SCI, may be inaccurate, although in most instances, the patient's neurologic condition improves as spinal shock resolves.[15–17] The primary injury creates edema and hemorrhage in the spinal cord that may propagate and evolve, resulting in deteriorating neurologic function, particularly within the zone of partial preservation; the several spinal segments caudal to the last normal neurologic level where there is less than normal motor and sensory function.

Although it is most common to observe neurologic improvement in the incompletely injured cervical spine patient,[18] deterioration, particularly the loss of one or two grades of motor power within the zone of partial preservation, is common in those with complete injuries and will often recover over time.[3,16,19] If deterioration is recognized, urgent evaluation is necessary to ensure that there is no potentially correctable cause such as persistent soft tissue or bony spinal cord compression as a result of disc herniation, hematoma, fracture fragments, or malalignment of the spinal canal.

This highlights the importance of neurologic monitoring in the spinal cord–injured individual, particularly in the first hours and days following SCI.[20] Once SCI is recognized in a patient, the patient must be transferred to a subspecialty SCI unit where highly trained allied health staff are able to monitor neurologic vital signs reliably and frequently. Staff caring for these patients must be trained to reliably perform the American Spinal Injury Association (ASIA) standard neurologic examination and must record these findings so that subsequent examiners may reliably identify neurologic deterioration. If this form of clinical neurologic monitoring is not available, the patient should be transferred to a unit or hospital where it can be performed. The failure to diagnose neurologic deterioration in a timely fashion and to investigate it fully may have catastrophic and permanent consequences.

INTERVENTION-RELATED DETERIORATION OF NEUROLOGIC FUNCTION

Iatrogenic neurologic deterioration may occur during endotracheal intubation of an individual with an unstable cervical spine or may be due to traction, immobilization, or closed reduction of the acutely injured spine.[1,3,5,19,21–23]

Airway protection is a major area of concern in the acutely traumatized patient. The risk for causing or exacerbating a cervical SCI is very real and carries with it a significant morbidity and

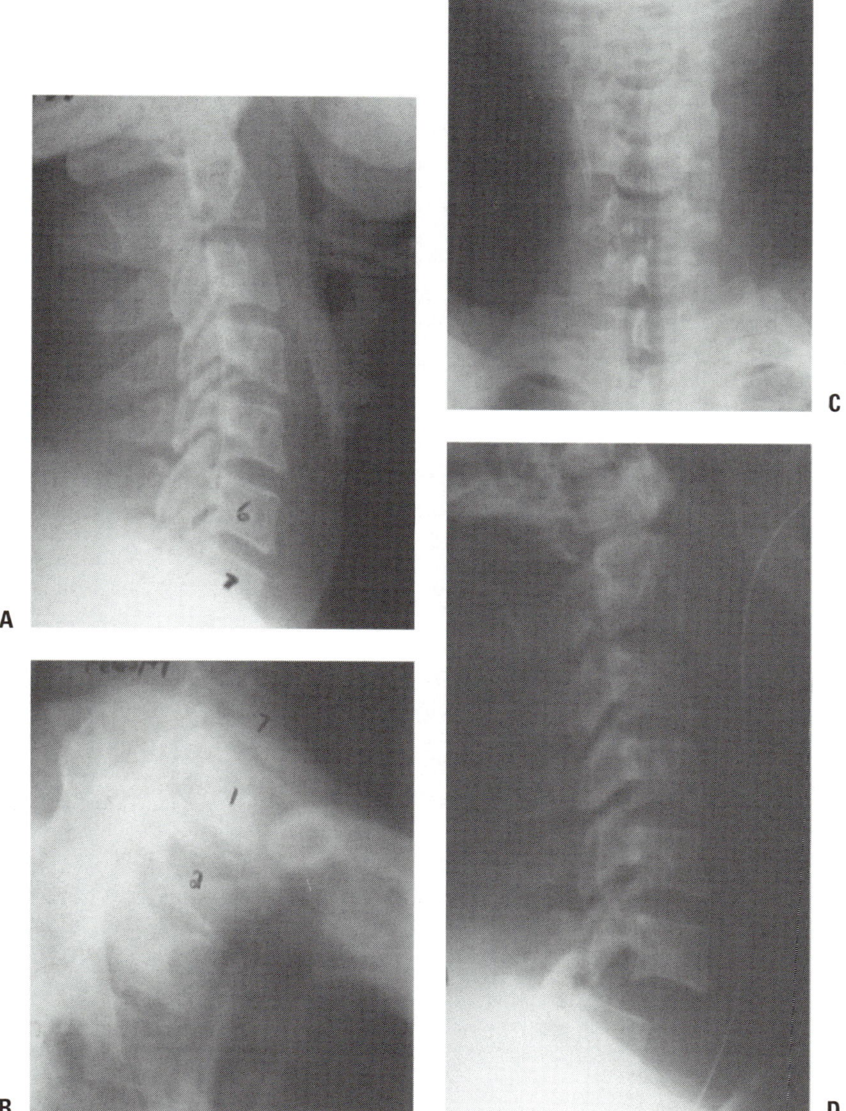

FIGURE 34.1. **A.** Lateral cervical spine radiograph. **B.** Swimmers view. **C.** Anteroposterior view. All three views show normal alignment and no bony injury. The computed tomography scan was normal in this obtunded patient. Several days postinjury, he developed marked neurologic deterioration and was noted to have a pure ligamentous bilateral facet dislocation at C6-C7. **D.** The only abnormal imaging finding before his dislocation and neurologic deterioration was soft tissue swelling in the retropharyngeal space on the original plain radiograph.

possibly mortality. In experienced hands, the overall risk for cervical spine injury from endotracheal intubation appears to be small, with one study reporting a 1.3% rate of neurologic deterioration after elective intubation of 150 cervical spine–injured adults.[24] Another paper retrospectively reviewed 81 cervical spine–injured patients who required urgent intubation in the emergency department. In-line cervical stabilization was used, and there were no cases of neurologic injury reported.[25] Intubation has not been shown to increase the probability of neurologic deterioration in cervical spine–injured patients admitted to hospital.[26,27] Acknowledging the fact that maintaining a patent airway and appropriate ventilation take precedence over other issues, it appears that intubation of the cervical spine–injured patient while maintaining in-line stabilization is a safe procedure. Application of manual or tong traction during intubation maneuvers may occasionally be inappropriate, particularly in the presence of occipitocervical injuries in which traction may increase the deformity and displacement.[28]

Several case series have described neurologic deterioration occurring during nonsurgical interventions commonly instituted during conservative care. Harrop et al.[5] described five patients who suffered neurologic deterioration within 24 hours of their cervical spine injuries. Four of the five experienced neurologic deterioration in association with halo vest, traction, and cervical spine collar application. The fifth patient in the series who deteriorated within 24 hours had bilateral vertebral artery injuries that resulted in fatal brainstem ischemia, which we shall discuss later in this chapter. Similarly, Marshall et al.[1] reported on nine patients who suffered neurologic deterioration with the use of a Rotorest bed, Stryker frame, halo vest, and application of skeletal traction. Although the application of traction and immobilization devices is generally considered to be safe,[29] there is a measurable risk of neurologic deterioration of up to 10% with nonsurgical treatment of spinal column injuries.[21,22]

The techniques of closed cervical reduction using skull tongs or halo rings present their own unique risk profile. Gardner-Wells tongs used to reduce cervical fractures carry with them a low 1.3% rate for neurologic injury.[30,31] Certain radiologic findings, such as unilateral or bilateral locked facets in association with traumatic intervertebral disc herniation may represent a much higher risk of neurologic injury with traction.[32–34] In the case series reported by Doran et al.,[32] 3 of 9 patients (33%) with unilateral or bilateral locked facets and herniated intervertebral disc material experienced neurologic deterioration with attempted closed reduction.[32] It is beyond the scope of this chapter to discuss the protocol for magnetic resonance imaging (MRI), proceeding with closed reduction, or contemplating anterior cervical discectomy and open reduction/fusion in patients with cervical fracture dislocations; however, we do recognize that there is a measurable risk of adverse neurologic outcome with each of these treatment options, including the nonsurgical options.

Other factors also increase the risk for neurologic deterioration, such as the presence of a flexion-based injury, multilevel cervical spondylosis, and ankylosing spondylitis.[3] The presence of ankylosing spondylitis in a patient with a cervical spine injury dramatically increases the likelihood of neurologic deterioration. Harrop et al.[5] had two patients in their series with ankylosing spondylitis, and both died secondary to neurologic deterioration. Colterjohn and Bednar[3] also found the presence of spondylitis to be a major risk factor for secondary neurologic deterioration after cervical spine injury. Other risk factors associated with neurologic deterioration in Colterjohn's study were the presence of disseminated idiopathic skeletal hyperostosis and multilevel cervical spondylosis, both conditions that stiffen the spine. The case series of Farmer et al.[4] also had three patients with a diagnosis of ankylosing spondylitis, and all three died from neurologic deterioration following cervical spine trauma. It is clear from the literature that the presence of a cervical fracture in an ankylosed spine carries a significant risk for neurologic morbidity and mortality. Early definitive surgical stabilization may present a lower risk than prolonged traction and bracing in this complex patient population.

SUBACUTE DETERIORATION FOLLOWING CERVICAL SPINE INJURY

Subacute neurologic deterioration, defined as neurologic deterioration occurring between 24 hours and 20 days after injury, is most commonly associated with secondary SCI (ascending myelopathy) or with carotid or vertebral arterial dissection. It is in this group of patients that identifying a cause for the deterioration is often critical. Potentially correctable causes include hypotension and persistent spinal cord compression by bone, soft tissue (disc), or hematoma.

ASCENDING MYELOPATHY

Harrop et al.[4] identified 7 of 12 patients in their series who deteriorated during this period and recognized that episodes of hypotension and the existence of vertebral artery injuries appeared to be the cause. Other series also have identified episodes of hypotension to be a risk factor for secondary SCI.[4] Secondary SCI commonly presents as an ascending myelopathy beginning 4 to 9 days after a complete cervical SCI.[4,5] Castillo et al.[2] were the first to report an association among spinal cord edema, hypotension, and secondary SCI.[2] Their patient, an 18-year-old man, suffered a C4-C5 complete SCI and 10 days after injury experienced an episode of hypotension, after which his motor and sensory paralysis ascended, leaving him ventilator dependent. A myelogram performed before the onset of ascending myelopathy showed no obstruction; however, when repeated after the onset of clinical deterioration, diffuse cord swelling extending above and below the site of initial injury was found. MRI confirmed the presence of cord edema, and there was also noted to be a small area of hemorrhage within the cord. This pattern of deterioration, now known as secondary SCI, or ascending myelopathy, has been reported by other authors as well (Fig. 34.2).[35,36]

The cause of secondary SCI occurring several days after the initial injury is not known, but because of its relationship with episodes of hypotension, some authors think that it represents a manifestation of vascular insufficiency that gradually leads to cord swelling and infarction.[39] This may be due to gradual occlusion or thrombus propagation of an arterial injury. Alternatively, secondary SCI may be due to venous infarction. During episodes of hypotension the flow through injured veins at the site of SCI is reduced enough to promote venous thrombosis. Thrombosis can then propagate a short distance proximal and distal to the initial site of injury, causing cord edema and eventually infarction. Both the diffuse cord edema and the intrathecal hemorrhage seen on MRI shortly after the onset of neurologic deterioration can be explained by venous infarction. For this

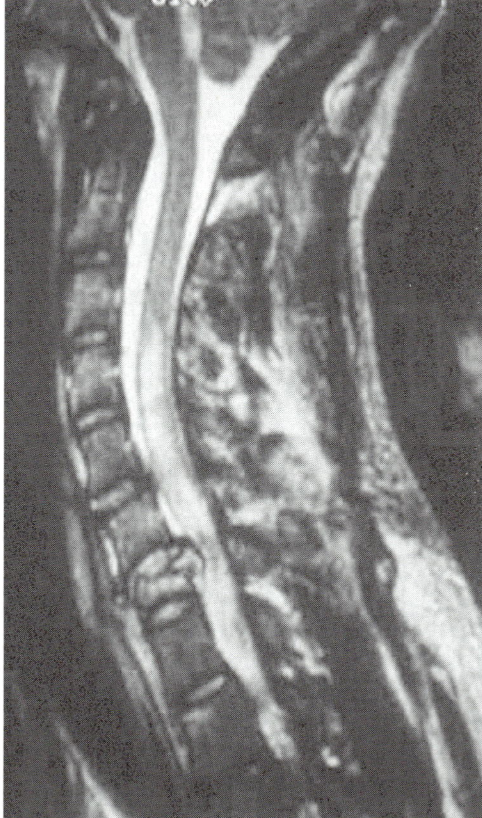

FIGURE 34.2. This 26-year-old male snowboarder presented with a C7 burst fracture and ASIA A complete quadriplegia. He developed ascending motor and sensory paralysis eventually ascending to a ventilator-dependent C4 last normal level. The magnetic resonance imaging scan shows extensive signal change within the spinal cord extending up to the C3 vertebral level.

reason some surgeons feel that patients should be kept normotensive or slightly hypertensive after acute cervical spine injury, and episodes of hypotension should be treated aggressively when detected, particularly around the time of surgery.[38] Inflammation and apoptosis have also been implicated in secondary SCI.[37] Unfortunately, there is no proven therapy for this pattern of neurologic deterioration, nor is there a reliable method for predicting its occurrence. Although there is little evidence to support various treatment approaches, when neurologic deterioration occurs, efforts to ensure that the patient is hemodynamically stable should be instituted. Some physicians also recommend the administration of a bolus of steroids, similar to the National Acute Spinal Cord Injury Study (NASCIS) II protocol. An urgent MRI is also recommended, and if residual cord compression is identified, consideration for surgical decompression should be undertaken.

Although the role and timing of surgical decompression in SCI is debated, it is generally accepted that when neurologic function is deteriorating in the presence of extrinsic spinal cord compression, this is an absolute indication for surgical decompression. Large traumatic disc protrusions (Fig. 34.3) and epidural hematomas (Fig. 34.4) are amenable to surgical decompression, often with dramatic neurologic improvement.

VERTEBRAL AND CAROTID ARTERIAL INJURY

Arterial injury is another well-recognized cause of delayed neurologic deterioration in the cervical spine–injured patient. Dissection, thrombosis, and pseudoaneurysm can occur in carotid and vertebral arteries after blunt trauma. These injuries can result in devastating strokes, which often occur days to weeks after the initial injury. Published reports have cited mortality rates up to 31% and severe neurologic deficits in up to 56% of patients with traumatic carotid or vertebral artery injury.[39] Physician awareness to the possibility of arterial injury is the key to making this diagnosis, because many patients are either asymptomatic or have the symptoms of arterial dissection masked by their associated injuries.

Carotid artery injury is diagnosed in 0.5% of patients admitted to hospital after blunt trauma.[40] Risk factors for carotid artery injury are an initial Glasgow Coma Scale (GCS) score of less than 8, head and anterior neck injury, facial fractures, and thoracic injury.[40] Cervical spine injury does not appear to be a strong predictor of carotid artery injury.[41] The mechanisms of

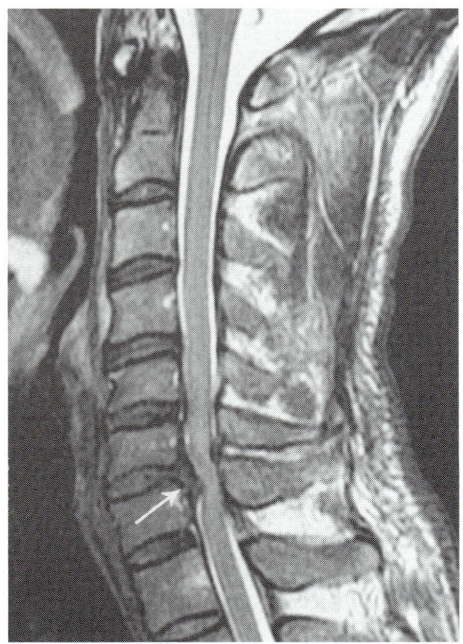

FIGURE 34.3. A 47-year-old man with a traumatic disc herniation after a cervical injury that occurred on a rollercoaster ride developed dramatic neurologic deterioration several days after the initial injury. Plain radiographs were normal; however, magnetic resonance imaging revealed a traumatic disc protrusion at C6-C7 *(arrow)*. He progressed to complete quadriplegia and has not recovered despite urgent surgical decompression.

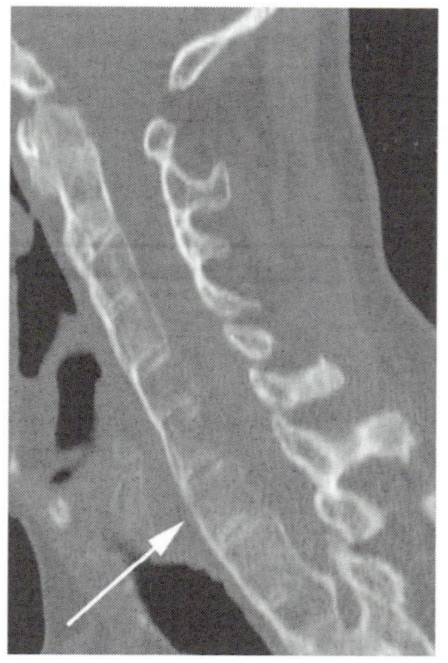

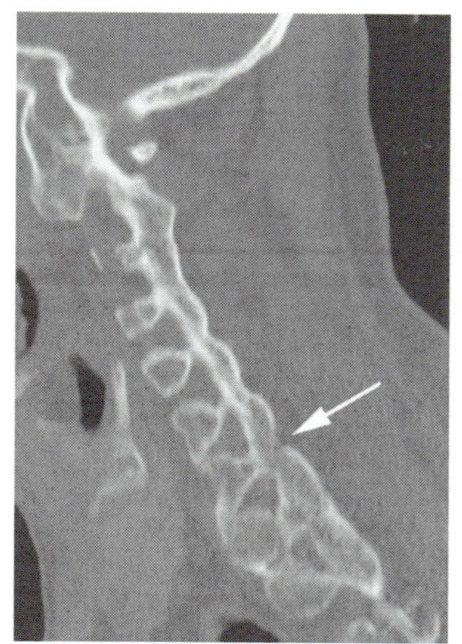

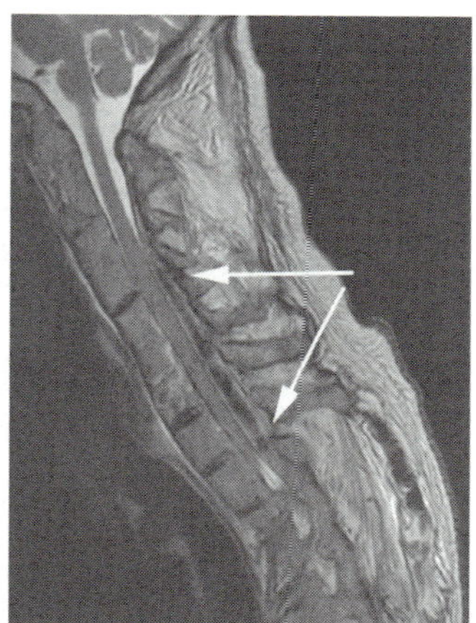

FIGURE 34.4. This 52-year-old man with known ankylosing spondylitis sustained a "trivial" injury to his neck when forcefully sitting down on a couch. Computed tomography revealed an undisplaced fracture at the level of the C7 vertebra (*arrows* in **A** and **B**). Several days after immobilization in a halo thoracic vest, he developed progressive quadriparesis. Urgent magnetic resonance imaging revealed an epidural hematoma significantly compressing the spinal cord from C4 to T1 (*white arrows* in **C**).

carotid artery dissection in blunt trauma are thought to be direct compression of the artery against the cervical spine or hyperextension of the neck, resulting in intimal tearing.[42] In two recent series, stroke or transient ischemic attack (TIA) was the presentation in 33%[39] and 34%[40] of patients with carotid artery dissection, indicating that a significant proportion of carotid artery dissections are still not diagnosed before neurologic deterioration. Consequently, carotid artery dissection should be investigated in any patient with severe chest, neck, or face trauma, head injury and neurologic deficit, or in patients with Horner syndrome and unexplained cranial nerve palsy.

The gold standard for diagnosis of carotid artery injury is cerebral angiography, but at many institutions, computed tomography (CT) angiography is the most common investigation used to diagnose carotid artery dissection because of accessibility, speed of acquisition, and the fact that most patients are in the CT scanner for evaluation of injuries. Once carotid artery dissection has been diagnosed, the most common treatment regimen includes anticoagulation with intravenous heparin followed by oral warfarin (Coumadin) therapy for 3 to 6 months. The rate of recurrent TIA or stroke is lower with anticoagulation than it is with antiplatelet therapy,[40,43,44] but the risk for hemorrhage in the multitrauma patient must be taken into account before treatment is initiated. Even with treatment, some studies have found a recurrence rate for stroke or TIA of 8% to 12%.[43] Carotid artery stenting is reserved for patients with large dissection flaps that appear unstable or are causing symptoms.

Once thought to be a relatively benign pathologic condition, vertebral artery injury is now recognized as a source of serious morbidity and mortality in the trauma patient. Vertebral artery injury occurs in approximately 0.4% of all blunt trauma patients.[40] Unlike carotid artery dissection, vertebral artery dissection has a strong association with cervical spine injury.[41,45] Willis et al.[46] studied the incidence of vertebral artery injury in 26 consecutive patients with cervical spine fractures or subluxations and found that 46% had vertebral artery injury as diagnosed on cerebral angiography.[46] The incidence of posterior circulation stroke with blunt vertebral artery injury is as high as 24%, and the mortality rate for patients with this injury attributable to vertebrobasilar ischemia is approximately 8%.[45]

Diagnostic options are similar to those noted in the earlier discussion. Vertebral artery dissection can occur anywhere along the length of the artery. Two common sites where dissection flaps are seen include the origin of the vertebral artery as it leaves the subclavian artery and at the artery's entry point into the foramen transversarium. Once vertebral artery dissection is diagnosed, the treating physician has the same treatment options as those presented earlier for carotid artery dissection. Antiplatelet therapy is frequently selected for patient with asymptomatic vertebral artery dissection. Patients with posterior circulation TIA or stroke may be given either antiplatelet agents or anticoagulation therapy at the treating physician's discretion.

LATE DETERIORATION FOLLOWING CERVICAL SPINE INJURY

Late neurologic deterioration occurring within the first year after SCI may occur in up to 3.6% of individuals, and after the first year, up to 12.1% experience neurologic deterioration.[47] The two principle causes associated with late neurologic deterioration are posttraumatic instability resulting in deformity and syringomyelia. As the life expectancy of spinal cord–injured patients improves, patients are diagnosed more frequently with late neurologic deterioration. Thus, radiologic surveillance of the spinal cord–injured patient has been considered.[48] Spinal alignment and biomechanical stability should be monitored with plain radiographs. A reasonable protocol would include a upright anteroposterior and lateral views when the patient first mobilizes postoperatively, again at discharge from rehabilitation, and at 3, 6, and 12 months after injury. Thereafter, the patient should be followed with radiographs every 1 to 3 years. Asymptomatic syringomyelia can be diagnosed with MRI, particularly on midsagittal T2-weighted imaging. Serial investigations performed every 2 to 5 years have been proposed to detect syrinx formation before it causes neurologic deterioration.[48]

Posttraumatic syringomyelia becomes symptomatic in 1.1% to 4.5% of patients with cervical SCI; radiologic or autopsy studies suggest an incidence as high as 22%.[49–51] Cervical SCIs, dislocations, increasing age, and spinal surgery are all independent risk factors for the development of symptomatic posttraumatic syringomyelia.[51]

Delayed posttraumatic instability in the patient with a cervical spine injury has been defined as the onset of clinical instability at least 20 days after trauma in a patient with adequate cervical spine radiographs initially judged to be normal or stable.[52] This diagnosis does not include patients whose cervical spine injuries were missed because of inadequate radiographs, nor does it include patients treated for cervical spine injuries whose primary treatment modality (surgery, halo vest) failed. Delfini et al.[52] published a case series of 25 patients with delayed posttraumatic cervical instability. They found that the mean duration from injury to diagnosis of instability was 41.5 days. The most common levels where biomechanical instability developed were at C4-C5 (32%) and C5-C6 (36%). The most common symptoms that prompted follow-up radiologic investigation included persistent pain in 11 patients (44%) and neurologic deterioration in 6 patients (24%). Again, all 25 patients in this case series had adequate radiographs performed during their initial presentation, and 10 of the 25 had either CT (6) or MRI (4) of the cervical spine as well. The most common explanation for the development of delayed posttraumatic instability is that ligamentous injury occurs at the time of injury and is not fully appreciated or recognized during the initial evaluation. When muscle spasm begins to settle, the lack of ligamentous integrity results in clinically relevant instability. What is truly remarkable is that in Delfini's series, four of the patients had MRI performed on initial presentation, but the diagnosis of ligamentous cervical spine instability remained elusive. Clearly, a high index of suspicion must be maintained to make the diagnosis of delayed posttraumatic instability before the development of neurologic deficit.

CONCLUSION

Neurologic deterioration of the cervical spine–injured patient is a catastrophic event that carries a 25% to 42% mortality rate. Survivors of secondary neurologic deterioration often lose at least one spinal level of function and may ascend to become respirator-dependent. Deterioration within the first 24 hours is most often due to iatrogenic intervention, including the application of traction and halo vest fixation. Intubation can also result in neurologic deterioration, so extreme caution must be exerted during this procedure. Deterioration occurring between postinjury days 1 and 20 is due to either secondary SCI or vertebral or carotid artery dissection or thrombosis. The pathophysiology of secondary SCI is poorly understood, but it appears to be a vascular phenomenon that can be exacerbated by episodes of hypotension. Lastly, deterioration occurring after postinjury day 20 may be due to delayed posttraumatic instability or syringomyelia. The diagnosis of delayed posttraumatic instability requires a high index of suspicion if it is to be recognized before it causes neurologic deterioration. Patients with conditions that result in stiffening of the spine, such as ankylosing spondylitis and diffuse idiopathic skeletal hyperostosis, are at a greatly increased risk for secondary neurologic deterioration, and extreme caution must be exerted when managing patients with these comorbidities.

REFERENCES

1. Marshall LF, Knowlton S, Garfin SR, et al. Deterioration following spinal cord injury: a multicenter study. *J Neurosurg* 1987;66:400–404.
2. Castillo M, Quencer RM, Green BA, et al. Acute, ascending cord ischaemia after mobilisation of a stable quadriplegic patient. *Lancet* 1988;1:759–760.
3. Colterjohn NR, Bednar DA. Identifiable risk factors for secondary neurologic deterioration in the cervical spine-injured patient. *Spine* 1995;20:2293–2297.
4. Farmer J, Vaccaro A, Albert TJ. Neurologic deterioration after cervical spinal cord injury. *J Spinal Disord* 1998;11:192–196.
5. Harrop JS, Sharan AD, Vaccaro AR, et al. The cause of neurologic deterioration after acute cervical spinal cord injury. *Spine* 2001;26:340–346.
6. Colterjohn NR, Bednar DA. Identifiable risk factors for secondary neurologic deterioration in the cervical spine-injured patient. *Spine* 1995;20:2293–2297.
7. Farmer J, Vaccaro A, Albert TJ, et al. Neurologic deterioration after cervical spinal cord injury. *J Spinal Disord* 1998;11:192–196.
8. Frankel HL, Hancock DO, Hyslop G, et al. The value of postural reduction in the initial management of closed injuries of the spine with paraplegia and tetraplegia. I. *Paraplegia* 1969;7:179–192.
9. Harrop JS, Sharan AD, Vaccaro AR, The cause of neurologic deterioration after acute cervical spinal cord injury. *Spine* 2001;26:340–346.
10. Heiden JS, Weiss MH, Rosenberg AW, et al. Management of cervical spinal cord trauma in Southern California. *J Neurosurg* 1975;43:732–736.
11. Katoh S, El Masry WS. Neurological recovery after conservative treatment of cervical cord injuries. *J Bone Joint Surg Br* 1994;76:225–228.
12. Katoh S, El Masry WS, Jaffray D, et al. Neurologic outcome in conservatively treated patients with incomplete closed traumatic cervical spinal cord injuries. *Spine* 1996;21:2345–2351.
13. Yablon IG, Ordia J, Mortara R, et al. Acute ascending myelopathy of the spine. *Spine* 1989;14:1084–1089.
14. Gerrelts BD, Petersen EU, Mabry J, et al. Delayed diagnosis of cervical spine injuries. *J Trauma* 1991;31:1622–1626.
15. Ditunno JF, Little JW, Tessler A, et al. Spinal shock revisited: a four-phase model. *Spinal Cord* 2004;42:383–395.
16. Fisher CG, Noonan VK, Smith DE, et al. Motor recovery, functional status, and health-related quality of life in patients with complete spinal cord injuries. *Spine* 2005;30:2200–2207.
17. Waters RL, Adkins RH, Yakura JS. Definition of complete spinal cord injury. *Paraplegia* 1991;29:573–581.
18. Dvorak MF, Fisher CG, Hoekema J, et al. Factors predicting motor recovery and functional outcome after traumatic central cord syndrome: a long-term follow-up. *Spine* 2005;30:2303–2311.
19. Bohlman HH. Acute fractures and dislocations of the cervical spine: an analysis of three hundred hospitalized patients and review of the literature. *J Bone Joint Surg Am* 1979;61:1119–1142.
20. Tominaga S. Periodical, neurological-functional assessment for cervical cord injury. *Paraplegia* 1989;27:227–236.
21. Katoh S, El Masry WS. Neurological recovery after conservative treatment of cervical cord injuries. *J Bone Joint Surg Br* 1994;76:225–228.
22. Katoh S, El Masry WS, Jaffray D, et al. Neurologic outcome in conservatively treated patients with incomplete closed traumatic cervical spinal cord injuries. *Spine* 1996;21:2345–2351.
23. Robertson PA, Ryan MD. Neurological deterioration after reduction of cervical subluxation: mechanical compression by disc tissue. *J Bone Joint Surg Br* 1992;74:224–227.
24. Suderman VS, Crosby ET, Lui A: Elective oral tracheal intubation in cervical spine-injured adults. *Can J Anaesth* 1991;38:785–789.

25. Scannell G, Waxman K, Tominaga G, et al. Orotracheal intubation in trauma patients with cervical fractures. *Arch Surg* 1993;128:903–905.
26. Hastings RH, Kelley SD. Neurologic deterioration associated with airway management in a cervical spine-injured patient. *Anesthesiology* 1993;78:580–583.
27. Meschino A, Devitt JH, Koch JP, et al. The safety of awake tracheal intubation in cervical spine injury. *Can J Anaesth* 1992;39:114–117.
28. Fisher CG, Sun JC, Dvorak M. Recognition and management of atlanto-occipital dislocation: improving survival from an often fatal condition. *Can J Surg* 2001;44:412–420.
29. Chan RC, Schweigel JF, Thompson GB. Halo-thoracic brace immobilization in 188 patients with acute cervical spine injuries. *J Neurosurg* 1983;58:508–515.
30. Cotler JM, Herbison GJ, Nasuti JF, et al. Closed reduction of traumatic cervical spine dislocation using traction weights up to 140 pounds. *Spine* 1993;18:386–390.
31. Grant GA, Mirza SK, Chapman JR, et al. Risk of early closed reduction in cervical spine subluxation injuries. *J Neurosurg Spine* 1999;90:13–18.
32. Doran SE, Papadopoulos SM, Ducker TB, et al. Magnetic resonance imaging documentation of coexistent traumatic locked facets of the cervical spine and disc herniation. *J Neurosurg* 1993;79:341–345.
33. Robertson PA, Ryan MD. Neurological deterioration after reduction of cervical subluxation: mechanical compression by disc tissue. *J Bone Joint Surg Br* 1992;74:224–227.
34. Ludwig SC, Vaccaro AR, Balderston RA, et al. Immediate quadriparesis after manipulation for bilateral cervical facet subluxation: a case report. *J Bone Joint Surg Am* 1997;79:587–590.
35. Aito S, El Masry WS, Gerner HJ, et al. Ascending myelopathy in the early stage of spinal cord injury. *Spinal Cord* 1999;37:617–623.
36. Yablon IG, Ordia J, Mortara R, et al. Acute ascending myelopathy of the spine. *Spine* 1989;14:1084–1089.
37. Tator CH, Fehlings MG. Review of the secondary injury theory of acute spinal cord trauma with emphasis on vascular mechanisms. *J Neurosurg* 1991;75:15–26.
38. Hadley MN, Walters BC, Grabb PA, et al. Guidelines for the management of acute cervical spine and spinal cord injuries. *Clin Neurosurg* 2002;49:407–498.
39. Kerwin AJ, Bynoe RP, Murray J, et al. Liberalized screening for blunt carotid and vertebral artery injuries is justified. *J Trauma* 2001;51:308–314.
40. Miller PR, Fabian TC, Bee TK, et al. Blunt cerebrovascular injuries: diagnosis and treatment. *J Trauma* 2001;51:279–285.
41. McKevitt EC, Kirkpatrick AW, Vertesi L, et al. Blunt vascular neck injuries: diagnosis and outcomes of extracranial vessel injury. *J Trauma* 2002;53:472–476.
42. Hughes KM, Collier B, Greene KA, et al. Traumatic carotid artery dissection: a significant incidental finding. *Am Surg* 2000;66:1023–1027.
43. Beletsky V, Nadareishvili Z, Lynch J, et al. Cervical arterial dissection: time for a therapeutic trial? *Stroke* 2003;34:2856–2860.
44. Dziewas R, Konrad C, Drager B, et al. Cervical artery dissection: clinical features, risk factors, therapy and outcome in 126 patients. *J Neurol* 2003;250:1179–1184.
45. Biffl WL, Moore EE, Elliott JP, et al. The devastating potential of blunt vertebral arterial injuries. *Ann Surg* 2000;231:672–681.
46. Willis BK, Greiner F, Orrison WW, et al. The incidence of vertebral artery injury after midcervical spine fracture or subluxation. *Neurosurgery* 1994;34:435–441.
47. Piepmeier JM, Jenkins NR. Late neurological changes following traumatic spinal cord injury. *J Neurosurg* 1988;69:399–402.
48. Bodley R. Imaging in chronic spinal cord injury: indications and benefits. *Eur J Radiol* 2002;42:135–153.
49. Anton HA, Schweigel JF. Posttraumatic syringomyelia: the British Columbia experience. *Spine* 1986;11:865–868.
50. Schurch B, Wichmann W, Rossier AB. Post-traumatic syringomyelia (cystic myelopathy): a prospective study of 449 patients with spinal cord injury. *J Neurol Neurosurg Psychiatry* 1996;60:61–67.
51. Vannemreddy SS, Rowed DW, Bharatwal N. Posttraumatic syringomyelia: predisposing factors. *Br J Neurosurg* 2002;16:276–283.
52. Delfini R, Dorizzi A, Facchinetti G, et al. Delayed post-traumatic cervical instability. *Surg Neurol* 1999;51:588–594.

CHAPTER 35

Venous Thromboembolism in Cervical Spine Trauma

Pradeep Thumbikat and Charles G. Fisher

INTRODUCTION

Deep vein thrombosis and pulmonary embolism are potentially avoidable problems that continue to cause mortality and morbidity among people with spinal cord injury (SCI), despite increased awareness in recent years. It has been reported that acute SCI is the highest risk factor for venous thromboembolism among hospitalized patients. A reduction in the incidence of venous thromboembolism and morbidity following it can be achieved only through a combination of a better appreciation of the nonspecific clinical presentation of venous thromboembolism in the spinal cord–injured population, effective prophylaxis, and a low threshold for investigation and treatment.

INCIDENCE

Getting a true estimate of the incidence of the problem is difficult because of the variability in the sensitivity of the tests that have been used to determine the presence or absence of either deep vein thrombosis or pulmonary embolism. In the absence of thromboprophylaxis, the incidence of deep vein thrombosis in the spinal cord–injured population has been reported to be as high as 67% to 100% using objective tests. There is evidence to show that among patients with SCI the incidence of fatal pulmonary embolism did not fall between the periods 1973 to 1977 and 1992 to 1998. In a recent multicenter study, 63% patients in a group receiving unfractionated heparin and intermittent pneumatic compression and 66% in the group receiving enoxaparin showed evidence of deep vein thrombosis on contrast venography, demonstrating that the problem of venous thromboembolism is still unsolved among patients with SCI and consequent multisystem problems.[1]

Significant morbidity and mortality result from the occurrence of deep vein thrombosis and pulmonary embolism. Additionally, considerable long-term disability can result because patients with SCI have low rates of venous recanalization following deep vein thrombosis and are subject to greater than usual bleeding complications following prolonged anticoagulation therapy.

Very few studies have looked at the incidence of venous thromboembolism in cervical trauma and cervical cord injuries separately. Among spinal cord–injured patients, it is generally accepted that the level of injury and the degree of completeness do not affect venous thromboembolism risk. In the spinal cord–injured population as a whole, pulmonary embolism is the third most common cause of death in the first postinjury year. It has been calculated that for those with acute SCI, the risk for death as a result of pulmonary embolism is 210 times greater than that of the normal population in the acute period, declining to 19.1 times normal for years 2 to 5 and further declining to 8.9 times normal for those who survive more than 5 years.

In the following discussion, those who sustain cervical trauma without a neurologic deficit need to be distinguished from those who do develop motor sensory impairment. Both groups have an increased susceptibility to venous thromboembolism following the trauma, but in the latter group the risk is enhanced because of the added immobility and paralysis. That trauma patients are at an increased risk of venous thromboembolism has been recognized for almost 100 years following a description by the pathologist McCartney, who noted the association between patients with fractures and death from pulmonary embolism.

The incidence of venous thromboembolism after any spinal injury depends on the population being studied, the nature of the injuries, the prophylactic measures used, and the method used to detect it. In patients at risk following all injuries, the incidence of deep vein thrombosis ranges from 10% to 20%, with pulmonary embolism rates between 1% and 2%. Among patients with pulmonary embolism, the mortality may be as high as 20% to 50%. In a recent study on the incidence of venous thromboembolism among high-risk trauma patients, Geerts et al.[2] used venography between 7 and 21 days after injury to detect deep vein thrombosis. Of the 349 patients in the study, 58% had clots, 18% being proximal. Seven (2%) of the patients developed pulmonary embolism, which was fatal in 3 patients.

RISK FACTORS

A large study on risk factors for venous thromboembolism after trauma used the American College of Surgeons National Trauma Data Bank to identify 1602 patients from a pool of 450,375 patients with venous thromboembolism.[3] It can be seen from the risk factors and odds ratios that some factors such as number of ventilator-dependent days, venous injury, and presence of SCI carry more risk than others (Table 35.1).

Other factors that increase the risk for venous thromboembolism in the general population also increase the susceptibility of the traumatized and paralyzed patient to a venous thromboembolism episode. These include an episode of previous venous thromboembolism, immobilization, malignant disease, heart failure, myocardial infarction, leg paralysis, obesity, varicose veins, estrogens, and pregnancy. Inherited abnormalities that increase a patient's risk for venous thromboembolism include antithrombin III deficiency, protein C deficiency, protein S deficiency, and dysfibrinogenemia. Apart from these, a significant association has also been reported between heterotopic ossification, delayed commencement of thromboprophylaxis, and deep vein thrombosis in spinal cord–injured patients.

TABLE 35.1 Risk Factors for Venous Thromboembolism

Risk Factor	Number at Risk	Odds Ratio (95% CI)
Age >40	178,851	2.29 (2.07–2.55)
Pelvic fracture	2707	2.93 (2.01–4.27)
Lower extremity fracture	63,508	3.16 (2.85–3.51)
Spinal cord injury with paralysis	2852	3.39 (2.41–4.77)
Head injury (AIS >3)	52,197	2.59 (2.31–2.90)
Ventilator days >3	13,037	10.62 (9.32–12.11)
Venous injury	1450	7.93 (5.83–10.78)
Shock on admissions: BP <90	18,510	1.95 (1.62–2.34)
Major surgical procedure	73,974	4.32 (3.91–4.77)

Adapted from Knudson MM, Ikossi DG, Khaw L, et al. Thromboembolism after trauma: an analysis of 1602 episodes from the American College of Surgeons National Trauma Data Bank. *Ann Surg* 2004;240:490–496, discussion 496–498, with permission.

PATHOGENESIS

Venous thromboembolism occurs when the constant balance in the body between thrombogenic and thrombolytic systems is disrupted. Pulmonary emboli in the vast majority of patients arise from thrombi in the deep veins of the legs, most clinically significant emboli being from the popliteal or more proximal deep veins of the legs. Less common sources include deep pelvic veins and more central veins. Approximately half of the patients who develop a proximal deep vein thrombosis go on to develop pulmonary emboli, many of them asymptomatic and clinically nonsignificant. Conversely, about 50% to 70% of patients with an objectively detected pulmonary embolism can be shown to have detectable deep vein thrombosis of the legs at the time of presentation. Whether or not a pulmonary embolus causes significant symptoms depends on the size of the embolus and the cardiorespiratory reserve of the patient.

CLINICAL FEATURES

Untreated or inadequately treated deep vein thrombosis can evolve to a chronic stage of postthrombotic syndrome characterized by chronic edema, induration, pain, and skin ulceration. The clinical diagnosis of venous thrombosis is highly nonspecific because none of the signs or symptoms is unique and each may be caused by nonthrombotic disorders. The clinical features commonly associated with deep vein thrombosis are leg pain, tenderness and swelling, a palpable cord along the course of superficial veins, discoloration, venous distention and prominence of the superficial veins, cyanosis, and, rarely, phlegmasia cerulea dolens. The signs and symptoms do not always correlate with the site and extent of the deep vein thrombosis. Other conditions that mimic deep vein thrombosis include muscle strain, a fracture in the paralyzed limb, hematoma, muscle tear, cellulitis, lymphangitis, knee derangements, heterotopic ossification, and Baker cyst. Untreated or inadequately treated deep vein thrombosis can evolve to a chronic stage of postthrombotic syndrome characterized by chronic edema, induration, pain, and skin ulceration.

Similarly, pulmonary embolism may manifest in one of several ways, depending on the size, location, and number of emboli and the patient's ability to compensate for altered cardiac and respiratory function, outlined as follows:

1. Transient dyspnea and tachypnea
2. Pulmonary infarction or congestive atelectasis causing pleuritic chest pain, cough, hemoptysis, pleural effusion, and pulmonary infiltrates on chest radiographs
3. Right heart failure with severe dyspnea and tachypnea
4. Cardiovascular collapse with hypotension, syncope, and coma
5. Vague and nonspecific presentation that may include confusion, pyrexia, wheezing, and unexplained cardiac rhythm abnormalities

Many of these signs and symptoms are often associated with other conditions that are also common in the spine-injured patient, such as chest sepsis. Several studies have shown that in more than half of all patients with clinically suspected pulmonary embolism, the diagnosis cannot be confirmed by objective testing. It is therefore necessary to have objective evidence before confirming or excluding pulmonary embolism.

DIAGNOSIS OF DEEP VEIN THROMBOSIS

In most patients, deep vein thrombosis after trauma is silent and can easily be missed. Leg swelling may be attributed to one of the other differential diagnoses discussed earlier, and fever and hypoxia can have multiple reasons, pulmonary embolism being only one of them. A lot of effort has therefore been targeted at more accurate methods for detecting deep vein thrombosis and pulmonary embolism.

A formal protocol to test a patient's clinical pretest probability of having deep vein thrombosis is recommended. This helps in the choice of tests that need to be carried out. The Wells model of clinical pretest probability of deep vein thrombosis is in widespread use and has been recommended by the working group of the Institute for Clinical Systems Improvement.[4] The scale divides patients into low risk, moderate risk, and high risk for having deep vein thrombosis. In the high-risk group, which includes patients with cervical trauma and SCI, the negative predictive value of ultrasound was only 82%; it is recommended that in this group, even if the ultrasound findings are negative, further tests should be considered. The algorithms devised by the same working group are helpful in the further assessment of a patient with suspected deep vein thrombosis or pulmonary embolism. The various tests used in the detection of deep vein thrombosis have specific advantages and some drawbacks, which are minimized by using a combination of tests where appropriate (Table 35.2).

Elevated D-dimer levels have been associated with the development of venous thromboembolism in medical patients. However, D-dimers, which are breakdown products of fibrin, are also elevated following trauma, especially in the first 48 hours after injury. The use of D-dimers as a screening tool in the trauma population has been questioned by studies that have shown poor correlation between D-dimer levels and the presence or absence of venous thromboembolism in the first few days following an injury. Wahl et al.[5] demonstrated that in the acute trauma population, the negative predictive value of a D-dimer test is only 92% but rises to 100% after 4 days and that the positive predictive value is 17%. It may, therefore, have a role following the acute period. A further confounding factor in the spinal cord–injured population is the persistent low level of systemic inflammation related to chest infections, tracheostomies, bacteruria consequent to introduction of intermittent or indwelling catheters, etc., and the effect that this may have on D-dimer levels. Algorithms developed for medical patients in a general hospital setting that use a combination of pretest probability scores and D-dimer levels have been shown to have a negative predictive value approaching 100, which implies that no episode of deep vein thrombosis is likely to be missed. These, however, are unlikely to be of great use in the recently spine-injured or traumatized patient because of the high false positivity rates.

Venography is considered the gold standard for detection of deep vein thrombosis, but its routine use is impractical because it is an invasive test that is expensive, time consuming, and technically

TABLE 35.2 Model of the Clinical Pretest Probability of Deep Vein Thrombosis

Score	Risk Factors
1	Active cancer (treatment ongoing or within previous 6 months or palliative)
1	Paralysis, paresis, or recent plaster immobilization of lower extremity
1	Recently bedridden for more than 3 days or major surgery within 4 weeks
1	Localized tenderness along the distribution of the deep venous system
1	Entire leg swollen
1	Calf swollen by more than 3 cm compared to asymptomatic leg (measured 10 cm below tibial tuberosity)
1	Pitting edema (greater in the symptomatic leg)
1	Collateral superficial veins (nonvaricose)
−2	Alternative diagnosis as likely or greater than that of deep vein thrombosis
If both legs are symptomatic, score the more severe side.	
High risk = scored 3 or more, moderate risk = 1 or 2, low risk = 0 or less	

Institute for Clinical Systems Improvement. Venous thromboembolism guidelines. April 2005. Available at: http:www.icsi.org.

exacting and cannot be used in all patients. Further, it is accompanied by a relatively high incidence of adverse effects, such as postvenographic phlebitis and allergic reactions. Gunduz et al.[6] reported as much as a 10% incidence of adverse sequelae following venography. Also, up to 10% of patients develop proven deep vein thrombosis after a negative venogram, either because the venogram initially missed seeing the deep vein thrombosis or because the contrast itself triggered deep vein thrombosis by causing endothelial injury. Extravasation into the dorsum of the foot and sloughing of tissue have also been reported. When used for diagnosis of deep vein thrombosis, the finding of a fully occlusive lesion or an outlined filling defect is conclusively positive, but a negative interpretation has less predictive power.

Radiolabeled fibrinogen scanning is very sensitive, but not specific. Todd et al.[7] found that fibrinogen scanning was positive in all of their patients, but the diagnosis of deep vein thrombosis was confirmed by another test in only half of the cases. Radiolabeled fibrinogen scanning is no longer employed routinely because it can take several days to yield results and also because fibrinogen is a human blood product with an unavoidable infection risk.

Color flow Duplex ultrasound is B mode ultrasound in which Doppler sampling is used to color code regions of the display based on flow direction and velocity or volume. It is noninvasive and has replaced venography as the initial imaging method of choice for patients with suspected lower extremity deep vein thrombosis. The drawback is that the test is neither as sensitive nor as specific as contrast venography. Veins that are normal compress easily under the pressure of the transducer head, whereas those containing thrombus resist compression. This difference in compressibility is exploited in the detection of a venous thrombus. The test is less useful below the popliteal trifurcation and above the saphenofemoral junction. The advantage of the test is that it is easy to perform and can be repeated as often as required, thus making it a good surveillance tool.[8] To conclude that a scan is negative requires centimeter-by-centimeter compression testing of the deep venous system, which can be time consuming and challenging.

Overall, no single test is completely applicable, accurate, and sensitive for the detection of deep vein thrombosis in the SCI population. The Consortium for Spinal Cord Medicine recommendations are that ultrasound be used for the study of patients with suspected deep vein thrombosis and venography be reserved for use when clinical suspicion is strong and the ultrasound examination findings are negative (Fig. 35.1).[9]

DIAGNOSIS OF PULMONARY EMBOLISM

The diagnosis of pulmonary embolism, much like the diagnosis of deep vein thrombosis, requires clinical suspicion combined with the careful interpretation of the results of objective tests. Arterial blood oxygen levels, alveolar arterial oxygen gradients, and pulse oximetry have no discriminative value in the diagnosis of pulmonary embolism, because patients may have other reasons for impaired gas exchange. Chest radiographs are also nonspecific and insensitive for pulmonary thromboembolism.

As in the case of suspected deep vein thrombosis, application of a formal protocol to determine the pretest probability of having a pulmonary embolism is helpful in determining the probability and in guiding subsequent investigative workup. Figure 35.1 outlines the Wells model for predicting clinical pretest probability for pulmonary embolism.

In patients with proven pulmonary embolism, an echocardiogram should be considered because the presence of right-sided heart strain is a strong predictor for subsequent death.

Ventilation-perfusion scanning of the lung is a relatively simple and noninvasive test that, unfortunately, is nondiagnostic in many patients. It is still used widely as the initial study of choice in many centers. If an embolus is present, it is seen as a perfusion defect in the affected area as opposed to the even distribution of blood flow from side to side and top to bottom that is seen in the normal lung. Small thrombi may not cause a defect, and even large or massive emboli may not be detected

Deep Vein Thrombosis (DVT) Diagnosis Algorithm

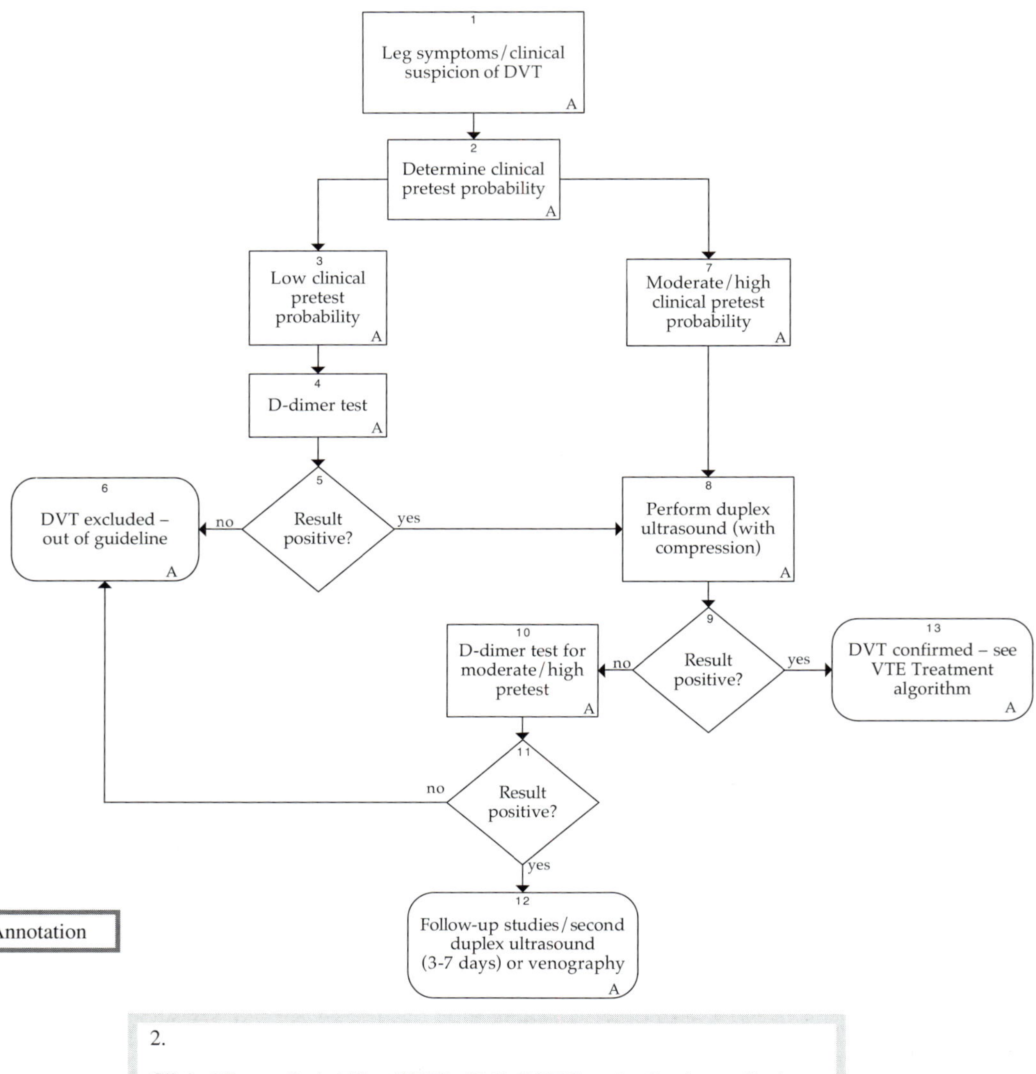

2.

Clinical Pretest Probability (CPTP - Wells DVT Score) – See Appendix A

Active cancer (on treatment for last 6 months or palliative)	1
Paralysis, paresis or plaster immobilization of lower limb	1
Immobilization previous 4 days	1
Entire leg swollen	1
Calf swollen by more than 3 cm	1
Pitting edema	1
Collateral superficial veins (non-varicose)	1
Probable alternative diagnosis	- 2

High DVT Risk = 3+
Moderate DVT Risk = 1-2
Low DVT Risk = < 1

If both legs are symptomatic, score the more severe leg.

FIGURE 35.1. Deep vein thrombosis diagnostic algorithm.[2] (Copyright 2009 by ICSI. Used with permission.)

if they are incompletely obstructing and do not asymmetrically sufficiently decrease regional perfusion to be detected on a perfusion scan (Fig. 35.2).

Pathologic processes other than pulmonary embolism, such as consolidation, can also cause perfusion defects. Ventilation scans when done in combination with perfusion scans increase the specificity but not the sensitivity of abnormal perfusion scans. Initially pulmonary embolism causes an area of blocked perfusion and normal ventilation—a V/Q mismatch. A ventilation defect smaller than the perfusion defect is more consistent with pulmonary embolism than with intrinsic pulmonary

Pulmonary Embolism Diagnosis Algorithm

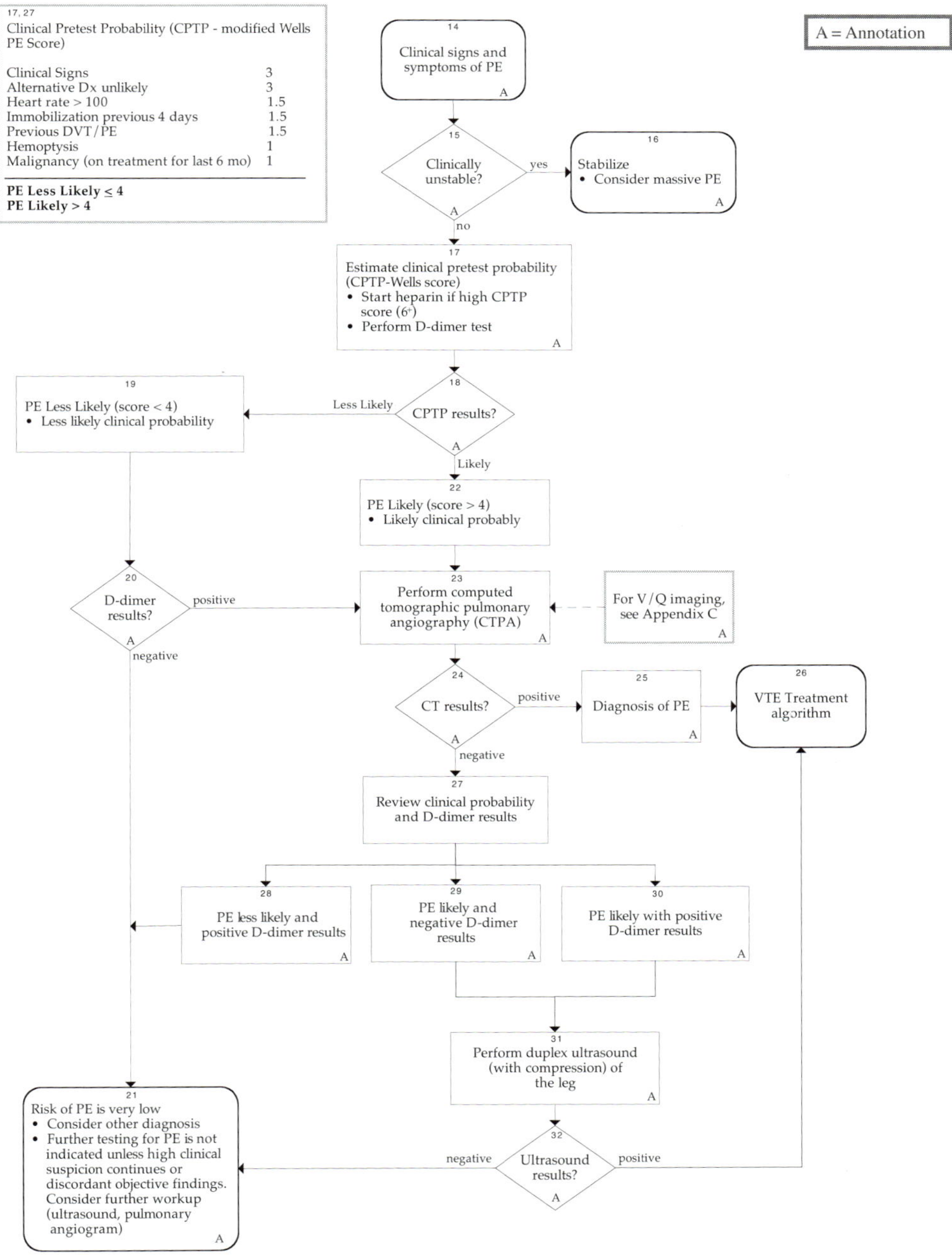

FIGURE 35.2. Pulmonary embolism diagnostic algorithm. (Copyright 2009 by ICSI. Used with permission.)

diseases. The V/Q scan is a relatively insensitive and nonspecific test, and excessive reliance should not be placed on the scan patterns. Further tests should be arranged where the scans are indeterminate and there is a high clinical probability of pulmonary embolism.

Pulmonary angiography is a reliable but invasive test for PE. A dye cutoff or a filling defect is confirmatory for pulmonary embolism in the appropriate clinical setting. Although it has for long been generally accepted as the gold standard in the diagnosis of pulmonary embolism, it is not infallible and may falsely diagnose pulmonary embolism in the presence of an intraluminal tumor or intraluminal mass. It may give a false-negative result when the thrombi are small and distal. When performed carefully, a positive pulmonary angiogram provides virtually 100% certainty that an obstruction to the pulmonary arterial blood flow does exist, and a negative pulmonary angiogram provides greater than 90% certainty in the exclusion of pulmonary embolism.

Many centers have now abandoned the use of these techniques in favor of computed tomography (CT) angiography of the pulmonary tree for the primary detection of a pulmonary embolism. The advantages of the technique as follows:

1. The spiral scanning technique is very rapid, and the entire lung can be imaged while the patient holds a breath.
2. It is relatively noninvasive and can be performed during the first pass of an injected bolus of venous contrast.
3. Enhancement of the obtained image is possible.
4. Other diagnoses can be established or excluded based on the evidence provided by the scan.

CT pulmonary angiography has high specificity and sensitivity for central clots, but specificity and sensitivity drop substantially for peripheral clots. The right protocols for acquisition of the image and the right technical equipment are very important for obtaining high-quality images. With improved techniques, familiarity, and equipment, the ability to exclude peripheral clots is increasing, but clinical probability must guide the decision to pursue further testing.

THROMBOPROPHYLAXIS IN CERVICAL SPINE TRAUMA

Patients with cervical spine injuries are a high-risk group for venous thromboembolism, which has been borne out by the extremely high incidence of deep vein thrombosis and pulmonary embolism in this group in various studies. It is important, therefore, that preventive strategies be adopted from the outset to minimize the occurrence of this complication. The strategies for venous thromboembolism prevention can be broadly divided into pharmacologic and mechanical measures. The best results are obtained when the two strategies are applied in combination (Table 35.3).

Some mechanical modalities are effective in reducing the incidence of deep vein thrombosis in acute SCI. These work by improving lower extremity venous return, which reduces stasis, an important cause for thrombus development in this population. Active and passive motion, centripetal massage, and rotating treatment tables have all been shown in limited studies to be of some benefit in reducing the incidence of deep vein thrombosis. These are relatively easy to carry out after the acute period and are associated with very few side effects.

Gradient elastic stockings reduce venous capacitance by applying a uniform distribution of pressure over the extremity. There are no studies demonstrating a difference in the incidence of deep vein thrombosis with thigh length versus calf length gradient elastic stockings. Complications with their use are rare, but can include peripheral neuropathy and skin problems when the stockings are not applied properly. Good fit can be a problem in obese patients. Electrical stimulation is a modality that works by stimulating dorsiflexors and plantar flexors of the ankle at a preset frequency for most of the day. It is not widely used in routine practice because the stimulation is painful in sensate patients and difficult in patients with lower extremity edema. Technical difficulties with equipment maintenance can also be a problem. External pneumatic compression is an effective way of augmenting lower extremity venous return and is popular in the acute phase. The external sleeves come in

TABLE 35.3 Deep Vein Thrombosis and Pulmonary Embolism Prophylaxis

Mechanical strategies
- Frequent turns, early mobilization
- Graduated elastic stockings
- Electrical stimulation
- Venous pump
- Intermittent external pneumatic compression

Pharmacologic strategies
- Unfractionated heparin, fixed or adjusted dose
- Low molecular weight heparin: enoxaparin, dalteparin
- Warfarin, other vitamin K antagonists
- Newer agents: fondaparinux, direct thrombin inhibitors

Vena caval filters

Patient education, information, general measures

both thigh length and calf length, and the mode of compression may be either graded sequential, multicompartmental uniform, or single-chamber uniform pressures. Although the multichambered sequential pressure devices show improved flow velocity, flow rate, shear stress, residual volume, and stimulation of fibrinolysis, they have not been demonstrated to be superior in clinical use. Combining external pneumatic compression pumps with gradient elastic stockings has a summative beneficial effect. Venous foot pumps are devices that act by rapidly flattening the plantar arches and increasing venous return. Experience with its use in patients with SCI is lacking.

ANTICOAGULANT PROPHYLAXIS

The results from currently available studies and the very high incidence of deep vein thrombosis and pulmonary embolism following SCI support the use of routine thromboprophylaxis in all patients with SCI. This should be started as early as possible, once primary hemostasis has been achieved. Where there is concern about bleeding at the injury site or elsewhere, mechanical prophylaxis as discussed previously should be started as soon as possible after hospital admission and anticoagulant prophylaxis initiated once the bleeding risk has decreased.[2] Mechanical thromboprophylaxis alone, however, is inadequate once the risk for bleeding has passed. The best results are obtained when mechanical prophylaxis is combined with pharmacologic anticoagulation. Pharmacologic options for the prevention of venous thromboembolism in patients with SCI include oral anticoagulants, unfractionated heparin, and low molecular weight heparin. Oral agents are impractical in patients with acute SCI because of the delayed and unpredictable onset of effective anticoagulation and the need for frequent laboratory monitoring. Unfractionated heparin has been the drug used historically in prophylaxis, but recent evidence suggests that low molecular weight heparin is more efficacious. In a comparison of enoxaparin 30 mg twice daily and low-dose unfractionated heparin in SCI initiated within 36 hours of the injury, Geerts et al.[2] demonstrated that there was a significantly higher incidence of venous thromboembolic episodes with unfractionated heparin. Further, the incidence of complications such as bleeding and heparin-induced thrombocytopenia was also higher. Others have shown that adjusted-dose heparin is more effective than fixed low-dose heparin and that tinzaparin, a low molecular weight heparin, is better at preventing thromboembolism than a high fixed dose of unfractionated heparin. Large studies in other surgical patient populations have not, however, demonstrated a difference in efficacy between low molecular weight heparins and unfractionated heparin, although there was a tendency toward fewer bleeding complications with the low molecular weight heparins. The dosage that is commonly used is 30 mg twice daily of enoxaparin or equivalent. The low molecular weight heparins are all smaller molecules than unfractionated heparin, but they differ in their molecular structure. Their efficacy in preventing venous thrombosis and their bleeding complications may not be equivalent. In a prospective comparison of enoxaparin 30 mg twice daily and dalteparin 5000 units daily among spinal cord–injured patients, Chiou-Tan et al.[10] found no difference in efficacy or bleeding rates between them. However, dalteparin was more cost-effective and patients expressed a preference for the once-daily dosing. There is less evidence available for the use of other low molecular weight heparins in the traumatized patient. The recommendations from the Consortium for Spinal Cord Medicine are that either low molecular weight heparin or adjusted-dose unfractionated heparin should be started as soon as possible, preferably within 72 hours of the injury in the absence of active bleeding or coagulopathy. Aspirin is not recommended for use in thromboprophylaxis.

Patients with SCI remain at risk for thromboembolism even after the acute phase. The duration of prophylaxis after SCI is controversial and has to some extent remained arbitrary. The risk for thromboembolism decreases in the medium and long term; the reason for this is unclear in paralyzed patients, in whom the risk related to paralysis and immobility continues to operate. Many practitioners continue anticoagulation for a period of 3 months or more following the injury. This may be done either with low molecular weight heparin or an oral vitamin K antagonist such as warfarin. If the latter is used, the international normalized ratio (INR) should be maintained around 2.5 (range 2 to 3). Some evidence exists to suggest that use of warfarin to maintain a therapeutic INR range may be associated with a reduced incidence of venous thromboembolism, but can result in a greater number of bleeding-related complications because of the greater degree of anticoagulation.

A decision to prolong therapy beyond 3 months should be individualized based on the need, medical condition, functional status, support services, and risk level of the patient. Factors such as limited participation in therapy programs, recurrent infections, heterotopic ossification, or history of thromboembolism may require that therapy be continued beyond 3 months. A rebound increase in the incidence of venous thromboembolism has also been observed in some studies following the discontinuation of anticoagulation.

General measures such as comprehensive patient education, exercise, weight loss, cessation of smoking, good elastic support, avoidance of constricting garters, leg bag straps, etc., should be adequately emphasized and should be an integral part of the prevention program.

The insertion of inferior vena caval filters has been advocated by some investigators. These devices are unlikely to be necessary when appropriate prophylaxis is used.[11] Their use is associated with complications and significant financial cost. However, they may have a role in patients who cannot undergo anticoagulation therapy because of concerns regarding bleeding or in the setting of a failure of prophylaxis. Although filters are highly effective in preventing pulmonary embolism, complications are associated with filter placement, including the induction of deep vein thrombosis, filter migration, and filter tilt, which may precipitate pulmonary embolism and caval thrombosis. Even with temporary filter placements, problems can be encountered with their removal, and concerns also exist about clot dislodgement and subsequent pulmonary embolism during removal.

TREATMENT OF DEEP VEIN THROMBOSIS AND PULMONARY EMBOLISM

General hospital treatment protocols in use for all patients should be used. Patients should be commenced on a full therapeutic dose of heparin or low molecular weight heparin if there is a strong suspicion of a thromboembolic episode. Once the diagnosis has been confirmed, they should be switched to an oral vitamin K antagonist and heparin maintained until therapeutic levels of anticoagulation have been achieved (INR >2). The period of anticoagulation required is a matter of debate, but a period of 6 months is the norm. In the event of a second thromboembolic episode, strong consideration should be given to lifelong treatment. Thrombolytics and surgical embolectomy have been advocated in the setting of a massive pulmonary embolism, but the rationale for these and their indications are beyond the scope of this chapter.

EMERGING STRATEGIES

Despite the best available surveillance and treatment, the incidence of venous thromboembolism has not decreased dramatically. To reduce mortality and morbidity and to reduce costs, the occurrence of venous thromboembolism must be reduced further. New drugs and strategies, including drugs that target other steps in the coagulation pathway, are being tested with this in mind. Fondaparinux is a nonheparin pentasaccharide compound structurally identical to the antithrombin III binding site of heparin, and thus exhibits selective antithrombin III–mediated inhibition of factor Xa. It has demonstrated a greater ability to reduce recurrent venous thromboembolism in large orthopaedic trials than enoxaparin and has less effect on the immune system, which may be a desirable property when used in patients who are at risk for multiorgan failure and sepsis. It also does not seem to induce heparin-induced thrombocytopenia. Idraparinux is a drug that can be injected subcutaneously once weekly and is being tried as a replacement for warfarin. Other drugs that directly inhibit thrombin are undergoing evaluation in the elective orthopaedic population, including recombinant hirudin, hirulog, melagatran, and the oral agent ximelagatran. Initial data suggest that they are more effective than enoxaparin and they, like enoxaparin, do not require blood monitoring. Their role in the trauma population is yet to be defined.

New techniques are also being investigated in the diagnosis of venous thromboembolism. Magnetic resonance angiographic techniques with and without enhancement are being tested in the diagnosis of both deep vein thrombosis and pulmonary embolism. Although these have not reached the point of being accepted into regular clinical practice, it is an area that holds a lot of promise. Magnetic resonance angiography will do away with the need for iodine-based contrast dyes and will also reduce radiation exposure.

REFERENCES

1. Spinal Cord Injury Thromboprophylaxis Investigators. Prevention of venous thromboembolism in the acute treatment phase after spinal cord injury: a randomized, multicenter trial comparing low-dose heparin plus intermittent pneumatic compression with enoxaparin. *J Trauma* 2003,54:1116–1126.
2. Geerts WH, Pineo GF, Heit JA, et al. Prevention of venous thromboembolism: the Seventh ACCP Conference on Antithrombotic and Thrombolytic Therapy. *Chest* 2004;126(suppl 3):S338S–S400 [review].
3. Knudson MM, Ikossi DG, Khaw L, et al. Thromboembolism after trauma: an analysis of 1602 episodes from the American College of Surgeons National Trauma Data Bank. *Ann Surg* 2004;240:490–496, discussion 496–498.
4. Institute for Clinical Systems Improvement. Venous thromboembolism guidelines. April 2005. Available at: http:www.icsi.org.
5. Wahl WL, Ahrns KS, Zajkowski PJ, et al. Normal D-dimer levels do not exclude thrombotic complications in trauma patients. *Surgery* 2003;134(4):529–532, discussion 532–533.
6. Gündüz S, Oğur E, Möhür H, et al. Deep vein thrombosis in spinal cord injured patients. *Paraplegia* 1993;31(9):606–610.
7. Todd JW, Frisbie JH, Rossier AB, et al. Deep vein thrombosis in acute spinal cord injury: a comparison of 1251 fibrinogen leg scanning, impedance plethysmography and venography. *Paraplegia* 1976;14(1):50–57.
8. Kadyan V, Clinchot DM, Colachis SC. Cost-effectiveness of duplex ultrasound surveillance in spinal cord injury. *Am J Phys Med Rehabil* 2004,83:191–197.
9. Consortium for Spinal Cord Medicine. Clinical Practice Guidelines: Prevention of Thromboembolism in Spinal Cord Injury, 2nd ed. Washington, DC: Consortium for Spinal Cord Medicine, 1999.
10. Chiou-Tan FY, Garza H, Chan KT, et al. Comparison of dalteparin and enoxaparin for deep venous thrombosis prophylaxis in patients with spinal cord injury. *Am J Phys Med Rehabil* 2003;82:678–685.
11. Anonymous. Deep venous thrombosis and thromboembolism in patients with cervical spinal cord injuries. *Neurosurgery* 2002;50(suppl 3):S73–S80 [review].

CHAPTER 36

Surgery-Related Neurologic Deterioration

John E. O'Toole, Kurt M. Eichholz, Russ P. Nockels, and Richard G. Fessler

INTRODUCTION

Neurologic deterioration after spinal cord injury (SCI) affects approximately 1.8% to 10% of spinal cord–injured patients.[1–5] Risk factors for neurologic decline include traction and halo application, ankylosing spondylitis, vertebral artery injury, and intubation.[1,2,4,5] Neurologic complications related directly to surgery for spinal trauma make up only a portion of these cases. Nevertheless, some of the causes are preventable, and awareness of the causes, manifestations, diagnoses, and treatments for these complications may reduce morbidity and enhance outcomes in this unfortunate patient population.

HISTORICAL CONTEXT

The history of spinal surgery provides the modern surgeon with some perspective on neurologic complications associated with trauma surgery. Until the nineteenth century, the surgical treatment of spinal trauma relied almost exclusively on external reduction techniques. Paul of Aegina in the seventh century AD was the sole exception in performing the first recorded procedure for SCI: a laminectomy for spinal cord compression after spinal fracture.[6] Hippocrates popularized the use of prone distraction frames and orthogonal force application on the apex of deformities, in what would presage the three-point bending moments of internal fixation devices.[7,8] As one might expect, however, neurologic outcomes and treatment complications for patients with spinal trauma remained grim.

The nineteenth century saw more frequent attempts at posterior decompressions, but mortality often was reported to be as high as 100%.[7] The first attempts at open interspinous wiring began in the late nineteenth century,[8] and in 1911 Albee[9] and Hibbs[10] introduced bone grafting into spinal surgery. Despite these advances, a majority of the patients who survived went on to suffer neurologic decline from progressive kyphosis.

The latter half of the twentieth century brought the advent of reliable internal spinal fixation devices, including anterior cervical plates and dorsal cervical fixation systems that over time have dramatically reduced progressive spinal deformity by permitting successful fusion.[11] This, in conjunction with better imaging techniques, operative instruments, and perioperative care, has allowed spinal surgeons to offer treatments for spinal trauma with the relatively low rates of iatrogenic injury that we witness today.

TIMING OF NEUROLOGIC DETERIORATION

Neurologic decline in the surgically treated patient with cervical spine trauma can be categorized in terms of cause (mechanical injury, vascular alterations, spinal instability, and intrinsic cord changes) or in terms of pathoanatomy (primary spinal cord versus root injury). However, it may be most helpful to think of surgery-related neurologic deterioration within a framework of the timing of the decline relative to surgical intervention (Table 36.1).

INTRAOPERATIVE CAUSES

Anesthesia-Related Causes

Neurologic injury may occur during any of the typical anesthesia-related events that prepare the cervical spine trauma patient for surgery. Forced hyperextension or hyperflexion of the neck during intubation or during positioning may lead to spinal cord compression. Fiberoptic intubations should prevent injurious head movements, and prepositioning and postpositioning somatosensory and motor evoked potential monitoring may detect spinal cord impingement because of head

TABLE 36.1 Timing and Causes of Postoperative Neurologic Deterioration

Intraoperative
Anesthesia-related complications
Intubation
Positioning
Hypotension
Reduction-related complications
Disc herniation
Epidural hematoma
Technique-related complications
Technical errors
Hardware misplacement
Approach-related
Postoperative
Immediate
Epidural hematoma
Reduction-related disc herniation or hematoma
Graft extrusion
Early delayed
Hypotension
Spinal instability, graft, hardware complications
Venous thrombosis or congestion
Hyperperfusion and reperfusion injury
Subacute posttraumatic ascending myelopathy
C5 radiculopathy
Late delayed
Spinal instability
Syrinx formation
Adjacent-level disease

position that can be reversed before initiating surgery.[12] Perhaps the most critical anesthetic factor during surgery is the maintenance of blood pressure.[4] Many of the primary and secondary mechanisms of SCI are caused or exacerbated by vascular ischemia or congestion.[1,13] The *Guidelines for the Management of Acute Cervical Spine and Spinal Cord Injuries* (hereafter *The Guidelines*) recommends at the Option level that systolic blood pressures less than 90 mm Hg should be avoided and that mean arterial blood pressure at 85 to 90 mm Hg should be sustained for the first 7 days after SCI.[14] This proves even more essential, and difficult, in the patient with multi–organ system trauma.

Reduction-Related Causes

Both closed and open attempts at reduction of traumatic spinal deformities have been associated with neurologic injury. This is most often a concern in the patient with a subaxial cervical fracture-dislocation and associated disc herniation, but neurologic deterioration has also been reported with external immobilization of a hangman fracture with a concomitant large ventral epidural hematoma that required operative decompression.[15] Although ideal management remains controversial, *The Guidelines* found that the permanent neurologic complication rate for closed reduction is 1% or less and the rate of transient deficits is 2% to 4%.[16] Although disc herniations may be seen in as many as half of all prereduction magnetic resonance imaging scans, no consistent correlation has been demonstrated between their radiographic presence and postreduction neurologic deterioration.[16] Therefore, *The Guidelines* recommend, at the Option level, early closed reduction in awake patients, prereduction MRI in patients whose examination cannot be followed, MRI for closed reduction failures, and no closed reduction in patients with an additional rostral injury.[16]

Technique-Related Causes

Precise neurologic complication rates resulting from surgical technique are difficult to glean from the literature.[17] In general, however, there seems to be approximately a 0.5% to 2% risk for direct surgical injury to the spinal cord or roots during cervical spine operations.[17–19] Radiculopathy and/or myelopathy may be caused by placement of instruments into a tight cervical canal or foramen that has not been decompressed, use of monopolar cautery near neural elements, unshielded drilling near neural elements, and inadequate visualization of anatomical structures.[18,20,21]

Intraoperative misplacement of instrumentation is another cause of neurologic decline. Although rare, excessively long screws in anterior cervical plating may penetrate the spinal canal and cord. This may be avoided by choosing screw length accurately from intraoperative fluoroscopy (e.g., by comparing the length of Caspar distraction posts to the depth of the vertebral body) and by using active fluoroscopy during placement of bicortical screws when indicated. Careful measurement of potential screw length can also be made off a lateral plain radiography once consideration for magnification is taken into account. Dorsal cervical wiring techniques, both sublaminar and interspinous, have been associated with a 1% to 17% neurologic complication rate resulting from encroachment on the spinal canal.[18,22,23] They have generally been abandoned in the subaxial spine and have been replaced with stranded, flexible cables in occipitocervical and atlantoaxial applications. Lateral mass screw placement may threaten the exiting nerve roots (manifesting as radiculopathy) or the vertebral artery (manifesting as posterior circulation ischemia or stroke). Heller et al.[24] demonstrated a 0.6% per screw nerve root injury rate and a 0% vertebral artery injury rate in 78 consecutive patients undergoing lateral mass fixation. These neurovascular violations may be avoided by careful selection of screw entry point and sufficiently superior trajectory to avoid the nerve root and lateral trajectory to avoid the vertebral artery.[18,24,25]

Individual surgical approaches to the cervical spine each carry unique risks for neurologic injury. Beginning at the craniocervical junction, particularly during lateral exposures, the lower cranial nerves, medulla, vertebral artery, and spinal cord may be damaged by excessive manipulation or by other mechanical or thermal disruption.

Dorsal approaches to the atlantoaxial complex carry increased risk for SCI in the presence of preoperative myelopathy, irreducible dislocation, or significant instability.[23] Specific complications from C1-C2 fixation include occipital neuralgia and numbness, hypoglossal injury, and vertebral artery laceration or occlusion (Fig. 36.1). The hypoglossal nerve runs ventral to the arch of C1 and approximately 2 to 3 mm lateral to the center of the lateral mass.[26] Therefore, proper medial angulation of screw trajectory, bicortical purchase of the C1 anterior arch, and avoidance of

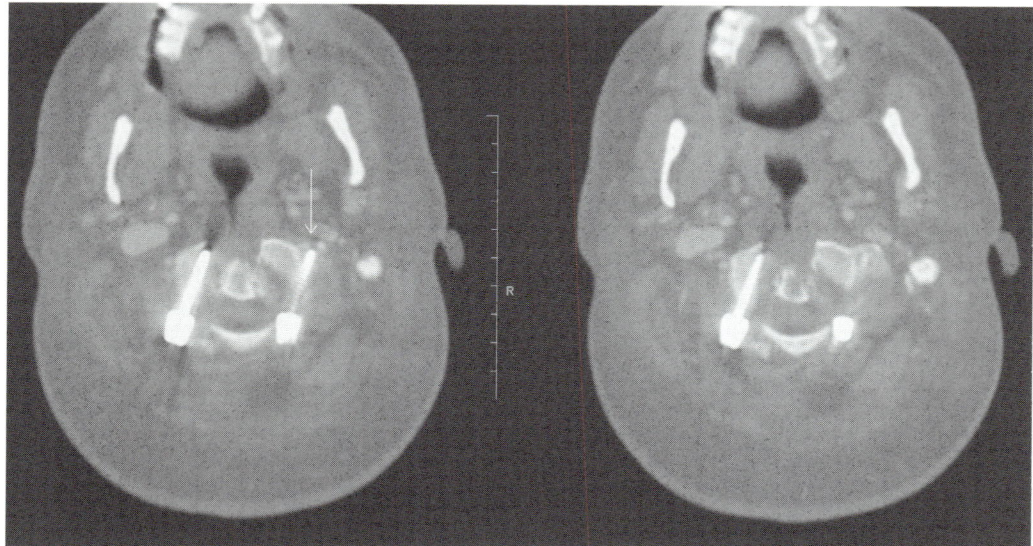

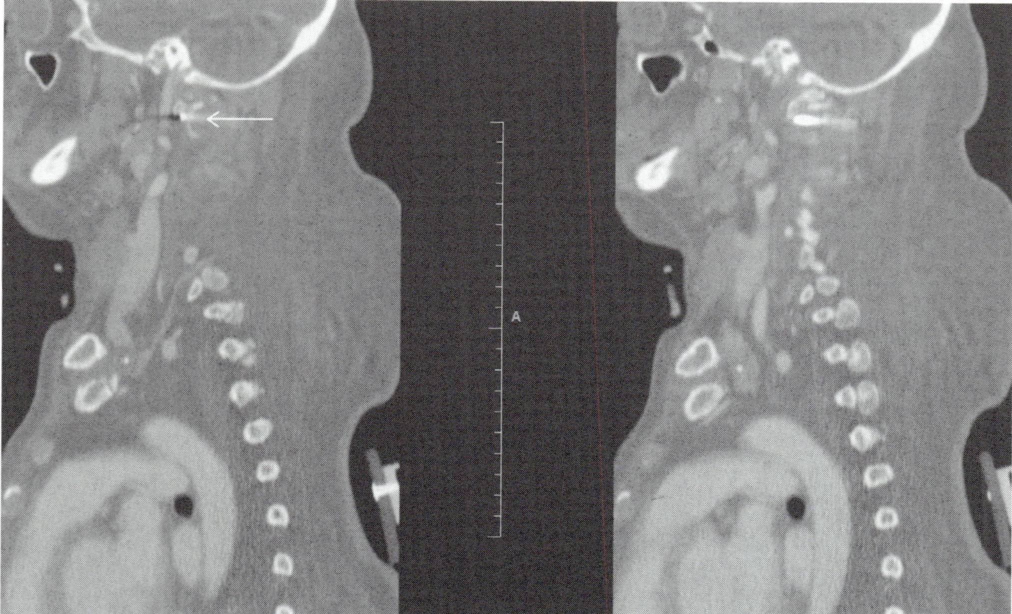

FIGURE 36.1. A. Axial computed tomography (CT) scan demonstrating errant placement of a C1 lateral mass screw into the left foramen transversarium *(arrow)*. **B.** Sagittal CT reconstruction after contrast injection demonstrates patency of the vertebral artery *(arrow)* despite the presence of the screw in the foramen transversarium.

excessive screw length should prevent this complication. With regard to vertebral artery injury, up to 18% of patients will have at least unilaterally unfavorable anatomy for transarticular screw placement.[18,27] Wright and Lauryssen[28] in their survey of American Association of Neurological Surgeons (AANS)/Congress of Neurological Surgeons (CNS) members on C1-C2 transarticular screw fixation found a 2.2% per screw risk of vertebral injury, but only 3.7% of these patients suffered neurologic deficits. This translated into a 0.1% per screw risk of neurologic deficit and 0.1% risk of death.[28] If brisk bleeding is encountered after drilling or tapping the screw path, most authors advocate insertion of the screw or simply packing the hole to tamponade bleeding from what is likely an unsalvageable artery.[29,30] Furthermore, if a vertebral artery laceration is suspected on placement of the first transarticular screw, no attempt should be made to place one on the contralateral side, in order to avoid bilateral injury.[31] Symptomatic vertebral artery injuries should be evaluated with emergent angiography and balloon occlusion followed by intensive care unit monitoring and hemodynamic support. The treatment of asymptomatic injuries is less well defined, but in most cases careful observation suffices[28] after angiographic evaluation to rule out pseudoaneurysm formation that might require anticoagulation and eventual endovascular obliteration.[32] Of note, follow-up evaluation by conventional or computed tomography (CT) angiography has been reported to reveal delayed arteriovenous fistula formation necessitating endovascular treatment.[30]

Ventral approaches to the cervical spine carry the unique risks for injury to critical peripheral nervous structures. These include the superior laryngeal nerve running obliquely across the field deep to the superior thyroid artery at the C3-C4 level; the recurrent laryngeal nerve on the right side coursing medially in the field in the tracheoesophageal groove at the C6-C7 level; and the sympathetic chain running along the lateral surface of the longus colli muscle (Fig. 36.2). The hoarseness accompanying damage to the laryngeal nerves recovers within several months in the majority of cases. Injury to the sympathetic chain producing Horner syndrome also most often resolves with time.

Dorsal approaches to the subaxial cervical spine carry the risks for positioning, hypotension, and technical errors as discussed earlier. In addition, "uneven" operative decompressions of stenotic

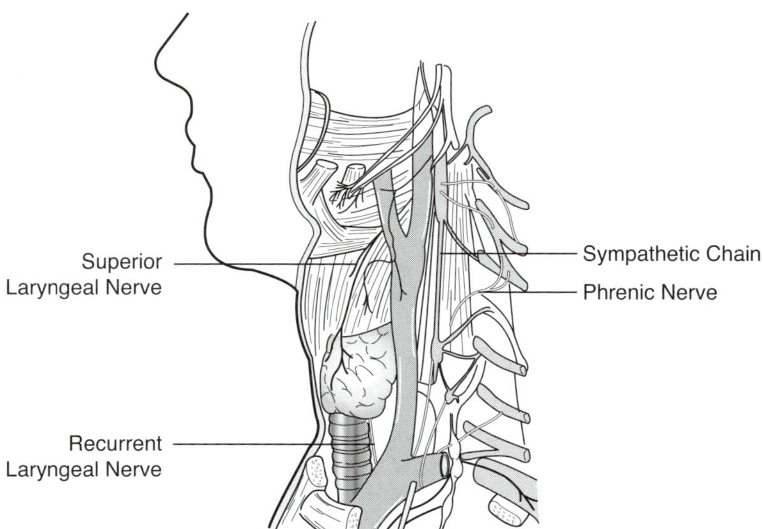

FIGURE 36.2. Anatomic drawing depicting the relationships of the relevant peripheral nerves of the neck that may be encountered during anterior cervical approaches.

segments as described by Yonenobu et al.[19] may also predispose to intraoperative cervical SCI. Posterior decompressions that are neither wide nor long enough may produce focal constrictions or "kinking" of the spinal cord, producing iatrogenic myelopathy.[18,33] Preoperative surgical planning must take into account the extent of bony removal beyond focal points of compression to avoid this complication.

Postoperative Causes

Neurologic deterioration in the postoperative period can further be divided into events that occur immediately (within hours), in an early delayed fashion (hours to weeks), and in a late delayed fashion (weeks to years).

Immediate. One of the most dreaded postoperative complications in cervical spine surgery is the development of an epidural hematoma at the operative site. Usually manifesting within hours or at most 1 to 2 days, neurologic deterioration can be rapid and dramatic from spinal cord compression.[34] With hematomas from anterior cervical approaches, neurologic symptoms may be preceded by dysphagia, Horner syndrome, and, most important, airway obstruction, necessitating intubation or emergent tracheotomy. An acute clinical decline requires emergent hematoma evacuation either at the bedside or on rapid return to the operating room. More gradual changes in examination findings may allow for urgent radiographs, CT, or MRI to determine the reason for the clinical change. Obviously, careful attention to hemostasis and the judicious use of closed-suction drainage help avoid these problems

As mentioned previously, reduction-related disc herniation or hematoma, although rare, may produce acute neurologic deficits. Posttraumatic epidural hematomas are reported to occur in 0.5% to 7.5% of spinal fractures.[15] The clinical changes associated with these lesions warrant immediate radiologic investigation and appropriate decompression.

Acute graft extrusion within the first 24 hours after anterior cervical reconstruction may cause significant cord injury but has become much less common with the routine use of anterior instrumentation systems.[35] Careful graft selection and endplate preparation also serve to prevent this complication that requires immediate reoperation.

Early Delayed. As mentioned at the outset, neurologic deterioration in the subacute period is a recognized problem in patients with spinal trauma. Although often attributed to instability,[1,36] spinal cord dysfunction in the first several days to weeks after injury has many possible causes, both spontaneous and iatrogenic.

Sustained hypotension postoperatively (as intraoperatively) places the patient with spinal trauma at increased risk for ischemic SCI. Because of the sensitivity of the gray matter to impaired perfusion, this typically manifests as a central cord syndrome,[1,13] which can take a few days to clinically evolve.[37] Again, *The Guidelines* recommend that mean arterial blood pressure should be maintained at 85 to 90 mm Hg for 7 days after injury to maintain adequate cord perfusion.[38]

Spinal instability from graft and hardware complications remains a concern in this period as well, particularly as patients begin to be mobilized. Unrealistic expectations for implants or unrecognized deficiencies in nonfixated columns of the spine may lead to graft collapse or extrusion and hardware pullout or fracture, any of which may produce compression of neural elements. Careful reconstructive techniques and adjunctive external rigid immobilization may reduce the frequency of these adverse events.

Infectious, inflammatory, and vascular events not directly related to surgery may also produce neurologic deterioration in the postoperative patient. For example, venous thrombosis and congestion as well as hyperperfusion or reperfusion injury have been postulated as potential mechanisms for delayed changes in spinal cord function.[1,4,39,40] Subacute posttraumatic ascending myelopathy has been defined as the loss of function of one or more spinal segments above an originally stable

SCI, developing typically 1 to 2 weeks after injury and accompanied by characteristic intramedullary hyperintense T2 signal changes on MRI.[1,36] Recent evidence has linked cellular apoptosis to the pathogenesis of subacute posttraumatic ascending myelopathy,[1,41,42] but further research is necessary to understand this entity.

Most commonly associated with surgery for cervical spondylotic disease, C5 radiculopathy is a well-known complication after 2% to 20% of major cervical decompressive operations.[43] The characteristic specific motor weakness of the C5 myotome and shoulder pain without sensory loss may appear from 6 hours to 4 weeks postoperatively, and generally resolves over months to years.[17,43] The C5 nerve root is susceptible because of its unique anatomy, specifically, shortest length and most obtuse takeoff angle of any cervical root.[44] Conservative measures do not seem to alter the clinical course, but operative foraminal decompression for affected patients may provide an opportunity for faster recovery.[43]

Late Delayed. Instability and progressive kyphotic deformity may produce neurologic deficit over time as a result of cord impingement and root compression.19,45 Inadequate constructs, pseudarthrosis, and failed internal fixation or external immobilization may all contribute to insufficient spinal integrity in the weeks and months after spinal trauma surgery.

Although not directly related to surgical intervention, posttraumatic syringomyelia is an unusual but well-known cause of delayed neurologic deterioration in SCI. Approximately 1% of patients will develop a symptomatic syrinx and present with worsening myelopathy, autonomic dysfunction, and pain 2 to 15 years after injury.[45] At least 50% of patients will improve with surgical fenestration or shunting.[45,46]

Finally, late-onset myelopathy or radiculopathy may develop resulting from formation or progression of spondylotic disease at segments adjacent to fused cervical segments. This adjacent-level disease theoretically develops in response to iatrogenic local tissue changes as well as augmented biomechanical stresses applied by the fused segments.[47–51] Radiographic rates of adjacent level degeneration after cervical fusion vary from 25% to 60%, but symptomatic disease is present in only 7% to 17%, and surgical intervention is needed in 6% to 15% of patients who have undergone fusion.[47–51] Average onset of symptoms from adjacent-level disease is approximately 5 years and has an annual incidence around 3%.[49–51] However, causative correlations between the presence of the fusion and development of spondylosis have not been reliably proven to date. Goffin et al.[48] demonstrated a 60% rate of adjacent-level spondylotic changes over 5 to 9 years after fusion for cervical fractures and dislocations in 25 patients. However, none of the patients became symptomatic or required operation for the adjacent-level degeneration. One of the most consistent risk factors for the development of adjacent-level degeneration is radiographic evidence of degeneration at the adjacent level at the time of the initial arthrodesis.[49–51] Ultimately, therefore, adjacent-level degeneration may simply be an acceleration of the natural history of the spondylotic disease, and would therefore have a lower annual incidence and require much longer follow-up to discover in the younger trauma population than in an older spondylotic patient cohort. Nevertheless, adjacent-level degeneration remains a diagnostic concern in patients who demonstrate neurologic deterioration several years after surgery.

CONCLUSION

Dramatic progress has been made over the last few decades in allowing spine surgeons to thoughtfully and effectively reconstruct traumatic deformations of the spinal column. This, in turn, has permitted earlier mobilization and rehabilitation of such patients. And although significant recovery for severely spinal cord–injured patients is still elusive, minimizing the recognizable causes of iatrogenic neurologic deterioration in the surgical patient will remain the cornerstone of improved outcomes in the future.

REFERENCES

1. Al-Ghatany M, Al-Shraim M, Levi AD, et al. Pathological features including apoptosis in subacute posttraumatic ascending myelopathy: case report and review of the literature. *J Neurosurg Spine* 2005;2:619–623.
2. Farmer J, Vaccaro A, Albert TJ, et al. Neurologic deterioration after cervical spinal cord injury. *J Spinal Disord* 1998;11:192–196.
3. Fehlings MG, Tator CH. An evidence-based review of decompressive surgery in acute spinal cord injury: rationale, indications, and timing based on experimental and clinical studies. *J Neurosurg* 1999;91:1–11.
4. Harrop JS, Sharan AD, Vaccaro AR, et al. The cause of neurologic deterioration after acute cervical spinal cord injury. *Spine* 2001;26:340–346.
5. Marshall LF, Knowlton S, Garfin SR, et al. Deterioration following spinal cord injury: a multicenter study. *J Neurosurg* 1987;66:400–404.
6. Gurunluoglu R, Gurunluoglu A. Paul of Aegina: landmark in surgical progress. *World J Surg* 2003;27:18–25.
7. Alberstone CD, Naderi S, Benzel EC. History. In: Benzel EC, ed. *Spine Surgery: Techniques, Complication Avoidance, and Management.* Vol. 1. 2nd ed. Philadelphia: Elsevier, 2005:1–21.
8. Montane I. Historical perspectives of spinal trauma. In: Errico TJ, Bauer RD, Waugh T, eds. *Spinal Trauma.* Philadelphia: JB Lippincott, 1991:1–9.
9. Albee FH. Transplantation of a portion of the tibia into the spine for Pott's disease: a preliminary report. *JAMA* 1911;57:885–886.
10. Hibbs PA. An operation for progressive deformity. *N Y State J Med* 1911;93:1013.
11. Houten JK, Errico TJ. History of spinal instrumentation: the modern era. In: Benzel EC, ed. *Spine Surgery: Techniques, Complication Avoidance, and Management.* Vol. 1. 2nd ed. Philadelphia: Elsevier, 2005:22–32.
12. Kombos T, Suess O, Da Silva C, et al. Impact of somatosensory evoked potential monitoring on cervical surgery. *J Clin Neurophysiol* 2003;20:122–128.
13. Hall ED, Springer JE. Neuroprotection and acute spinal cord injury: a reappraisal. *NeuroRx* 2004;1:80–100.
14. American Association of Neurological Surgeons/Congress of Neurological Surgeons Guidelines Committee. Blood pressure management after acute spinal cord injury. *Neurosurgery* 2002;50:S58–S62.
15. Buchowski JM, Riley LH 3rd. Epidural hematoma after immobilization of a "hangman's" fracture: case report and review of the literature. *Spine J* 2005;5:332–335.
16. American Association of Neurological Surgeons/Congress of Neurological Surgeons Guidelines Committee. Initial closed reduction of cervical spine fracture-dislocation injuries. *Neurosurgery* 2002;50:S44–S50.
17. Yonenobu K, Hosono N, Iwasaki M, et al. Neurologic complications of surgery for cervical compression myelopathy. *Spine* 1991;16:1277–1282.
18. Malone DG, McLain RF, Caruso JR. Neurologic complications. In: Benzel EC, ed. *Spine Surgery: Techniques, Complication Avoidance, and Management.* Vol. 2. 2nd ed. Philadelphia: Elsevier, 2005:1970–1977.
19. Yonenobu K, Okada K, Fuji T, et al. Causes of neurologic deterioration following surgical treatment of cervical myelopathy. *Spine* 1986;11:818–823.
20. Callahan RA, Johnson RM, Margolis RN, et al. Cervical facet fusion for control of instability following laminectomy. *J Bone Joint Surg Am* 1977;59:991–1002.
21. Graham JJ. Complications of cervical spine surgery: a five-year report on a survey of the membership of the Cervical Spine Research Society by the Morbidity and Mortality Committee. *Spine* 1989;14:1046–1050.
22. Lundy DW, Murray HH. Neurological deterioration after posterior wiring of the cervical spine. *J Bone Joint Surg Br* 1997;79:948–951.
23. Smith MD, Phillips WA, Hensinger RN. Complications of fusion to the upper cervical spine. *Spine* 1991;16:702–705.
24. Heller JG, Silcox DH, 3rd, Sutterlin CE 3rd. Complications of posterior cervical plating. *Spine* 1995;20:2442–2448.
25. Fehlings MG, Cooper PR, Errico TJ. Posterior plates in the management of cervical instability: long-term results in 44 patients. *J Neurosurg* 1994;81:341–349.
26. Ebraheim NA, Misson JR, Xu R, et al. The optimal transarticular C1-2 screw length and the location of the hypoglossal nerve. *Surg Neurol* 2000;53:208–210.
27. Nogueira-Barbosa MH, Defino HL. Multiplanar reconstructions of helical computed tomography in planning of atlanto-axial transarticular fixation. *Eur Spine J* 2005;14:493–500.
28. Wright NM, Lauryssen C. Vertebral artery injury in C1-2 transarticular screw fixation: results of a survey of the AANS/CNS section on disorders of the spine and peripheral nerves. American Association of Neurological Surgeons/Congress of Neurological Surgeons. *J Neurosurg* 1998;88:634–640.
29. Gluf WM, Brockmeyer DL. Atlantoaxial transarticular screw fixation: a review of surgical indications, fusion rate, complications, and lessons learned in 67 pediatric patients. *J Neurosurg Spine* 2005;2:164–169.
30. Gluf WM, Schmidt MH, Apfelbaum RI. Atlantoaxial transarticular screw fixation: a review of surgical indications, fusion rate, complications, and lessons learned in 191 adult patients. *J Neurosurg Spine* 2005;2:155–163.
31. Coric D, Branch CL Jr, Wilson JA, et al. Arteriovenous fistula as a complication of C1-2 transarticular screw fixation: case report and review of the literature. *J Neurosurg* 1996;85:340–343.

32. Mendez JC, Gonzalez-Llanos F. Endovascular treatment of a vertebral artery pseudoaneurysm following posterior C1-C2 transarticular screw fixation. *Cardiovasc Intervent Radiol* 2005;28:107–109.
33. Stoops WL, King RB. Neural complications of cervical spondylosis: their response to laminectomy and foramenotomy. *J Neurosurg* 1962;19:986–999.
34. Hans P, Delleuze PP, Born JD, et al. Epidural hematoma after cervical spine surgery. *J Neurosurg Anesthesiol* 2003;15:282–285.
35. Epstein NE. Reoperation rates for acute graft extrusion and pseudarthrosis after one-level anterior corpectomy and fusion with and without plate instrumentation: etiology and corrective management. *Surg Neurol* 2001;56:73–80, discussion 80–71.
36. Belanger E, Picard C, Lacerte D, et al. Subacute posttraumatic ascending myelopathy after spinal cord injury: report of three cases. *J Neurosurg* 2000;93:294–299.
37. Levy WJ, Dohn DF, Hardy RW. Central cord syndrome as a delayed postoperative complication of decompressive laminectomy. *Neurosurgery* 1982;11:491–495.
38. American Association of Neurological Surgeons/Congress of Neurological Surgeons Guidelines Committee. Management of acute central cervical spinal cord injuries. *Neurosurgery* 2002;50:S166–S172.
39. Seichi A, Takeshita K, Kawaguchi H, et al. Postoperative expansion of intramedullary high-intensity areas on T2-weighted magnetic resonance imaging after cervical laminoplasty. *Spine* 2004;29:1478–1482, discussion 1482.
40. Tator CH, Fehlings MG. Review of the secondary injury theory of acute spinal cord trauma with emphasis on vascular mechanisms. *J Neurosurg* 1991;75:15–26.
41. Emery E, Aldana P, Bunge MB, et al. Apoptosis after traumatic human spinal cord injury. *J Neurosurg* 1998; 89:911–920.
42. Yamaura I, Yone K, Nakahara S, et al. Mechanism of destructive pathologic changes in the spinal cord under chronic mechanical compression. *Spine* 2002;27:21–26.
43. O'Toole JE, Olson TJ, Kaiser MG. Surgical management of dissociated motor loss following complex cervical spine reconstruction. *Spine* 2004;29:E56–E60.
44. Shinomiya K, Okawa A, Nakao K, et al. Morphology of C5 ventral nerve rootlets as part of dissociated motor loss of deltoid muscle. *Spine* 1994;19:2501–2504.
45. Gleason TF, Massey TH. Late sequelae of spinal trauma. In: Errico TJ, Bauer RD, Waugh T, eds. *Spinal Trauma.* Philadelphia: JB Lippincott, 1991:563–570.
46. Asano M, Fujiwara K, Yonenobu K, et al. Post-traumatic syringomyelia. *Spine* 1996;21:1446–1453.
47. Azmi H, Schlenk RP. Surgery for postarthrodesis adjacent-cervical segment degeneration. *Neurosurg Focus* 2003;15:E6.
48. Goffin J, van Loon J, Van Calenbergh F, et al. Long-term results after anterior cervical fusion and osteosynthetic stabilization for fractures and/or dislocations of the cervical spine. *J Spinal Disord* 1995;8:500–508, discussion 499.
49. Hilibrand AS, Carlson GD, Palumbo MA, et al: Radiculopathy and myelopathy at segments adjacent to the site of a previous anterior cervical arthrodesis. *J Bone Joint Surg Am* 1999;81:519–528.
50. Hilibrand AS, Robbins M. Adjacent segment degeneration and adjacent segment disease: the consequences of spinal fusion? *Spine J* 2001;4:190S–194S
51. Ishihara H, Kanamori M, Kawaguchi Y, et al. Adjacent segment disease after anterior cervical interbody fusion. *Spine J* 2004;4:624–628.

CHAPTER 37

Pulmonary and Airway Considerations

James S. Harrop, Laura A. Snyder, Alexander R. Vaccaro, and Robert Heary

INTRODUCTION

Trauma patients require a primary evaluation to establish a patent airway that can be maintained, adequate oxygenation, and a functioning circulatory system. Once a patient is considered hemodynamically stable, a thorough secondary evaluation with a detailed neurologic examination is essential. If a cervical spine or spinal cord injury is suggested, further precautions to detect and prevent airway difficulties and pulmonary injuries is essential. Impairment of oxygenation and impairment of the pulmonary system resulting from a cervical spinal injury are the leading causes of in-hospital morbidity and mortality in these patients. This chapter will discuss pulmonary complications related to cervical spinal trauma and their recommended management.

INITIAL AIRWAY MANAGEMENT

Securing the patient's airway is the first priority after any traumatic injury and particularly after a cervical spine or spinal cord injury. Typically, if there is concern over the patient's airway or the ability to protect the airway, endotracheal intubation should be initiated. One spinal injury subpopulation for which physicians should have an early or low threshold for intubation is cervical spinal cord–injured patients (loss of motor or sensation). Patients with complete motor paralysis, particularly above the C5 level, have been shown to have a higher morbidity when there are delays in establishing a secure airway.[1]

The benefit of providing tracheal intubation to maintain a patient's airway is that it maximizes patient oxygenation and, therefore, cardiopulmonary function. Unfortunately, the placement of an endotracheal tube is typically performed with the patient's neck in a hyperextended position to provide for visualization of the vocal cords. In emergent situations, when the spine has not been fully evaluated or "cleared," intubation should be performed with the neck stabilized using manual in-line traction. In elective procedures, the use of fiberoptic visualization has been shown to cause less mobilization of the spinal column and, therefore, possibly prevent further spine or spinal cord injury.[2]

Although there are numerous benefits to the initiation of endotracheal intubation, unfortunately, with prolonged intubation (defined as >7 days) adverse consequences such as laryngeal trauma and tracheal stenosis may develop.[3] The alternative technique of prolonged nasotracheal intubation should also be avoided because it has been correlated with increased frequency of sepsis and sinusitis, along with increased morbidity.[4,5] For these reasons, it may be beneficial to proceed with tracheostomy placement if prolonged intubation is expected.

OCCIPITOCERVICAL FRACTURES

Cervical spinal trauma may result in vertebral ligamentous disruption, prevertebral soft tissue edema, and possibly hematoma formation (Fig. 37.1). Anatomically, the upper airway and trachea are in close proximity to the cervical vertebral column (Fig. 37.2), and, therefore, any injury in this region may result in significant retropharyngeal edema causing compression or deformation of the upper airway (Fig. 37.3). In the adult population, the typical uninjured prevertebral soft tissue measurements on a lateral plain radiograph are illustrated in Table 37.1. Following cervical trauma, resulting prevertebral edema may produce stenosis of the airway, inability to clear secretions, and possibly airway obstruction.

Neurologically injured patients have the highest incidence of pulmonary and airway issues. However, patients with isolated cervical spine injuries without neurologic injury must also be closely monitored because of the potential of prevertebral swelling and airway obstruction. The treatment by closed traction reduction of a traumatic dislocation has been illustrated to safely reestablish spinal alignment with the potential of restoring neurologic function. This technique provides for serial incremental changes in the patient's alignment while monitoring neurologic function. Unfortunately, cervical spine hyperflexion, some injury patterns such as displaced odontoid fractures, and compression of the soft palate and trachea against the spine may further compromise an airway already traumatized by edema. Harrop et al.[6] correlated closed reduction and postural manipulation of posteriorly displaced odontoid fractures and the potential for respiratory distress.[9]

Immobilization of cervical fractures can be accomplished through application of a hard collar halo vest or with surgical stabilization. The use of a halo apparatus, while providing more stability than a collar and being less invasive than surgical intervention, may contribute to airway and ventilatory difficulties. Mercer[7] illustrated that halo immobilization may contribute to respiratory failure

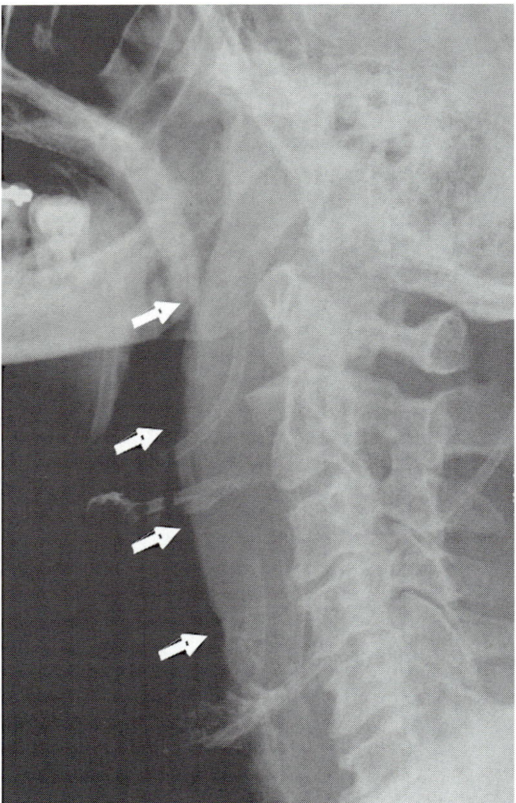

FIGURE 37.1. Ligament disruption and edema in a 45-year-old man suffering hyperextension injury from falling down stairs.

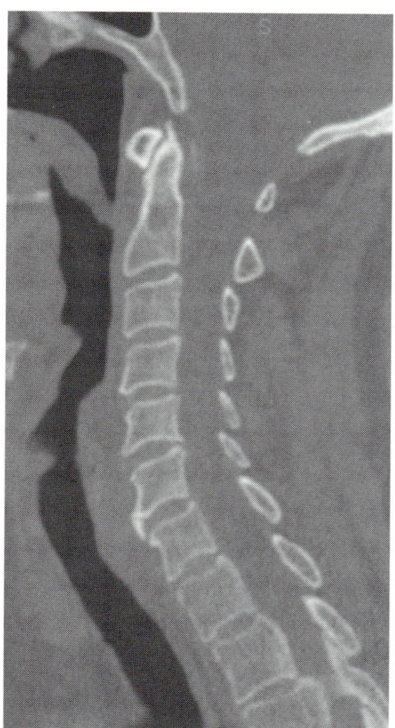

FIGURE 37.2. The upper airway and trachea are close to the cervical vertebral column even when there is no injury.

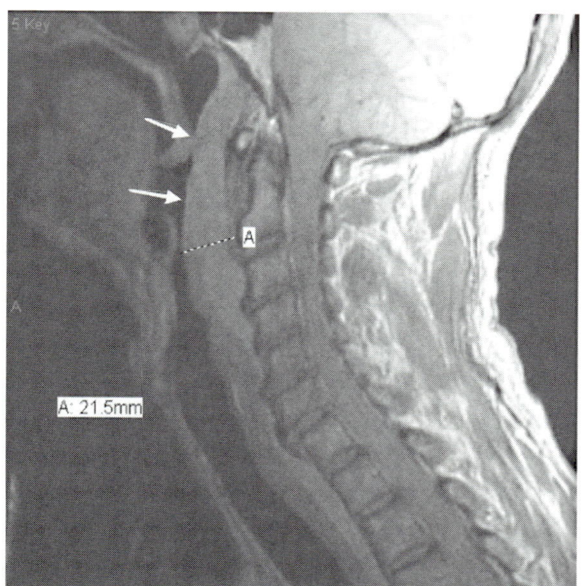

FIGURE 37.3. Retropharyngeal edema causing airway compression in a cervical spinal cord–injured patient.

TABLE 37.1 Uninjured Prevertebral Soft Tissue Measurements on a Lateral Plain Radiograph in the Adult Population

Cervical Spine Level	Prevertebral Soft tissue (mm)
C1	10
C2-C4	5–7
C5-C7	22

after tracheal extubation as a result of difficulties with chest excursion and ventilation. In addition, orotracheal mask application may also be difficult in patients with halo immobilization because of the difficulty with access to the patient's face.

PROLONGED AIRWAY MANAGEMENT

Endotracheal or nasotracheal intubation has been established as a means to provide an initial secure airway following cervical trauma. An alternative to prolonged intubation, because of its adverse effects, may be a tracheostomy. Tracheostomies are beneficial because they reduce the airway length of endotracheal and nasotracheal tube contact and, therefore, reduce airway resistance and dead air space. In neurologically compromised patients, this may be significant because tracheostomy may provide these patients breathing strength to overcome airway resistance and, thus, provide for shortened periods of ventilatory support.[8,9] While tracheostomies provide a faster and more efficient wean from ventilators, they also provide psychological benefits in that patients may be able to mouth words, possibly speak, and have greater mobility.

PROLONGED PULMONARY MANAGEMENT

Monitoring and assessing pulmonary issues after cervical spine trauma can provide certain challenges. These challenges are determined by the patient's level of spinal injury, concurrent traumatic injuries, neurologic status, age, and general medical comorbidities. Patients with cervical spinal cord injury (SCI) with a preexisting medical condition (diabetes mellitus, hypertension, coronary artery disease), pneumonia, or lung disease (chronic obstructive pulmonary disease or asthma) have a higher incidence of prolonged pulmonary dysfunction, as well as a greater need for initial and prolonged ventilatory support.

Neurologically compromised patients, following trauma, especially involving the cervical region, often have significant compromise to their pulmonary systems. Harrop et al.[10] illustrated that a higher level of complete cervical SCI is more likely to require prolonged ventilation and tracheostomy. Specifically, the incidence of tracheostomy for a C2 or C3 American Spinal Injury Association (ASIA) A patient was 100% as opposed to zero in a patient with a C8 ASIA A injury.[10] A complete SCI with a neurologic level rostral to the C5 level may be a predictor for the necessity of prolonged mechanical ventilation.[10,11] Often, patients with high cervical cord–level injuries will initially maintain ventilation but appear to fatigue and require delayed intubation and ventilation. This may be as a result of simple fatigue or slight rostral neurologic decline. In patients with a high cervical CSI level, the diaphragm (phrenic nerve–C3-C5) may be the only functioning muscle of respiration. This muscle is typically small in neurologically intact patients, and its usual ventilatory requirements are minimal as a result of the support of the intercostals muscles. In higher cervical motor–complete patients, this muscle will strengthen and hypertrophy with continued exertion and may assist in eventual mechanical ventilatory weaning. Cord-injured patients are commonly treated with high-dose methylprednisolone, which may have a deleterious effect on diaphragm muscle function (myopathy), increasing the need for ventilatory support. Furthermore, an increased mortality (presumably from pulmonary causes) is seen when steroids are continued for more than 24 hours.

MAINTAINING VENTILATION

The inability of patients with cervical SCIs or other neurologic dysfunction to protect their airway and clear secretions has been associated with an increased risk for early-onset pneumonia.[12] In the patient with SCI, impaired motor strength limits the ability to cough, protect the airway reflexes, and clear secretions. If these patients contract pneumonia, this will result in prolongation of their intubation. The patients not only have to strengthen their respiratory musculature, but they also have to mount an immune response to the pulmonary infection. These infections result in a prolonged inflammatory response that limits the reserve capacity of the injured pulmonary system and the ability of the patient to wean off the mechanical ventilator. Despite these difficulties, even high-tetraplegic patients (C4 and above) can be successfully weaned from mechanical ventilation. Oo et al.[13] noted that 21% of patients with initial diaphragm paralysis and high cervical SCI were able to breathe independently after 4 to 14 months, with an additional 15% having some diaphragm recovery.

AGE AS A PRIMARY RISK FACTOR

As the general population ages in North America, spine and spinal cord injuries in the elderly are a more common occurrence. Not only are elderly patients more susceptible to medical illnesses, but they are also at a greater risk for respiratory distress because of a sixfold decrease in their ability to protect their airway reflexes.[14] In addition, with advanced age there is a decrease in pulmonary function through a decrease in the vital capacity, compliance, reserve volumes, and respiratory muscle strength. The occurrence of a traumatic cervical spinal injury compromises an already tenuous respiratory system, thereby creating the potential for further respiratory dysfunction. The most vulnerable patient population is those with a motor complete cervical SCI. This group, particularly the elderly, has been shown to be at an increased risk for pulmonary difficulties and tracheostomy requirement.[10] Increased age has also been shown to correlate with an increased incidence of pneumonia and to negatively correlate with long-term survival.[15] Pulmonary venous thromboembolism is also more likely to develop in older patients.[16]

DEEP VEIN THROMBOSIS AND PULMONARY EMBOLISM

Patients with SCI are one of the populations at highest risk for deep vein thrombosis and pulmonary embolism. If untreated, these patients are likely to develop thrombosis in their immobile appendages. The greatest risk for deep vein thrombosis occurs during the acute care stay, but remains high through the rehabilitation process.[16] During the acute care hospitalization, the use of low-dose unfractionated heparin, intermittent pneumatic compression, and elastic (graduated compression) stockings does not provide satisfactory protection. The optimal treatment to prevent deep vein thrombosis is prophylactic anticoagulation in combination with mechanical compression devices. The timing to initiate anticoagulation in these trauma patients, many of whom are in the perioperative period, has yet to be fully defined. The authors recommend initiation of fractionated heparin 48 hours after trauma or surgery. Placement of a vena caval filter may be a prudent consideration, but data documenting its effectiveness in this population are lacking. During the rehabilitation process, anticoagulation (unfractionated heparin or full-dose warfarin) in combination with other mechanical means is recommended.

CONCLUSION

Respiratory distress commonly occurs in cervical spine and spinal cord injury patients as a result of a multitude of factors. These patients require vigilant surveillance of their airways, breathing, and oxygenation in accordance with their spinal level of injury and neurologic status. When determining treatment options, it must be noted that traction and immobilization techniques can potentiate further airway obstruction. Because airway and pulmonary dysfunction is a frequent problem and concern in this patient population, patients with SCI who manifest any signs or symptoms of respiratory distress should be managed with early airway access through intubation and possibly tracheostomy.

REFERENCES

1. Velmahos GC, Toutouzas K, Chan L, et al. Intubation after cervical spinal cord injury: to be done selectively or routinely? *Am Surg* 2003,69:891–894.
2. Rudolph C, Schneider JP, Wallenborn J, et al. Movement of the upper cervical spine during laryngoscopy: a comparison of the Bonfils intubation fibrescope and the Macintosh laryngoscope. *Anaesthesia* 2005;60:668–672.
3. Whited RE. A prospective study of laryngotracheal sequelae in long-term intubation. *Laryngoscope* 1984;94: 367–377.
4. Deutschman CS, Wilton P, Sinow J, et al. Paranasal sinusitis associated with nasotracheal intubation: a frequently unrecognized and treatable source of sepsis. *Crit Care Med* 1986;14:111–114.
5. Salord F, Gaussorgues P, Marti-Flich J, et al. Nosocomial maxillary sinusitis during mechanical ventilation: a prospective comparison of orotracheal versus the nasotracheal route for intubation. *Intensive Care Med* 1990;16: 390–393.
6. Harrop JS, Vaccaro AR, Przybylski GJ. Acute respiratory compromise associated with flexed cervical traction after C2 Fractures. *Spine* 2001;26:50–54.
7. Mercer M. Respiratory failure after tracheal extubation in a patient with halo frame cervical spine immobilization–rescue therapy using the combitube airway. *Br J Anesth* 2001;86:886–891.
8. Davis K Jr, Campbell RS, Johannigman JA, et al. Changes in respiratory mechanics after tracheostomy. *Arch Surg* 1999;134:59–62.
9. Diehl JL, El Atrous S, Touchard D, et al. Changes in the work of breathing induced by tracheotomy in ventilator-dependent patients. *Am J Resp Crit Care Med* 1999;159:383–388.
10. Harrop JS, Sharan AD, Scheid EH Jr, et al. Tracheostomy placement in complete cervical spinal cord injuries: American Spinal Injury Association Grade A. *J Neurosurg* 2004;100(suppl Spine 1):20–23.
11. Claxton AR, Wong DT, Chung F, et al. Predictors of hospital mortality and mechanical ventilation in patients with cervical spinal cord injury. *Can J Anesth* 1998;45:144–149.
12. Berrouane Y, Daudenthun I, Riegel B, et al. Early onset pneumonia in neurosurgical intensive care unit patients. *J Hosp Infect* 1998;40:275–280.
13. Oo T, Watt JW, Soni BM, et al. Delayed diaphragm recovery in 12 patients after high cervical spinal cord injury: a retrospective review of the diaphragm status of 107 patients ventilated after acute spinal cord injury. *Spinal Cord* 1999;37:117–122.
14. Pantoppidan H, Beecher HK. Progressive loss of protective reflexes in the airway with the advance of age. *J Am Med Assoc* 1960;174:77–81.
15. DeVivo MJ, Kartus PL, Rutt RD, et al. The influence of age at time of spinal cord injury on rehabilitation outcome. *Arch Neurol* 1990;47:111–114.
16. Green D, Hartwig D, Chen D, et al. Spinal cord injury risk assessment for thromboembolism (SPIRATE Study). *Am J Phys Med Rehab* 2003;82:950–956.

CHAPTER 38

Posttraumatic Syringomyelia

Rishi N. Sheth, Glen Manzano, and Allan D. Levi

INTRODUCTION

Syringomyelia (from the Greek word *syrinx*, tube and *myelos*, marrow) is defined as dilatation of the central canal of the spinal cord. The clearest definition distinguishes between hydromyelia, which is an abnormal dilation of central canal, and the term syringomyelia, which is reserved for central cavities not connected to the central canal. Some authors have viewed the two entities as a continuum of the same pathologic disease.[1]

Abnormal cavitation of the spinal cord has been recognized for well over four centuries. The first description of this entity was in 1564 by Etienne, when he described a cystic lesion in the spinal cord. It was not until 1827 that the term *syringomyelia* was first coined by Ollivier d'Angers.[2] Until the twentieth century the diagnosis of posttraumatic syringomyelia was challenging. Physicians had to rely on the clinical presentation; however, since the advent of magnetic resonance imaging (MRI), this has changed. Patients are now diagnosed early in the disease process, before the development of symptomatology.

As the life span of patients with spinal cord injury (SCI) increases as a result of better medical care and improvements in noninvasive imaging such MRI, physicians will be increasingly encountering the associated long-term complications of SCI, such as syrinx formation.[3,4] Treatment of syringomyelia remains controversial. Treatment modalities directed toward specific pathologic conditions have generated a wide range of surgical interventions. This chapter will discuss possible causes of posttraumatic syringomyelia and their treatment options.

TYPES OF SYRINGOMYELIA

In 1973, Barnett[3] classified syringomyelia based on clinical and experimental data as follows:

Type I. Syringomyelia with obstruction of the foramen magnum and dilatation of the central canal (communicating)
- A. Associated with Chiari I malformation
- B. Associated with other anomalies of the foramen magnum

Type II. Syringomyelia with spinal cord lesions (noncommunicating)
- A. Associated with intramedullary spinal cord tumors
- B. Associated with spinal arachnoiditis
- C. Following trauma to the spine
- D. Compressive myelomalacia secondary to spondylosis or tumor

Type III. Idiopathic syringomyelia

PATHOGENESIS OF POSTTRAUMATIC SYRINGOMYELIA

Despite advances in diagnostic tools, our knowledge of the pathophysiology of syrinx formation remains relatively poor. Theories have been put forward to explain the cause of the formation of these cysts. Many of the theories proposed attempt to explain the formation of a syrinx in association with abnormalities of the posterior fossa; such explanations have limited relevance to posttraumatic syringomyelia. The precise pathogenesis of syrinx formation after trauma to the spine is unknown. Our limitations in gaining a basic understanding of the pathophysiology of this entity are due to the lack of reliable animal models for syringomyelia associated with trauma.

The incidence of syringomyelia varies depending on the individual study. Incidence rates range between 1.1% and 10%.[4–7] With the advent of MRI, higher incidence rates have been quoted.[8] The time lapse between the occurrence of symptoms and trauma is reported to be as early as 2 months to as late as 34 years.[9,10] The most common location of the cyst is at the epicenter of the initial fracture and dissects the avascular plane between the dorsal columns and the central gray mater. In a large autopsy study of 105 cases, Milhorat et al.[11] showed that the histopathology of a posttraumatic syrinx is different compared to other etiologies. The posttraumatic syrinx involves the parenchyma asymmetrically, reaches the pial surface, and is not associated with the central canal. There is irreversible damage to the gray and white matter of spinal cord with focal necrosis and wallerian degeneration.[11] The cyst can be a single cavity or have septations within it containing cerebrospinal fluid (CSF) with high protein content. The cyst is surrounded by reactive gliosis.

Certain factors have been proposed to cause the initial cyst formation, including ischemic damage, necrosis resulting from intracellular release of lysosomes and enzymes, resolution of hematoma, and mechanical destruction of the cord.[12–15] Sgouros and Williams[16] referred to these as primary cysts because of the initial impact on the spinal cord.

The factors responsible for expansion of the cyst are also a matter of controversy. Williams' theory of alteration in CSF flow dynamics is most favored. There is evidence supporting the connection between the syrinx and subarachnoid space leading to local alteration in CSF flow dynamics that eventually causes expansion of the cyst, supporting Williams' theory of CSF dynamics.[17–20]

How does CSF shunting into the syrinx occur? The presence of arachnoid adhesions within the subarachnoid space around the location of the primary SCI is well known and is evident when performing surgery in these patients. The role of arachnoiditis following SCI in the formation of a syrinx has been supported by experimental evidence. Cho et al.[22] found that the frequency of cyst formation was higher in animals that were exposed to trauma followed by local kaolin injection rather than trauma alone. Recently, Stoodley et al.[23] demonstrated that CSF flows from the subarachnoid space into the central canal of normal rat spinal cord via Virchow-Robin spaces. It is hypothesized that this normal flow may be accentuated by the abnormal arachnoid strands acting in a valvelike fashion. Finally, in the setting of posttraumatic syrinx, cine MRI frequently demonstrates obstruction of flow around the injury epicenter.

CLINICAL PRESENTATION

Deterioration of neurologic function in a patient with previous SCI should alert the treating physician about the possibility of syringomyelia. A baseline neurologic examination should be documented so that comparison can be made with future examinations. Assessment of pain level, motor and sensory reflexes, and autonomic functions should be made. Because some of the spinal cord cyst can extend into the brainstem, examination of lower cranial nerves, cerebellum, and long tracts should be included.

The signs and symptoms of syringomyelia can be highly variable, including pain; motor, sensory, and autonomic involvement; or a combination of these.[24,25] Pain is the most frequent initial presentation.[4] It varies in characteristics and can be neuropathic, local, musculoskeletal, or radiating. Motor deficits and spasticity are the next most common presentations. If the syrinx starts in the thorax, ascending motor deficits can be seen in the arms and hands. Dissociated sensory loss, autonomic dysreflexia, hyperhidrosis, and sphincter dysfunction are included in the wide range of presentations.[26–28] Because of asymmetric involvement of the cord parenchyma, presentation can be unilateral or bilateral. Schaller et al.[29] found a positive correlation between the severity of symptoms and incomplete reduction of spine fracture and the degree of arachnoid scarring in the preoperative radiologic studies.

IMAGING

Until a few decades ago, the diagnosis of posttraumatic syringomyelia was based on careful clinical examination of these patients. This was challenging to the physician given the insidious onset and slow variable course of signs and symptoms. The classic description of segmental dissociated sensory loss with hand atrophy may not be present in all cases.[30]

Since the mid-1980s, MRI has become the gold standard for diagnosing syringomyelia from any cause.[31–34] The entire extent of the cyst should be visualized, including the craniocervical junction on T1- and T2-weighted images (Fig. 38.1). The addition of gadolinium contrast helps to rule out intramedullary tumors and may help delineate the extent of scar tissue at the injury site.[35] In assessing the results of surgical intervention, MRI scans are helpful in following the size of the cyst.

Even though computed tomography (CT)-myelogram has fallen out of favor, it can be helpful in patients who are unable to undergo MRI because of the presence of a pacemaker, metallic foreign body, or spinal instrumentation causing significant artifact.[36,37] Electrophysiologic studies show prolongation of F-wave latencies in patients with syrinx.[4]

Clinically, it may be difficult to distinguish posttraumatic syringomyelia from progressive posttraumatic myelomalacia myelopathy, which has different surgical implications. MRI has been helpful in this situation. The myelomalacic spinal cord has irregular, poorly defined margins and may be tethered to the dural sac on MRI. On the other hand, syringomyelia of the cord is a cystic cavity on MRI and follows CSF signal intensity. This distinction can be further confirmed by ultrasound study of the spinal cord intraoperatively.[38]

Cine MRI gives real-time motion picture–like analysis of CSF flow dynamics in and around the spinal cord cyst. The pulsatile flow of CSF is impeded at the site of tethering and the syrinx (Fig. 38.2). This vital information helps in planning the site of surgical intervention. Cine MRI can be

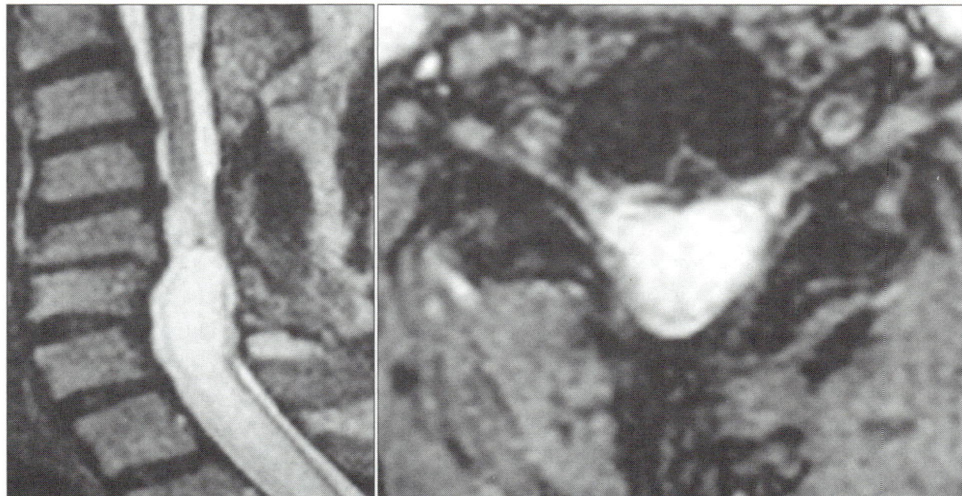

FIGURE 38.1. Sagittal **(A)** and axial **(B)** T2-weighted magnetic resonance imaging demonstrates a cystic cavity filled with cerebrospinal fluid and consistent with a posttraumatic syrinx.

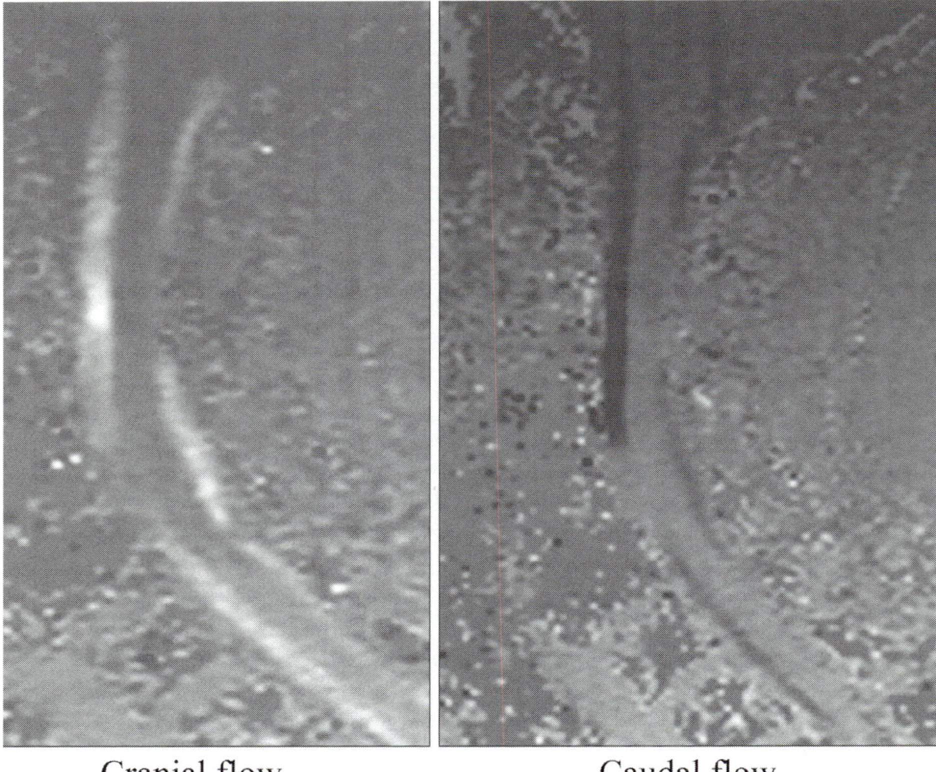

FIGURE 38.2. Cine magnetic resonance imaging shows the dual direction of flow of cerebrospinal fluid (CSF) around the spinal cord. The scans demonstrate the obstruction of CSF flow at the level of spinal cord tethering.

used postoperatively to assess the surgical results and confirm the restoration of normal CSF flow around the damaged spinal cord.

TREATMENT

The treatment of posttraumatic syringomyelia remains controversial. There is a lack of systematic studies comparing the various treatments. Experience is somewhat limited because of the small number of patients that actually are treated surgically.[26,39] Finally, the location of the syrinx, extent of scarring, and baseline neurologic deficit before treatment are quite variable from patient to patient.

In many institutions, patients who undergo surgical treatment demonstrate progressive signs or symptoms of neurologic deterioration and have MRI evidence of a cystic cavity in the spinal cord. The aim of treatment in most instances is to restore CSF flow around the spinal cord. Surgical intervention involves performance of a laminectomy at the site of the cyst epicenter and/or the site of tethering. With the help of transverse and longitudinal views, ultrasound can precisely delineate the location and extent of the cyst (Fig. 38.3). The initial dural opening is made away from the site where the cord is tethered so as not to injure it. The spinal cord is released from the adjoining dura carefully, paying close attention to the evoked potentials. In addition, nerve root adhesions are released. There may be associated arachnoid adhesions, some of which may form cystic pockets containing CSF. Arachnoid cyst walls associated with trauma tend be thicker and firmly adherent to adjacent dura compared to congenital ones. The cyst wall along with its adhesions is meticulously

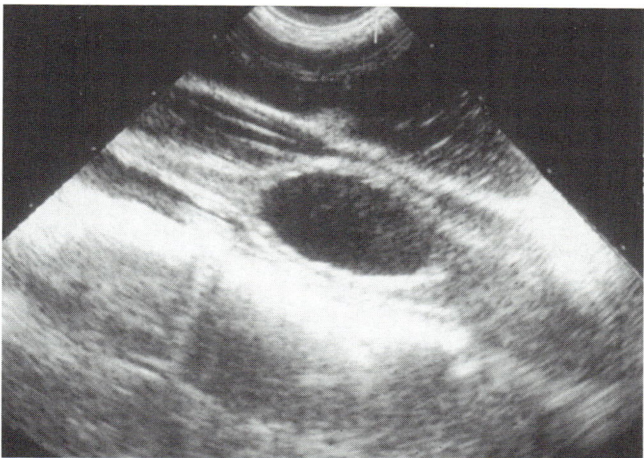

FIGURE 38.3. Sagittal intraoperative ultrasound view of the lower thoracic spinal cord demonstrating a large syrinx.

taken down from its dural and cord attachments. We use intraoperative somatosensory evoked potentials (SSEPs) and motor evoked potentials (MEPs) to monitor spinal cord function during surgery. Steroids or hypothermia are administered if the intraoperative electrophysiologic monitoring significantly deteriorates.

Untethering alone may be sufficient to reduce the cyst size and alleviate the signs and symptoms of posttraumatic cystic myelopathy.[26] If the spinal cord cyst does not collapse or if it has a significant rostrocaudal extension, many surgeons prefer to shunt to the extramedullary space. A 2-mm midline myelotomy using a No. 11 blade is made at the caudal part of the cyst. A Spetzler tube is then inserted slowly and directed rostrally as far as it goes without resistance. Intraoperative ultrasound is also useful in locating the optimal site for midline myelotomy and to visualize any septations within the cyst cavity. The distal end of the tube is left in the subarachnoid space away from the site of adhesions and scar. The tube is anchored to the pial surface with a 7-0 Prolene suture. Alternatively, the syrinx can be shunted to extraspinal spaces such as the pleural or peritoneal cavities.[39,40] Shunting is not without risks. Shunt tube obstruction, dislocation, infection, granuloma formation, peritoneal pseudocyst, low CSF pressure, and delayed tethering are among the many potential complications. Failure rates of up to 50% have been reported with shunting alone.[9,41,42]

Ultrasound images are obtained at the end of the untethering procedure to confirm that the spinal cord is freely floating in the subarachnoid space without any adhesions and to see the normal pulsation of cord with respirations free of any arachnoid loculations. It also helps to confirm the proper placement of the catheter in the cyst and subsequent collapse of the syrinx. Achieving thorough homeostasis is important because blood may predispose to further scar formation and eventual retethering of the spinal cord.

Finally, a duraplasty is performed using cadaveric dura to keep the subarachnoid space widened, which maintains free flow of CSF around the cord to avoid retethering[10] (Fig. 38.4). A lumbar drain may be inserted, if a satisfactory dural closure has not been achieved, to avoid a CSF leak or a delayed pseudomeningocele.

Other techniques for treating posttraumatic syringomyelia include transection of the spinal cord at the level of syrinx in paraplegic patients, myelopediculotomy (i.e., multiple fenestrations through the cyst wall using a laser), use of a neuroendoscope to break down septae within an established syrinx, and fetal spinal cord transplantation.[43–46]

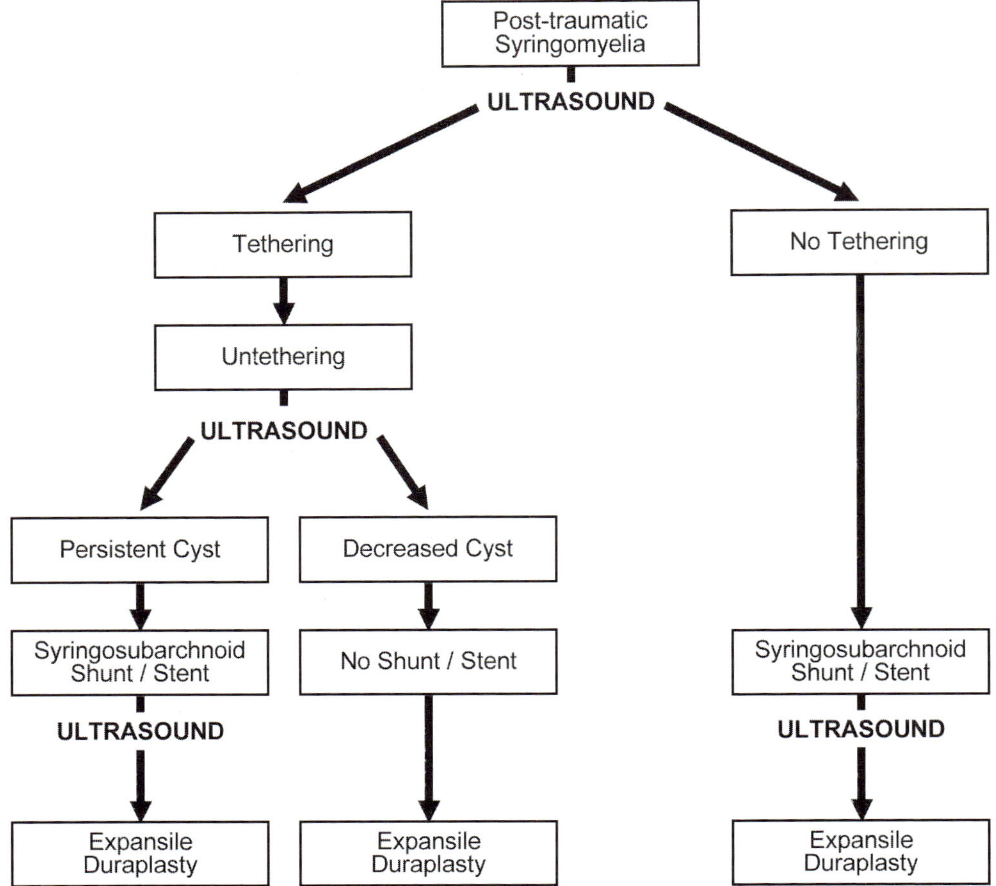

FIGURE 38.4. Treatment algorithm for patients with progressive posttraumatic cystic myelopathy. (From Lee TT, Alameda GJ, Gromelski EB, et al. Outcome after surgical treatment of progressive posttraumatic cystic myelopathy. *J Neurosurg* 2000;92[suppl 2]:149–154.)

The results of surgical intervention are variable. Pain relief and motor improvement are more common than reversal of sensory loss. Depending on the study, pain relief ranges from 55.6% to 100% and motor improvement ranges from 8% to 89%. The variability in studies arises from the different length of follow-up and different modalities of treatment.[4,26,39,40]

Prevention of cyst formation should also be a goal of the treating surgeon. The results of a retrospective study demonstrated that patients with 15 degrees of posttraumatic kyphosis and 25% stenosis were twice as likely to develop a syrinx, and the probability of developing posttraumatic syringomyelia was directly proportional to the degree of stenosis and kyphosis at the site of initial injury. The authors suggested that surgical reconstruction of the spinal canal via decompression or correction of kyphosis should be considered at the time of injury to relieve the chronic mechanical stress to the spinal cord.[47]

CONCLUSION

There is growing awareness of the long-term complications in patients with chronic SCI, such as posttraumatic syrinx. Patients with SCI are living longer. This, in combination with the advent of sensitive diagnostic tools such as MRI, has resulted in an increasing number of patients being diagnosed with posttraumatic syringomyelia. Cine MRI is a useful tool in delineating the degree of CSF obstruction at the site of SCI. Spinal cord untethering should be considered as a primary treatment modality in cases in which significant adhesions exist between the spinal cord and the dural sac because significant problems still exist with shunting alone procedures.

REFERENCES

1. Finlayson AI. Syringomyelia and related conditions. In: Joynt RJ, ed. *Clinical Neurology*. Vol. 3. Philadelphia: JB Lippincott, 1989:1–17.
2. Foster JB, Hudgson P. Historical introduction. In: Barnett HJM, Foster JB, Hudgson P, eds. *Syringomyelia.* London: WB Saunders, 1973:3–10.
3. Barnett HJM. The epilogue. In: Barnett HJM, Foster JB, Hudgson P, eds. *Syringomyelia.* London: WB Saunders, 1973:302–313.
4. Rossier AB, Foo D, Shillito J, et al. Posttraumatic cervical syringomyelia: incidence, clinical presentation, electrophysiological studies, syrinx protein and results of conservative and operative treatment. *Brain* 1985;108: 439–461.
5. Schurch B, Wichmann W, Rossier AB. Post-traumatic syringomyelia (cystic myelopathy): a prospective study of 449 patients with spinal cord injury. *J Neurol Neurosurg Psychiatry* 1996;60:61–67.
6. Griffiths ER, McCormick CC. Post-traumatic syringomyelia (cystic myelopathy). *Paraplegia* 1981;19:81–88.
7. Bursell JP, Little JW, Stiens SA. Electrodiagnosis in spinal cord injured persons with new weakness or sensory loss: central and peripheral etiologies. *Arch Phys Med Rehabil* 1999;80:904–909.
8. Backe HA, Betz RR, Mesgarzadeh M, et al. Post-traumatic spinal cord cysts evaluated by magnetic resonance imaging. *Paraplegia* 1991;29:607–612.
9. Hida K, Iwasaki Y, Imamura H, et al. Posttraumatic syringomyelia: its characteristic magnetic resonance imaging findings and surgical management. *Neurosurgery* 1994;35:886–891.
10. Levi AD, Sonntag V. Management of posttraumatic syringomyelia using an expansile duraplasty: a case report. *Spine* 1988;23:128–132.
11. Milhorat TH, Capocelli AL, Anzil AP, et al. Pathological basis of spinal cord cavitation in syringomyelia: analysis of 105 autopsy cases. *J Neurosurg* 1995;82:802–812.
12. Fairholm DJ, Turnbull IM. Microangiographic study of experimental spinal shock injuries. *J Neurosurg* 1971;35:277–286.
13. Kao CC, Chang LW. The mechanism of spinal cord cavitation following spinal cord transaction. I: A correlated histochemical study. *J Neurosurg* 1977;46:197–209.
14. Kao CC, Chang LW, Bloodworth JMB. The mechanism of spinal cord cavitation following spinal cord transaction. II: Electron microscope observation. *J Neuropathol Exp Neurol* 1977;36:140–156.
15. Woodard JS, Freeman LW. Ischemia of the spinal cord: an experimental study. *J Neurosurg* 1956;13:63–72.
16. Sgouros S, Williams B. Management and outcome of posttraumatic syringomyelia. *J Neurosurg* 1996;85: 197–205.
17. Savoiardo M. Syringomyelia associated with postmeningitic spinal arachnoiditis: filling of the syrinx through a communication with the subarachnoid space. *Neurology* 26: 551–554, 1976.
18. McLean DR, Miller JDR, Allen PBR, et al. Posttraumatic syringomyelia. *J Neurosurg* 1973;39:485–492.
19. Williams B. The distending force in the production of "communicating syringomyelia." *Lancet* 1969;2:189–193.
20. Williams B. Pathogenesis of syringomyelia. *Acta Neurochir (Wien)* 1993;123:159–165.
21. Williams B, Terry AF, Jones HWF, et al. Syringomyelia as a sequel to traumatic paraplegia. *Paraplegia* 1981;19:67–80.
22. Cho KH, Iwasaki Y, Imamura H, et al. Experimental model of posttraumatic syringomyelia: the role of adhesive arachnoiditis in syrinx formation. *J Neurosurg* 1994;80:133–139.
23. Stoodley MA, Jones NR, Brown CJ. Evidence for rapid fluid flow from the subarachnoid space into the spinal cord central canal in the rat. *Brain Res* 1996;707:155–164.
24. El Masry WS, Biyani A. Incidence, management, and outcome of post-traumatic syringomyelia: in memory of Mr. Bernard Williams. *J Neurol Neurosurg Psychiatry* 1996;60:141–146.
25. Yarkony GM, Sheffler LR, Smith J, et al. Early onset posttraumatic cystic myelopathy complicating spinal cord injury. *Arch Phys Med Rehabil* 1994;75:102–105.
26. Lee TT, Alameda GJ, Gromelski EB, et al. Outcome after surgical treatment of progressive posttraumatic cystic myelopathy. *J Neurosurg* 2000;92(suppl 2):149–154.
27. Edgar R, Quail P. Progressive post-traumatic cystic and non-cystic myelopathy. *Br J Neurosurg* 1994;8:7–22.
28. Honan WP, Williams B. Sensory loss in syringomyelia: not necessarily dissociated. *J R Soc Med* 1993;86: 519–520.

29. Schaller B, Mindermann T, Gratzl O. Treatment of syringomyelia after posttraumatic paraparesis or tetraparesis. *J Spinal Disord* 1999;12:485–488.
30. Adams RD, Victor M, Ropper AH. *Principles of Neurology*. 6th ed. New York: McGraw-Hill, 1997:1269–1273.
31. Sherman JL, Farkovich AJ, Citrin CM. The MR appearance of syringomyelia: new observations. *AJR Am J Roentgenol* 1987;148:381–391.
32. Pojunas K, Williams AL, Daniels KL, et al. Syringomyelia and hydromyelia: magnetic resonance evaluation. *Radiology* 1984;153:679–683.
33. Batzdorf U. Chiari I malformation with syringomyelia: evaluation of surgical therapy by magnetic resonance imaging. *J Neurosurg* 1988;68:726–730.
34. Backe HA, Betz RR, Mesgarzadeh M, et al. Post-traumatic spinal cord cysts evaluated by magnetic resonance imaging. *Paraplegia* 1991;29:607–612.
35. Slasky BS, Bydder GM, Niendorf HP, et al. MR imaging with gadolinium-DTPA in the differentiation of tumor, syrinx, and cyst of the spinal cord. *J Comput Assist Tomogr* 1987;11:845–850.
36. Stoaniemi KA, Pyhtinen J, Myllyla VV. Computed tomography in the diagnosis of syringomyelia. *Acta Neurol Scand* 1983;68:121–127.
37. Quencer RM, Green BA, Eismont FJ. Post traumatic spinal cysts: clinical features and characterization with metrizamide computed tomography. *Radiology* 1983;146:415–423.
38. Falcone S, Quencer RM, Green BA, et al. Progressive post-traumatic myelomalacic myelopathy (PPMM): imaging and clinical features. *AJNR Am J Neuroradiol* 1994;15:747–754.
39. Falci SP, Lammertse DP, Best L, et al. Surgical treatment of posttraumatic cystic and tethered spinal cords. *J Spinal Cord Med* 1999;22:173–181.
40. Barbaro NM, Wilson CB, Gutin PH, et al. Surgical treatment of syringomyelia: favorable results with syringoperitoneal shunting. *J Neurosurg* 1984;61:531–538.
41. Batzdorf U, Klekamp J, Johnson JP. A critical appraisal of syrinx cavity shunting procedures. *J Neurosurg* 1998;89:382–388.
42. Sgouros S, Williams B. A critical appraisal of drainage in syringomyelia. *J Neurosurg* 1995;82:1–10.
43. Dunward QJ, Rice GP, Ball MJ, et al. Selective spinal cordectomy: clinicopathological correlation. *J Neurosurg* 1982;56:359–367.
44. Edgar R, Quail P. Progressive post-traumatic cystic and non-cystic myelopathy. *Br J Neurosurg* 1994;8:7–22.
45. Huewel N, Perneczky A, Urban V, et al. Neuroendoscopic technique for the operative treatment of septated syringomyelia. *Acta Neurochir Suppl (Wien)* 1992;54:59–62.
46. Thompson FJ, Reier PJ, Uthman B, et al. Neurophysiological assessment of the feasibility and safety of neural tissue transplantation in patients with syringomyelia. *J Neurotrauma* 2001;18:931–945.
47. Abel R, Gerner HJ, Smit C, et al. Residual deformity of the spinal canal in patients with traumatic paraplegia and secondary changes of the spinal cord. *Spinal Cord* 1999;37:14–19.

SECTION XII

Controversies

CHAPTER 39

Management of Multiple Trauma

Charles Davis and Steven Ludwig

INTRODUCTION

The management of a patient with multiorgan system trauma is complex. Timing of the management of spinal injuries must be coordinated with a multidisciplinary trauma team. Many times, definitive treatment must be delayed until the patient is stabilized and life-threatening injuries are treated. Injuries caused by blunt high-impact trauma are common and frequently involve several systems. For example, flexion-distraction injuries of the lumbar spine are associated with a 50% incidence of intra-abdominal injuries. Moreover, common injury patterns are sometimes observed in patients who have fallen from a height. This mechanism of injury can present with associated head, intra-abdominal, and thoracic injuries; pelvic and lower extremity fractures; and lumbar burst fractures. Therefore, patients experiencing polytrauma must be evaluated with an awareness of the possibility of associated injuries and must be managed in a time-relevant fashion.

Immediate treatment goals for patients who have experienced polytrauma differ from those of patients with isolated spinal column injury. Because of the need for addressing immediate life-threatening injuries, spinal column fractures often are missed and definitive treatment of them might be delayed. In a retrospective study by Anderson et al.,[1] 24% of 181 trauma patients experienced delay in diagnosis of thoracolumbar injury. Compared with other patients, those in the delayed diagnosis group had lower Glasgow Coma Scale scores and were more often hypotensive and had critical injuries. The most common reason for a spine injury to be missed is the inability of the patient to cooperate with a comprehensive spinal examination because of altered mental status. The altered mental status can occur secondary to head trauma, endotracheal intubation with pharmacologic paralysis, or intoxication. The clinical significance of a missed thoracolumbar injury under these clinical scenarios is debatable but potentially catastrophic. Moreover, understanding that noncontiguous traumatic injuries to the spinal column may occur in up to 20% of patients should increase a clinician's index of suspicion for scrutinizing radiographs of the entire spine.

On arrival at the trauma unit, the patient should be immobilized on a backboard with a cervical collar. The initial evaluation should follow a logical and thorough format for evaluation and treatment. The Advanced Trauma Life Support (ATLS) protocol clearly identifies the priorities for conducting a primary assessment of life-threatening injuries. The mnemonic "ABCDEF" can aid the clinician in the primary survey in following a logical approach to care of the patient who has experienced polytrauma. The initial trauma assessment, or primary survey, should be performed at the time of the patient's arrival at the trauma center. This survey includes rapid assessment of vital signs and patient status via blood pressure, pulse, respiratory rate, pulse oximetry, temperature, urinary output, and arterial blood gases. All values provide important and timely clues regarding the patient's overall status, particularly airway, breathing, and circulation.

Care of the spinal column is maintained throughout the ATLS protocol. It should be assumed that all of these patients have a spine injury until such an injury can be ruled out. Patients should have a cervical collar placed in the field and should be placed on a backboard for transport. Identifying a spinal column injury should be an important part of the primary survey when assessing motor and sensory deficits. Altered cognitive response at this time should alert the clinician to potential injury. Vital signs that reveal a patient to be hypotensive without the normal physiologic response of tachycardia might signify neurogenic shock. Moreover, during the initial survey, it is important to realize that a multiply injured patient with a spinal cord injury (SCI) resulting in neurogenic shock might have additional injuries causing massive bleeding and associated hypovolemic shock. Recognition and rapid treatment of these different causes of hemodynamic instabilities are paramount to the successful resuscitation of a patient who has undergone trauma.

Once the patent is stable, a complete evaluation can ensue and operative planning for spinal injuries should be performed. Timely stabilization of spinal injuries allows for early rehabilitation, better pulmonary care, and decreased risk for deep venous thrombosis in the neurologically intact patient. Early spine stabilization also might enhance neurologic recovery and prevent neurologic deterioration, although this is debatable. McLain and Benson,[2] in a review of 27 patients, showed that no difference in blood loss or perioperative complications was observed when operating on the spine early versus late in the setting of multiple trauma. Thus, surgery should progress when the patient is medically stable. One retrospective review of 138 patients with multiple traumatic injuries who required spinal decompression showed no significant difference in medical complications between patients operated on within 72 hours of injury and those operated on after 72 hours from the time of injury.[3] However, patients with cervical spine injuries and neurologic defects had less morbidity when operated on within 72 hours of injury.[3]

AIRWAY

The main priority in the assessment of a trauma patient is to evaluate and ensure the patency of the airway. This evaluation must be performed with constant care to protect the cervical spine until a concomitant injury has been ruled out. Along with cervical spine immobilization, administration of supplemental oxygen should be among the first interventions applied. Maintaining a blood saturation level of 100% is important for oxygen delivery to traumatized organs.

The upper airway should be cleared of any obstruction, including blood, secretions, and foreign bodies, and the mandible, larynx, and trachea should be quickly evaluated for fractures. The use of a chin lift or jaw thrust and a nasopharyngeal or oropharyngeal airway can help maintain a patent airway. Cervical spine precautions should be maintained until cervical instability is ruled out both clinically and radiographically.

Early radiographic evaluation of the cervical spine must include anteroposterior (AP), lateral, and open-mouth views of the cervical spine. It is imperative to obtain radiographs that clearly show the entire cervical spine to the C7-T1 junction. This can be accomplished by pulling downward on the upper extremities to help visualize the lower cervical spine or by obtaining a lateral swimmers view of the cervical spine. If a patient is awake and alert with no distracting injuries and has not received a large amount of narcotics, normal radiographic results and negative findings of a clinical examination could be all that is needed to clear the patient's cervical spine. However, if the radiograph does not show the cervicothoracic junction, computed tomography (CT) with coronal and sagittal reconstructions might be necessary to rule out spinal injury. In a patient who has altered mental status and negative radiographic findings, an occult discoligamentous injury cannot be ruled out. Under these circumstances, magnetic resonance imaging (MRI) can serve to rule out this type of injury.

BREATHING

After the airway is assessed, the breathing or adequacy of ventilation should be checked. The clinician should observe the chest for the rise and fall of normal breathing. Listening for bilateral normal breath sounds and percussing to evaluate for hemothorax or pneumothorax must be done. Palpating for crepitus or instability of the rib cage should also be done to rule out a flail chest. Supplemental oxygen should be maintained throughout the primary survey. The use of an orotracheal, nasotracheal, or surgical airway might be necessary if the airway cannot be maintained. Intubation must be performed with adequate control of the cervical spine. This involves in-line cervical stabilization and use of rigid laryngoscopes or flexible fiberoptic scopes. These modalities prevent further spinal column injury or neurologic ascension of a preexisting cervical injury.

CIRCULATION

Assessment of circulation and blood volume is the third step in the ATLS protocol. Diminished pulses, hypotension, and cool, pale skin can be indications of hypovolemia. Although hypotension in the trauma patient with SCI might stem from neurogenic shock, it is possible for cardiac shock, mediastinal shock (aortic transection, pericardial tamponade, cardiac rupture), hypothermia, and hypovolemic shock to occur simultaneously. Hemorrhage is the most frequent cause of hypotension, occurring in 95% of cases of blunt trauma. If hemorrhage is ruled out, other causes must be investigated. Decreased blood pressure and bradycardia can indicate neurogenic shock. A core temperature of less then 95° C indicates hypothermia. Any ST segment elevations on an electrocardiogram or abnormal wall motion or decreased ejection fraction as evaluated by echocardiography might warrant further investigation into cardiac shock. Mediastinal shock might have occurred if muffled heart sounds or an audible cardiac murmur are heard.

After blunt trauma, the location of blood loss must be identified. Blood loss can be internal or external. Internal blood loss can occur in the intrathoracic, intraperitoneal, or extraperitoneal areas or in the extremities in the case of long bone fractures. External hemorrhage is easily diagnosed, and initial management should consist of the application of external pressure, either manually or with the use of a compression dressing. Blood loss in the abdominal cavity (spleen and liver), thoracic cavity (aortic disruption), retroperitoneal cavity (pelvic fractures), and extremities can be more difficult to diagnose. Significant intrathoracic bleeding usually can be identified by decreased breath sounds during physical examination or by visualization on plain films and advanced imaging studies of these regions. Free intraperitoneal blood can be evaluated by radiography, ultrasonography, lavage, and physical examination. Long bone fractures can be identified through physical examination and radiography. Extraperitoneal hemorrhage can be inferred from the presence of pelvic fractures. Pelvic fractures might cause life-threatening retroperitoneal hemorrhage and mandate immediate intervention.

If the possibility of intra-abdominal hemorrhage is suspected, further studies must be conducted. The use of a diagnostic peritoneal lavage has historically been used by trauma centers to rule out such injuries (sensitivity 100%, specificity 84%). Other modalities are now used that are currently replacing diagnostic peritoneal lavage. These include CT if the patient is stable enough to withstand transport to the scanner (sensitivity 95%, specificity 95%).[4] Another screening tool that is used is ultrasonography, especially focused assessment with sonography for trauma (FAST) ultrasonography (sensitivity 90%, specificity 95%). This modality might be the study of choice at certain centers. However, the efficacy of ultrasound depends on the experience of the operator, and significant injuries can be missed.

During the primary assessment, the trauma team must initiate resuscitation of the patient. Two large-caliber (12 to 18 gauge) intravenous catheters should be placed, preferably in the upper extremities, for administration of fluid therapy. If peripheral intravenous access is not possible, or if the patient's hemodynamic status warrants, central venous access might be necessary.

Once intravenous access has been established, blood should be drawn for a complete blood count, serum electrolyte chemistries, coagulation panel, typing and cross-matching, pregnancy test, and toxicology screens. Lactic acid levels also are useful measurements, because the lactate concentration rises with anaerobic metabolism related to inadequate tissue perfusion. This might indicate inadequate resuscitation or undiscovered, uncorrected injury. An arterial blood gas value provides the clinician with feedback regarding the patient's metabolic and oxygenation status.

Initially, resuscitation of patients with multiple injuries might include crystalloid isotonic solutions, such as lactated Ringer's or PlasmaLyte A solutions. Several liters might be required to increase the mean arterial pressure to a goal of 90 mm Hg for adequate tissue and spinal cord perfusion. If blood loss is greater than 20% of the patient's total blood volume or if the crystalloid infusion provides minimal or no hemodynamic response, the use of Rh-negative type O or type-specific blood might be indicated. If readily available, cross-matched blood should be used to replace lost blood, as indicated. Fresh-frozen plasma can be used in patients who are coagulopathic, and platelets can be used in patients who have thrombocytopenia (platelet count below 50,000/mm^3) with bleeding diathesis.

In the acute setting, urinary output is not the most accurate indicator of volume status and organ perfusion. All patients with SCIs should have a Foley catheter placed to maintain volume status. In the normotensive or stabilized patient, urinary output of 0.5 to 1.0 mL/kg per hour is a good indicator of adequate renal perfusion.

DISABILITY

The primary survey should include a basic neurologic examination. The Glasgow Coma Scale is useful as a quick neurologic tool that affords some prognostic value when performed serially. Altered levels of consciousness might be related to the patient's ventilation or circulatory status, including hypoxia, hypercarbia, hypovolemia, and hypothermia. Depressed consciousness otherwise might be related directly to central nervous system trauma or substances (drugs and/or alcohol).

Gross neurologic assessment can be performed at this juncture. The patient should be carefully log-rolled with continued stabilization of the cervical spine. The spine should be palpated in its entire length, palpating for stepoffs or crepitation. If the patient is interactive and appropriate, motor and sensory function can be ascertained.

The importance of a detailed and accurate neurologic examination of the patient with an SCI cannot be overlooked. The Glasgow Coma Scale score is a good measure of a patient's level of consciousness; however, a detailed examination that includes motor sensory and reflex assessment is important for the diagnosis and treatment of a patient with a spinal column injury. Complete versus incomplete neurologic injury must be assessed, in addition to the status of spinal shock. Spinal shock rarely lasts longer than 24 to 48 hours, and the return of the anal wink and a positive bulbocavernosus reflex is indicative of the end of spinal shock. Neurologic status is one of the main clinical factors influencing the treatment of the patient with spinal injury. Through the efforts of the American Spinal Injury Association, a consistent and reproducible system has been devised (Fig. 39.1). Key muscle groups should be evaluated (Table 39.1) and graded according to strength. The motor score is based on 10 key muscles bilaterally. The sensory score is assessed by light touch and pin-prick on each of the 28 dermatomes. Absent sensation is graded as 0; hypoesthesia or hyperesthesia is graded as 1; and normal sensory findings are graded as 2. The level of neurologic injury is defined as the most caudal level with full intact sensation and greater than antigravity strength as revealed by a motor examination. The examination must establish complete or incomplete injury. The presence of any motor or sensory function caudal to the level of injury, especially in the sacral area, defines an incomplete injury.

Incomplete injuries can be classified into clinical syndromes that might be prognostic for recovery. These are Brown-Séquard, central cord, anterior cord, and posterior cord syndromes. Ninety percent of incomplete lesions produce Brown-Séquard syndrome, central cord syndrome, or anterior cervical cord syndrome.

Brown-Séquard syndrome consists of a unilateral lesion that usually is the result of a penetrating trauma or unilateral pedicle or lamina fracture. It is characterized by ipsilateral loss of motor function and contralateral loss of pain and temperature. Prognosis for this injury is very good, with significant improvement occurring.

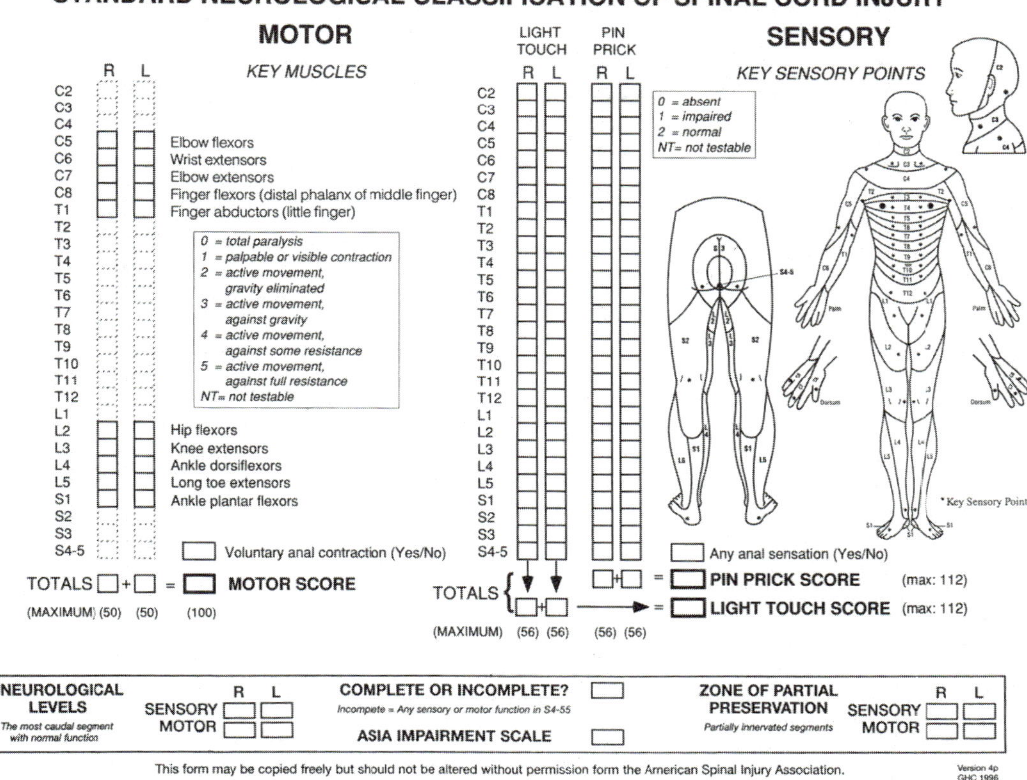
STANDARD NEUROLOGICAL CLASSIFICATION OF SPINAL CORD INJURY

MOTOR

R L KEY MUSCLES

C2
C3
C4
C5 Elbow flexors
C6 Wrist extensors
C7 Elbow extensors
C8 Finger flexors (distal phalanx of middle finger)
T1 Finger abductors (little finger)
T2
T3
T4
T5
T6
T7
T8
T9
T10
T11
T12
L1
L2 Hip flexors
L3 Knee extensors
L4 Ankle dorsiflexors
L5 Long toe extensors
S1 Ankle plantar flexors
S2
S3
S4-5 Voluntary anal contraction (Yes/No)

0 = total paralysis
1 = palpable or visible contraction
2 = active movement, gravity eliminated
3 = active movement, against gravity
4 = active movement, against some resistance
5 = active movement, against full resistance
NT= not testable

TOTALS □+□ = □ MOTOR SCORE
(MAXIMUM) (50) (50) (100)

LIGHT TOUCH R L | PIN PRICK R L

SENSORY

KEY SENSORY POINTS

C2 C3 C4 C5 C6 C7 C8 T1 T2 T3 T4 T5 T6 T7 T8 T9 T10 T11 T12 L1 L2 L3 L4 L5 S1 S2 S3 S4-5

0 = absent
1 = impaired
2 = normal
NT= not testable

Any anal sensation (Yes/No)

TOTALS □+□ = PIN PRICK SCORE (max: 112)
□+□ = LIGHT TOUCH SCORE (max: 112)
(MAXIMUM) (56) (56) (56) (56)

• Key Sensory Points

NEUROLOGICAL LEVELS — The most caudal segment with normal function — R L SENSORY MOTOR

COMPLETE OR INCOMPLETE? — Incomplete = Any sensory or motor function in S4-S5

ASIA IMPAIRMENT SCALE

ZONE OF PARTIAL PRESERVATION — Partially innervated segments — R L SENSORY MOTOR

This form may be copied freely but should not be altered without permission form the American Spinal Injury Association.

Version 4p GHC 1996

FIGURE 39.1. American Spinal Injury Association scoring system.

TABLE 39.1 Key Muscle Groups

Level	Muscle Group
C5	Elbow flexors (biceps, brachialis)
C6	Wrist extensors (extensor carpi radialis longus and brevis)
C7	Elbow extensors (triceps)
C8	Finger flexors (flexor digitorum profundus to the middle finger)
T1	Small finger abductors (abductor digiti minimi)
L2	Hip flexors (iliopsoas)
L3	Knee extensors (quadriceps)
L4	Ankle dorsiflexors (tibialis anterior)
L5	Long toe extensors (extensor hallucis longus)
S1	Ankle plantar flexors (gastrocnemius, soleus)

Central cord syndrome is the most common of these clinical syndromes and occurs almost exclusively in the cervical region. It produces sacral sensory sparing with decreased motor function in both upper and lower extremities bilaterally. The motor deficit to the upper extremity often is more significant than the lower extremity deficit. Frequently, the patient experiences immediate partial recovery after being placed in traction. The prognosis is variable; however, more than 50% of patients experience return of bowel and bladder control, become ambulatory, and enjoy improved hand function.

Anterior cord syndrome usually is caused by a flexion-type injury in which a fragment of bone or disc impinges on the anterior spinal artery. It is characterized by complete motor loss and loss of pain and temperature, with preservation of deep touch, proprioception, and vibratory sensation. The prognosis for this syndrome is poor.

Posterior cord syndrome involves the dorsal columns and is characterized by loss of proprioception and vibratory sensation, with the preservation of motor function and the remaining sensory functions. This syndrome often occurs in patients with displaced fractures of the posterior elements, such as the lamina.

EXPOSURE

Adequate visual exposure of the patient is essential for a thorough examination, particularly to ensure evaluation of the body for areas of bleeding or deformity. Imaging studies are a necessary adjunct in evaluation of the trauma patient but should not interfere with resuscitation. The primary radiographs, which should be obtained in all trauma patients concurrent with the primary survey, include an AP view of the chest, an AP view of the pelvis, and a lateral view of the cervical spine. As indicated by physical examination, additional anatomy-specific or protocol-based radiographic studies can be obtained as part of the secondary survey. In addition, the diagnosis of a spinal injury warrants imaging of the entire spinal column to rule out a noncontiguous injury.

SECONDARY SURVEY

The secondary survey should involve a complete head-to-toe evaluation of the patient. Continued reevaluation often is overlooked, which can contribute to a poor outcome. Often, overwhelming injuries mask other injuries that, if left unrecognized and untreated, can cause significant morbidity.

As previously stated, patients with polytrauma have a higher incidence of missed spinal injuries. The spinal injuries can be missed because of failure to obtain images of the entire spine or because of unreliable examination results if the patient has an altered mental status from a head injury, intoxication, or intubation. Sengupta[5] reported an incidence of 2% to 30% for missed spinal injuries. This occurred more in the cervical spine at the occipital cervical and cervicothoracic junction. Poonnoose et al.[6] reviewed 569 traumatic spinal injuries and showed a 9.1% incidence of missed spinal injuries. Thirty-four patients had received inappropriate treatment, and 26 patients had experienced neurologic deterioration. Their review emphasized the importance of the possibility of discoligamentous injuries in patients with normal radiographs.

Fixation of unstable fractures of the pelvis, femur, and tibia should be performed within the first 24 hours after injury if medically feasible. Early fracture fixation with the use of internal or external fixation allows for a decreased incidence of fat embolism syndrome, a decreased incidence of acute respiratory distress syndrome (ARDS), and early mobilization of the patient. Early fracture fixation reduces the length of time required in the intensive care unit and the overall hospital stay. Bone et al.[7] found that patients managed with early stabilization averaged 2.8 days in the intensive care unit and 17.3 days in the hospital, compared with 7.6 days in the intensive care unit and 26.6 days in the hospital for the group that had delayed stabilization. The average hospital cost was 66% higher for the delayed stabilization group.

Care must be taken to maintain spinal precautions while immediate life-saving procedures are being performed. In patients with cervical spine injuries, intraoperative stabilization with a cervical collar or the application of Gardner-Wells tongs for cervical traction might be necessary to maintain spinal stability. For patients with multiple extremity injuries but no abdominal or thoracic trauma, the application of a halo might provide provisional stability or even definitive care to the injured cervical spine. It is mandatory that patients with spinal column injuries undergo repeat radiographic and neurologic evaluations to ensure that no change has occurred if multiple transfers are occurring.

Patients with multiple injuries and a dislocated cervical spine who are awake, alert, and cooperative can undergo attempted reduction with the use of serial traction and radiographic evaluation. However, for obtunded patients or patients for whom attempted traction reduction has failed, MRI or CT myelography to rule out the presence of a traumatically herniated disc is warranted. Patients with an intracranial pressure monitor or Swan-Ganz catheter are unable to undergo MRI. For these patients, CT myelography is required.

Patients with associated spinal column injuries who are awaiting definitive operative stabilization because of hemodynamic instability can benefit from a Rotorest bed. Use of this bed allows for rotational mobilization, prevention of decubitus ulcer formation, and routine skin care while maintaining spinal stability.

Isolated stable thoracolumbar spine injuries typically are treated with some means of external immobilization. This can be in the form of a thoracolumbar sacral orthosis (TLSO), Jewett brace, or extension cast. However, in those patients who have thoracolumbar injuries with multiorgan system involvement, external bracing might be difficult to apply and maintain. In this patient population, an operative stabilization procedure may be indicated. Minimally invasive surgical techniques have evolved and might allow for a less invasive means of stabilizing the spine.

FAT EMBOLISM SYNDROME

After musculoskeletal trauma, marrow fat from the fracture site or sites can embolize and become concentrated in the pulmonary vascular bed. This embolization activates a complex series of interactions, including the coagulation cascade, increased platelet function, and release of vasoactive substances. The clinical manifestation is acute hypoxia, mental status changes, and infiltration on the chest radiograph. This usually occurs within the first 72 hours. Isolated long bone fractures are associated with a low incidence of fat embolism syndrome, 0.5% to 2.0%, whereas long bone fractures in the patient who has experienced polytrauma are associated with an incidence of fat embolism syndrome approaching 15%.[8]

Studies have shown that early fracture stabilization results in a decreased incidence of fat embolism syndrome. Riska and Myllynen[8] compared two groups of multiply injured patients and found that the incidence of fat embolism syndrome was 1.4% in those treated with early fracture stabilization and 22% in those treated without it. Similarly, in a prospective randomized series of early versus delayed stabilization of femoral shaft fractures, Bone et al.[7] found no cases of fat embolism syndrome in the early stabilization group.

ACUTE RESPIRATORY DISTRESS SYNDROME

ARDS is characterized clinically by diffuse infiltrates observed on the chest radiograph and refractory hypoxemia. An extended period of intubation usually is needed. Late sepsis, multiorgan system failure, and high mortality rates are commonly associated with ARDS.[9,10] Many studies have shown that early fracture stabilization can reduce the incidence of ARDS. In a large retrospective review, Johnson et al.[9] found that delaying fracture stabilization for more than 24 hours was associated with a fivefold increase in the incidence of ARDS, particularly in more severely injured patients. When such patients were treated with delayed stabilization, the incidence of ARDS was 75%; when managed with early stabilization, it was 17%.

CONCLUSION

After the patient has been hemodynamically stabilized and all immediate life-threatening injuries have been cared for, a plan for definitive treatment of the spinal column injury must be formulated. Determining the stability of an injury based on plain and advanced-imaging radiographs will indicate the need for operative stabilization. The goals of treatment should be determined. These include maintaining normal neurologic function, improving neurologic function, preventing late pain and deformity, and allowing for rapid mobilization with early aggressive rehabilitation. Once the initial interventions for resuscitation have ceased, evaluation of the operative goals and how these goals can be achieved with the least morbidity can be made. With the exception of a patient progressively losing neurologic function, spinal injury management rarely requires emergent intervention. However, the spine surgeon should be involved in the care of the multiply injured patient from admission through rehabilitation. Early appropriate spinal intervention may afford the benefits of decreased mortality, increased hemodynamic stability, decreased pulmonary complications, early mobilization, decreased complications of recumbency, decreased narcotic requirements, and a greater likelihood of a less morbid outcome.

ACKNOWLEDGMENT

We thank Dori Kelly, MA, for expert editing of the manuscript.

REFERENCES

1. Anderson S, Biros MH, Reardon RF. Delayed diagnosis of thoracolumbar fractures in multiple-trauma patients. *Acad Emerg Med* 1996;3:832–839.
2. McLain RF, Benson DR. Urgent surgical stabilization of spinal fractures in polytrauma patients. *Spine* 1999;24: 1646–1654.
3. Schlegel J, Bayley J, Yuan H, Fredricksen B. Timing of surgical decompression and fixation of acute spinal fractures. *J Orthop Trauma* 1996;10:323–330.
4. Liu M, Lee CH, P'eng FK. Prospective comparison of diagnostic peritoneal lavage, computed tomographic scanning, and ultrasonography for the diagnosis of blunt abdominal trauma. *J Trauma* 1993;35:267–270.
5. Sengupta DK. Neglected spinal injuries. *Clin Orthop Relat Res* 2005;431:93–103.
6. Poonnoose PM, Ravichandran G, McClelland MR. Missed and mismanaged injuries of the spinal cord. *J Trauma* 2002;53:314–320.
7. Bone LB, Johnson KD, Weigelt J, Scheinberg R. Early versus delayed stabilization of femoral fractures: A prospective randomized study. *J Bone Joint Surg Am* 1989;71:336–340.
8. Riska EB, Myllynen P. Fat embolism in patients with multiple injuries. *J Trauma* 1982;22:891–894.
9. Johnson KD, Cadambi A, Seibert GB. Incidence of adult respiratory distress syndrome in patients with multiple musculoskeletal injuries: effect of early operative stabilization of fractures. *J Trauma* 1985;25:375–384.
10. Bernard GR, Artigas A, Brigham KL, et al. The American-European Consensus Conference on ARDS: definitions, mechanisms, relevant outcomes, and clinical trial coordination. *Am J Respir Crit Care Med* 1994;149:818–824.

CHAPTER 40

Cervical Spine Injuries in the Athlete—Stingers, Burners, Transient Quadriparesis: Return to Play Criteria

David Magit, Michael DeLuca, and Jonathan N. Grauer

INTRODUCTION

Great controversy exists regarding the management of cervical spine injuries in athletes. This is of particular concern because 1 in 10 of the cervical spine injuries that occur in the United States originate from athletic injuries.[1]

These injuries are seen in athletes of all levels and in a variety of sporting venues, including diving, surfing, skiing, football, boxing, lacrosse, wrestling, soccer, rugby, ice hockey, and gymnastics. Tator et al.[2] identified diving accidents as the cause in 11% of patients in Toronto with acute spinal cord injuries.[3] Hockey accounted for 28 spinal cord injuries in Canada between 1976 and 1983.[3] Over the past 25 years, 223 American football players have sustained cervical spinal cord injuries (SCIs) without full neurologic recovery.[4]

The sequelae of such cervical spine injuries vary significantly. These can range from minor cervical strains to complete quadriplegia. The incidence of complete quadriplegia among high school and college football athletes has been reported as high as 2.5 per 100,000 in 1976 and as low as 0.5 per 100,000 in 1991.[5] Improved coaching and tackling techniques, rule changes banning the use of spear tackling, and improved equipment are credited for this decline in catastrophic quadriplegia. In fact, Cantu and Mueller[4] recently noted that teaching the fundamental techniques of the game, equipment standards, and improved medical care both on and off the playing field have led to a 270% reduction in permanent SCI from a peak of 20 per year during the period 1971 to 1975 to 7.2 per year during the past 10 years.

Despite this decrease, the incidence of noncatastrophic cervical spine injuries such as cervical stingers or burners and transient quadriplegia remain prevalent. This chapter details these injuries and addresses the current approach to return to play in athletes with cervical spine injuries.

ON-FIELD MANAGEMENT

Management of athletes with acute cervical spine injuries requires a corroborative effort among medical staff personnel, including team trainers and physicians, as well as local emergency medicine technicians. Coaches, referees, and players must also be aware of potential injuries and treatment protocols.

For lesser injuries, reporting is important to make sure potential treatment can be initiated. For more significant and potentially catastrophic injuries, comprehensive plans of action should be in place.

A designated medical team leader and clarification of the responsibilities of each team member should be decided before the start of the game. Emergency equipment, including all the necessary tools for airway and cardiopulmonary management, should be present and held accounted by a team member. Other essential equipment includes proper age-appropriate backboards and cervical immobilization equipment. For example, Waninger et al.[6] showed that backboard immobilization of helmeted ice hockey and lacrosse players appropriately limited cervical motion during transportation.

In the event of an acute cervical spine injury, the player should be immediately taken from play. A complete history and physical examination should be performed. Treatment should be initiated as warranted.

For collision spots, helmets and shoulder pads should not be removed unless absolutely necessary. Several studies demonstrated that significant cervical alignment changes occur with removal of either the helmet or the shoulder pads.[7–10] In the subaxial spine, increased cervical extension results from removal of the helmet with the shoulder pads left in place. Likewise, removal of the shoulder pads without removal of the helmet results in an increase in cervical flexion. Conversely, in the case of a C1-C2 injury, helmet removal causes flexion and distraction.[11] Any of these motions can threaten an already compromised spinal cord. Authors have thus concluded that, because of the increased motion associated with equipment removal, patients with cervical spine injuries should have helmets and shoulder pads removed only in a carefully monitored setting with multiple trained medical personnel available to assist.

STINGERS OR BURNERS

Stingers, also know as burners, are transient neuropraxias of the brachial plexus or cervical nerve roots. After impacting the neck or shoulder, athletes describe temporary episodes of unilateral upper extremity burning dysesthesias which may be associated with motor weakness. Symptoms usually persist for minutes to hours, but patients may report symptoms for days to weeks after injury.[12–14]

These injuries are common in collision or contact sports and are the most frequent cervical spine–related injury in football. Incidence is reported to be 7.7% per year and as high as 65% during a player's career.[15,16] In general, stingers are reported to occur in as many as 50% of athletes participating in collision sports.[17,18]

Several mechanisms have been postulated for the cause of symptoms associated with stingers. The first is compression of the nerve root caused by neck extension and rotation and/or lateral bending toward the side of injury. This mechanism of injury is thought to be responsible for approximately 85% of all stingers and usually occurs in relatively older athletes.[14] This may be due to the relative narrowing of the associated foramen. Accordingly, these findings may be associated with chronic recurrent stingers, more significant neuropraxia, and axonotmesis.[12]

Alternatively, stingers may be caused by traction on the brachial plexus. This occurs with depression of the shoulder and lateral bending of the neck away from the side of injury. Because these injuries are generally directly related to a specific traction maneuver, as opposed to underlying neural element compression, they are less likely to be recurrent unless related to a specific type of play. These injuries are also less likely correlated with neck pain or loss of cervical motion.[19]

Lastly, stingers can occur from a direct blow to the brachial plexus. Markey et al.[13] studied cervical spine injury mechanisms in 261 football players from the United States Military Academy. The authors determined that stingers could result from compression of the fixed brachial plexus between the player's shoulder pad and the superior-medial scapula as the pad is pushed into the area of Erb's point (point of fixation of the upper trunk of the brachial plexus to the transverse process).[13] C5 and C6 nerve roots are most commonly affected.

It has been hypothesized that the Torg ratio might be associated with the occurrence of stingers. This is measured as a distance from the midpoint of the posterior aspect of the vertebral body to the nearest point on the corresponding spinolaminar line divided by the anterior posterior width of the vertebral body.[20] This provides a measure of cervical stenosis. It has been suggested that a ratio of less than 0.8 corresponds with significant spinal stenosis, compared to a control group of 1.00 or more. In the setting of cervical stenosis, forced hyperextension may result in root compression and the transient loss of motor or sensory function associated with stingers. However, this is most likely from foraminal stenosis and is probably not the best application of this ratio (compared to transient quadriplegia, which is more directly related to central stenosis).

Meyer et al.[14] evaluated the relationship of the Torg ratio with the occurrence of stingers in 266 collegiate football players. The authors identified 40 players with stingers, 34 resulting from an extension-compression mechanism and 6 from a brachial plexus traction mechanism. In 47.5% of the stinger group, the Torg ratio was less than 0.8 at one or more levels. Conversely, no player with a brachial plexus injury mechanism had a Torg ratio less than 0.8. Overall, players with a Torg ratio less than 0.8 had three times the risk for experiencing stingers than those without. This may correlate with decreased area for the neural elements.

Castro[21] could not demonstrate this correlation of Torg ratio with first-time stingers. Castro performed a prospective review of 165 college football players and noted a 7.7% incidence of first-time stingers. The average Torg ratio for all players was 0.92 ± 0.12 (with the seventh cervical level corresponding to the narrowest level). The author determined that initial stinger experience depended on position played and body type, but was not predicted by the Torg ratio. However, the author did find a relationship between Torg ratio and multiple stingers, reporting that players with multiple stingers had a significantly smaller Torg ratio than players who experienced only one incident (0.75 versus 0.87).

TRANSIENT QUADRIPARESIS

Transient quadriparesis is a form of cord neurapraxia. Sensory changes include burning pain and loss of sensation. Motor changes range from weakness to complete paralysis of two or four extremities. This has been reported to occur in approximately 1.3 per 10,000 college football athletes.[22]

It is generally thought that this results from hyperextension, or possibly hyperflexion, of the neck in the setting of a congenitally or developmentally narrowed cervical canal. In addition to potential cord compression, the vascular supply of the cord may be compromised, contributing to the temporary neurologic sequelae. Most of the time, symptoms related to this injury last for only 10 to 15 minutes, but these can extend beyond 48 hours. Patients generally experienced a gradual, complete return of function with full, painless cervical spine motion.

The Torg ratio described previously with regard to stingers is also applied to transient quadriplegia. Torg et al.[22] did find that a Torg ratio of 0.80 or less correlated with a high sensitivity (93%) for transient neurapraxia. However, the positive predictive value of the Torg ratio for this injury was low (0.2%). This was thus not found to be a good screening tool for determining the suitability of an athlete for participation in contact sports.

Similar results have been found by others.[23] It has thus been concluded that cervical stenosis does not directly predispose an individual to permanent catastrophic neurologic injury and should not preclude an athlete from participation in contact sports.

Brigham and Warren[24] pointed out that many professional football players have a straight or kyphotic cervical spine on the neutral lateral radiograph (loss of normal lordosis know as spear tacklers' spine) and that this might be of concern if lordosis could not be achieved on extension. In addition, the authors noted that because of the large size of the athletes and their proportionately large vertebral bodies, these unique athletes often have a relatively small Torg ratio without true stenosis as defined by a decreased cord space.

RETURN TO PLAY CRITERIA

Return to play guidelines for various cervical spine injuries and abnormalities is a hotly debated topic. The problem stems from the difficulty in determining true sensitivity and specificity of any criteria for predicting future injury for a wide variety of sports and types of play. There is also the concern that any increased chance for significant cervical injury may not be acceptable. Conversely, there is pressure from players, coaches, etc., to allow continued participation. Unfortunately most of these decisions are difficult to determine definitively, and most clinicians make recommendations based on personal experiences and support of a limited body of knowledge.

Stingers are often of very short duration and limited deficit and thus are underreported. Nonetheless, it is important for the player and medical personnel to understand that the player should not return to play until symptoms have completely resolved and there is painless range of motion. Certainly any persistent symptoms will warrant further investigation. Recurrent stingers or symptoms lasting longer than expected warrant further investigation.

In terms of transient quadriparesis, Torg et al.[25] retrospectively reviewed 110 cases of cervical cord neuropraxia in an attempt to make recommendations for return to play. No contraindication to play was noted if there was a Torg ratio of 0.8 or less in an asymptomatic athlete. Relative contraindication to play was noted if there was a Torg ratio of 0.8 or less with one episode of cervical cord neuropraxia. In stating this to be a relative contraindication, it was meant that return to play must be carefully considered by the patient, family, and coach, all of whom understood the associated risks with continued play. Absolute contraindication to play was noted with a documented episode of cervical cord neurapraxia associated with ligamentous instability, symptoms of neurologic findings lasting more than 36 hours, and/or multiple episodes.

Certainly any persistent pain or neurologic deficit after an episode of transient quadriparesis should be considered a ligamentous or bony injury until proven otherwise. Cervical cord neurapraxia associated with magnetic resonance imaging (MRI) evidence of a spinal cord defect or cord edema was considered to be an absolute contraindication to return to play.

Beyond the group of patients with episodes of neurologic dysfunction discussed previously, several authors have attempted to categorize conditions with no contraindications, relative contraindications, and absolute contraindications for return to play for contact or collision sports.[26,27] Most of these have no more than Class III data to support their inclusion but may act as general guidelines.

Contraindications to return to play have been categorized as follows:

No Contraindications

1. Healed anterior, lateral, or posterior disc herniation treated conservatively
2. Type II Klippel-Feil lesions involving fusion of one or two interspaces at C3 or below in an individual with full cervical motion and absence of occipitocervical anomalies, instability, disc disease, or degenerative changes
3. Spinal bifida occulta
4. Disc herniations requiring intervertebral discectomy and interbody fusion for a lateral or central herniation in the setting of a solid, asymptomatic fusion
5. Patients with healed stable nondisplaced fractures without sagittal malalignment

Relative Contraindications

1. Provided that the patient is pain free, has full cervical range of motion, and has no abnormal neurologic signs
   - **A.** Healed nondisplaced Jefferson fracture
   - **B.** Healed type I and type II odontoid fractures
   - **C.** Healed lateral mass fractures of C2
2. Healed, stable, minimally displaced vertebral body compression fracture without sagittal malalignment
3. Healed stable fracture of the posterior elements, excluding spinous process fractures
4. Presence of minimal residual facet instability after surgical or conservative treatment of cervical disc disease
5. After a healed two- or three-level cervical fusion

Absolute Contraindications

1. Odontoid anomalies, including odontoid agenesis, odontoid hypoplasia, os odontoideum
2. Atlano-occipital fusion alone or associated with other abnormalities
3. Type I Klippel-Feil anomaly consisting of a mass fusion of the cervical and upper thoracic vertebrae
4. Type II Klippel-Feil anomaly with fusion of one or two interspaces with associated limited motion and/or associated occipitocervical anomalies or instability
5. Atlantoaxial instability with disruption of the transverse and/or alar ligament as demonstrated by an abnormal atlanto-dens interval on lateral flexion-extension views
6. Atlantoaxial rotatory fixation
7. Injuries involving the upper cervical spine involving a fracture or ligamentous injury
8. Atlantoaxial fusion
9. Subaxial spinal instability defined by lateral radiographs that show 3.5 mm or more of horizontal displacement of one vertebra over the other or more than 11 degrees of rotational difference compared with the adjacent vertebrae as measured on lateral flexion or extension plain radiographs
10. Acute fracture of either the body or posterior elements with or without ligamentous instability
11. Healed subaxial vertebral body fractures with sagittal malalignment
12. Acute fracture of the vertebral body with associated posterior arch fractures and/or ligamentous laxity
13. Residual bony canal compromise from retropulsed bony fragments
14. Continued pain, abnormal neurologic findings, or limited motion from a healed cervical fracture
15. Symptomatic acute soft or chronic disc herniation with associated neurologic findings, pain, or motion loss
16. After a successful one-level fusion in the presence of diffuse congenital narrowing of the cervical canal.

Despite attempts to unify return to play criteria, there is still much disagreement. This was highlighted by a questionnaire study performed by Morganti et al.[28] Ten cases of cervical spine injuries were reviewed by over 100 physicians specializing in sports medicine or spine care. Published guidelines were not strictly adhered to, and there was a marked lack of consensus regarding postinjury management of these injuries.

CONCLUSION

Clearly, the cervical spine represents a potentially devastating area of injury for the athlete. Injuries can range from strains to quadriplegia. Measures have been taken to minimize the incidence of cervical spine injury in the athlete. For example, in 1976, spear tackling was outlawed by the National Federation of State High School Associations and the National Collegiate Athletic Association because of convincing data that the majority of cervical spine injuries were due to axial loading.[29] This lead to a precipitous decline in the number of cervical injuries. There were 34 cases of tetraplegia in 1976 and only 5 cases in 1984.[5] Also, 42% of fatalities were due to cervical injury from 1965 to 1974. This rate decreased to 14% and 5% over the next two decades.[30] Other measures have also been considered. Many players now wear cowboy collars or other devices to prevent cervical hyperextension. Emphasis on teaching of tackling fundamentals and proper mechanics, improved shoulder pad construction, and off-season neck strengthening programs aim to prevent injury.[31] Return to play criteria have been defined, but certainly these are subject to opinion and interpretation of limited data.

REFERENCES

1. Maroon JC, Bailes JE. Athletes with cervical spine injury. *Spine* 1996;20:2294–2299.
2. Tator CH, Edmonds VE, New ML. Diving: a frequent and potentially preventable cause of spinal cord injury. *Can Med Assoc J* 1981;125:1323–1324.

3. Tator CH, Ekong CE, Rowed DW, et al. Spinal injuries due to hockey. *Can J Neurol Sci* 1984;11:34–41.
4. Cantu RC, Mueller FO. Catastrophic spine injuries in American football, 1977–2001. *Neurosurgery* 2003;53: 358–362.
5. Clarke KS. Epidemiology of athletic neck injury. *Clin Sports Med* 1998;17:83–97.
6. Waninger KN, Richards JG, Pan WT, et al. An evaluation of head movement in backboard-immobilized helmeted football, lacrosse, and ice hockey players. *Clin J Sport Med* 2001;11:82–86.
7. Swenson TM, Lauerman WC, Blanc RD, et al. Cervical spine alignment in the immobilized football player: radiographic analysis before and after helmet removal. *Am J Sports Med* 1997;25:226–230.
8. Gastel JA, Palumbo MA, Hulstyn MJ, et al. Emergency removal of football equipment: a cadaveric cervical spine injury model. *Ann Emerg Med* 1998;32:411–417.
9. Palumbo MA, Hulstyn MJ, Fadale PD, et al. The effect of protective football equipment on alignment of the injured cervical spine: radiographic analysis in a cadaveric model. *Am J Sports Med* 1996;24:446–453.
10. Laprade RF, Schnetzler KA, Broxterman RJ, et al. Cervical spine alignment in the immobilized ice hockey player: a computed tomographic analysis of the effects of helmet removal. *Am J Sports Med* 2000;28:800–803.
11. Donaldson WF, Lauerman WC, Heil B, et al. Helmet and shoulder pad removal from a player with suspected cervical spine injury: a cadaveric model. *Spine* 1998;23:1729–1732.
12. Levitz CL, Reilly PJ, Torg JS. The pathomechanics of chronic, recurrent cervical nerve root neurapraxia: the chronic burner syndrome. *Am J Sports Med* 1997;25:73–76.
13. Markey KL, DiBenedetto M, Curl WW. Upper trunk brachial plexopathy: the stinger syndrome. *Am J Sports Med* 1993;21:650–655.
14. Meyer SA, Schulte KR, Callaghan JJ, et al. Cervical spinal stenosis and stingers in collegiate football players. *Am J Sports Med* 1994;22:158–166.
15. Castro FP. Stingers, cervical cord neurapraxia, and stenosis. *Clin Sports Med* 2003;22:483–492.
16. Sallis RE, Jones K, Knopp W. Burners: offensive strategy in an under-reported injury. *Phys Sports Med* 1992;20: 47–55.
17. Clancy WG, Brand RL, Bergfeld JA. Upper trunk brachial plexus injuries in contact sports. *Am J Sports Med* 1977;5:209–216.
18. Cantu RC. Stingers, transient quadriplegia, and cervical spine stenosis: return to play criteria. *Med Sci Sports Exerc* 1997;29:S233–S235.
19. Kelly JD. Brachial plexus injuries: evaluating and treating "burners." *J Musculoskel Med* 1997;14:70–80.
20. Pavlov H, Torg JS, Robie B, et al. Cervical spinal stenosis: determination with vertebral body ratio method. *Radiology* 1987;164:771–775.
21. Castro FP. Stingers, the Torg ratio, and the cervical spine. *Am J Sports Med* 1997;25:603–608.
22. Torg JS, Pavlov H, Genuario SE, et al. Neuropraxia of the cervical spinal cord with transient quadriplegia. *J Bone Joint Surg Am* 1986;68:1354–1370.
23. Herzog RJ, Dillingham MF, Sontag MJ. Normal cervical spine morphometry and cervical spine stenosis in asymptomatic professional football players: plain film radiography, multiplanar computed tomography, and magnetic resonance imaging. *Spine* 1991;16S:S178–S186.
24. Brigham CD, Warren R. Head to head on spear tackler's spine: criteria and implications for return to play. *J Bone Joint Surg Am* 2003;85:381–382.
25. Torg JS, Corcoran TA, Thibault LE, et al. Cervical cord neuropraxia: classification, pathomechanics, morbidity, and management guidelines. *J Neurosurg* 1997;87:843–850.
26. Torg JS, Rasmsey-Emrhein JA. Suggested management guidelines for participation in collision activities with congenital, developmental, or postinjury lesions involving the cervical spine. *Med Sci Sports Exerc* 1997;29:S256–S272.
27. Vaccaro AR, Klein GR, Ciccoti M, et al. Return to play criteria for the athlete with cervical spine injuries resulting in stinger and transient quadriplegia/paresis. *Spine J* 2002;2:351–356.
28. Morganti C, Sweeney CA, Albanese SA, et al. Return to play after cervical spine injury. *Spine* 2001;26:1131–1136.
29. Torg JS, Quedenfeld TC, Burstein A, et al. National football head and neck injury registry: report on cervical quadriplegia, 1971 to 1975. *Am J Sports Med* 1979;7:127–132.
30. Torg JS, Truex R Jr, Quedenfeld TC, et al. The National Football Head and Neck Injury Registry: report and conclusions *JAMA* 1978;241:1477–1479.
31. Eddy D, Congeni J, Loud K. A review of spine injuries and return to play. *Clin J Sport Med* 2005;15:453–458.

INDEX

Page numbers followed by *f* or *t* indicate material in figures or tables, respectively.

B

Q

T